Dysphagia

Clinical Management in Adults and Children

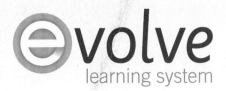
evolve
learning system

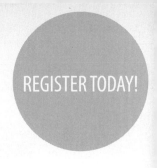

To access your free Evolve Resources, visit:

http://evolve.elsevier.com/Groher/dysphagia

Evolve Student Learning Resources for Groher & Crary: *Dysphagia: Clinical Management in Adults and Children*, first edition, offers the following features:

- **Video Clips**

  More than 50 video clips that highlight selected content within chapters and critical thinking cases on Evolve.

- **Bonus Full-Length Video**

  An introduction to adult swallowing disorders.

- **Critical Thinking Cases**

  Provide opportunities for students to test their application and critical thinking skills.

- **Glossary**

  Serves as a valuable reference tool for students beginning their studies in this specialty area.

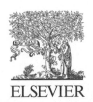
ELSEVIER

Dysphagia

Clinical Management in Adults and Children

MICHAEL E. GROHER, PHD, FASHA

Professor
Truesdail Center for Communicative Disorders
University of Redlands
Redlands, California

MICHAEL A. CRARY, PHD, FASHA

Professor, Communicative Disorders
Director, Swallowing Research Laboratory
College of Public Health and Health Professions
University of Florida
Gainesville, Florida

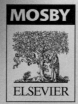

MOSBY

ELSEVIER

3251 Riverport Lane
Maryland Heights, Missouri 63043

DYSPHAGIA: CLINICAL MANAGEMENT IN ADULTS
AND CHILDREN ISBN: 978-0-323-05298-6

Copyright © 2010 by Mosby, Inc., an affiliate of Elsevier Inc.

Library of Congress Cataloging-in-Publication Data
Groher, Michael E.
Dysphagia : clinical management in adults and children / Michael E. Groher, Michael
A. Crary.—1st ed.
      p. ; cm.
    Includes bibliographical references and index.
    ISBN 978-0-323-05298-6 (pbk. : alk. paper)
    1. Deglutition disorders. I. Crary, Michael A., 1952- II. Title.
    [DNLM: 1. Deglutition Disorders. WI 250 G874d 2010]
RC815.2.G76 2010
616.3'23—dc22

2009035166

Vice President and Publisher: Linda Duncan
Executive Editor: Kathy Falk
Managing Editor: Jolynn Gower
Publishing Services Manager: Patricia Tannian
Project Manager: Carrie Stetz
Designer: Karen Pauls

Printed in the United States of America

Last digit is the print number: 9 8 7 6

Contributors

Jo Puntil-Sheltman, MS, CCC, BRS-S

Board-Recognized Dysphagia Specialist
Developmental Specialist
Dixie Regional Medical Center
St. George, Utah

HELENE M. TAYLOR, MA, CCC-SLP, CLE

Speech-Language Pathologist
Dysphagia and Craniofacial Clinic Team Member
Primary Children's Medical Center
Salt Lake City, Utah

Dedication

This book is dedicated to the individuals who have influenced our own work, many of whom were pioneers in the development and support of the multidisciplinary concept of dysphagia management. The clinical and translational research that each has provided has built the foundation for a subspecialty that undoubtedly will continue to grow and benefit the patients we treat:

Joan Arvedson, Ian Cook, Nick Diamant, Olle Ekberg, Michael Feinberg, Susan Langmore, George Larsen, Maureen Lefton-Greif, Jeri Logemann, Arthur Miller, Robert Miller, JoAnn Robbins, Reza Shaker

And to the members of the first multidisciplinary dysphagia team at a major teaching hospital, Johns Hopkins:

Jim Bosma, David Bucholtz, Martin Donner, Bronwyn Jones, Haskins Kashima, Patti Linden, Bill Ravich

And finally, to those who represent a new generation of clinical scientists, many of whom have influenced our efforts and others with whom we have worked directly. These individuals and many others whose work we have read and respect will continue to provide us with important insights:

Margareta Bülow, Susan Butler, Giselle Carnaby-Mann, Julie Cichero, Ichiro Fujishima, Maggie Lee Huckabee, Paula Leslie, Rosemary Martino, Gary McCulloch, Bonnie Martin-Harris, Cathy Pelletier, David Smithard, Catriona Steele, Koji Takahashi, and more....

Clinical science can be a slow science. It requires not only dedication to time and effort, but true commitment to the patients who will eventually benefit from these efforts. Clinical science is not without setbacks, pitfalls, and flaws. So to those who engage in clinical science in the name of helping others, we attempt to remember the words of two prominent world citizens, and we apologize if we convey their words incorrectly:

First they ignore you, then they laugh at you, then they argue with you, then you win.
Mahatma Gandhi
It is common sense to take a method and try it. If it fails, admit it frankly and try another. But above all, try something.
Franklin D. Roosevelt

With best wishes to all,

M. G. & M. C.

This text is for the clinician who wants to establish a basic and comprehensive foundation in managing infants, children, and adults with swallowing disorders. The focus is on the processes of providing diagnostic and treatment services for persons with dysphagia, and on the research that supports those services. Because of the comprehensive approach, some details of diagnosis and treatment will not be fully appreciated after the first reading by novice clinicians but will be useful for journeyman clinicians. It is our opinion that the organization of this text will be an aid to the professor who is providing instruction in dysphagia management at a basic and advanced level. Aids in teaching include access to an extensive image library of instrumental swallowing examinations (on the companion Evolve Web site); a liberal use of short, clinically based examples of myriad problems associated with dysphagia; critical thinking case examples (Clinical Corner boxes in the chapters); and cases that require students to analyze their own decision-making skills as they integrate historical, clinical, and instrumental results using a series of prompts that probe their problem-solving skills (on the Evolve Web site). In addition, we have tried to infuse our own biases and insights with anecdotal stories (Practice Notes in the chapters) given to us by the hundreds of patients we have treated.

It is our opinion that dysphagia management is best taught by illustrating approaches to problem solving. To this end we have tried to avoid being prescriptive in favor of an emphasis on discovering available options for care and in weighing the risks and benefits of those options. Too often prescriptive approaches in clinical care take away one's options to solve patient care problems.

The successful management of persons with dysphagia is accomplished only through the cooperation of numerous specialists (see Chapter 1). Although it is well known that a multidisciplinary approach with these patients is best, this approach also may suffer from failure to coordinate care. Often, the coordination of that care is accomplished by the speech-language pathologist. In this text we have emphasized the role of the speech-language pathologist. The roles of other disciplines are explained largely in the clinical case presentations within each chapter.

Ultimately, this is a text that highlights the problems of persons with dysphagia and how professionals might ameliorate their swallowing difficulties. It will become apparent that swallowing difficulty may be secondary to a large number of medical and sometimes nonmedical (psychogenic) disorders, and that swallowing problems are more than a physiologic change in the swallowing mechanism. The text takes the perspective that being unable to swallow normally might result in major consequences to one's medical and psychological health. Secondary medical problems such as aspiration pneumonia, undernutrition, and dehydration may predispose the patient to other complications such as immunocompromise, mental confusion, or death. Because of this, dysphagia specialists must develop a strong background of general medical knowledge. The reader should be able to understand or be alerted to key medical concepts relating to the dysphagic circumstance within each chapter, but may have to go beyond this text for more detailed explanations of some concepts.

Being unable to ingest one's favorite foods safely, or being unable to eat normally in public, understandably will affect one's quality of life with the potential for secondary episodes of depression, anxiety, and social withdrawal. Preparation of special diets is time consuming and in some cases economically challenging. In short, our lifestyles frequently revolve around mealtimes. Interruptions to these normal routines are potentially devastating. Therefore treatments are geared not only to the restoration of physiologic function, but ultimately to a state of psychosocial normalcy that was disturbed as a result of a failure to swallow normally. Care of persons with dysphagia should be viewed as an attempt to rehabilitate lost function as well as prevent future medical complications by retaining learned rehabilitative strategies.

Managing persons with dysphagia has become a subspecialty for many health care professionals. For the speech-language pathologist it is a specialty that has emerged only within the last 30 years. As clinicians have become more familiar with the issues involved in the care of dysphagic persons, clinical and basic science investigators have helped answer and ask questions that have helped improve the quality of that care. Many of these efforts have come together in a journal *(Dysphagia)* devoted exclusively to dysphagia, a research society that meets annually (The Dysphagia Research Society), and the largest special interest division, number 13 (Dysphagia), within the American Speech, Language, and Hearing Association. There also has been a steady increase of texts with contributions from many disciplines aimed at the pathology, diagnosis, and treatment of persons with swallowing disorders. It is our hope that this text will not only add to that number, but also inspire those researchers and clinicians interested in dysphagia to continue the quest to improve the lives of persons with swallowing disorders.

Contents

Dysphagia

Clinical Management in
Adults and Children

Chapter 1

Dysphagia Unplugged

MICHAEL E. GROHER AND JO PUNTIL-SHELTMAN

OBJECTIVES

1. Define dysphagia and its ramifications.
2. Discuss the epidemiology of dysphagia.
3. Discuss the medical and social consequences of dysphagia.
4. Provide an overview of the clinical management of dysphagia.
5. Discuss the role of persons who manage dysphagia.
6. Discuss the types of settings in which dysphagic patients might be seen and how this might affect their management.

1

WHAT IS DYSPHAGIA?

Dysphagia takes its name from the Greek root *phagein*, meaning to ingest or engulf. Combined with the prefix *dys-*, it connotes a disorder of or difficulty with swallowing. It is correctly pronounced with a long or short "a." The final syllable, "ja," requires a hard pronunciation rather than the soft "dja" to avoid confusion with the communicative language disorder, *dysphasia*.

Taber's *Cyclopedic Medical Dictionary*[1] defines five subcategories of dysphagia:

1. *Constricta:* narrowing of the pharynx or esophagus
2. *Lusoria:* esophageal compression by the right subclavian artery
3. *Oropharyngeal:* difficulty with propulsion from the mouth to the esophagus
4. *Paralytica:* Paralysis of muscles of mouth, pharynx, or esophagus
5. *Spastica:* Dysphagia from spasm of the pharynx or esophagus

In clinical practice, only oropharyngeal dysphagia from this list is used with any frequency.

Interestingly, medical students learn that dysphagia is a swallowing problem primarily associated with disease of the esophagus. However, when used properly the term should refer to a swallowing disorder that involves any one of the three stages of swallowing: oral, pharyngeal, or esophageal. It is not a primary medical diagnosis but rather a **symptom** of underlying disease and therefore is described most often by its clinical characteristics (**signs**). Complaints such as coughing and choking during or after a meal, food sticking, **regurgitation, odynophagia,** drooling, unexplained weight loss, and nutritional deficiencies all may be associated with dysphagia. Because dysphagia is a symptom of underlying disease that is not necessarily specific to the swallowing tract, it can be associated with varied diagnoses. These diagnoses are summarized in Box 1-1. Throughout this

---

Practice Note 1-1

While acting as a consultant to a food production company, I asked them what they thought the extent of their market would be, indicating that to my knowledge we only had gross estimates of how many persons with dysphagia would benefit from specialized foods. They told me that they had been working with a firm that did an extensive analysis on this topic and had prepared a detailed report on the potential market. I asked them to send me a copy because I was interested in data that documented the incidence of dysphagia in the United States. Two weeks later I received a package with a copy of the data. To my surprise, there were at least 15 pages of references. On closer inspection of the first page, I noticed that the firm they had hired had used the key word dysphasia, not dysphagia. I broke the news to them that what they had paid for was an extensive review of the literature on language disorders after neurologic injury, not swallowing disorders. What a difference a few letters can make!

BOX 1-1 Summary of Conditions That May Contribute to Dysphagia

NEUROLOGIC DIAGNOSES
Stroke
Traumatic brain injury
Dementia
Motor neuron disease
Myasthenia gravis
Cerebral palsy
Guillain-Barré syndrome
Poliomyelitis
Infectious disorders
Myopathy
Progressive disease:
    Parkinsonism
    Huntington's disease
    Progressive supranuclear palsy
    Wilson's disease
Age-related changes

CONNECTIVE TISSUE/RHEUMATOID DISORDERS
Polydermatomyositis
Progressive systemic sclerosis
Sjögren's disease
Scleroderma
Overlap syndromes

STRUCTURAL DIAGNOSES
Any tumor involving the alimentary tract

IATROGENIC DIAGNOSES
Radiation therapy
Chemotherapy
Intubation or tracheostomy
Postsurgical cervical spine fusion
Postsurgical coronary artery bypass grafting
Medication-related

OTHER OR RELATED DIAGNOSES
Severe respiratory compromise
Psychogenic condition(s)

CLINICAL CORNER 1-1

L. G. was admitted to the hospital for a left brain stroke. On admission he was nonresponsive and a nasogastric feeding tube was placed to provide nutrition and hydration. As his responsiveness improved, the nasogastric feeding tube was removed and he began oral feeding. As he fed himself, it was noted that he choked on most attempts and dysphagia was suspected. The clinical evaluation noted a weak tongue and poor laryngeal elevation. The instrumental examination showed signs of tracheal aspiration. The diagnosis of dysphagia secondary to stroke was confirmed.

CRITICAL THINKING:

1. Why might a nasogastric tube be placed on admission?
2. Should the nasogastric tube have been removed? Why do you think it was removed?

CLINICAL CORNER 1-2

M. M. was admitted to the burn unit with severe burns to the head, neck, and upper torso. Because of associated pain he was heavily sedated. As his condition improved and before he was allowed to eat orally, a request for a swallowing evaluation was made because it was noticed he was not swallowing his secretions well. The evaluation of swallowing revealed normal strength of the swallowing musculature; however, he was disoriented and could not maintain his alertness level for more than 30 seconds. Because of his poor mental status and alertness level he was not allowed to eat and was considered to be at risk for dysphagia.

CRITICAL THINKING:

1. How might medications contribute to dysphagia?
2. Could poor mental status result in choking? Give some examples.

text, most of these diagnoses will receive individualized attention. See Chapter 7 for a full discussion of symptoms and signs associated with dysphagia.

Dictionary-based definitions of dysphagia imply that it is the result of a physiologic change in the muscles needed for swallowing. Physiologic change often leads to the two hallmarks of dysphagia: delay in the propulsion of a **bolus** as it transits from the mouth to the stomach and/or misdirection of a bolus. *Misdirection* can be defined as bolus material entering the upper airway and/or lungs or material that enters the mouth, pharynx, or esophagus during swallowing attempts but fails to reach the stomach. In these circumstances, classification of dysphagia by either clinical or instrumental examination seems warranted and straightforward.

However, not all patients with physiologic abnormalities of the swallowing mechanism show obvious delay in bolus flow or misdirection of bolus flow. The question that may arise for the clinician (and often for the researcher who has selected a cohort of patients with dysphagia) is the degree of severity of physiologic changes in the swallowing musculature needed before a patient is classified as having dysphagia. For instance, physiologic changes in the swallowing musculature have been described in older persons[2]—such as reduction in tongue strength or esophageal motility—both of which may delay the delivery of food or liquid to the stomach. However, only when such changes result in perceptible changes in eating habits or associated medical complications such as **under-**

CLINICAL CORNER 1-3

L. T. was admitted to the psychiatry unit with symptoms of acute schizophrenia. When eating, it was noted he would take excessive time to finish, with intermittent choking episodes. The speech pathologist who evaluated him for signs and symptoms of dysphagia found that the oropharyngeal swallowing musculature was intact. As she watched the patient eat, she noted a rapid feeding rate with inappropriate bite sizes. She also noted excessive talking while eating, and the choking episodes occurred during these talking periods. The patient was classified as dysphagic as a result of emotional and behavioral abnormalities.

CRITICAL THINKING:

1. What other types of behavioral disorders might contribute to dysphagia?
2. Why did this patient choke while eating and talking?

nutrition or **aspiration pneumonia** is a person classified as truly having dysphagia. Because swallowing is a dynamic process, persons may not exhibit signs and symptoms of dysphagia with every swallow and every bolus type. In these cases, they may be considered to be at risk for dysphagia or, alternatively, operationally defined as dysphagic. It is also possible that the swallowing musculature is normal but the patient is not alert enough to use that musculature because of his or her decompensated medical condition. In such cases it is assumed that attempts to swallow would result in dysphagic complications. In these cases, the patient may be classified as at risk for dysphagia. Patients may demonstrate abnormalities of behavior that interfere with the normal swallowing process; these may cause dysphagic signs and symptoms or put the patient at risk for dysphagia. Therefore dysphagia is defined not only by abnormalities of the mechanics of the swallowing musculature, but also by the consequences of failure, or potential failure, of that musculature owing to factors not always specifically related to swallow mechanics. For this reason the authors prefer the definition of dysphagia offered by Tanner[3]: "Dysphagia: [an] impairment of emotional, cognitive, sensory, and/or motor acts involved with transferring a substance from the mouth to stomach, resulting in failure to maintain hydration and nutrition, and posing a risk of choking and **aspiration**" (p. 152).

A *swallowing disorder* should be distinguished from a feeding disorder. A feeding disorder is impairment in the process of food transport outside the alimentary system. A *feeding disorder* usually is the result of weakness or incoordination in the hand or arm used to move the food from the plate to the mouth. In the United Kingdom and the United States a feeding disorder, particularly in the context of infants and children, may be the same as a swallowing disorder. Persons with feeding disorders (motor transfer problems) also may be dysphagic, such as those with cerebral palsy whose neurologic disability affects both feeding (motoric transfer) and swallowing. It is not known whether a feeding disorder that might require assistance with food transport also affects the subsequent act of swallowing, perhaps by interfering with timing of swallowing events.

A swallowing disorder also is to be distinguished from an *eating disorder* such as **anorexia** or **bulimia nervosa**. Whereas patients with dysphagia, bulimia, and anorexia may have difficulty with poor appetite, changes in dietary selections, and problems with the oral preparation of the bolus, patients with bulimia and anorexia rarely have demonstrable changes in or complaints of swallowing difficulty.[4]

INCIDENCE AND PREVALENCE

The *incidence* of a disorder is the reported frequency of new occurrences of that disorder over a long time (usually at least 1 year) in relation to the population in which it occurs. The *prevalence* of a disorder is the number of cases in a population during a shorter, prescribed period, usually in a specific setting. Exact measures of the incidence and prevalence of swallowing disorders in large and various populations are impossible because of differences in accepted definitions of dysphagia, the setting in which it is measured (**acute**, **rehabilitation**, **chronic**), and differences in the measurement tools across studies to detect it.[5] For instance, asking a patient if she or he has a swallowing disorder to determine the prevalence is a very different method of detection compared with the use of an instrumental examination such as **videofluoroscopy.** Most demographic data that are reported relating to swallowing disorders are prevalence data. The importance of knowing the prevalence of a disorder can help guide clinicians in the detection of that disorder and therefore helps plan how resources might be devoted to that disorder. For instance, if an examiner knew that a certain abnormality was found in less than 1% of that population, the examiner may not

---

CLINICAL CASE EXAMPLE 1-1

The hospital's chief of staff was reviewing a request from the dysphagia team to hire an additional speech pathologist and dietitian to screen and treat patients on the hospital's new stroke and acute geriatric units. Part of the rationale for the request was based on recent published guidelines from the Centers for Medicare & Medicaid Services that screening for dysphagia on a stroke unit was prudent because of evidence that early detection may prevent associated **morbidity** and **mortality,** both of which would increase costs for the health care system and, by implication, the hospital. Furthermore, prevalence data from five studies were submitted indicating that at least half of the patients on the stroke unit and a similar number on the acute geriatric unit may have dysphagia. The financial officer estimated that early detection and treatment of dysphagia would result in a cost savings that far exceeded the cost of the two new employees who would be assigned to those units. After integrating the request from the dysphagia team, the evidence from the literature on prevalence, and the potential cost savings to the medical center, the chief of staff approved the request.

spend time looking for that abnormality because its expected frequency of occurrence would be low. If, however, a particular abnormality was found in more than 50% of the persons with a particular disorder, the examiner would be alerted to expect the occurrence of deficits associated with that disorder. Therefore if the data suggested that 50% of patients who have had an acute stroke could have dysphagia, and that 20% of that group might have silent aspiration, an examiner would expect that half of the patients with acute stroke would have swallowing impairment and about half of those are at high risk for silent aspiration. Furthermore, pneumonia develops in 37% of acute stroke patients with aspiration.[6] Knowledge of these prevalence data provides valuable assistance to medical personnel who initially screen for and manage the medical complications after acute stroke (see Chapter 4).

The American Speech-Language-Hearing Association (ASHA) estimates that 6 to 10 million Americans show some degree of dysphagia, although it is not known how these estimates were made.[7] Kuhlemeier[8] reported that the incidence of reported dysphagia in the state of Maryland rose from 3 in 1000 in 1979 to 10 in 1000, probably as a result of better reporting methods. Using these estimates, approximately 25,000 persons in Maryland in 1989 had dysphagia as either a primary or secondary diagnosis.

Prevalence by Setting

Estimates of prevalence of dysphagia vary by setting because certain age groups (older adults and newborns) and diagnoses (neurogenic) are more likely to demonstrate dysphagia. For instance, patients entering a rehabilitation setting may not have as many accompanying medical problems and dysphagia as those entering a nursing home. Conversely, infants born prematurely may have many medical problems that may secondarily result in dysphagia. In a survey of the entire population of an acute general hospital, fewer patients with dysphagia would be found in the general population compared with a survey of a special section of that hospital, such as the stroke unit.

Community

Estimates of the prevalence of dysphagia among older persons living in the community range from 16% to 22%.[9,10] One study reported on the prevalence of dysphagia in a younger cohort (14- to 30-year-olds) living in the community who had been referred for complaints of dysphagia.[11] In this selected group, 70% had demonstrable pathologic conditions that accompanied their symptoms.

Acute and Chronic Geriatric Care

Of the 211 patients admitted to an acute geriatric unit in Singapore, the prevalence of dysphagia was 29% on admission and 28% at discharge.[12] In a nursing home in Maryland (chronic care), as many as 60% of residents had a combination of swallowing and/or feeding difficulty.[13] One study found that when feeding and swallowing difficulty were combined, as many as 87% of the residents in a home for the aged were at risk for inadequate oral intake.[14] Follow-up data of nursing home residents with oropharyngeal dysphagia indicate a mortality rate of 45% at 1 year.[15]

Acute General Hospitals

Using the Fleming Index of Dysphagia, a tool to identify dysphagia, Layne et al.[16] found that nearly one third of their patients had a diagnosis consistent with dysphagia. These findings were nearly 18% higher than those provided by Groher and Bukatman,[17] who reported a 13% prevalence rate in similar settings. The discrepancy in prevalence was explained by the fact that patients who were dehydrated in the study by Layne et al. were classified as dysphagic, whereas this was not a marker for dysphagia used in the collection of the Groher and Bukatman data.

Acute Rehabilitation Unit

Of 307 consecutive admissions to an acute rehabilitation facility, one third of patients were dysphagic.[18] Of this group, half had dysphagia as a result of a stroke, followed by traumatic brain injury (20%), spinal cord injury and brain tumor (7%), and progressive neurologic disease (5%). On admission, the patients with the most severe dysphagia were those with traumatic brain injury, followed by stroke. The least severe dysphagia occurred in those with brain tumors.

Special Populations

Some primary medical diagnoses are more likely to precipitate dysphagic symptomatology, such as diseases that affect the central and peripheral nervous system and disorders affecting the structures of the alimentary tract, such as cancer. An estimated 300,000 to 600,000 persons in the United States each year are affected by dysphagia from neurologic disorders alone; most cases occur after a stroke.[5] If these data are reliable, dysphagia is a common symptom after a stroke.

Stroke. Prevalence reports of dysphagia after stroke depend on when in the course of recovery the detection of a swallowing impairment was made. For instance, in acute stroke (less than 5 days after onset) the prevalence of dysphagia may be as high as 50%, whereas 2 weeks after stroke only 10% to 28% of patients may be dysphagic. Recognizing these discrepancies, Smithard et al.[19] provided follow-up of 121 (untreated) acute stroke patients for 6 months using a clinical dysphagia examination and videofluoroscopy to detect swallowing deficits. Immediately after stroke, 51% were believed to be at risk for aspiration. After 7 days, only 27% were still considered to be at risk. At 6 months, 3% of the survivors had persistent difficulty, whereas 3% who previously were not dysphagic were now considered at risk. These results suggest that early detection is important in preventing dysphagic complications and that a significant number of patients will improve without intervention specific to their dysphagia. Similarly, comparable prevalence figures for dysphagia on admission (43% to 51%) were found by Gordon et al.[20] and Mann et al.,[21] although the latter group noted a higher prevalence of dysphagic symptoms at 6 months (50%) than other studies with prevalence rates that ranged from 3% to 9%.[19,21] Daniels et al.[22] found that 36 (65%) of 55 patients with acute stroke had dysphagia. Of these 36, more than half aspirated. Of these, two thirds did so silently, suggesting that events of aspiration could be detected only by videofluoroscopy, not the bedside examination. In long-term follow-up, 94% of these patients returned to oral intake. Interestingly, the presence or absence of **silent aspiration** did not discriminate between patients who returned to successful oral feeding.

Head/Neck Cancer. Surprisingly, there have been no large studies of the prevalence or incidence of swallowing disorders in unselected patients after treatment for head/neck cancer, although it is well known that dysphagia is a frequent complication. Dysphagia can be result from the removal of tissue, with subsequent sensory and motor loss, and the effects of **radiation therapy** and **chemotherapy**. Before patients in their study received treatment, Pauloski et al.[23] found that 59% had symptoms consistent with dysphagia. In a large multicenter treatment trial of patients with laryngectomies who were treated with either surgery and radiation or radiation and chemotherapy, approximately 33% had some type of swallowing-related difficulty at 2-year follow-up.[24] In a series of 46 patients treated by **supraglottic laryngectomy**, 60% had dysphagia after their hospital stay.[25] Evidence suggests that patients with pharyngeal tumor resections and those with tumors involving the tongue base are more likely to have dysphagia.[26]

Head Injury. Dysphagia is common after severe head injury. Data report that the incidence of dysphagia ranges from 4.5% (9 of 199) of consecutive admissions in an acute care setting[27] to an incidence of 78% (31 of 40) in a similar setting.[28] Discrepancies in reporting may be attributable to the initial severity of the injury and the method used to detect and define dysphagia. Incidence data are available for patients who survive head injury and enter a rehabilitation setting; the incidence ranges from 27% to 30%[27,29] to 42% (218 of 524).[30] In a mixed group (type of injury and time after onset), Lazarus and Logemann[31] found that approximately half of the patients they examined with videofluoroscopy showed evidence of dysphagia. Among patients with head injuries entering a rehabilitation setting, Winstein[29] found that 27% were dysphagic on admission to rehabilitation and that only 6% were dysphagic after 5 months of rehabilitation. Of 62 consecutive patients receiving outpatient rehabilitation, Yorkston et al.[28] reported that 13% remained dysphagic. In general, the more severe the initial injury, the higher the incidence of dysphagia. Some patients remain comatose and are unable to eat, whereas others require extensive neurosurgical procedures with prolonged **intubation** and mental status changes, all of which may preclude attempts at oral ingestion. However, once patients enter the rehabilitation setting, their chances of returning to oral feeding are good.

Progressive Neurologic Disease. Progressive neurologic diseases that frequently result in dysphagia include **Parkinson's disease** and its variants, **amyotrophic lateral sclerosis**, **multiple sclerosis**, **myasthenia gravis**, and diseases of **systemic rheumatic** origin, such as **dermatomyositis, polymyositis, rheumatoid arthritis, scleroderma,** and **Sjögren's syndrome**. Systemic rheumatic disorders are far rarer than Parkinson's disease or multiple sclerosis but merit consideration in a discussion of dysphagia and neurologic disease. Because of the progressive nature of these disease processes, the point in disease progression at which dysphagic symptoms occur is never certain. For instance, some patients report dysphagia as the initial symptom of the disease, whereas others may never mention dysphagia. In general, however, as disease severity increases, so does dysphagia. Complications from dysphagia, particularly those that threaten pulmonary function, may lead to aspiration pneumonia and death.

Parkinson's Disease. Although dysphagia secondary to Parkinson's disease appears to be common, accurate measurements are restricted by subject selection bias and dysphagia detection methods. However, most authors agree that dysphagia occurs in at least 50% of patients with Parkinson's disease.[32-34] In 72 patients with Parkinson's disease of varying severity, Leopold and Kagel[35] found that as many as 82% reported swallowing difficulty. The prevalence of dysphagia may be higher in patients with Parkinson's disease who also have significant dementia.[36]

Amyotropic Lateral Sclerosis. When amyotrophic lateral sclerosis (ALS) affects the **bulbar musculature**, dysphagia may be one of the first symptoms of the disease. In studies of patients with ALS at first diagnosis, 25% to 30% have evidence of bulbar symptomatology.[37,38] It can be assumed that at least one third of patients with a diagnosis of ALS will have some difficulty swallowing, particularly as the disease progresses. Known characteristics of disease progression that affect the bulbar musculature result in progressively severe dysphagia symptomatology.[39]

Multiple Sclerosis. Hartelius and Svensson[40] found that more than 33% of a large series of patients with multiple sclerosis (MS) had either chewing or swallowing problems. Dysphagic complaints in patients receiving follow-up care in an outpatient clinic ranged between 30% and 40%.[41] Similar to those with ALS, not all patients with MS will have dysphagia unless the bulbar musculature is involved, and symptoms are more likely to appear as the disease progresses. After evaluating 143 consecutive patients with primary and secondary progressive MS, Calcagno et al.[42] confirmed dysphagic symptoms in 34%. Their study showed a positive relation between dysphagia and disease severity and between dysphagia and brainstem involvement. After surveying 309 patients with MS, DePauw et al.[43] found that 24% had chronic swallowing difficulty and another 5% admitted to transitory difficulty. As patients became more disabled according to a scale of disability measurement, the prevalence of dysphagia increased to 65%.[43]

Myasthenia Gravis. In selected populations of patients with myasthenia gravis, approximately one third will be dysphagic.[44] The prevalence of dysphagia depends largely on the extent of muscle fatigue and other medical complications such as respiratory impairment secondary to an acute exacerbation of muscle weakness.

Muscular Dystrophy. There are no published reports of the prevalence of dysphagia in muscular dystrophy, although there are reports of swallowing dysfunction secondary to peripheral oropharyngeal and esophageal muscle weakness in those with oculo-pharyngeal, Duchenne, and myotonic muscular dystrophy.[45-47]

Polymyositis and Dermatomyositis. The prevalence of dysphagia after the diagnosis of either polymyositis or dermatomyositis is not known. As with other progressive neurologic conditions, with these disorders the course and response to medical therapy may differ; therefore the presence of dysphagia is variable. Because of their predilection to involve the **proximal muscle**, swallowing can be affected in these disorders.

Rheumatoid Arthritis. Geterude et al.[48] found that 8 of 29 patients with rheumatoid arthritis (RA) had complaints of dysphagia. In a series of 31 patients with dysphagia and RA, Ekberg et al.[49] documented pharyngeal dysfunction in 20.

Scleroderma. As many as 90% of patients with scleroderma have swallowing-related complaints.[50] Accompanying **erosive esophagitis** was found in 60% of 53 patients with scleroderma.[51] In these patients, dysphagia was always an accompanying complaint. In patients with scleroderma, dysphagic complaints usually are confined to the esophagus, although secondary effects on the oral and pharyngeal stages resulting from esophageal dysmotility should be considered.

Sjögren's Syndrome. As many as 75% of patients with Sjögren's syndrome have dysphagia.[52] The potential of this syndrome to involve all stages of swallowing function is well known.

Premature Infants. The incidence of infants born prematurely in the United States has increased to more than 12% of all live births and 18% of African-American births.[53] A growing concern has been the incidence of emotional and neurodevelopmental disabilities in the very low birth weight population (less than 26 weeks' gestation). Estimates indicate that as many as 90% of low birth weight infants may be prone to disorders of feeding.[54]

CONSEQUENCES OF DYSPHAGIA

Because dysphagia frequently accompanies many medical diagnoses, it is important to appreciate its potential impact on patient care. It is well recognized that dysphagia is a symptom of disease, but it also has the potential to secondarily precipitate morbidity and mortality. As such, its impact on health can be substantial. Additionally, it can affect the patient's overall quality of life.

Medical Consequences

A potential complication of patients with oropharyngeal dysphagia is aspiration pneumonia. The treat-

CLINICAL CASE EXAMPLE 1-2

A request for services was sent to the speech pathologist to evaluate a 70-year-old man for suspected dysphagia. He had lived in the nursing home for 2 years after a left brain stroke that left him with aphasia and poor mobility. He spent most of his day sitting in a wheelchair or in bed watching TV and was beginning to show evidence of **decubitus ulcers** on his coccyx. The nurses reported he was showing increased disinterest in his soft mechanical diet and was choking at most meals on his liquids. He rarely finished a meal. A review of his medical record revealed a consultation from the dietitian who noted that his **albumin** was 3.0 g/dL, he had lost 5% of his body weight in the past 2 weeks, and he was **hypernatremic**. Based on these parameters the dietitian concluded that the patient was undernourished and dehydrated and wondered if his previous history of dysphagia was contributory. The patient was examined in bed. He was able to follow one-step commands and name simple objects but was not oriented to time or place. During the examination the patient fell asleep every minute and the speech pathologist had to continually awaken him to maintain his attention and cooperation. An examination of his oral peripheral speech mechanism revealed a mild right facial weakness but otherwise was normal. Test swallows with various food items were delayed but without overt coughing. Tests with liquids revealed numerous choking episodes. Based on his physical examination and the results of his laboratory tests it was concluded that his swallow may improve if he were properly hydrated and nourished, and that it was unlikely that hydration and nourishment could be accomplished by mouth because his alertness level was poor. Furthermore, his nutritional and hydration requirements would have to be elevated because of fluid loss from the decubitus ulcers. It also was likely that his ulcers would not heal unless his protein stores were improved. For this reason, a **nasogastric tube** was recommended with regular reevaluation of his laboratory values and mental status to make recommendations for possible return to oral feeding. It was hypothesized that since he had been eating normally before this acute change that the dysphagia was most consistent with a change in metabolic status and not related to a change in his neurologic presentation.

ment of aspiration pneumonia is costly, and it is associated with increased length of stay in the hospital,[55] greater disability at 3 and 6 months,[55,56] and poorer nutritional status during hospitalization.[55] One study[55] found an increased mortality risk in stroke patients for whom swallowing was considered unsafe at 6 months' follow-up, whereas another study did not find this relation at 3 months.[56] Dehydration is a frequent adjunct in those with dysphagia after stroke.[55-57] Dehydration can lead to increased mental confusion and generalized organ system failure, both of which lead to greater decompensation of swallowing.[58] Dysphagia may lead to undernutrition, which adversely affects energy levels (ability to sustain a swallow), and if severe or chronic, compromises the immune system. Compromise to the immune system potentially delays healing and increases susceptibility to infection, **sepsis**, and death.[58]

Psychosocial Consequences

Oral ingestion of food and liquid is a pleasurable activity for most people. Social interactions often revolve around sharing a meal. "Let's have lunch, are you free for dinner, or can we meet for an early breakfast?" Having a piece of wedding cake, being offered an hors d'oeuvre at a party, enjoying a midnight snack, and going to one's favorite restaurant are all examples of common situations that require the ability to swallow. Swallowing difficulty therefore may limit the extent to which a person might socialize, leading to major changes in a normal lifestyle. Fear of overt choking episodes and the associated discomfort might contribute to social isolation and accompanying depression. Spouses and family members are equally affected because of the potential social limitations dysphagia may precipitate. Even making subtle changes in dietary preferences to compensate for dysphagia may lead to feelings of discontent. Eating may no longer be pleasurable. It becomes an activity performed only for nourishment. The need for special preparations at mealtime provides additional stress. Special dietary supplements may be costly, often posing financial burdens.

Clinical Management

The care of patients in whom dysphagia is suspected usually begins with a basic process of identification in an attempt to answer the question of whether dysphagia is present. This process can be the result of a simple screening, such as watching a patient eat or drink small amounts of food. Such a screening might be done after a patient has had an acute neurologic event such as a stroke. Some patients begin to eat without screening because the risk factors for dys-

I first met George at the New York Hospital in the outpatient clinic. He obviously was a man of means as he told stories of extensive travel. His swallowing evaluation that day revealed it was not safe for him to eat orally because of a specific muscle weakness, and a gastrostomy tube was recommended. He was noticeably upset by this recommendation. Because he was only 35 years old, we suspected that this might put an end to his life as a world traveler; however, George was not convinced. After his gastrostomy was placed, to my surprise he told me he had made arrangements for a 3-week trip to Spain and Portugal. He had arranged to ship cases of formula for his tube to each hotel on his travel itinerary before his departure. When he arrived in Spain, his formula was waiting. Normally he would have dined on bouillabaisse and fresh fish with a fine Chablis. Instead, he self-administered six cans of a liquid formula per day into his gastrostomy tube and continued to enjoy the ambience of Europe. He was determined not to let his severe pharyngeal dysphagia interfere with other aspects of his life.

phagia are not present. An example might be a patient who has not had any swallowing difficulty in the past but required a feeding tube immediately after an operation for medical purposes and who has been cleared by the physician to return to oral ingestion. As patients return to eating, either the medical staff or the patient notices swallowing difficulty. Outpatients may report to their general practitioner that they are having swallowing difficulty. In all these situations a clinical evaluation of swallowing will be initiated.

Clinical Examination

The clinical evaluation should include a thorough review of the medical and psychosocial history (see Chapter 9). This is followed by a physical evaluation that includes a screening of mental status, an evaluation of the musculature of the head and neck and, if appropriate, trial swallows of liquid, semisolid, and solid materials. If the clinical examination fails to adequately explain the patient's symptoms or requires more in-depth visualization of any phase of the swallowing sequence, an instrumental examination may be necessary. The clinical indicators for use of instrumental assessment techniques have been published by ASHA.[59]

Instrumental Examination

The instrumental assessment of the **aerodigestive tract** most commonly is done by barium x-ray studies, direct visualization, and measurement of pressures within the aerodigestive tract during swallowing attempts. The most common x-ray technique that assesses the oral, pharyngeal, and cervical esophageal phases of swallowing is the *modified barium swallow* (videofluoroscopy). ASHA provides a statement of guidelines for speech-language pathologists (SLPs) who perform this procedure.[60] A standard barium swallow (**esophagram**) may be used to evaluate the esophagus. Direct visualization of the pharyngeal, laryngeal, and esophageal compartments is done by **endoscopy**. Guidelines for the performance and interpretation of the endoscopic evaluation of swallowing by SLPs are provided by ASHA.[61] Patient preparation and positioning for each of these studies vary according to focus of the anatomic region being examined. Pressure measurements during swallowing (**manometry**) are more routinely done for clinical purposes in the esophagus than in the mouth or pharynx. A full discussion of these and other instrumental techniques used in the evaluation of swallowing is provided in Chapters 10 and 11.

Treatment Options

Ideally, the clinical and/or instrumental evaluations will lead to a treatment plan. The goal of most treatment plans is to ensure that the patient can consume enough food and liquid to remain nourished and hydrated and that the consumption of these materials does not pose a threat to airway safety resulting in aspiration pneumonia. If treatment is indicated, four main areas are considered: behavioral, dietary, medical, and surgical.

Behavioral interventions include engaging the patient in some change in swallowing behavior. Changes make take the form of simple compensations, such as a change in posture or eating rate, or in rehabilitative strategies, such as teaching a patient a new way to swallow, or in strengthening muscles. Dietary interventions might include modifications of texture, taste, or volume. Medical interventions may include a change in medication negatively affecting mental status and swallow or the placement of a nasogastric feeding tube. Surgical interventions might include mobilization of a weak vocal fold or the placement of a gastrostomy tube. Combinations of these options are common; however, the timing of each intervention is patient dependent. A full discussion of treatment planning, including options and details of rationale and use, is presented in Chapters 12 through 14.

WHO MANAGES DYSPHAGIA?

Patients who have disruptions in swallowing potentially involve many members of the medical community. Those whose dysphagia is related to the head and neck may see an otolaryngologist, dentist, SLP, or neurologist. To further define the disorder, these specialists often need the services of a radiologist. Those whose swallowing disorder may be of esophageal origin may require the services of a gastroenterologist. If the swallowing disorder is related to an acute respiratory condition, a patient may be under the care of a pulmonologist, pulmonary physical therapist, and respiratory therapist. If the swallowing disorder is related more to the process of feeding, an occupational therapist frequently is involved. If the swallowing disorder results in compromise to the nutritional system, a dietitian is consulted. While the patient is in the hospital, the nurse frequently is involved in the identification and treatment of the patient's swallowing disorder. In short, patients with swallowing disorders require the attention of many specialists who must work in concert to achieve swallowing safety and nutritional stability. The prominence of individual roles at any given time depends on the patient presentation.

Ideally, health care professionals who are concerned about the patient's swallowing safety and nutritional adequacy will work together toward the mutual goal of improving the patient's swallowing performance. Coordination of effort is important if timely results are to be achieved. Some medical centers have designated swallowing teams and swallowing team leaders. In many hospitals, the SLP assumes the role of swallowing team leader. The role each specialist plays on the team will vary across settings. For instance, some gastroenterologists diagnose and treat swallowing problems that involve the esophagus, but disorders of the esophagus are not their special interest. Specific interest in the swallowing-impaired patient also will vary. For instance, few radiologists have a specific interest in patients who report dysphagia. The result of this variance in interest and focus is that not all swallowing disorder teams are the same, and in some cases not all potential members will be represented.

Speech-Language Pathologist

SLPs have taken a leading role in the management of patients with dysphagia related to poor oral and pharyngeal swallowing mechanics. In most centers, they coordinate the swallowing team and are frequently the first professional to perform a history and physical examination that is specific to oropharyngeal dysphagia. Based on these data they consult other members of the dysphagia team, obtain approval from the patient's attending physician for any additional testing or referrals, and integrate the rehabilitative components of the dysphagia treatment program. Only within the past 20 years have specific practice guidelines for managing dysphagia by SLPs been developed. These include an outline of the knowledge and skills needed to treat oropharyngeal dysphagia and the need to understand the esophageal components of swallowing to make appropriate medical referrals.[62]

SLPs were evaluating and treating articulation disorders of children with cerebral palsy as early as the 1940s. Because of the decompensation of the oromotor system in children with cerebral palsy, both speech and swallowing were affected; however, treatments specific to swallowing were not a routine part of care by the SLP. Working in a medical setting studying patients with Parkinson's disease in the late 1960s, Dr. Jeri Logemann found that videofluoroscopy was ideally suited to study patients' speech and swallowing skills. Soon this technique was used to study the effects of cancer in the head and neck on swallowing performance, and in 1976 at the American Speech and Hearing Association National Convention she presented one of the first papers by an SLP on the diagnosis and treatment of swallowing disorders after surgical procedures for cancer in the head and neck. That the paper was accepted at the convention was a monumental achievement because there was no rec-

---

Practice Note 1-3

I well remember the reaction of ASHA in the 1970s and early 1980s to the acceptance of the role of the SLP in managing patients with dysphagia. It was the "new guard" versus the traditionalists. Letters to the editor flew back and forth, most arguing that this area of practice was potentially life threatening and SLPs did not have the medical background necessary to be competent. Treating patients with dysphagia labeled one as borderline heretic with threats of a breach of ethics. Today, patients with dysphagia dominate the caseloads of SLPs working in medical settings, and children with dysphagia are being managed in the public school setting. And both ASHA and the medical community have embraced the role of the SLP in these efforts.

ognized category for a paper on swallowing, and evaluating and treating patients with swallowing disorders was not within the accepted scope of practice for an SLP. This radical departure from the traditional role of the SLP raised more than a few eyebrows.

As Logemann was beginning her distinguished career in dysphagia management, Dr. George Larsen, also working in a medical setting with adults, began to develop treatments specific to patients with neurogenic swallowing disorders. Because so many of his patients with speech and language disorders had accompanying swallowing dysfunction, he began to search the literature for relevant treatment approaches. He discovered a literature full of descriptions of how a person swallows but no mention of how to treat the impairment. Using his background in neurology and physiology, he began to develop treatment approaches and reported them in the literature. He wrote about appropriate postures[63] and need for some patients to bring the swallowing sequence under volitional control.[64] He was convinced that the most successful approaches would result from a team effort, and he described the use of trained feeding volunteers as part of the process.[63] The momentum to evaluate and treat swallowing disorders in children and adults grew

throughout the 1980s. The momentum was sustained by the publication of two texts by SLPs summarizing empirical evidence supporting the role of the SLP and emphasizing the need for collaboration among various medical professionals.[65,66] Both texts have undergone revisions. Today, SLPs have assumed a leadership role in providing care to children and adults with oropharyngeal dysphagia. SLPs are at the forefront of providing the research and educational components that support their clinical efforts. Miller and Groher[67] have described a more detailed history of the involvement of the SLP in the management of swallowing disorders.

Otolaryngologist

The otolaryngologist is skilled in the evaluation of the upper digestive tract. In particular, the use of endoscopy by otolaryngologists for direct visualization of the structures of the nasopharynx, oropharynx, pharynx, and larynx adds information relative to the structural, sensory, and motor aspects of the pharyngeal stage of swallowing. In patients with head/neck cancer who require surgery, otolaryngologists provide surgical and postsurgical management. In this regard, they must be sensitive not only to issues of cancer control, but also to the preservation of speech and swallowing functions. The otolaryngologist may be involved with the surgical placement and removal of a patient's **tracheostomy tube**. Because these tubes may interfere with normal swallowing, these specialists work with the dysphagia team to remove the tubes as soon as medically feasible.

Gastroenterologist

The gastroenterologist who participates on the swallowing disorders team usually has a special interest in the esophagus. Because primary esophageal disorders that precipitate dysphagia can have secondary effects on the pharyngeal and oral stages of swallowing, it is important to include the gastroenterologist in the evaluation of the patient who may appear to only have symptoms that relate to the oral or pharyngeal stages of swallowing (see Chapter 7). The gastroenterologist is familiar with the management of **gastroesophageal reflux disease** (GERD), or heartburn, a symptom that may be related to dysphagia. The gastroenterologist may use special sensors that measure the amount of acid content in the alimentary tract using a test called **24-hour pH monitoring**. The gastroenterologist may use manometry to measure esophageal motility and prescribe medications to improve esophageal motility or to control GERD. The use of esophageal endoscopy to make visual observations of the esophageal mucosa to rule out a stricture

---

CLINICAL CORNER 1-4

Dr. Miller and I followed Dr. Larsen to a patient with occult hydrocephalus who could not initiate a swallow. Results of examination of his oral peripheral mechanism were normal, and Dr. Larsen suggested that we needed to stimulate laryngeal elevation. The following day we watched in disbelief as Dr. Larsen approached the patient with a probe tip wrapped in gauze, dipped in saline solution, and attached to a primitive facial nerve stimulator. As he applied the electric current to the thyroid notch, a swallow was initiated and the patient continued to swallow without the assistance of the stimulation. Our collective elation that "treatment" could be so easy was quickly dampened when Dr. Larsen warned it could be dangerous to use such a technique with every patient because it could trigger laryngospasm and death. We learned two things that day: not all treatments are for every patient, and some treatments carry accompanying risk.

CRITICAL THINKING:
1. Why might an electrical current facilitate swallowing?
2. Name other types of medical treatments that carry risk.

or cancer is a role of the gastroenterologist. The gastroenterologist is responsible for the nonsurgical placement of a feeding tube in the stomach called a **percutaneous endoscopic gastrostomy** (PEG) tube.

Radiologist

The radiologist who may be a regular member of the swallowing disorders team often has a special interest in the gastrointestinal tract. Radiologists provide both dynamic (videofluorographic) and static (**plain films**) imaging of the aerodigestive tract and lung fields. Often these studies provide the diagnostic information that guides swallowing treatment. Special tests such as computed tomography performed after static images of the aerodigestive tract are done by a radiologist. The SLP frequently works in conjunction with the radiologist in performing the modified barium swallow (see Chapter 10). The interpretation of the modified barium swallow study is often done concurrently by the SLP and the radiologist.

Neurologist

Because the majority of patients with oropharyngeal dysphagia have swallowing impairment as a result of neurologic disease, the neurologist has an important role in the identification and subsequent management of swallowing problems. It is critical that patients with symptoms of dysphagia without a known cause be considered for evaluation by the neurologist. Some neurologic diseases that precipitate dysphagia can be treated with medication. Finding a cause also is important in providing the patient with an explanation for the dysphagia and in providing a prognosis for future complications.

Dentist

Patients with dysphagic symptoms may be identified first by the dentist during routine dental care. Of particular interest to the dentist are any oral-stage manifestations of swallowing disorders, such as problems with chewing, bolus formation, or dental disorders such as **osteoradionecrosis** that would make swallowing painful. The dental prosthodontist is skilled at making appliances for the oral cavity that can facilitate swallowing in patients who have had oral structures removed because of cancer. In Japan, the dentist is often the team leader in the care of patients with dysphagia.

Nurse

The nurse has 24-hour responsibility for monitoring the patient's swallowing problem. Monitoring the amount of intake and recording it in the medical record is an important role for the nurse. Not only do nurses often identify problems during eating in patients in whom dysphagia is not suspected, but they also provide the guidance necessary to help the patient with identified dysphagia use recommended swallowing strategies. Other responsibilities include administering tube feedings, maintaining good oral hygiene, and assigning volunteers to assist selected patients at mealtime.

Dietitian

The dietitian assesses the patient's nutritional and hydration needs and monitors the patient's response to those needs. Because dysphagia frequently affects a patient's nutrition and hydration status, and because the result of poor nutrition and hydration affects a patient's overall medical stability, it is important to involve the dietitian in the care plan for patients with dysphagia. Because dietitians frequently monitor mealtime activities, they may be the professional who initially detects a swallowing disorder. If specialized dysphagic diets are ordered for the patient, the dietitian may communicate with the food service to ensure that the special diet is prepared properly. If a patient is unable to eat orally, the dietitian may make a recommendation for a tube feeding. Guidelines for the amount and rate of tube feeding frequently are recommended by the dietitian.

Occupational Therapist

The occupational therapist is skilled in retraining the patient to self-feed. If the patient is unable to self-feed because of weakness or incoordination, the occupational therapist needs to be involved in the patient's care. Special adaptive feeding devices, such as a **plate guard** or built-up utensils for easier grasping, are ordered by the occupational therapist to assist the patient in achieving feeding independence. In some medical centers, the SLP and occupational therapist work closely with infants in the neonatal intensive care unit.

Neurodevelopmental Specialist

The neonatal intensive care unit (NICU) setting can influence the infant's brain development and organization as well as the parent-infant relationship. The neurodevelopmental specialist (NDS) is keenly aware of this relationship and will tailor the infant's care to individual needs. An NDS may be a speech pathologist or occupational therapist who has specialized in assisting the premature infant in developmental growth by fostering supportive care during the infant's nervous system development. Neurodevelopmental care includes, but is not limited to, proper infant positioning to support neurodevelopmental tone and maturation. Often it is important to regulate to tolerance the infant's visual, tactile, and auditory stimulation. Feeding is one of the most difficult tasks in which a premature infant can succeed. The NDS provides continued assessment regarding the timing and safety of the infant's oral feedings by breast or bottle. The NDS also monitors the infant's physiologic and behavioral responses to the environment and fosters a positive outcome.

Pulmonologist/Respiratory Therapist

Although the pulmonologist may not be a regular member of the dysphagia team, patients of pulmonologists frequently have swallowing disorders that require management by the swallowing team. Patients with respiratory disorders that require tracheostomy and ventilatory support (respirators) often have accompanying swallowing difficulty. Working with the respiratory therapist and pulmonologist to improve pulmonary toilet is an important step toward **decannulation**. Removing a patient's respiratory supports often is a prerequisite for improving the swallowing response.

LEVELS OF CARE

The prevalence, cause, and type of swallowing disorder that might be encountered depend in part on the setting in which the patient is seen. Correspondingly, the role of each professional may be different, or access to some medical specialties may not be available. For instance, it is rare for a gastroenterologist to have a full-time appointment in a nursing home facility or that a radiologist would be on staff in that facility. Traditionally, levels of care are divided into five categories: acute, **subacute**, rehabilitation, **skilled nursing**, and **home health**.

Acute Care Setting

In a survey of two acute care hospitals, Groher and Bukatman[17] found the prevalence of swallowing-related disorders to be 13%. The majority of these patients were found in the intensive care units and the neurology and neurosurgery units. Owing to the acute nature of their illness, patients in the acute care setting frequently have multiple medical complications, require **intubation** tubes connected to ventilators, have tracheostomy tubes in place, require feeding tubes for nutrition, and have frequent changes in their physical and mental status. Because their stay in the hospital may be short (2 to 5 days), their swallowing needs must be addressed rapidly. Frequently there is not sufficient time or patient cooperation

CLINICAL CASE EXAMPLE 1-3

The SLP was called by the thoracic surgeon to the intensive care unit for a consultation. Her patient had just undergone cardiac bypass surgery and had respiratory complications requiring the placement of a tracheostomy tube. The patient was now medically stable and was ready to resume oral feeding. The SLP consulted with the respiratory therapist, who mentioned that the patient still required some oxygenation by facial mask for short periods during the day. After noting those times, the SLP returned when the mask was not in use because it might potentially interfere with the evaluation. On physical evaluation the patient had reduced tongue strength and could make a weak, breathy voice only when the tracheotomy tube was occluded. She had a nasogastric tube in place for nutritional purposes. During the evaluation the dietitian came in and told the SLP that the patient was not tolerating the feeding given by nasogastric tube and that it would be beneficial for the patient to begin to eat orally because some of those complications could be avoided. The SLP gave the patient small amounts of ice chips and water, as well as gelatin and pudding. The patient showed delayed swallowing of all materials and a weak cough on the liquids. The SLP believed that the patient may be at risk for aspiration because of pharyngeal weakness that may have involved the true vocal fold. She believed an instrumental evaluation to allow her to observe the pharyngeal stage of swallow would be appropriate and that swallowing endoscopy would be the test of choice because it can be accomplished at the patient's bedside. She received approval for the study from the consulting physician and the test was performed the same day. Swallowing endoscopy revealed that during the coughing episodes the patient was protecting her airway; however, there appeared to be some weakness in the left true vocal fold. She recommended that the patient start a special dysphagic diet and communicated that to the dietitian, who made the arrangements. The otolaryngologist was consulted for his opinion on whether any intervention would be appropriate for the vocal fold weakness. The SLP designed specific swallowing instructions and shared them with the patient and nursing staff. This case is a good example of how many disciplines can be involved in caring for a patient who has dysphagia.

because of mental status to order sophisticated laboratory tests. In this circumstance, the clinician may have to rely on the history and clinical evaluation to make a diagnosis and establish a treatment plan. If an instrumental evaluation is recommended, care must be given to scheduling. If the patient is able to cooperate with laboratory testing and is a candidate to proceed for further rehabilitation, his or her future care is facilitated if the acute care clinician can document the swallowing disorder with an instrumental technique such as videofluoroscopy or endoscopy.

Neonatal Care Unit

Children born prematurely often must stay in the hospital for extended periods in the neonatal intensive care unit (NICU). Specialized interventions for premature newborns such as improved systems of delivering respiratory support have resulted in higher survival rates of low birth weight infants. In the 1980s, the concept of integrated developmental care was introduced to minimize the potential for emotional and neurodevelopmental disorders after discharge. This type of care emphasizes the coordinated efforts of nurses, physicians, therapists, and other care providers toward common goals, with each discipline supporting the other. This type of care also recognizes issues of parent-child separation and the atypical environment of a hospital on the child's development.

More recently, infants admitted to the NICU are managed by "cluster care." Before the availability of cluster care, infants received medical care at any hour during the day. However, the cluster care concept allows infants to sleep for 3 hours, after which time they are awakened for all their care, including feeding, diaper changes, and needed tests. Cluster care allows the infant to regularize his or her schedule, similar to what would occur outside the hospital environment.

Subacute Care Setting

Patients admitted to subacute care usually are not ready for a strenuous rehabilitation program. They may require additional medical monitoring but not the type of costly care of an acute admission associated with intensive care. If a swallowing treatment goal was formulated in the acute setting, the action plan to achieve that goal is implemented in the subacute unit. For instance, if the goal was to try to wean a patient from the tracheostomy tube as a way to ensure swallowing safety, the swallowing team would work toward that goal. If a patient continued to require tube feeding after leaving the acute care unit, a goal of the swallowing team in the subacute unit might be to begin restoring oral **alimentation**. Patients may stay in the subacute unit from 5 to 28

days. After this admission, they may be discharged home, to a rehabilitation facility, or to a skilled nursing facility.

Rehabilitation Setting

Patients who enter rehabilitation settings usually are judged to have the physical stamina needed to complete a full day of tasks oriented toward restoring lost function. In most cases, the patient also will be able to learn new information. For those with swallowing impairment, it may mean they need to learn or solidify their learning of new swallowing strategies. The role of the speech pathologist is to teach the patient swallowing strategies (see Chapters 12 to 14). This may include special maneuvers or postures. It also may entail specialized diets. Frequently, the goal in the rehabilitation setting as it pertains to swallowing is to return the patient to a dietary level that is as near to normal as possible while ensuring swallowing safety. Swallowing safety may be defined as the maintenance of nutrition and **hydration** without medical complications. Not only is it considered medically unsafe for a patient to get food or fluid in the lungs, but it is also unsafe to not get sufficient nutrition and hydration to maintain normal bodily functions. For instance, lack of proper nutrition and hydration can lead to excessive fatigue, mental status changes, poor wound healing, anorexia, and a greater chance of developing infections. After a 1-month period of successful rehabilitation, the patient usually is discharged home. Those in whom medical complications develop during rehabilitation or who do not improve to a level of partial independence may be discharged to a skilled nursing facility.

Skilled Nursing Facility

Patients who enter skilled nursing facilities usually have either not responded to attempts at rehabilitation, are not candidates for rehabilitation after their acute hospitalization, are too ill to be at home, or have chronic medical conditions that require monitoring in a structured environment. The prevalence of swallowing disorders in this setting has been reported to be as high as 60%.[13] The high prevalence in this setting is because the patients have multiple medical problems that predispose them to dysphagia. The majority, for instance, may have a neurologic disease that has compromised the swallowing musculature or has interfered with the cortical controls needed to complete the swallowing sequence. Their swallowing disorders are chronic. Some patients will have seen some recovery in their dysphagia, whereas others will continue to rely on tube feedings. For those who recover, it is important to help them maintain their skills. Those who must rely on tube feedings after their hospital stay will require reevaluation for the possibility of returning to oral feeding. For some, returning to oral alimentation will not be possible. Because of the potential for patients in this setting to be medically fragile, it is easy to decompensate their swallowing skills by a slight change in medical status, rather than a new, major event such as stroke. An example of this phenomenon might be a patient who is not swallowing a sufficient amount of liquids, who may then develop a urinary tract infection that results in a fever with generalized fatigue, anorexia, and a disinterest in eating. In this situation, the patient may not be ingesting enough calories to be able to sustain the strength needed to produce a safe swallow throughout the entire meal. As a consequence of fatigue, the patient is more likely to show signs of dysphagia.

Another example might be a patient who has been eating well but whose medications were changed. The unwanted side effect from the medication change could negatively affect the nervous system to create a problem with motor movement, and swallowing is secondarily affected. For example, medications that create sedative effects are capable of decompensating an already fragile swallow by slowing motor movement and interfering with the cortical controls necessary to complete an entire meal. The potential for fluctuations in metabolism in this patient population often make it difficult to establish a single factor that precipitated the dysphagia.

It is known that patients in skilled nursing facilities usually are in older age cohorts. Not only do they endure the effects of diseases that result in dysphagia commonly found in older persons (e.g., stroke, Parkinson's disease), but they also have impairments in swallowing as a result of the aging process. Change in taste perception and in the strength and speed of the swallowing muscles are examples of these alterations. The speech pathologist working in the skilled nursing facility is kept busy managing the large number of patients with swallowing disorders. Many patients with dysphagia are able to eat safely only if they are at the proper dietary level and only if they are following the recommended feeding strategies. Any change in baseline metabolism or any new neurologic insult may decompensate their swallowing skills so that they are at risk for developing medical complications. Many times the focus of therapeutic effort for the SLP working in the skilled nursing facility is one of prevention—attempting to keep patients as safe as possible while eating, even in the circumstance of suspected dysphagia. Such preventive efforts not only may require direct intervention with behavioral and dietary treatment strategies, but also entail monitoring of mealtime activities to ensure that patients who are at risk of aspiration are following the prescribed dysphagia treatment plan.

Often the mental or physical status of patients in the skilled nursing environment interferes with their ability to cooperate with a formal dysphagia evaluation. Clinicians must rely on a combination of the medical history and detailed observations of each meal to establish the treatment plan. If the patient is not eating orally, the clinician often must rely on the physical examination and on his or her judgment of how well the patient managed attempts at oral ingestion as part of that examination. The examination will be limited further by poor access to modified barium swallow studies or other laboratory investigations. Transportation of patients to receive these tests presents another challenge because chronically ill patients are difficult to move.

The chronic medical conditions of patients in skilled nursing facilities often are life threatening. For this reason, patients and their families may execute an advance directive (see Chapter 15). The *advance directive* is a statement executed by the patient or family (if they hold medical power of attorney) of their desires and wishes regarding their medical care in life-threatening situations, such as whether the patient would want to be resuscitated for cardiac arrest. Part of this directive may pertain to their wishes to sustain nutrition, especially when the support for nutrition may involve feeding tubes. Patients may elect to not be fed by a feeding tube despite the risk of aspiration and life-threatening pneumonia. In these cases, the role of the swallowing clinician is to recommend the safest mode of ingestion, making sure that the patient and family understand the potential risks.

Home Health

Patients who have left the hospital or the rehabilitation setting for home may require additional monitoring or direct treatment from therapists who perform their responsibilities in the patient's home environment. Patients who are unable to swallow should receive regular reevaluations for attempts at oral feeding unless oral feeding is contraindicated by the medical care team. Most often, the clinician responsible for managing the swallowing disorder in the home environment is ensuring that the patient is following the swallowing strategies or has improved to a point at which consideration should be given to changing the dietary level. These changes often are made in consultation with the patient and family and are based on the physical examination and observations of eating.

CLINICAL CORNER 1-5

An 86-year-old man who had been living in a nursing home was admitted to the hospital with a suspected right brain stroke. He was confused on admission, and the attending physician did not think it was safe for him to eat orally so a nasogastric tube was placed. At the nursing home he was eating a modified soft diet because his teeth were in poor repair. He had a past history of GERD and **Barrett's esophagitis**. After 2 days a swallowing evaluation was ordered before he was allowed to resume oral feeding.

CRITICAL THINKING:

1. How many medical disciplines might become involved with this patient? Who and why?
2. What are the chances that he will be dysphagic based on his history? Are age and prior living setting considerations in this case? How might these facts affect the diagnosis and treatment?
3. Are there any special issues revolving around which side of the brain was injured that might relate to dysphagia?

TAKE HOME NOTES

1. Dysphagia is a symptom of a disease, not a primary disease. It is characterized by a delay or misdirection of something swallowed as food moves from the mouth to the stomach. It has both medical and psychosocial consequences on a patient's quality of life.
2. A feeding disorder usually refers to the process of food transport. An eating disorder may not be related to a swallowing disorder.
3. The prevalence of dysphagia is highest in patients with neurologic disease.
4. Patients in acute care intensive care units and those in skilled nursing facilities tend to be at highest risk for dysphagia.
5. There may not be a clear link between dysphagic symptoms and the patient's primary medical diagnosis in patients who reside in skilled nursing facilities.
6. Patients in skilled nursing facilities are medically fragile, and their swallowing response can be easily decompensated by fatigue or an acute medical condition such as an infection.
7. Aspiration of liquid and food is the consequence of those materials entering the airway below the level of the vocal folds.

8. Aspiration of liquid or food may or may not produce a lung infection known as *aspiration pneumonia*.
9. Respiratory impairments such as those requiring an endotracheal tube or tracheostomy tube also interfere with swallowing.
10. The SLP frequently is the coordinator of the swallowing team and therefore needs to have an understanding of each team member's perspective of the dysphagic patient. Many specialists could become involved in the care of a patient with dysphagia.
11. The evolution of the NICU has provided advanced technologies to maintain survival for infants as young as 23 weeks' gestational age. The feeding specialist in the NICU often is skilled in neurodevelopmental studies.

References

1. *Taber's cyclopedic medical dictionary*, Philadelphia, 1993, F.A. Davis.
2. Achem SR, Devault KR: Dysphagia in aging, *J Clin Gastroenterol* 39:357, 2005.
3. Tanner DC: *Case studies in communicative sciences and disorders*, Columbus, OH, 2006, Pearson Prentice Hall.
4. Barofsky I, Fontaine KR: Do psychogenic dysphagia patients have an eating disorder? *Dysphagia* 13:24, 1998.
5. Agency for Health Care Policy and Research: *Diagnosis and treatment of swallowing disorders (dysphagia) in acute-care stroke patients (evidence report/technology assessment No. 8)*, Rockville, MD, 1999, Agency for Health Care Policy and Research.
6. Doggett DL, Tappe KA, Mitchell MD et al: Prevention of pneumonia in elderly stroke patients by systematic diagnosis and treatment of dysphagia: an evidenced-based comprehensive analysis of the literature, *Dysphagia* 16:279, 2001.
7. American Speech-Language-Hearing Association: *Ad Hoc Committee on Dysphagia Report*, April, 57, 1987. Available at www.asha.org.
8. Kuhlemeier K: Epidemiology and dysphagia, *Dysphagia* 9:209, 1994.
9. Bloem BR, Lagaay AM, van Beek W et al: Prevalence of subjective dysphagia in community residents aged over 87, *Br Med J* 300:721, 1990.
10. Lindgren S, Janzon L: Prevalence of swallowing complaints and clinical findings among 50-70 year old men and women in an urban population, *Dysphagia* 6:187, 1991.
11. Lundquist A, Olsson R, Ekberg O: Clinical and radiologic evaluation reveals high prevalence of abnor-

malities in young adults with dysphagia, *Dysphagia* 13:202, 1998.

12. Lee A, Sitoh YY, Lien PK et al: Swallowing impairment and feeding dependency in the hospitalized elderly, *Ann Acad Med Singapore* 28:371, 1999.

13. Siebens H, Trupe E, Siebens A et al: Correlates and consequences of eating dependency in the institutionalized elderly, *J Am Geriatr Soc* 34:192, 1986.

14. Steele CM, Greenwood C, Ens I et al: Mealtime difficulties in a home for the aged: not just dysphagia, *Dysphagia* 12:43, 1997.

15. Croghan JE, Burke EM, Caplan S et al: Pilot study of 12 month outcomes of nursing home patients with aspiration on videofluoroscopy, *Dysphagia* 9:141, 1994.

16. Layne KA, Losinski DS, Zenner PM et al: Using the Fleming Index of Dysphagia to establish prevalence, *Dysphagia* 4:39, 1989.

17. Groher ME, Bukatman R: The prevalence of swallowing disorders in two teaching hospitals, *Dysphagia* 1:3, 1986.

18. Cherney LR: Dysphagia in adults with neurologic disorders: an overview. In Cherney LR, editor: *Clinical management of dysphagia in adults and children*, Gaithersburg, MD, 1994, Aspen.

19. Smithard DG, O'Neill PA, England R et al: The natural history of dysphagia following a stroke, *Dysphagia* 12:188, 1997.

20. Gordon C, Langton HR, Wade DT: Dysphagia in acute stroke, *Br Med J* 295:411, 1987.

21. Mann G, Hankey GJ, Cameron D: Swallowing function after stroke—prognosis and prognostic factors at 6 months, *Stroke* 30:744, 1999.

22. Daniels SK, Brailey K, Priestly DH et al: Aspiration in patients with acute stroke, *Arch Phys Med Rehabil* 79:14, 1998.

23. Pauloski BR, Rademaker AW, Logemann JA et al: Pretreatment swallowing function in patients with head and neck cancer, *Head Neck* 22:474, 2000.

24. Hillman RE, Walsh MJ, Wolf GT et al: Functional outcomes following treatment for advanced laryngeal cancer, *Ann Otol Rhinol Laryngol* 107:2, 1998.

25. Beckhardt RN, Murray JG, Ford CN et al: Factors influencing functional outcome in supraglottic laryngectomy, *Head Neck* 16:232, 1994.

26. McConnel FM, Logemann JA, Rademaker AW et al: Surgical variables affecting postoperative swallowing efficiency in oral cancer patients: a pilot study, *Laryngoscope* 104:87, 1994.

27. Field LH, Weiss CJ: Dysphagia with head injury, *Brain Injury* 3:19, 1989

28. Yorkston KM, Honsinger MJ, Matsuda PM et al: The relationship between speech and swallowing disorders in head-injured patients, *J Head Trauma Rehabil* 4:1, 1989.

29. Winstein CJ: Neurogenic dysphagia: frequency, progression, and outcome in adults following head injury, *Phys Ther* 63:1992, 1983.

30. Cherney LR, Halpern AS: Recovery of oral nutrition after head injury in adults, *J Head Trauma Rehabil* 4:42, 1989.

31. Lazarus C, Logemann JA: Swallowing disorders in closed head trauma patients, *Arch Phys Med Rehabil* 68:79, 1987.

32. Lieberman AN, Horowitz L, Redmond P et al: Dysphagia in Parkinson's disease, *Am J Gastroenterol* 74:157, 1980.

33. Edwards LL, Pfeiffer RF, Quigley EMM et al: Gastrointestinal symptoms in Parkinson's disease, *Mov Disord* 6:151, 1991.

34. Bushmann M, Dobmeyer SM, Leeker L et al: Swallowing abnormalities and their response to treatment in Parkinson's disease, *Neurology* 39:1309, 1989.

35. Leopold NA, Kagel MC: Prepharyngeal dysphagia in Parkinson's disease, *Dysphagia* 11:14, 1996.

36. Bine JE, Frank EM, McDade HL: Dysphagia and dementia in subjects with Parkinson's disease, *Dysphagia* 10:160, 1995.

37. Caroscio JT, Mulvihill MN, Sterling R: Amyotrophic lateral sclerosis: its natural history, *Neurol Clin* 5:1, 1987.

38. Mulder DS: *The diagnosis and treatment of amyotrophic lateral sclerosis*, Boston, 1980, Houghton Mifflin.

39. Hillel AD, Miller RM: Bulbar amyotrophic lateral sclerosis: patterns of progression and clinical management, *Head Neck* 11:51, 1989.

40. Hartelius L, Svensson P: Speech and swallowing symptoms associated with Parkinson's disease and multiple sclerosis: a survey, *Folia Phoniatr Logop* 46:9, 1994.

41. Restivo DA, Marchese-Ragona R, Patti F: Management of swallowing disorders in multiple sclerosis, *Neurol Sci* 4:338, 2006.

42. Calcagno P, Ruoppolo G, Grasso M et al: Dysphagia in multiple sclerosis—prevalence and prognostic factors, *Acta Neurol Scand* 105:40, 2002.

43. DePauw A, Dejaeger E, D'hooghe B et al: Dysphagia in multiple sclerosis, *Clin Neurol Neurosurg* 104:345, 2002.

44. Murray JP: Deglutition in myasthenia gravis, *Br J Radiol* 35:43, 1962.

45. Restivo DA, Marchese R, Staffieri A et al: Successful botulinum toxin treatment of dysphagia in oropharyngeal myotonic dystrophy, *Gastroenterology* 199:1416, 2000.

46. Nozaki S, Umaki Y, Sugishita S et al: Videofluorographic assessment of swallowing function in patients with Duchenne muscular dystrophy, *Clin Neurol (Rinsho Shinkeigaku)* 47:407, 2007.

47. Bellini M, Biagi S, Stasi C et al: Gastrointestinal manifestation in myotonic muscular dystrophy, *World J Gastroenterol* 12:1821, 2006.

48. Geterude A, Bake B, Bjelle A: Swallowing problems in rheumatoid arthritis, *Acta Otolaryngol* 111:1153, 1991.

49. Ekberg O, Redlund-Johnell I, Sjoblom KG: Pharyngeal function in patients with rheumatoid arthritis, *Acta Radiol* 28:35, 1987.

50. Fulp SR, Castell DO: Scleroderma esophagus, *Dysphagia* 5:101, 1990.

51. Zamost BJ, Hirschber J, Ippoliti AF et al: Esophagitis in scleroderma: prevalence and risk factors, *Gastroenterology* 92:421, 1987.

52. Grande L, Lacima G, Ros E, Fint J, Pera C. Esophageal motor function in primary Sjögren's syndrome, *Am J Gastroenterol* 88:378, 1993.

53. Martin JA, Hamilton BE, Sutton P et al: *Births: final data for 2002* (national vital statistics report, vol 52, no 10), Hyattsville, MD, 2003, National Center for Health Statistics.

54. Arvedson J, Brodsky L: *Pediatric swallowing and feeding: assessment and management*, ed 2, San Diego, 1993, Singular.

55. Smithard DG, O'Neill PA, Park C et al: Complications and outcome after acute stroke. Does dysphagia matter? *Stroke* 27:1200, 1996.

56. Kidd D, Lawson J, Nesbitt R et al: The natural history and clinical consequences of aspiration in acute stroke. *Q J Med* 88:409, 1995.

57. DePippo KL, Holas MA, Reding MJ et al: The Burke Dysphagia Screening Test, *Stroke* 24:173, 1993.

58. Andreoli TE, Carpenter CCJ, Griggs RC et al: *Cecil essentials of medicine*, ed 6, Philadelphia, 2004, WB Saunders.

59. American Speech-Language-Hearing Association: *Clinical indicators for instrumental assessment of dysphagia: guidelines, ASHA 2002 Desk Reference*, Rockville Pike, MD, 2002, ASHA.

60. American Speech-Language-Hearing Association: Guidelines for speech-language pathologists performing videofluoroscopic swallowing studies, *ASHA Supplement*, 24:178, 2004.

61. American Speech-Language-Hearing Association: *The role of the speech-language pathologist in the performance and interpretation of endoscopic evaluation of swallowing, technical report*, Rockville Pike, MD, 2005, ASHA.

62. American Speech-Language-Hearing Association: Knowledge and skills for speech-language pathologists providing services to individuals with swallowing and/or feeding disorders, *ASHA Supplement* 22:81, 2002.

63. Larsen GL: Rehabilitation of dysphagia: mechanica, paralytica, pseudobulbar, *J Neurosurg Nurs* 8:14, 1976.

64. Larsen GL: Rehabilitation for dysphagia paralytica, *J Speech Hear Disord* 37:187, 1972.

65. Logemann JA: *Evaluation and treatment of swallowing disorders*, San Diego, 1983, College-Hill Press.

66. Groher ME, editor: *Dysphagia: diagnosis and management*, Stoneham, MA, 1984, Butterworth.

67. Miller RM, Groher ME: Speech-language pathology and dysphagia: a brief historical perspective, *Dysphagia* 8:180, 1993.

Chapter 2

Normal Swallowing in Adults

MICHAEL E. GROHER

CHAPTER OUTLINE

OBJECTIVES

1. Define the key anatomic structures involved in swallowing.
2. Define the groups of muscles that participate in swallowing.
3. Define the peripheral and central neurologic controls for swallowing.
4. Discuss the key physiologic components that occur when moving a bolus from the mouth to the stomach.
5. Discuss how normal swallowing is affected by bolus type and delivery.
6. Describe swallowing associated with normal aging.

Normal swallowing includes an integrated, interdependent group of complex feeding behaviors emerging from interacting cranial nerves of the brainstem and governed by neural regulatory mechanisms in the medulla, as well as in sensorimotor and **limbic cortical systems**. Healthy individuals simultaneously perform the sequential sensory and motor patterns of mastication and swallowing with little effort and conscious awareness. For purposes of simplification, such sensory-guided discriminatory feeding and sensory-cued, stereotyped swallowing behaviors usually are divided into four stages (Practice Note 2-1): (1) the oral preparatory stage, in which food is masticated in preparation for transfer; (2) the oral stage, which entails the transfer of material from the mouth to the oropharynx; (3) the pharyngeal stage, in which material is transported away from the oropharynx, around an occluded laryngeal vestibule, and through a relaxed cricopharyngeus muscle into the upper esophagus; and (4) the esophageal stage, in which material is transported through the esophagus into the gastric **cardia**. An additional stage of swallowing that precedes the oral stage has been proposed by Leopold and Kagel,[1] who argue that visual appreciation of the bolus before its placement in the oral cavity may send a cognitive message that may help stimulate saliva during bolus preparation.

Knowledge of the anatomic and physiologic aspects of this interdependent group of voluntary and involuntary behaviors requires detailed study if the goal is to rehabilitate persons with dysphagia, which may be caused by a wide array of neurologic and structural impairments resulting from injury or disease affecting the central nervous system, cranial nerves, and muscles.

Practice Note 2-1

A single bolus of varying texture and size can be chewed and swallowed while a person carries on a conversation, and at the same time a beverage may be imbibed while various portions of the more solid food are held in the mouth. With relaxation of the pharyngeal constrictors, a sword can be passed from the pharynx through the cricopharyngeal muscle (not recommended without practice) and, with effort, a person can swallow solids while standing on his or her head!

NORMAL ANATOMY

The oral cavity extends from the lips anteriorly to the nasopharynx posteriorly and contains the tongue, gums, and teeth. The oral cavity is separated from the nasal cavity by the bony palate and velum (soft palate). It is composed of a highly mobile lower jaw, or mandible, consisting of a U-shaped body containing important ridges for muscle attachments. The upper jaw, or maxilla, meets the zygomatic or cheek bone and is adjoined by the L-shaped palatine bones, lying posterior to the nasal cavity. The perpendicular part of the palatines forms the back of the nasal cavity, whereas the horizontal part forms the back of the bony palate. The velum and posterior nasopharyngeal wall seal and open communication between the nasal and oral cavities during swallowing and respiratory behaviors, respectively. The nasopharynx lies above the velum, and the oropharynx lies posterior to the mouth. The pharynx extends below to the esophagus; its inferior portion is called the *hypopharynx* and is separated from the esophagus by the cricopharyngeal muscle (Figure 2-1). The cartilaginous larynx lies anterior to the hypopharynx at the upper end of the trachea, suspended by muscles attached to the hyoid bone. The cricoid cartilage lies above the trachea, with the thyroid cartilage above it. Both are suspended from muscles attached to the hyoid bone, which itself is suspended between the jaw, tongue, and sternum by suprahyoid and infrahyoid musculature.

The respiratory system is protected during pharyngeal swallow by occlusive muscular constriction of the laryngeal vestibule and downward displacement of the epiglottis. The true vocal cords are at the inferior margin of the laryngeal ventricle and are attached anteriorly at the thyroid cartilage and posteriorly at the arytenoid cartilages. The vestibular (false) vocal folds separate the ventricle and the vestibule. The epiglottis extends from the base of the tongue into the pharyngeal cavity.

The valleculae are lateral recesses at the base of the tongue on each side of the epiglottis. The piriform sinuses are lateral recesses between the larynx and the anterior hypopharyngeal wall (Figure 2-2). These recesses serve as important anatomic landmarks in the videoradiographic assessment of pharyngeal swallow. Figure 2-3 shows a lateral view of the key anatomic structures in the region of the head and neck.

Oral Preparatory Stage

The mandibular branch of the trigeminal nerve (cranial nerve [CN] V) innervates the principal muscles for chewing behaviors. The primary muscles of

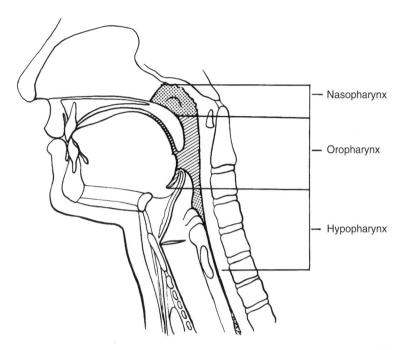

FIGURE 2-1. Lateral view of the anatomy of the head and neck with demarcations of three major regions: nasopharynx, oropharynx, and hypopharynx.

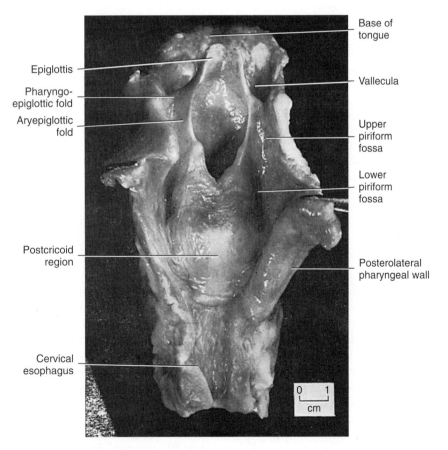

FIGURE 2-2. Anatomic specimen of the pharyngeal compartment as it surrounds the airway. The bolus flows into the vallecular spaces and around the epiglottis inferiorly into the piriform fossa before entering the esophagus.

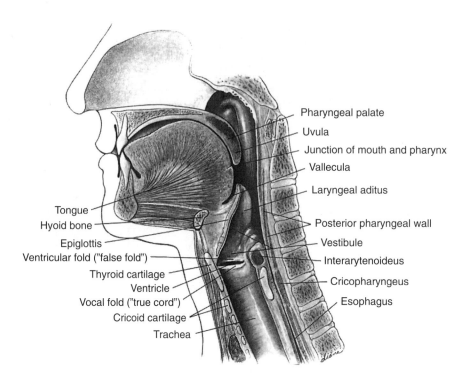

FIGURE 2-3. Lateral view of the anatomy of the head and neck pertinent to swallowing. (From Bosma JF, Donner MW, Tanaka E et al: Anatomy of the pharynx, pertinent to swallowing, *Dysphagia* 1:24, 1986.)

TABLE 2-1				
Muscles of Mastication				
Muscle	**Origin**	**Insertion**	**Nerve**	**Action**
Temporalis	Temporal fossa of skull	Ramus and coronoid process of mandible	Trigeminal	Elevates or closes mandible; retracts mandible
Masseter	Zygomatic arch	Ramus of mandible	Trigeminal	Elevates or closes mandible
Medial pterygoid	Palatine bone, lateral pterygoid plate, tuberosity of maxilla	Ramus of mandible	Trigeminal	Elevates or closes mandible
Lateral pterygoid	Great wing of sphenoid and lateral pterygoid plate	Neck of condyle of mandible	Trigeminal	Depressor or opener of mandible; protrudes mandible; permits side-to-side movement of mandible

chewing are the masseter, temporalis, and pterygoid muscles, which attach to the sphenoid wing of the temporal bone. The masseter closes the jaw while the temporalis moves it up, forward, or backward (Table 2-1). The medial pterygoid muscles work bilaterally to elevate the mandible while they shift the jaw to the opposite side unilaterally. The lateral pterygoid muscles work together, pulling down or forward while moving the jaw or chin to the opposite side unilaterally. Both sets of pterygoid muscles cooperate to grind in mastication.

The facial nerve (CN VII) innervates lower facial muscles attached to the maxillae and mandible of the skull. These include the buccinator muscles, which compress the lips and flatten the cheeks in the movement of food across the teeth (Table 2-2). The buccinator fibers blend with those of the orbicularis oris, the sphincter of the lips.

The hypoglossal nerve (CN XII) innervates the tongue, which contains four separate intrinsic muscle masses that have different effects on the shape, contour, and function of the tongue.

Oral/Pharyngeal Stage

The pharyngeal cavity of the neck, which is suspended from the base of the skull and anchored to the top of

TABLE 2-2

Muscles of the Face

Muscle	Origin	Insertion	Nerve	Action
Orbicularis oris	Neighboring muscles, mostly buccinators; has many layers of tissue around the lips	Skin around lips and angles of the mouth	Facial	Closes, opens, protrudes, inverts, and twists lips
Zygomaticus minor	Zygomatic bone	Orbicularis oris in upper lip	Facial	Draws upper lip upward and outward
Levator labii superior	Below infraorbital foramen in maxilla	Orbicularis oris in upper lip	Facial	Pulls up or elevates upper lip
Levator labii superior alaeque nasi	Process of maxilla	Skin at mouth angle, orbicularis oris	Facial	Raises angle of the mouth
Zygomaticus major	Zygomatic bone	Fibers of the orbicularis oris, angle of the mouth	Facial	Draws upper lip upward; draws angle of mouth upward and backward; the smiling muscle
Levator anguli oris	Canine fossa of maxilla	Lower lip near angle of the mouth	Facial	Pulls down corners of mouth
Depressor anguli oris	Outer surface and above lower border of mandible	Skin of cheek, corner of mouth, lower border of mandible	Facial	Draws lower lip down; draws angle of mouth down and inward
Depressor labii inferior	Lower border of the mandible	Skin of lower lip, orbicularis oris	Facial	Depresses lower lip
Mentalis	Incisor fossa of mandible	Skin of chin	Facial	Pushes up lower lip; raises chin
Risorius	Platysma, fascia over the masseter skin	Angle of mouth, orbicularis oris	Facial	Draws corners or angle of mouth outward; causes dimples; gives expression of strain to face
Buccinator	Alveolar process of maxilla, buccinators ridge of mandible	Angle of mouth, orbicularis oris	Facial	Flattens cheek; holds food in contact with teeth; retracts angles of the mouth

the sternum, is formed by 26 pairs of striated muscles innervated by six cranial and four cervical nerves. The horseshoe-shaped hyoid bone in the neck serves as a fulcrum that provides a mechanical advantage for pharyngeal musculature associated with swallowing behaviors of the posterior tongue, pharynx, and larynx.

In the nasopharynx, five muscles adjust the position of the velum with respect to the food bolus: the palatoglossal and levator veli palatini muscles (pharyngeal plexus and accessory nerve), which elevate the soft palate and seal the nasopharynx; the tensor veli palatini (mandibular branch of the trigeminal nerve), which tenses the palate and dilates the orifice of the eustachian tube; the palatopharyngeal muscle (pharyngeal plexus and spinal accessory nerve), which depresses the soft palate, approximates the palate or pharyngeal folds, and constricts the pharynx; and the muscularis uvula (spinal accessory nerve), which shortens the soft palate (Table 2-3).

The hypoglossal (CN XII), trigeminal (CN V), and facial (CN VII) nerves innervate the suprahyoid group of muscles. The hypoglossal nerve supplies the geniohyoid, which draws the hyoid bone up and forward, depressing the jaw, and the trigeminal nerve supplies the mylohyoid, which elevates the hyoid bone and tongue and depresses the jaw (Table 2-4). The digastric muscles contain anterior and posterior bellies. The anterior belly is innervated by the mandibular branch of the trigeminal nerve (CN V) and depresses the jaw or raises the hyoid bone, whereas the posterior portion is innervated by the facial nerve (CN VII) and elevates or retracts the hyoid. The facial nerve (CN VII) innervates the stylohyoid muscle, which elevates the hyoid bone during swallowing. In addition, the hyoglossus and the genioglossus serve as laryngeal elevators, as well as extrinsic tongue muscles, and are designed to depress the tongue or help elevate the hyoid bone when the tongue is fixed. The accessory nerve (CN XI), in association

TABLE 2-3

Muscles of the Palate

Muscle	Origin	Insertion	Nerve	Action
Levator veli palatini	Apex of temporal bone	Palatine aponeurosis of soft palate	Vagus and accessory	Raises soft palate
Tensor veli palatini	Fossa of sphenoid bone	Palatine aponeurosis of soft palate	Trigeminal	Stretches soft palate
Palatoglossus	Undersurface of soft palate	Side of tongue	Vagus and accessory	Raises back of tongue during the first stage of swallowing
Palatopharyngeus	Soft palate	Pharyngeal wall	Vagus and accessory	Shuts off nasopharynx during second stage of swallowing
Uvulae	Posterior nasal spine and palatine aponeurosis	Into uvula to form its chief bulk or content	Vagus and accessory	Shortens and raises uvula

TABLE 2-4

Suprahyoid Muscles

Muscle	Origin	Insertion	Nerve	Action
Mylohyoid (anterior belly digastric)	Inner surface of mandible	Upper border of hyoid bone	Trigeminal	Elevates tongue and floor of mouth; depresses jaw when hyoid bone is in fixed position
Digastric (anterior belly)	Intermediate tendon by loop of fascia to hyoid bone	Lower border of mandible	Trigeminal	Raises hyoid bone if jaw is in fixed position; depresses jaw if hyoid bone is in fixed position
Geniohyoid	Mental spine of mandible	Hyoid bone	Cervical (C1 and C2) through hypoglossal	Draws hyoid bone forward; depresses mandible when hyoid bone is in fixed position
Stylohyoid	Stylohyoid process of temporal bone	Body of hyoid at greater cornu	Facial	Elevates hyoid and tongue base
Hyoglossus	Greater cornu of hyoid	Into tongue sides	Hypoglossal	Tongue depression
Genioglossus	Upper genial tubercle of mandible	Hyoid, inferior tongue, and tip of tongue	Hypoglossal	Protrusion and depression
Styloglossus	Anterior border of styloid process	Into side of tongue	Hypoglossal	Elevates up and back
Palatoglossus	Anterior surface of soft palate	Dorsum and side of tongue	Glossopharyngeal, vagus, and accessory	Narrows fauces and elevates posterior tongue

with the hypoglossal (CN XII) nerve, innervates the styloglossus, which draws the tongue up and back during swallowing. The glossopharyngeal (CN IX) and accessory (CN XI) nerves also cause the palatoglossus to raise the back of the tongue and lower the velum. The styloglossus and palatoglossus raise the back of the tongue and lower the sides of the soft palate.

The vagus nerve (CN X) and the spinal accessory nerve (CN XI) innervate the muscular pharynx, whose superior, middle, and inferior constrictor muscles constitute its external circular layer and work together to transport a bolus of food toward the esophagus during swallowing. Three other muscles constitute the internal longitudinal layer of the pharynx: the palatopharyngeus, stylopharyngeus, and salpingopharyngeus. The stylopharyngeus (glossopharyngeal nerve) elevates the pharynx, and to some extent the larynx, during swallowing, and the salpingopharyngeus (accessory nerve and pharyngeal plexus) draws

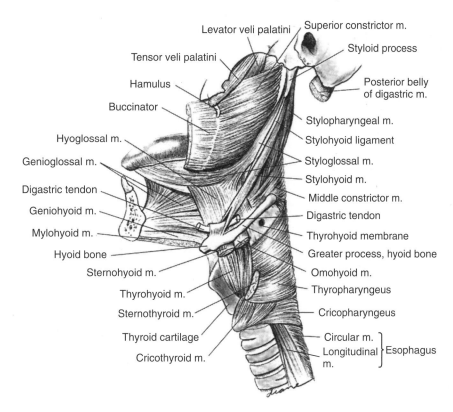

FIGURE 2-4. Lateral view of the key muscles of the head and neck used in swallowing. (From Bosma JF, Donner MW, Tanaka E et al: Anatomy of the pharynx, pertinent to swallowing, *Dysphagia* 1:24, 1986.)

the lateral walls of the pharynx up. The palatopharyngeus muscle draws the velum down.

The cricopharyngeal muscle is an important single muscle that lies at the transition level between the pharynx and the esophagus. Functionally, it is separate from both the pharynx and the esophagus and acts as a sphincter, relaxing during passage of the bolus from the pharynx into the esophagus. It is innervated by both pharyngeal branches of the vagus and sympathetic fibers from the middle and inferior cervical ganglia. The key muscles used in the oral and pharyngeal stages of swallowing are shown in Figure 2-4.

Esophageal Stage

The esophagus is a distensible tube, approximately 21 to 27 cm (10 inches) long, connecting the pharynx (at C6) and stomach (at T12). It is separated from the pharynx by the pharyngeal esophageal segment (PES) and from the stomach by the lower esophageal sphincter (LES). Under resting conditions, the esophageal **lumen** is collapsed, creating a potential space that can easily distend up to 3 cm to accommodate swallowed air, liquids, or solids. The esophagus is lined with a protective, stratified, squamous epithe-

lium that covers an inner layer of circular fibers and an outer layer of longitudinal fibers. At its proximal end (upper fourth) the muscle is **striated**, whereas the distal two thirds are composed of **smooth muscle**. The middle third, in the region of the aorta, is a combination of smooth and striated muscle. As it courses through the thorax at the level of the **carina**, the esophagus runs lateral and posterior to the left ventricle of the heart, creating a natural bend as it courses anteriorly toward the diaphragmatic hiatus. After passing the diaphragmatic hiatus, it connects to the body of the stomach at the level of the LES. The smooth muscle of the LES is arranged in a specialized spiral configuration as it joins the inner oblique muscle zone of the stomach. The relation of the esophagus to the heart and tracheobronchial tree, as well as its path through the diaphragmatic hiatus, is shown in Figure 2-5.

NORMAL PHYSIOLOGY

Many studies have examined the normal aspects of the oropharyngeal swallow sequence. The rationale usually given for such studies is that clinicians must be able to compare normative data with patient data

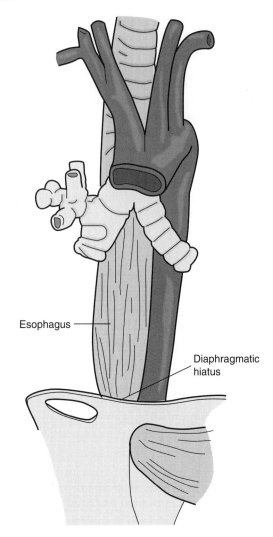

Esophagus

Diaphragmatic
hiatus

FIGURE 2-5. The esophagus courses through the chest cavity and through a hiatus in the diaphragm, ending at the level of the stomach.

Practice Note 2-2

Try experiencing the effects of an open valve (the lips) and a closed nasal passage on your own swallowing performance. First swallow your saliva. Then try to swallow your saliva with your lips open, noticing the differences in effort expended. Do the same thing with the nose open and then pinch the nostrils closed and swallow.

functional swallow in the context of his or her swallowing complaint, past medical history, and the results of physical and instrumental examinations.

Normal swallowing performance depends on the rapid transfer of the bolus from the oral cavity to the stomach. A liquid bolus may pass through the pharynx within 2 seconds and enter the stomach in less than 5 seconds. Efficient movement is accomplished by the strength of the neuromuscular contraction exerted on the bolus and on the forces of gravity. Efficient bolus movement is accomplished when coordinated neuromuscular contractions and relaxations create zones of high pressure on the bolus and zones of negative pressure below the level of the bolus. Some parts of the swallowing chain, such as the esophagus, remain under negative pressure because of their location. Creating zones of high and low pressure is largely accomplished by the coordination and strength of the swallowing valves: lips, velum, airway closure, PES opening and closing, and upper esophageal sphincter (UES) opening and closing. A patent nasal airway also may be important (Practice Note 2-2). The tongue provides the initial positive driving force. The tongue's posterior deflection provides the basis for laryngeal elevation by applying traction to the hyoid bone. Efficient (i.e., timely and strong) laryngeal elevation helps create a negative zone of pressure in the pharynx, particularly in the region of the PES. This allows the bolus to move rapidly, and therefore safely, from a zone of high pressure into a zone of negative pressure. Moving from a zone of high pressure into another zone of high pressure caused by a pathologic condition (e.g., muscle weakness or incoordination) inhibits bolus flow and results in **stasis** and residue that may be aspirated into the airway.

Oral Preparation

Food or liquid in the mouth stimulates taste, temperature, and pressure (touch) receptors. The primary receptors of taste are located on the tongue, on the hard and soft palate, in the pharynx, and in the

to determine whether an abnormality exists. Although this approach to detection has heuristic appeal, studies of the normal swallow have revealed significant variability among normal (healthy) subjects, particularly in the oral preparatory and oral stages of swallowing.[2-5] Part of this variability is attributable to subject selection, bolus type, and the tools used to measure swallow performance. Other variability seems inherent in the swallowing process. It appears that the mechanism for swallowing must be variable to accommodate the variations of bolus type and amount for successful ingestion in different circumstances of eating, such as eating while talking, in varied environments, and at various rates. The astute clinician will not ignore those aspects of normal swallow performance that have been empirically evaluated but should also be imminently cognizant of placing a person's supralaryngeal region. The receptors are activated by saliva. Saliva is produced by the activation of the submandibular, submaxillary (autonomic aspects of CN VII), and parotid glands (autonomic aspects of CN IX). Activation of these glands is achieved by the actions of the jaw, tongue, and hyoid bone during bolus preparation and by the inherent taste of the bolus. The primary sensory receptors on the dorsum of the tongue responsible for the perception of salt, sweet, sour, and bitter are activated by saliva. In addition to facilitating taste and bolus formation, saliva is important in the maintenance of adequate oral hygiene by controlling microorganisms, in the regulation of the acidity levels in the stomach and esophagus because of it bicarbonate composition, and in the breakdown of carbohydrates. The number of times a person swallows saliva in 1 hour can vary between 18 and 400 and largely depends on the rate of salivary flow.[6]

Sensations of taste are carried by the chorda tympani branch of CN VII on the anterior two thirds of the tongue and through the greater petrosal branch on the hard and soft palate. Taste on the posterior third of the tongue is mediated by CN IX. Sensations of taste are sent to the nucleus tractus solitarii (NTS) in the medulla of the brainstem (see sections on neurologic controls), where they are transmitted to the sensorimotor cortex by the thalamus. Taste receptors in the region of the **laryngeal aditus** are carried to the NTS by the superior laryngeal branch of CN X. Appreciation of taste depends largely on smell. Smell sensations are carried by direct stimulation of the nasal cavity and by smell elicited by chewing, during which odors travel posteriorly into the nasopharynx. Interpretation of smell is ultimately accomplished through the thalamus to the frontal and temporal cortices by information carried by CN I. Information (memories) relating to smell may be stored in the **hippocampus**.

The coordinated action of the tongue and jaw moves a bolus laterally onto the molar table for deformation. Further deformation is accomplished by variable contacts of the tongue to the hard palate. Although the tongue may play a large role in containing the bolus in the oral cavity before swallow, evidence indicates that during solid bolus mastication, material is allowed to collect in the vallecular recesses at the tongue base before swallow initiation.[5] The ultimate role of the tongue is to manipulate, shape, hold, and then transfer the bolus into the oropharynx, signaling the onset of the oral stage of swallow as the swallowing sequence transitions into the pharyngeal stage with the passage of the bolus through the oropharyngeal port. The exact nature of the

sensory cues that signal a bolus is ready for swallowing is not completely understood; however, studies have shown that the superior laryngeal nerve branch of the vagus is important in swallow initiation[7] and in the sensory protective mechanisms of the upper airway.[8] The mechanics of bolus preparation can be appreciated with **videofluoroscopy**. The first images are taken as the patient faces the camera and chews a piece of cracker (Video 2-1). The undulating and varied movements of the tongue and jaw are apparent. In the lateral view, the tongue can be seen touching the hard palate as material is pushed toward the tongue base, filling the valleculae before the swallow (Video 2-2).

Oral Stage

Once the bolus is prepared, the tongue tip is elevated to occlude the anterior oral cavity at the alveolar ridge, and the bolus is held against the hard palate. The edges of the tongue dorsum contain the bolus laterally. The tongue tip and dorsum appear to work longer in containment activity than the posterior tongue after the oral stage is initiated; however, the posterior tongue is more responsible for delivering the bolus into the pharynx.[9] Before—but almost simultaneous with—the first posterior movement of the tongue, respiration ceases (see following section on respiration), followed by arytenoid cartilage approximation precipitating true vocal fold adduction. Retraction of the tongue is primarily accomplished by extrinsic tongue muscles: digastricus (CN V), mylohyoid (CN V), and the geniohyoid (CN XII). The tongue base applies positive pressure to the tail of the bolus by its contact with the velum and posterior pharyngeal wall, which allows the bolus to move rapidly through the pharynx into an open PES. As the tongue propels the bolus posteriorly, the palatopharyngeal folds are pulled medially to form a slit through which the bolus can pass. The levator veli palatinii muscles help elevate the velum to seal the nasopharyngeal opening. The combined action of the tongue's contact to the velum and posterior pharyngeal wall and sealing the nasopharynx contribute to the maintenance of positive pressure on the bolus as it moves toward zones of negative pressure in the hypopharynx. By the tongue's connections to the hyoid bone, and the hyoid bone's connections to the thyroid and cricoid cartilages, the larynx is pulled up and forward, resting under the tongue base that now partially covers the opening to the airway. As the larynx rises, the cartilaginous epiglottis makes its descent over the top of the airway, completing an elaborate system of airway protection that allows the bolus to be directed toward the esophagus rather than into the trachea.

The extent of epiglottic descent depends on anterior hyoid displacement, tongue base retraction force, and bolus size.[10] Rapid and complete laryngeal elevation (2 to 3 cm on average) aids in creating negative pressure in the region of the hypopharynx. As the bolus enters the pharynx, it is divided by the **vallecular spaces** at the level of the tongue base, helping deflect it away from the airway as an additional component of airway protection.

Respiration and Swallow

Protection of the upper airway through the oropharyngeal phase of swallowing is crucial to swallowing safety. Respiration and swallowing are linked by their anatomy (common conduits of mouth and pharynx) and their neuroanatomic relations in the medulla of the brainstem. This relation is expressed functionally because respiration is inhibited by swallowing, and disorders of respiration often affect swallow safety (see Chapter 8). The period of airflow inhibition (swallow apnea) in most normal adults begins before the onset of the oral stage of swallow.[11,12] During mastication, respiratory patterns are modified from normal tidal patterns; however, apnea does not occur until the bolus collects at the vallecular level.[13] A short exhalation cycle precedes shallow apnea. As the tail of the bolus passes through the PES, the larynx descends and respiration continues on the exhalation cycle slightly before the PES closes.[12] Exhalation is accompanied by a buildup of subglottic pressure that separates the vocal folds apart. This release of pressure is heard as an audible burst by using a stethoscope placed at the laryngeal level.[14] This burst of exhalation is considered a protective feature in case any swallowed material is lodged in the upper airway. This explosion of exhaled air is encouraged with the Heimlich maneuver. The pattern of exhalation-swallow-exhalation may change in normal aging[15,16] and in disease (Clinical Corner 2-1).[17] The duration of swallow apnea in normal subjects varies from 0.75 to 1.25 seconds depending on the subject's age and bolus size.[18] In general, the larger the bolus size, the longer the duration of swallow apnea.[16] During swallow apnea the true vocal folds move medially but do not fully approximate.[12] It is possible that the cessation of respiration during swallowing is not physiologically tied to vocal fold movement because patients with laryngectomy show similar periods of swallow apnea compared with normal subjects.[19]

Pharyngeal Stage

The pharyngeal stage begins when the bolus arrives at the level of the valleculae and ends when the PES closes.[20] When the bolus enters the pharynx, the

---

CLINICAL CORNER 2-1

While dining one evening a couple noticed someone at an adjoining table suddenly jump up and complain loudly that something was sticking in his throat. He seemed quite uncomfortable and was starting to sweat. Because of the commotion the waiter rushed over and began the Heimlich maneuver by pressing his hands around the diner's waist, forcefully pushing on his diaphragm with rapid thrusts. Unfortunately, this did not relieve his customer's symptoms and he continued to complain that something was stuck.

CRITICAL THINKING

1. Why didn't the Heimlich maneuver relieve the customer's symptoms?
2. What might have been the problem?

---

hyoid bone continues its superior and anterior movement toward the edge of the mandible, tilting the larynx under the retracting tongue base to protect the bolus from entering the upper airway. The false vocal folds offer further protection in conjunction with the closure of the laryngeal aditus by the aryepiglottic folds. As a result of contraction of the thyroepiglottic ligament and posterior tongue contraction, the epiglottic cartilage descends from its erect position over the laryngeal aditus. Thus many mechanisms are active in preventing the bolus from entering the upper airway. These include (1) cessation of active respiration, (2) approximation of the true and false vocal folds, (3) closure of the laryngeal aditus, (4) deflection of bolus material by the tongue base over a rising larynx, and (5) division of the bolus through the valleculae that direct the bolus around the superior aspect of the airway entrance.

As the bolus enters the pharynx, the superior, middle, and inferior constrictor muscles are activated sequentially to narrow and shorten the pharynx, contributing to peristalsis-like movements in the posterior pharyngeal wall that aid in bolus propulsion into the esophagus. The duration of pharyngeal muscle contraction is unaffected by bolus size.[21]

The forward movement of the hyoid bone is important in applying traction forces on the PES to achieve maximum opening.[22] Before the bolus arrives in the pharynx, muscles in the region of the PES that had been closed before swallow are relaxed by parasympathetic signals carried by CN IX to the brainstem. After relaxation, the PES is pulled open during hyolaryngeal movements. As the bolus continues its descent toward the region of the PES, it remains divided as it passes

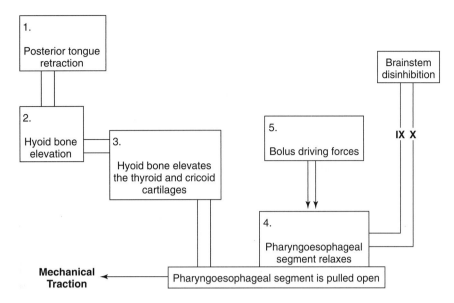

FIGURE 2-6. Schematic representation of the three mechanisms of the pharyngoesophageal segment (*PES*) opening. They include mechanical traction (*1*, *2*, and *3*), brainstem disinhibition (relaxation) (*4*), and bolus driving forces (*5*).

lateral to the larynx into the piriform recesses of the hypopharynx, where the bolus is rejoined as it enters the esophagus. Preference for bolus flow through the pharynx has been found in healthy normal patients. Seta et al.[23] studied the preference of bolus flow in 167 normal patients. Although all patients had bolus flow in both halves of the pharynx, 58% showed no difference, 35% had left dominance, and 7% showed right dominance.[23] In addition to PES relaxation and mechanical traction, the PES is distended by the driving force of the bolus. The neurologic and biomechanical processes required for distention and closing of the PES are summarized in Figure 2-6.

As the tail of the bolus passes the region of the PES, primary esophageal peristalsis begins as the PES closes. The airway reopens and the hyoid bone returns to its resting position. These activities signal the end of the pharyngeal phase of swallow. The timing of oropharyngeal swallowing events from the beginning of vocal fold closure to the reopening of the vocal folds at the end of the swallowing sequence is depicted in Figure 2-7. (For more detail on the activity of the PES during swallowing, see Chapter 7.) The structural and biomechanical aspects of the oral and pharyngeal phases of swallowing seen in the lateral and anteroposterior planes can be appreciated in a narrated version of a videofluoroscopic examination of swallowing (Video 2-3). Video 2-4 provides a narrated version of the normal swallow as seen by endoscopy.

Esophageal Stage

Before the bolus enters the esophagus, the esophageal lumen remains closed within the chest cavity under negative pressure. Pressures generated in the closed UES vary from 30 to 110 mm Hg depending on patient age and the type of **manometric** catheter used to gather the data.[24] Esophageal swallowing tasks require an ordered pattern of function that depends on coordinated activities in three distinct zones: the proximal, striated muscle zone; the body; and the specialized smooth muscle of the distal zone. Bolus movement through these zones is characterized by an orderly, ringlike progression of contractions until the bolus enters the LES and the stomach. Liquid boluses, depending on viscosity, often precede this wave of contractions. The cervical portion of the esophagus works in conjunction with the hypopharynx, allowing the PES to fully relax and distend to accommodate bolus size. As the bolus enters the esophagus, a primary contraction wave (primary peristalsis) is triggered in the proximal, striated portion by vagal (CN X) efferent activity. This activity may be inhibited by multiple swallow attempts if the pharynx fails to clear its contents.[25] The motor activity in the cervical esophagus is rapid and gradually slows as it approaches the mid (level of the aortic arch) and distal esophageal regions.[26] Typically, the contraction force in the cervical esophagus is the strongest and is accompanied in time by a drop in pressure (relaxation) in the LES to allow the bolus to enter the stomach. Esophageal

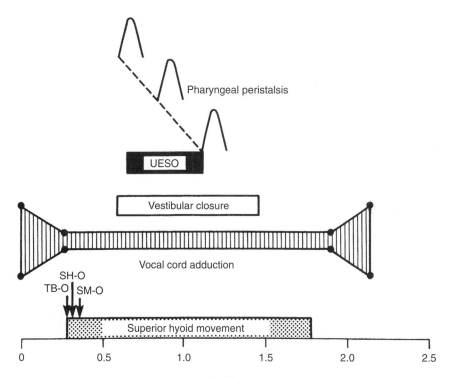

FIGURE 2-7. The relation of the time of vocal fold closure and hyoid bone elevation during a 5-mL barium swallow. Bolus transit through the pharynx and across the upper esophageal sphincter *(UES)* begins and ends while the vocal folds are at maximal adduction. *SH-O,* Onset of superior hyoid movement; *SM-O,* onset of submental myoelectrical activity; *TB-O,* onset of tongue base movement; *UESO,* UES opening. (From Shaker R, Dodds WJ, Dantas RO et al: Coordination of deglutitive glottic closure with oropharyngeal swallowing, *Gastroenterology* 98:1478, 1990.)

smooth muscle contraction (distal two thirds) has a sequential behavior by which proximal activity successively inhibits the next most distal portion of the esophagus.[27] The bolus propagation pressures generated in the esophagus are typically measured by manometric techniques. A visual representation of primary peristalsis is presented in Figure 2-8. The radiographic representation of esophageal peristalsis is presented in Video 2-5. The patient is standing while swallowing a liquid and a semisolid bolus. The ringlike contraction waves of the esophageal lumen can be appreciated, as can the bolus entering the stomach through the LES. The primary peristaltic wave on the liquid bolus is followed by a secondary wave. It is apparent that the semisolid bolus flows at a slower pace.

Primary peristalsis is followed by secondary peristalsis. The secondary peristaltic wave follows the primary wave and is propagated by the bolus distending the esophagus. Its propagation may begin at any point in the esophageal body and often assists in primary transport of solid food boluses because the primary wave may fail to push the bolus to the level of the LES. Primary and secondary peristalsis are accompanied by longitudinal muscle contraction, resulting in shortening of the esophagus by its proximal attachments to the hypopharynx and distal attachments to the stomach (see Chapter 7 for a discussion of Zenker's diverticulum and esophageal shortening).

Tertiary contractions of the esophagus are random contractions that are not peristaltic (orderly) in nature and are inefficient in assisting in bolus transport. In general, they occur independent of swallowing activity but have been reported to occur more frequently in older adults.[28] Tertiary contractions may be the result of air trapped in the esophagus, or they may result from irritation of the esophageal lumen such as from gastroesophageal reflux.

BOLUS AND DELIVERY VARIATION

Altering volume, texture, taste, and delivery method may affect the biomechanics of the normal swallow. Dietary modifications are frequently used in the treatment of patients with dysphagia (see Chapters 12 to 14) to assist in compensating for their deficits. The prescribed modifications in volume, texture (viscos-

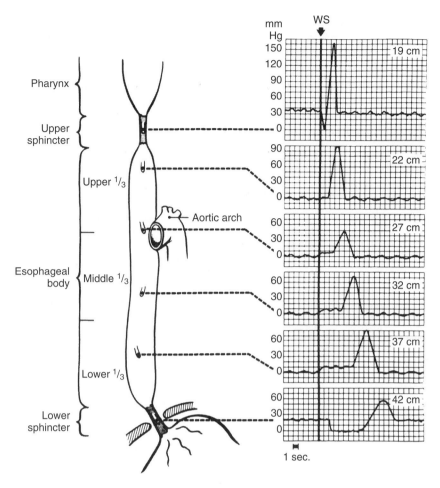

FIGURE 2-8. A manometric tracing of primary esophageal peristalsis. Pressure catheters are placed at various levels of the esophagus (19 cm from the incisors to 42 cm). Their representative measures of pressure are seen as peaks of activity on the *right* of the figure. Before the first pressure wave, a drop in pressure is seen from approximately 40 mm Hg (closed sphincter) to 0. This drop in pressure represents the opening and relaxation of the upper esophageal sphincter. The first primary esophageal contraction is the highest and therefore the strongest. As the bolus reaches the level of the aortic arch, the pattern of contraction is reduced because of the bending of the esophagus around the arch and the transition from striated to smooth muscle. Note that as the primary peristaltic wave begins, there is a corresponding drop in the pressure of the lower esophageal sphincter from approximately 25 mm Hg to 0 as it relaxes to await the oncoming bolus. A positive wave in the lower esophageal sphincter after this drop in pressure can be seen as a consequence of the sphincter closing.

ity), and taste to facilitate normal swallowing are based on studies on the effects of these parameters on normal swallowing. Results from such studies are not uniform because of subject variability, measurement tool(s) used (e.g., intramuscular and surface electromyography, ultrasound, manometry, videofluoroscopy), subject instructions, and definitions of when specific biomechanical events begin and end. There are no published outcomes data on the precise effects of volume, texture, and taste modification in patients with dysphagia, although these parameters are routinely modified in clinical care.

Volume and Biomechanics

Studies have shown that the normal amount of a liquid taken per swallow attempt may range from 10 to 25 mL depending on the test instructions, gender, type of cup, and body size.[29,30] Most studies that examine the effects of volume on swallowing biomechanics have studied bolus volumes that range from 1 to 20 mL. These studies have focused on the effects of volume on the movement of the hyoid bone. Movement parameters can include maximal displacement and the duration of movement, documenting total time and velocity. Some investigators have found minimal effects of hyoid displacement between small and larger boluses,[31,32] whereas others have documented larger total displacement with an incremental increase in bolus volume more prominent in men.[33,34] One study found that larger volumes had a greater effect on superior, rather than anterior hyoid, movement.[35] Other studies have not focused specifically on hyoid mechanics but rather on the biomechanical and pressure changes associated with oral and pharyngeal transit, duration of swallow apnea, and PES mechanics.

Lingual swallowing pressures with varying bolus volumes were unaffected as bolus size was increased,[36] suggesting that increased effort in oral-stage transit is not needed as the size of a liquid bolus increases. However, the tongue changed its contour to contain larger boluses before swallow onset.[36] Ekberg and Nylander[27] found no change in the speed of pharyngeal transit between small and large boluses.

A direct relation appears to exist between bolus size and the length of time the PES stays open and the onset time of relaxation. Cook et al.[37] studied 21 normal volunteers using concurrent videofluoroscopy, surface electromyography, and manometry with four different bolus sizes ranging from 2 to 20 mL. In general, as the bolus size increased the PES stayed open longer, and the onset of relaxation was closer to the onset of the anterior movement of the hyoid bone. These results suggest a possible relation between the sensory aspects of the oral stage of swallow (bolus volume) and the mechanics of the PES. These results provide further evidence of the interdependence of the stages of swallowing.

Viscosity

Studies of the effects of viscosity, taste, and bolus delivery on swallowing have focused on the changes in biomechanical effort that may be needed as these variables are changed. Measurement of swallowing effort is accomplished best with manometric techniques, allowing the investigator to document changes in swallow-generated pressures.

In general, researchers agree that swallow-generated pressures are more sensitive to changes in viscosity than are changes in volumes of the same consistency. As the consistency of the bolus becomes thicker, greater tongue pressures are needed to transport it from the oral cavity[36]; studies have shown no differences between men and women.[38] This increase in generated force was highest at the point where the anterior tongue made contact with the hard palate.

Pelletier and Dhanaraj[39] studied the effects of sweet, salty, sour, and bitter on swallowing pressures in 10 healthy, young subjects. Subjects were also

CLINICAL CORNER 2-2

A 75-year-old patient with respiratory disease was evaluated for difficulties swallowing liquids. Physical evaluation revealed that he had generalized weakness in the lips and tongue. He could take his liquids from a cup without any coughing episodes, but he had some coughing while using a straw. The patient reported that he was more comfortable using a straw and preferred it to the cup. The speech pathologist cut the straw in half and the patient then took his liquids with the straw without any difficulty.

CRITICAL THINKING
1. Why might this patient have more difficulty using a straw than a cup?
2. Why might shortening the length of the straw improve his swallowing performance?

asked to judge the palatability of each test substance from "extremely like" to "dislike." Although palatability judgments did not affect swallowing pressures, higher pressures (compared with water) were generated with the moderate-sucrose, high-salt, and high–citric acid test samples.

Straw drinking is a typical method to deliver a liquid bolus (Video 2-6). The patient takes multiple sips by straw. There are brief periods between each swallow when the airway opens briefly. Successful straw drinking requires adequate lip strength and intraoral pressures to draw the fluid into the oral cavity from the cup. In general, the airway must remain closed during sequential swallow attempts; therefore the biomechanical requirements may differ from single or multiple swallows from a cup. Daniels and Foundas[40] identified three distinct airway protection patterns during sequential straw drinking in 15 healthy young males, suggesting variation in how the upper airway is protected during sequential swallows using a straw with variations in the length of time the laryngeal vestibule remained closed (Clinical Corner 2-2).

SWALLOW AND NORMAL AGING

In persons older than 65 years, some demonstrable changes in swallowing performance are attributable to age alone. These changes may interact to decompensate swallowing. Some of these changes may appear as early as age 45 years.[41] These changes may be attributable to peripheral alterations in sensory perception, such as smell and taste, and decreased muscle strength secondary to changes in mass and contractility. Loss of muscle strength (force) and speed in older persons results in increased, but normal, swallow durations compared with younger cohorts.[42] Increased swallow durations were also found in healthy older adults who had more **periventricular white matter** lesions compared with healthy older adults without them.[43] Other structures involved in swallowing that may show changes in mass and contractility include the tongue, lips, jaw, velum, and lungs. Loss of elasticity in lung tissue coupled with reduced respiratory capacity and control may indirectly affect swallow because of the known interactions between breathing and swallowing. Although these changes may not directly precipitate dysphagia, they may exacerbate conditions that are primary causative factors (e.g., neurologic disease). It is safe to assume that some aspects of swallowing are decompensated by normal aging and that the degree of compensation may enhance these effects in the diseased state. Robbins et al.[41] found that the ability of older persons to sustain isometric tasks involving the tongue may be different than in younger cohorts. These findings suggest that normal swallowing biomechanics may change under conditions of stress, such as might be imposed by hospitalization. Separating the effects of normal aging on swallowing from those in which disease is considered the primary causative factor presents a difficult clinical challenge.

Oral Stage and Aging

Tongue **hypertrophy** from fatty deposits and an increase in connective tissue results in a reduction of tongue mobility and tongue force as measured manometrically.[44] Some investigators have not found a significant difference in tongue pressure generation between normal, healthy older adults and younger cohorts,[38,45] although the time to reach maximum swallow pressures during swallowing was slower in older adults.[45] Significant differences are observed when comparing younger and older cohorts on their ability to generate maximum tongue pressures on nonswallowing tasks.[45] The difference between maximum isotonic pressures and the maximum pressure needed to complete a normal swallow seen in older persons, but not in younger cohorts, was discussed by Logemann et al.[46] They noted that the difference between these two measures in older persons represents a lack of pressure reserve and speculated that the difference may be important only when older persons need to rely on a pressure reserve, such as during illness.

Sensory changes related to aging include decrements in smell and taste,[47,48] although it is not clear whether these changes are attributable to primary loss of sensory receptors, poor oral hygiene, poor health, medications that reduce salivary flow, impaired nutritional status, or a combination of these factors.[49] Alterations in the ability to discriminate between materials with varying viscosity have been reported, although whether this is the result of primary sensory changes or a loss in the cortical representation of viscosity discrimination is not clear.[50]

Alterations in dentition necessitating the use of dentures may affect oral-stage mechanics. Ill-fitting dentures affect oral-stage preparation and may also interfere with access to the sensory receptors on the hard palate. For bolus materials that require mastication, older persons require additional time because of decreased jaw biting force.[51]

Pharyngeal Stage and Aging

Cinefluorography has shown that a decrease in the connective tissue in the suprahyoid musculature that supports laryngeal elevation may result in inadequate anterior laryngeal movement that secondarily reduces the opening of the PES.[52] Radiographic studies of healthy older persons show that pharyngeal constriction is normal compared with younger cohorts.[53] The restriction of PES opening is also evident on manometric studies, as evidenced by higher hypopharyngeal and intrabolus pressures in addition to increased pharyngeal contraction pressures.[44] In videofluoroscopic recordings of normal older and younger men, the older men showed significantly reduced anterior hyoid bone movement, resulting in less distention of the PES.[54] Failure of the PES to adequately distend results in shorter PES relaxation times and may explain increased higher pharyngeal contraction pressures as a compensation for shorter opening times.[55] High intrabolus pressures may be consistent with a restriction of flow through the PES and in selected older patients may explain reports of cervical dysphagia (see Chapter 7). Resting pressures within the PES are lower in older cohorts and may affect the competency of that barrier of swallowed contents that may move from the esophagus to the posterior pharynx.[56]

Videofluoroscopic swallowing studies comparing older and younger male cohorts revealed more instances of airway penetration after age 50 years.[57] Even though these threats to airway protection were evident, no subject demonstrated evidence of aspiration as a consequence of material entering the upper airway.

Studies have shown that the duration of the airway closure time in older persons is longer compared with younger cohorts.[41,58] This difference may be related to documented slower oral- and pharyngeal-stage transit times in older cohorts, resulting in a physiologic compensation to maintain airway closure and swallow safety. Changes in sensitivity in the protective reflexes in the upper airway may occur with aging. When calibrated puffs of air were delivered to the supraglottic larynx of older and younger subjects, laryngeal reflex (closure) responses were not as evident in the older subjects until the puffs of air achieved higher pressure levels.[59] Aviv et al.[59] suggest that this weaker response may indicate that the sensory mechanisms involved in upper airway protection may decompensate with normal aging.

Esophagus and Aging

In general, radiographic studies and manometrics document that esophageal motor activity decreases with age, but aging alone does not always explain dysphagic complaints. Reduction in the amplitude of esophageal contractions caused by smooth muscle thickening has been reported,[52] as well as delay in esophageal emptying and an increase in nonperistaltic contractions resulting in increased esophageal dilation and stasis.[60]

NEUROLOGIC CONTROLS OF SWALLOWING

Neuroregulation of swallowing involves the activation of multiple levels of afferent and efferent pathways at different levels of the nervous system,

---

CLINICAL CORNER 2-3

An 82-year-old man went to his primary care physician and reported that it had become more difficult to swallow solids foods over the past few months. Six months previously he started taking an antidepressant because he was not adjusting well to his wife's recent death. He denied choking episodes, so his doctor ordered a **barium esophagram**. The radiologist noted that with solid boluses there was a mild delay of bolus flow at the level of the aortic arch and no evidence of a stricture.

CRITICAL THINKING

1. Did the patient's physician believe the swallowing problem represented new disease or normal aging?
2. Speculate on why the patient did not have a swallowing problem 1 year ago.

---

including the cranial nerves, brainstem, cerebellum, subcortex, limbic cortex, and **neocortex**. Some aspects of swallowing appear to operate at a purely reflexive level, but it is more likely that swallowing does not represent a truly reflexive, brainstem-mediated response because food items are rarely swallowed the same way each time regardless of similarity in bolus type and size. As such, swallowing is believed to represent a more patterned type of neurologic response that can be influenced by control centers above the level of the brainstem. The peripheral muscles of swallowing contract sequentially but can be altered to accommodate the feeding activity. Therefore swallowing relies on both peripheral and central neurologic control systems that are activated differentially depending on the feeding circumstance. For instance, a person normally does not volitionally "think" about starting a swallowing response when eating but can "think" about swallowing when trying to swallow a pill. Although the mechanism is not totally understood, the act of swallowing potentially involves nervous system connections at multiple levels.

Peripheral and Medullary Controls

Pharyngeal swallow is initiated by sensory impulses transmitted as a result of stimulation of receptors on the fauces, tonsils, soft palate, base of the tongue, posterior pharyngeal wall, and anterior surface of the epiglottis.[61] These sensory impulses reach the NTS of the medulla primarily through the seventh, ninth, and tenth CNs. The efferent function is mediated through the ninth, tenth, eleventh, and twelfth CNs by the nucleus ambiguus (NA) (Tables 2-5 and 2-6; Figure 2-9). The highly integrated activities of swallowing depend on a combination of voluntary and involuntary control of the position of the lips, teeth, jaw, cheeks, and tongue—all mediated by multiple cranial nerves. Through innervation by the fifth CN, the masseter and pterygoid muscles provide the control of leverage, stabilization, and centering of the movable parts of the buccal cavity. Mastication depends primarily on CN V, whereas the muscles of the lips and cheeks depend on motor functions of CN VII. The extrinsic muscles of the tongue depend on the motor function of the CNs V and XII, except for the palatoglossus (elevator of the tongue root), which is innervated by CNs X and XI. All the intrinsic tongue muscles are innervated by CN XII. All the muscles of the soft palate are innervated primarily by CN X except the tensor veli palatini, which is innervated by CN V. The stylopharyngeus, a longitudinal muscle, widens the pharynx and is innervated by CN IX, whereas the palatopharyngeus is innervated primarily

TABLE 2-5	
Afferent Controls Involved in Swallowing	
Sensory Function	**Innervation (Cranial Nerve)**
General sensation, anterior two thirds of the tongue	Lingual nerve, trigeminal (V)
Taste, anterior two thirds of the tongue	Chorda tympani, facial (VII)
Taste and general sensation, posterior third of the tongue	Glossopharyngeal (IX)
Mucosa of valleculae	Internal branch of superior laryngeal nerve (vagus; X)
Primary afferent	—
Secondary afferent	Glossopharyngeal (IX)
Tonsils, pharynx, soft palate	Pharyngeal branch of vagus (X)
Pharynx, larynx, viscera	Glossopharyngeal (IX) Vagus (X)

TABLE 2-6	
Efferent Controls Involved in Swallowing	
Efferent/Stage	**Innervation (Cranial Nerve)**
Oral	
Masticatory, buccinators, floor of mouth	Trigeminal (V)
Lip sphincter	Facial (VII)
Tongue	Hypoglossal (XII)
Pharyngeal	—
Constrictors and stylopharyngeus	Glossopharyngeal (IX)
Palate, pharynx, larynx	Vagus (X)
Tongue	Hypoglossal (XII)
Esophageal	
Esophagus	Vagus (X)

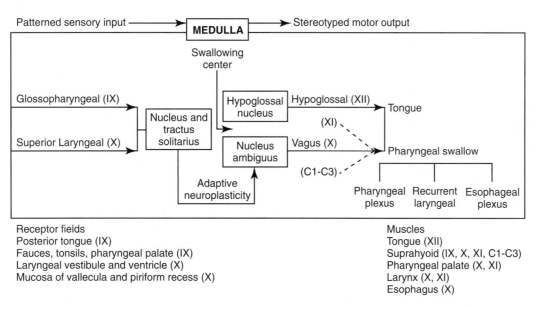

FIGURE 2-9. Conceptualization of the components of pharyngeal swallow as sensory-cued, stereotyped behaviors.

by CNs X and XII. The maxillary and mandibular sensory divisions of CN V are primarily involved in providing sensation pertaining to the lips, palate, teeth, inner mouth, and proprioceptive aspects of the muscles of mastication. The gag reflex and nasal regurgitation depend on the function (or dysfunction) of the glossopharyngeal and vagus nerves. Some controversy exists over the origin of the PES (cricopharyngeal) resting tone, which may not rely solely on the cervical sympathetic nervous system but may depend more heavily on vagal input for both contraction and relaxation.[62]

The literature refers to a swallowing center composed of key nuclei involved in afferent and efferent swallow control functions with interneuronal connections to respiratory centers in the medulla at the level of the obex of the fourth ventricle. This swallowing center has been defined as the dorsal NTS and ventral NA and the adjacent reticular formation.[63] This concept probably is an oversimplification. Based on current evidence, it is more likely that major contributions from neural activity in supramedullary structures, such as pons, mesencephalon, and limbic and cerebral cortices, are involved in modulation of oral and pharyngeal swallowing and voluntary and involuntary behaviors.

The brainstem coordinates efferent impulse flow by way of the trigeminal, vagus, and hypoglossal cranial nerves to the muscles of the oropharynx, by way of CN X to the muscles of the hypopharynx, by way of CNs V and XII to the extrinsic muscles of the larynx, and by way of CN X to the intrinsic muscles of the larynx and esophagus. The cervical esophagus may receive two vagal efferent supplies from nerves within the neck. One comes from the recurrent laryngeal nerve and another from the pharyngoesophageal nerve that rises proximal to the **nodose ganglion** or from an esophageal branch of the superior laryngeal nerve (SLN). Such double innervation of the cervical esophagus in human beings has not been proved but might provide a margin of safety to prevent esophageal distention and reflux.

Sequentially timed discharges from the medulla result in movement of a bolus through successive levels of the esophageal musculature. Esophageal smooth muscle contractions have a sequential behavior by which proximal activity successively inhibits the next most distal portion of the esophagus.[64] Esophageal distention is signaled on visceral afferent nerves passing in the upper five or six thoracic sympathetic roots, presumably to the thalamus and inferior postcentral gyrus, where they may cause symptoms described as pressure, burning, gas, or aching. When such symptoms are described as *pain,* the referral patterns are based on sensory impulses from tissues innervated by somatic nerves that cross the corresponding spinal levels.

Motor fibers originating in the NA innervate the pharyngeal, laryngeal, and upper esophageal striated muscles. By way of the dorsal vagal nucleus, the NA also innervates the heart, lungs, and gastrointestinal tract smooth muscle.[65] Rootlets emerging from the medulla form the peripheral vagus, which exits the skull through the jugular foramen. Above the nodose ganglion, the vagus nerve sends branches to the pharyngeal plexus, which supplies the mucosa and musculature of the pharynx, larynx, and PES (Figure 2-10).[65]

The highly important branch of the vagus—the SLN—is sensory to the laryngeal mucosa and motor to the cricothyroid muscle. The vagus terminates as the recurrent laryngeal nerve (RLN) that loops around the aorta and returns to the larynx and hypopharynx. The RLN supplies muscles intrinsic to the larynx and is believed not to supply the cricopharyngeus, which apparently derives its innervations from the pharyngeal plexus.[66]

CLINICAL CASE EXAMPLE 2-1

An 86-year-old man recently had heart surgery. After surgery he had a stroke affecting the premotor cortex of the left hemisphere. The man has a past history of depression treated with an antidepressant. He also had a history of Bell's palsy that affected CN VII in the upper and lower half of the left side of his face. He presented to the clinician with dysphagia. On examination the patient reported difficulty chewing and stated that food did not taste good. He noted considerable choking and a feeling that food was sticking in his throat. Physical examination of CN function revealed weakened right facial musculature from the stroke and weakened left facial musculature from the previous Bell's palsy. He was unable to make a tight lip seal because of bilateral CN VII nerve weakness. His tongue deviated to the right on protrusion, and range of motion was reduced (CN XII). Inspection of the oral cavity revealed moderate **xerostomia**. His voice was hoarse and breathy, although the velum rose evenly during testing of the gag reflex. His swallowing study showed poor bolus preparation, limited laryngeal elevation, pharyngeal stasis on pudding textures, and aspiration of thin liquids at the moment of swallow. It was concluded that the patient's poor bolus preparation could have been caused by multiple factors: tongue weakness, poor motor control from the involvement of a cortical motor area known to be important to bolus preparation, lack of taste appreciation from xerostomia (medication side effect), and probable involvement of the chorda tympani branch of CN VII (on the left). It was further concluded that his pharyngeal symptoms were attributable to poor laryngeal elevation caused by tongue weakness. This resulted in reduced opening of the PES, thus making it difficult for pudding to enter the esophagus, which caused the feeling that food was sticking in his throat. Liquids were aspirated because the vocal folds could not close fast enough because of the involvement of the recurrent branch of CN X that may have been damaged during the heart surgery, combined with the failure of the larynx to forcefully elevate and tilt forward because the tongue was weak. The pharyngeal branch of CNs IX and X was unaffected as evidenced by an intact gag reflex.

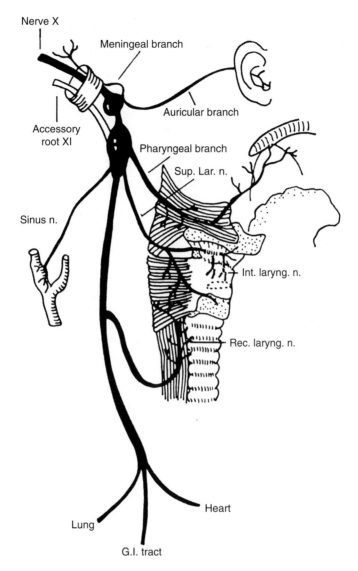

Nerve X

Meningeal branch

Auricular branch

Accessory
root XI

Pharyngeal branch

Sup. Lar. n.

Sinus n.

Int. laryng. n.

Rec. laryng. n.

Heart

Lung

G.I. tract

FIGURE 2-10. Schematic representation of the three peripheral branches of cranial nerve X: the pharyngeal branch to the region of the velum and pharynx; the internal and recurrent branches to the larynx; and the autonomic branch to the heart, lungs, and gastrointestinal tract. *Sup. Lar.*, Superior laryngeal nerve; *Int. laryng. n.*, internal laryngeal nerve; *Rec. laryng. n.*, recurrent laryngeal nerve.

The neural control systems that subserve pharyngeal swallow are initiated by the action of CN afferents, but isolated central activation is not possible even though voluntary components exist. It appears that afferent impulses competent to initiate swallowing must conform to highly codified stimulus patterns that enter the NTS of the brainstem by way of its fasciculus and are relayed into the reticular formation, where connections exist to motor neurons lying in the nuclei of the fifth, seventh, and twelfth CNs and the NA.

Other brainstem motor neurons of interest in the neuroregulation of swallowing include the salivatory

nuclei on either side of the genu of CNs VII and IX that provide saliva to the oral cavity and the dorsal motor nucleus of the vagus that innervates the esophageal smooth muscle (Figure 2-11).

The neuroregulatory brainstem mechanisms for pharyngeal swallow exist within the medullary reticular formation 1.5 mm from the midline on either side of the obex of the fourth ventricle. On each side of the midline is a site that communicates with the opposite side through cross-connections running behind the obex. As a result, bilateral symmetry of pharyngeal swallow is achieved. Each half of the medullary reticular formation exerts ipsilateral inhibition

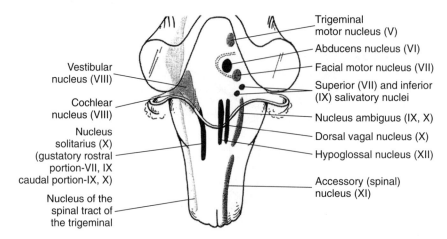

FIGURE 2-11. A view of the relations of the key brainstem nuclei involved in swallowing. Most nuclei are within close proximity in the dorsal and ventral parts of the medulla.

and excitation on appropriate motoneurons, with the exception of the inferior constrictor muscles, whose excitation is strictly contralateral.

Pharyngeal swallow involves a sequence of excitation and inhibition produced by several motor neuronal pools on each side of the brainstem.[63] Experimental unilateral destruction of the medulla eliminates swallowing in the ipsilateral musculature, except for the crossed pharyngeal constrictor muscle pathway. However, the responsiveness of the contralateral side to afferent input for the side of the lesion is still normal. For example, destruction of the left lateral medulla does not prevent right-sided swallowing if the left SLN is stimulated. This has immediate clinical relevance, especially in the case of unilateral destructive lesions to the brainstem.

The peripheral neural organization of swallowing has been largely elucidated by recording the electrical activity of involved muscles, beginning with onset of contraction in the mylohyoid and including concurrent activity in muscles innervated by CN V and those of the posterior tongue, superior constrictor, palatopharyngeus, palatoglossus, stylohyoid, and geniohyoid. These initiators constitute what has been called the *leading complex*.[67] Because the pharyngeal constrictor muscles form a continuous sheet of striated muscle, an overlapping "firing sequence" is observed beginning with the superior pharyngeal constrictor (the principal muscle), the middle pharyngeal constrictor, and the inferior pharyngeal constrictor, with distinct rostral (thyropharyngeus) and caudal (cricopharyngeus) components. The superior constrictor is active at the same time as the leading complex activity. A reconstruction of firing patterns leads to the conclusion that inhibition probably sur-

rounds or brackets (in a time sense) the excitation of swallowing.[67]

The convergent supranuclear afferent systems (rostral to the brainstem) include the maxillary branch of CN V and CNs IX and X. These lead to the descending or spinal trigeminal system and the fasciculus and nucleus solitarii. The magnocellular part of the NTS receives input from the sensorimotor cortex and the ventromedial thalamus.[68] Some fibers of CNs IX and X project to the lateral cuneate nucleus (lateral portion of posterior spinal column), serving as a relay to the ventroposteromedial nucleus of the thalamus and limbic cortical system.

There are intrinsic and extrinsic neurologic controls for the esophageal components of swallowing. The extrinsic portion includes fibers that innervate the striated and smooth muscle portions of the esophagus. The striated (proximal third) portion of the esophagus is innervated by the recurrent branch of the vagus by the NA in the brainstem. Sympathetic and parasympathetic fibers leave the dorsal vagal nucleus in the brainstem, course through the NA, and innervate the smooth (distal two thirds) muscle of the esophagus. The intrinsic portion of esophageal nervous innervation is supplied by a neural network that lies between the circular and longitudinal esophageal musculature, referred to as the *mesenteric plexus*.

Supranuclear Swallowing Controls

Normal oral feeding appears to involve brainstem reflex initiation by way of several types of peripheral excitation as well as a central facilitation of its limbic and cortical sensorimotor pathways. The importance of peripheral afferent stimulation cannot be underestimated because a bolus appears to be required to sustain repetitive swallowing activity. It is difficult to conceive of the act of swallowing as either purely reflexive (brainstem mediated) or purely voluntary (supranuclear mediated) because the repetitive nature of motor activity and potential differences in sensory inputs undoubtedly need to be modulated by higher cortical structures. It is conceivable that supranuclear connections to the brainstem swallowing center are necessary to continue, modify, and monitor swallowing activity when necessary as well as respond appropriately to different sensory stimuli. Conceivably, supranuclear systems are organized so that repetitive and overlearned efferent response networks (such as chewing) are maintained by a series of feedback loops that connect jaw activity to frontal motor areas. These networks interact with interneurons that communicate with lower brainstem centers.[69] Other cortical centers appear to be reserved for modifications in swallowing activity depending on either the volitional nature of the task or changes in afferent information that may require alterations in motor performance. Kennedy and Kent[70] theorize that swallowing takes place at three different levels of nervous system organization: (1) a peripheral level that is linked to afferent bolus characteristics, (2) a subcortical level that organizes and executes learned patterns of efferent activity, and (3) a descending cortical portion that responds to any needed changes in motor activity based on perceived changes in the need to modify feeding behavior. Examples of volitional behaviors might include the need to eat faster, the need to expectorate an unwanted bolus, or perhaps the need to talk and masticate simultaneously. Investigations of these multiple pathways and centers have been conducted in human beings and animals with various laboratory techniques, including functional magnetic resonance imaging, electrical stimulation, ablation of suspected control centers, positron emission tomography, and transcranial magnetic stimulation. A complete understanding of the interrelations among centers during varying volitional and nonvolitional swallowing tasks remains speculative.

Regions of the cerebral cortex identified as active participants during swallowing are the anterior insular cortex with connections to the primary and **supplementary motor cortices**,[71] **orbitofrontal operculum**,[72] and the medial and superior portion of the **anterior cingulate gyrus**.[73] Interestingly, some of these areas appear to be active only for particular bolus types, such as water or a thicker liquid.[73] For instance, using functional magnetic resonance imaging, Shibamoto et al.[73] found that a swallow attempt with the combination of water and a capsule activated limbic and neocortical structures as well as the cerebellum. Other studies have shown activation of multiple cortical and subcortical sites, including the basal ganglia.[74,75] From preliminary data on a small number of subjects the right cortical hemisphere appears to be more active during volitional swallows, whereas the left is more active during reflexive activity.[76]

TAKE HOME NOTES

1. Swallowing is accomplished by a complex interaction of striated and smooth muscles whose sensory and motor components are carried by multiple cranial nerves.
2. The cranial nerves involved in swallowing send sensory information to the NTS. Motor components are organized in the NA. Together the NTS and NA comprise the "swallowing center" located in the medulla of the brainstem.
3. Higher cortical control centers are capable of influencing the brainstem swallowing center.
4. The preparation and movement of a bolus during swallowing can be theoretically conceived as a series of valves that must open and close in a coordinated manner. This activity creates zones of high pressure around the bolus and zones of negative pressure below the level of the bolus. These pressure mismatches, together with gravity, create bolus flow.
5. Respiration ceases during swallowing. Protection of the airway to achieve a safe swallow is multifaceted. It is accomplished by primary airway closure at the level of the true and false vocal folds, laryngeal elevation, tongue base retraction, and epiglottic tilt.
6. The process of aging alone does not create dysphagia but may contribute to it, especially during disease-related decompensation.

References

1. Leopold NA, Kagel MA: Dysphagia—ingestion or deglutition? A proposed paradigm, *Dysphagia* 12:202, 1997.

2. Stephan JR, Taves DH, Smith RC et al: Bolus location at the initiation of the pharyngeal stage of swallowing in healthy older adults, *Dysphagia* 20:266, 2005.

3. Kendall KA: Oropharyngeal swallowing variability, *Laryngoscope* 112:547, 2002.

4. Mishellany A, Woda A, Peyron MA: The challenge of mastication: preparing a bolus suitable for deglutition, *Dysphagia* 21:87, 2006.

5. Hiiemae KM, Palmer JB: Food transport and bolus formation during complete feeding sequences on foods of different initial consistency, *Dysphagia* 14:31, 1999.

6. Kapila YV, Dodds WJ, Helm JF et al: Relationship between swallow rate and salivary flow, *Dig Dis Sci* 29:528, 1984.

7. Ponderoux P, Logemann JA, Kahrilas PJ: Pharyngeal swallowing elicited by fluid infusion: role of volition and vallecular containment, *Am J Physiol* 270:G347, 1996.

8. Widdicombe JG: Airway receptors, *Resp Physiol* 125:3, 2001.

9. Wilson EM, Green JR: Coordinative organization of lingual propulsion during the normal adult swallow, *Dysphagia* 21:226, 2006.

10. Logemann JA, Kahrilas PJ, Cheng J et al: Closure mechanisms of the laryngeal vestibule during swallowing, *Am J Physiol* 262(2 Pt 1):G388, 1992.

11. Cook IJ, Dodds WJ, Dantas RO et al: Timing of videofluoroscopic, manometric events, and bolus transit during the oral and pharyngeal phases of swallowing, *Dysphagia* 4:8, 1989.

12. Martin-Harris B, Brodsky MB, Price CC et al: Temporal coordination of pharyngeal and laryngeal dynamics with breathing during swallowing: single liquid swallows, *J Appl Physiol* 94:1235, 2003.

13. Palmer JB, Hiiemae KM: Eating and breathing: interactions between respiration and feeding on sold food, *Dysphagia* 18:169, 2003.

14. Cichero JAY, Murdoch BE: What happens after the swallow? Introducing the glottal release sound, *J Med Speech Pathol* 11:31, 2003.

15. Shaker R, Li Q, Ren J et al: Coordination of deglutition and phases of respiration: effect of aging and tachypnea, bolus volume, and chronic obstructive pulmonary disease, *Am J Physiol* 263(5 Pt 1):G750, 1992.

16. Hiss SG, Treole K, Stuart A: Effects of age, gender, bolus volume, and trial on swallowing apnea duration and swallow/respiratory phase relationships of normal adults, *Dysphagia* 16:128, 2001.

17. Leslie P, Drinnan M, Ford G et al: Swallow respiration patterns in dysphagic patients following acute stroke, *Dysphagia* 17:202, 2002.

18. Klahn MS, Perlman AL: Temporal and durational patterns associating respiration and swallowing, *Dysphagia* 14:131, 1999.

19. Hiss SG, Strauss M, Treole K et al: Swallowing apnea as a function of airway closure, *Dysphagia* 18:293, 2003.

20. Kendall KA, McKenzie S, Leonard R et al: Timing events in normal swallowing: a videofluoroscopic study, *Dysphagia* 15:74, 2000.

21. Ekberg O, Olsson R, Sundgren-Borgstrom P: Relation of bolus size and pharyngeal swallow, *Dysphagia* 3:69, 1988.

22. Ishida R, Palmer JB, Hiiemae KM: Hyoid motion during swallowing: factors affecting forward and upward displacement, *Dysphagia* 17:262, 2002.

23. Seta H, Hashimoto K, Inada H et al: Laterality of swallowing in healthy subjects by anterior-posterior projection using videofluoroscopy, *Dysphagia* 21:191, 2006.

24. Castel JA, Castell DO: Modern solid state computerized manometry of the pharyngoesophageal segment, *Dysphagia* 8:270, 1993.

25. Bardan E, Xie P, Aslam M et al: Disruption of primary and secondary esophageal peristalsis by afferent stimulation, *Am J Physiol Gastrointest Liver Physiol* 279:G255, 2000.

26. Castell DO: Esophageal manometric studies: a perspective of their physiological and clinical relevance, *J Clin Gastroenterol* 2:91, 1980.

27. Ekberg O, Nylander G: Cineradiography of the pharyngeal stage of deglutition in 150 patients without dysphagia, *Br J Radiol* 55:253, 1982.

28. Ren J, Shaker R, Kusano M et al: Effect of aging on the secondary esophageal peristalsis: presbyesophagus revisited, *Am J Physiol* 268:G379, 1995.

29. Adnerhill I, Ekberg O, Groher ME: Determining normal bolus size for thin liquids, *Dysphagia* 4:1, 1989.

30. Lawless HT, Bender S, Oman C et al: Gender, age, vessel size, cup vs. straw sipping, and sequence effects on sip volume, *Dysphagia* 18:196, 2003.

31. Wintzen AR, Badrising UA, Ross RAC et al: Influence of bolus volume on hyoid movements in normal individuals and patients with Parkinson's disease, *Can J Neurol Sci* 21:57, 1994.

32. Ekberg O, Olsson R, Sundgren-Borgström P: Relation of bolus size and pharyngeal swallow, *Dysphagia* 3:69, 1988.

33. Leonard RJ, Kendall KA, McKenzie S et al: Structural displacements in normal swallowing: a videofluoroscopic study, *Dysphagia* 15:146, 2000.

34. Chi-Fishman G, Sonies BC: Effects of systematic bolus velocity and volume changes on hyoid movement kinematics, *Dysphagia* 17:278, 2007.

35. Jacob K, Kahrilas PJ, Logemann JA et al: Upper esophageal sphincter opening and modulation during swallowing, *Gastroenterology* 97:1469, 1989.

36. Miller JL, Watkin KL: The influence of bolus volume and viscosity on anterior lingual force during the oral stage of swallowing, *Dysphagia* 11:117, 1996.

37. Cook IJ, Dodds WJ, Dantas RO et al: Timing of videofluoroscopic, manometric events, and bolus transit during the oral and pharyngeal phases of swallowing, *Dysphagia* 4:8, 1989.

38. Youmans SR, Stierwalt JAG: Measures of tongue function related to normal swallowing, *Dysphagia* 21:102, 2006.

39. Pelletier CA, Dhanaraj GE: The effect of taste and palatability on lingual swallowing pressure, *Dysphagia* 21:121, 2006.

40. Daniels SK, Foundas AL: Swallowing physiology of sequential straw drinking, *Dysphagia* 16:176, 2001.

41. Robbins JA, Hamilton J, Lof G et al: Oropharyngeal swallowing in normal adults of different ages, *Gastroenterology* 103:823, 1992.

42. Robbins J: Normal swallowing and aging, *Semin Neurol* 16:309, 1996.

43. Levine R, Robbins JA, Maser A: Periventricular white matter changes and oropharyngeal swallowing in normal individuals, *Dysphagia* 7:142, 1992.

44. Shaker R, Lang IM: Aging and deglutitive motor function: effect of aging on the deglutitive oral, pharyngeal, and esophageal motor function, *Dysphagia* 9:221, 1994.

45. Nicosia M, Hind JA, Roecker EB et al: Age effects on the temporal evolution of isometric swallowing pressure, *J Gerontol A Biol Sci Med Sci* 55:634, 2000.

46. Logemann JA, Pauloski BR, Rademaker AW et al: Temporal and biomechanical characteristics of oropharyngeal swallow in younger and older men, *J Speech Lang Hear Res* 43:1264, 2000.

47. Murphy C, Shubert CR, Cruickshanks KJ et al: Prevalence of olfactory impairment in older adults, *JAMA* 288:2307, 2002.

48. Schiffman SS: Taste and smell losses in normal aging and disease, *JAMA* 278:1357, 1997.

49. Schiffman SS, Graham BG: Taste and smell perception affect appetite and immunity in the elderly, *Eur J Clin Nutr* 54:S54, 2000.

50. Smith CH, Logemann JA, Burghardt WR et al: Oral and oropharyngeal perceptions of fluid viscosity across the age span, *Dysphagia* 21:209, 2006.

51. Peyron MA, Blanc O, Lund JP et al: Influence of age on the adaptability of human mastication, *J Neurophysiol* 92:773, 2004.

52. Jones B, Donner MW: *Normal and abnormal swallowing: imaging in diagnosis and therapy*, New York, 1991, Springer-Verlag.

53. McKee GJ, Johnston BT, McBride GB et al: Does age or sex affect pharyngeal swallowing? *Clin Otolaryngol* 23:100, 1998.

54. Logemann JA, Pauloski BR, Rademaker AW et al: Temporal and biomechanical characteristics of oropharyngeal swallow in younger and older men, *J Speech Lang Hear Res* 43:1264, 2000.

55. Van Herwaarden MA, Katz PO, Gideon M et al: Are manometric parameters of the upper esophageal sphincter and pharynx affected by age and gender? *Dysphagia* 18:211, 2003.

56. Shaker R, Ren J, Podvrsan B et al: Effect of aging and bolus variables on pharyngeal and upper esophageal sphincter motor function, *Am J Physiol* 264:427, 1993.

57. Daggett A, Logemann JA, Rademaker AW et al: Laryngeal penetration during deglutition in normal subjects of various ages, *Dysphagia* 21:270, 2006.

58. Selley WG, Flack FC, Ellis RE et al: Respiratory patterns associated with swallowing. Part 1. The normal adult pattern and changes with aging, *Age Aging* 18:168, 1989.

59. Aviv JE, Martin JH, Jones ME et al: Age-related changes in pharyngeal and supraglottic sensation, *Ann Otol Rhinol Laryngol* 10:749, 1994.

60. Zboralske FF, Amberg JR, Soergel KH: Presbyesophagus: cineradiographic manifestations, *Radiology* 82:463, 1964.

61. Jean A: Brainstem organization of the swallowing network, *Brain Behav Evol* 25:109, 1984.

62. Mu L, Sanders I: Sensory nerve supply of the human oro- and laryngopharynx: a preliminary study, *Anat Rec* 258:406, 2000.

63. Jean A: Brain stem control of swallowing: neuronal network and cellular mechanisms, *Physiol Rev* 81:929, 2001.

64. Ekberg O, Nylander G: Cineradiography of the pharyngeal stage of deglutition in 150 individuals without dysphagia, *Br J Radiol* 55:253, 1982.

65. Rontal M, Rontal E: Lesions of the vagus nerve: diagnosis, treatment, and rehabilitation, *Laryngoscope* 87:72, 1977.

66. Mu L, Sanders I: Muscle fiber-type distribution patterns in the human cricopharyngeus muscle, *Dysphagia* 17:87, 2002.

67. Doty RW, Bosma JF: Electromyographic analysis of reflex deglutition, *J Neurophysiol* 19:44, 1956.

68. Bass N: The neurology of swallowing. In Groher, ME, editor: *Dysphagia: diagnosis and management*, ed 3, Boston, 1997, Butterworth-Heinemann.

69. Martin RE, Sessle BJ: The role of the cerebral cortex in swallowing, *Dysphagia* 8:195, 1993.

70. Kennedy JG, Kent RD: Physiologic substrates of normal deglutition, *Dysphagia* 3:24, 1988.

71. Daniels SK, Foundas AL: The role of the insular cortex in dysphagia, *Dysphagia* 12:146, 1997.

72. Martin RE, Kemppainen P, Masuda Y et al: Features of cortically evoked swallowing in the awake primate, *J Neurophysiol* 82:1529, 1999.

73. Shibamoto I, Tanaka T, Fujishima I et al: Cortical activation during solid bolus swallowing, *J Med Dent Sci* 54:25, 2007.

74. Hamdy S, Rothwell JC, Brooks DJ et al: Identification of the cerebral loci processing human swallowing with H2(15)O PET activation, *J Neurophysiol* 81:1917, 1999.

75. Suzuki M, Asada J, Ito K et al: Activation of cerebellum and basal ganglia on volitional swallowing detected by functional magnetic resonance imaging, *Dysphagia* 18:71, 2003.

76. Kern MK, Jaradeh S, Arndorfer RC et al: Cerebral cortical representation of reflexive and volitional swallowing in humans, *Am J Physiol* 280:G354, 2001.

Chapter 3

Normal Swallowing and Development in the Term and Preterm Infant

JO PUNTIL-SHELTMAN

OBJECTIVES

1. Identify and understand core concepts of newborn development.
2. Identify the difference between a nonnutritive suck and a nutritive suck.
3. Identify and understand the benefits of breast milk.
4. Identify and understand the major swallowing milestones between birth and age 12 months.

It is important for the feeding specialist to understand the acquisition of normal swallowing in infancy. Term infants have the appropriate time in utero to achieve mature neurologic and physiologic development, whereas preterm infant development is shortened. One characteristic of term infants is a natural physiologic flexion; this flexion occurs whether the infant is in the prone or supine position. This position helps the infant remain neurologically organized and stable in awake states and throughout the feeding process. Preterm infants need to develop the skills necessary to maintain physiologic stability outside the uterus.

EMBRYOLOGY AND FETAL DEVELOPMENT

Knowledge of embryology and fetal development is vital in understanding the acquisition of swallowing. There are approximately 23 stages of development from prenatal to fetal development. Early embryonic development is described in stages because of the **morphologic** characteristics. The *embryonic period* terminates at the end of the eighth week, when the beginnings of all essential human structures are present. The *fetal period* extends from 9 weeks to birth and is characterized by growth and elaboration of structures. Fetuses are viable at 23 weeks after fertilization. The survival rate of fetuses younger than 23 weeks is poor. *Gastrulation* is the formative process by which the three germ layers and axial orientation are established in embryos. Gastrulation begins with the formation of the primitive streak. Each of the three germ layers (ectoderm, endoderm, and mesoderm) gives rise to specific tissues and organs.[1]

The *embryonic ectoderm* gives rise to the epidermis, central and peripheral nervous systems, retina of the eye, and various other structures. The embryonic endoderm is the source of the epithelial linings of the respiratory and gastrointestinal tracts, including the glands opening into the gastrointestinal tract and glandular cells of associated organs such as the liver and pancreas. The *embryonic mesoderm* gives rise to the smooth muscular coatings, connective tissues, and vessels associated with tissues and organs. The mesoderm also forms most of the cardiovascular system and is the source of blood cells and bone marrow, the skeleton, striated muscles, and reproductive and excretory organs. This process occurs during the third week of gestation. By this time the central nervous system develops from the neural plate, which transforms into the neural tube.

Early in the fourth week after conception, the pharyngeal apparatus develops. At this point, the human embryo somewhat resembles the regions of the fish embryo at the comparable stage of development. This would explain the former use of the term *branchial apparatus* (from the Greek word *brancha*, meaning gill). Past literature references the term "branchial arch," whereas current literature refers to this important area as the *pharyngeal arch*. The pharyngeal apparatus consists of pharyngeal arches, pouches, grooves, and membranes. All these embryonic structures contribute to the formation of the head and neck. Most congenital anomalies in these regions originate during transformation of the pharyngeal apparatus into its adult derivatives. By the end of the fourth week, four pairs of pharyngeal arches are visible externally. The first pair of pharyngeal arches plays a major role in facial development. More specifically, the face, neck, nasal cavities, mouth, larynx, and pharynx, along with muscular attachments of the head and neck, are all derived from the pharyngeal arches. These arches include the muscular component that differentiates into the muscles of the head and neck and a nerve that supplies the mucosa and muscles derived from the arch. In the fourth week the development of the forebrain begins, producing a prominent elevation of the head and a C-shaped curvature of the embryo. Upper and lower limb buds are recognizable by the end of the fourth week. The respiratory and gastrointestinal systems are developing at this same embryonic time. Both systems develop from the laryngotracheal groove in the primitive pharynx. The laryngotracheal groove gives rise to the larynx, trachea, bronchi, lungs, and esophagus.[1]

The fourth to eighth weeks are crucial for neural and organ development. The 12 cranial nerves are formed during the fifth to sixth weeks of development. During these weeks, all major organs and systems of the body form three germ layers. The three germ layers differentiate into various tissues and organs so that by the end of the embryonic period, the beginnings of all the main organ systems have been established. The beginnings of the most essential external and internal structures are formed during the fourth to eighth weeks. This is the most critical period of development. Any disturbance during this period may cause major congenital anomalies of the embryo.

From the ninth to twelfth weeks the head constitutes half the **crown-heel length** of the fetus. Growth in body length accelerates rapidly. At nine weeks the liver is the major site for the formation of red blood cells, whereas urine formation begins between the ninth and twelfth weeks and is discharged into the amniotic fluid. Nonnutritive sucking occurs between the eleventh and twelfth weeks. Between the twelfth and thirteenth weeks the fetus is capable of swallowing amniotic fluid. The fetus grows rapidly from the thirteenth to sixteenth weeks. Limb movements become coordinated by week 14. The sex of the external genitalia can be recognized at 12 to 14 weeks, and at 17 to 20 weeks the mother first detects movement of the fetus. By week 18 the gag reflex is present. The skin is covered with a cheeselike material, and the body of a 20-week fetus is completely covered with fine hair. Rapid growth occurs between weeks 20 and 25. This period gives rise to rapid eye movements, the lungs are beginning to secrete **surfactant**, and fingernails are present. Between 25 and 29 weeks the fetus can survive outside the womb with medical support. The central nervous system has matured to direct rhythmic breathing movements and attempts to control body temperature. Eyes are opened at this time, and hair is noted on the head. From 30 to 34 weeks the fetus continues to grow and can survive if born prematurely, likely with less medical intervention. The rooting reflex is noted by 32 weeks' gestation, although the coordination of the suck-swallow-breathe bursts is usually more developed by 34 weeks.

NORMAL DEVELOPMENTAL MILESTONES

It is important that the feeding specialist develop an appreciation for normal developmental milestones in systems other than swallowing. Poor development, or lack of development, often may be seen in multiple systems and provides clues as to the child's level of functioning. The normal development of sensory systems such as hearing, vision, taste, and smell may be crucial in understanding the child's disordered feeding ability.

Auditory Development

The critical period for auditory development begins around 24 weeks' gestation and continues until 3 to 4 years of age. The fetus is protected from high-frequency sounds by tissue absorption. The fetus hears low-frequency sounds through fluid and bone conduction. The fetus is now aware of the mother's voice. The auditory system of the fetus is vulnerable to injury by exposure to intense low-frequency noise. After the birthing process, sound exposure shifts from fluid- and tissue-conducted sound to air-conducted, which adds high-frequency sounds. It is vital to protect the auditory system of a preterm infant, especially from 24 to 32 weeks' gestational age. The infant should be protected from any noise above 45 dB.[2] Hearing in preterm infants from 32 to 34 weeks' gestational age demonstrates rapid maturation of the cochlea and auditory nerve. Hearing in the infant older than 34 weeks shows an increase in speed of conduction and an increasing ability to localize and discriminate sound. It is recommended that the combination of continuous background sound and transient sound in any isolette not exceed an hourly average of 55 dB. Transient sounds produced by voices or equipment should not exceed 70 dB. Typically sounds from a ventilator or from bubbling tubing noise range from 60 to 80 dB. The American Academy of Pediatrics recommends that noise in the neonatal intensive care unit (NICU) be maintained at levels below 60 dB to prevent cochlear damage.

Visual Development

High noise levels, bright lights, sleep deprivation, and long-term sedation can affect the processes of early visual development. From conception to 20 weeks, the brain's structural development and genetic mapping for vision occur. Gross structures are in place by 23 to 24 weeks. A critical period is from 20 weeks' gestation to 3 years of age, when neuronal and cell realignment is being laid. At 24 to 28 weeks the fetus's eyelids unfuse, the lens is cloudy, and the cornea is hazy until 27 weeks. At 25 weeks, vascularization begins and the retina demonstrates rod differentiation. During this same time the cortex is undergoing rapid dendritic growth. The infant demonstrates no pupillary response and is very **myopic**. From 30 weeks' gestation to approximately 3 to 4 months the infant develops ocular dominance columns. At 31 to 34 weeks' gestation these ocular dominance column formations include the maturity of the retina, the lateral geniculate nucleus, cortical radiations, and waves of endogenous retinal stimulation (during rapid eye movement sleep). The infant needs rapid eye movement sleep to build ocular columns. Visual column development occurs at approximately 40 weeks' gestation (term) to 7 months. These include ocular dominance, lines and patterns, movement, depth, color, visual mapping, and complex visual processing.[3] It is imperative that the infant's visual system is protected, especially from 23 to 32 weeks of age. At 34 weeks to term the infant's eyes begin to track, show visual preferences, and spontaneously orient toward soft light. By 40 weeks the eyes attend to form, objects, and faces. Infants begin to visually track and can see objects at 2 feet but attend best at 8 to 12 inches.

Development of Taste and Smell

Oral chemoreception (taste) develops early in utero. Stimulation of the trigeminal nerve and activation of taste buds develop at approximately 12 to13 weeks' gestation. Receptors are noted at 16 weeks and reach their adult number by 40 weeks. *Nasal chemoreception* (smell) occurs by the eleventh week. Trigeminal nerve endings respond at 7 to 10 weeks. The basic structures are developing between the eleventh and fifteenth weeks. Fetal breathing movements displace amniotic fluid by 22 weeks. Some of the sources of fetal chemoreceptor stimulation are fragrant molecules in the blood and amniotic fluid. These receptors penetrate mucus receptors, eliciting a response. At this time, the infant is swallowing with different taste perceptions. Chemoreception in preterm infants responds to odorants by at least 28 to 29 weeks. Taste preferences begin to differentiate by at least 28 to 29 weeks. Chemoreception in term infants is developed so that they can detect, localize, and discriminate a variety of distinct odors. They especially have an attraction to the mother's scent and breast odors.

Motor Reflex Development

Normal reflexive and motor milestones are precisely integrated with the infant's ability to feed successfully. By 28 weeks' gestational age the rooting, sucking, **Moro** (startle), **crossed extension**, **flexor withdrawal**, and **plantar grasp** reflexes are all present. These reflexes help establish stability throughout the body for movement, protection, and feeding. By 35 weeks' gestational age the neonatal neck and body righting, positive support, tonic neck, and **proprioceptive placing** are established. These reflexes assist in weight bearing in the upright position, the ability to support weight on the forearms, and the ability to rotate the head. By 1 month of age the infant normally has better control of these tasks. As the infant grows, the limbs, trunk, head, and neck provide support for successful feeding and movement.

NORMAL INFANT SWALLOWING

Swallowing begins in utero at approximately the twelfth to thirteenth week. After birth the infant needs to learn to coordinate the suck-swallow-breathe process. Successful feeding is a complex motor and sensory activity. Feeding involves the infant's ability to (1) engage and remain engaged in a physiologically and behaviorally challenging task, (2) organize oral motor movements to achieve long-term functional benefits, (3) coordinate breathing with swallowing to avoid prolonged apnea or aspiration of fluids, and (4) regulate the depth and frequency of breathing to maintain physiologic stability.[4] Feeding is a marker for neurologic maturation. Coordinated feedings require sensory-motor integration of a suck, swallow and ventilation. Preterm infants demonstrate a disorganized pattern of sucking bursts and pauses.[5] They demonstrate a more stable pattern of rhythmic sucking and swallowing by 34 to 36 weeks' gestation. This coordinated pattern is essential for the prevention of aspiration. Infants use the rooting reflex to find the mother's nipple (or nipple from a bottle) and proceed to latch. Fluid is expressed from the nipple by a combination of intraoral suction and external pressure. The fluid moves because of changes in pressure. These changes include positive pressure from the jaw (compression)—pushing the fluid out—and negative pressure from the tongue and oral cavity (suction) that *draws* fluid out of the nipple.[6]

Normal Anatomy

The oral motor components needed for successful feeding are the lips, jaw, tongue, buccal mucosa, and the hard and soft palate. The lips form an anterior seal around the nipple or areola, which helps keep the nipple midline. The jaw provides stability for other structures and assists in creating negative pressure by working with the tongue. The infant's tongue is large compared with the oral cavity. The tongue creates a seal by forming a central tongue groove to wrap the edges around the nipple and together with the jaw create the negative pressure to express milk. The hard palate provides a surface against which the tongue compresses, providing the positive pressure needed to extract or express the milk; it also stabilizes the nipple. The soft palate, in conjunction with the tongue, creates the posterior seal to the oral cavity. It also elevates during the swallow to allow passage of the bolus into the pharynx and seals the nasal cavity to prevent nasal regurgitation. When the posterior part of the tongue is depressed, the buccal mucosa moves inward and then outward during the compression phase; this mucosa is supported by the buccinator muscles and fat pads.[7]

The pharynx of an infant differs from that of an adult. The hyoid is high in the neck with the thyroid cartilage almost continuous with the hyoid bone. Consequently, there is less laryngeal elevation during swallowing compared with an adult. In infants, the pharynx shows a gentle curve from the nasopharynx to the distal pharynx. As the infant grows, the gentle curve gradually changes to form close to a 90-degree angle between the nasopharynx and oropharynx as seen in adults.[8] This relation explains why infants are obligatory nasal breathers. The oral cavity grows larger in a downward, forward movement as the tongue and larynx descend in the first year of life to accommodate communication. The larynx continues to grow until approximately 3 years of age, when its growth slows until the onset of puberty when it has another period of growth.

Nonnutritive and Nutritive Sucking

Nonnutritive sucking consists of rhythmic movements on a pacifier or finger. It is described as rapid sucking intervals. However, at times these intervals are irregular and vary in length. Infants continue to breathe when they suck on a pacifier, finger, or thumb. Nonnutritive sucking is very soothing to premature infants because it helps calm them and promotes generalized peristalsis in the gastrointestinal system.[9]

Nutritive sucking is usually very rhythmic and occurs at a suck/swallow ratio of 1:1. Infants suck and swallow in this sequence between 10 and 30 times before they take a breath and continue feeding. Healthy infants swallow six times per minute while awake and six times per hour while asleep.[6] Nutritive sucking may begin at 32 weeks' gestational age, although most success for feeding is initiated at 34 weeks. During nutritive sucking there is an apneic period during the swallow. The swallow-respiratory pattern is usually completed as an inspiration-swallow-expiration pattern, although Selley et al.[10] also have reported that inspiration-expiration-swallow-expiration is another common pattern. Infants eventually integrate precisely coordinated suck-swallow-breathe bursts within the first 2 months of life. Premature infants initially have a difficult time coordinating this process. Preterm infants demonstrate disorganized sucking patterns such as lack of rhythm of the total sucking activity. These infants lack the ability to increase or decrease sucking pressures in relation to milk flow. Disorganized feeding issues in a preterm infant can last up to 45 weeks after term if the infant is medically fragile.

Suckle Versus Sucking

There are two distinct differences in early infant feeding between suckle and suck. The initial type of feeding pattern to be established is the *suckle*. This pattern is first seen between the second and third trimester. The infant is able to express milk from a nipple by using a backward-forward movement. The tongue rarely passes the lips, and the lips are loosely fit around the areola or nipple. At 6 months of age the infant integrates the suckle pattern into an integrated sucking pattern. During this process, the tongue moves in an up-and-down motion. The lips have a stronger seal caused by the shifting of the tongue motion. The tongue has more room to move up and down due to the downward and forward movement of the oral cavity. The similarity of these two types of sucks is the movement of the jaw and tongue to express the milk from the nipple. The difference is that the tongue moves from a forward-backward motion to an up-and-down motion. The term *suck* is a generic term to describe the organized expression of liquid from a nipple.

Breastfeeding

Human milk is universally accepted as the best food for a normal, healthy term infant. Breast milk intake should be encouraged for the first 12 months of life.[11] Research shows that milk from a premature infant's mother may be particularly suited for the infant's special needs and that human milk is easier to digest than formula because of its fat, protein, and carbohydrate composition. The milk of a mother who gives birth prematurely is different from breast milk expressed after a term birth. This preterm milk contains higher concentrations of nitrogen, sodium, chloride, magnesium, and iron, minerals that are essential for a premature infant. Breast milk has natural infection-fighting components that are most beneficial for the preterm infant.

Breast milk is produced by pumping; thus frequent pumping is essential to lay down the receptors so that the breast lactates. Pumping should be started once the infant is delivered and should continue every 2 to 3 hours until successful breastfeeding is established. Proper positioning and latching on are crucial to successful breastfeeding. *Latching on* refers to the way the infant takes the breast into the mouth. When a baby is latched on well, the nipple is in the posterior portion of the mouth. If the baby is positioned appropriately (either **cross-cradle** or football hold) in a developmentally supportive manner, the latch is more successful. The exact technique of getting the infant on to the breast is not always simple. Each baby behaves differently, and each mother's breasts may be different. Initially the mother brings the infant to the breast and allows the rooting reflex to occur to find the nipple. As a general rule, the infant should have both the nose and chin latched on, covering most of the areola with the lower lip, rather than the upper lip. The lips are turned outward with the chin and nose touching the breast. If the latch is successful, the sucking reflex is initiated once the breast makes contact with the hard palate. The infant sucks continuously to facilitate the mother's "let down" of milk. The milk flows quickly so that the infant can achieve a rhythmic sucking pattern. If an infant latches on in this manner, the lower gums are under the milk sinuses and can extract milk from the breast more efficiently. The infant's body is rotated slightly upward so the infant can look at the mother. A good latch with abundant milk supply will lead to weight gain, pain-free nursing, and short feeding times (about 10 minutes per breast).[11] These steps are important to successful breastfeeding. Breastfeeding is a natural bonding process between mother and infant.

Early Infancy

During the first 2 to 3 months of life, the infant's primary goal is to achieve homeostasis with the environment.[6] At this time, primitive neurologic reflexes are all present. The infant's neurodevelopmental milestones play an important role in the normal process of feeding. The infant is usually in physiologic flexion, which promotes the proper posture for eating. Infants feed until **satiety** and then provide cues or signs of fullness. These signs are crucial to recognize the infant's system of self-regulation.

Transitional Feeding

Transitional feedings are the steps from liquid intake to chewing semisolids. The transition to soft solid foods, such as rice cereal or pureed fruit, should not be provided earlier than 4 months or later than 7 months depending on the infant's maturity. The major changes in the infant's anatomy at this age are the downward and forward growth of the mandible and the presence of teeth. The tongue no longer fills the entire oral cavity. Infants initially have difficulty transporting the bolus to the posterior cavity. They may sputter, cough, choke, and spit out food. At times they will show sucking movements rather than biting. If developmentally stable, the 5- to 7-month-old infant should be introduced to spoon feeding and approximately 1 month later to cup drinking (see Chapter 4). At this time the infant has better head and trunk control that provides postural stability for

sitting with support. The infant also begins to vocalize and interacts with the caregiver during feedings.

Six to Twelve Months

Between 6 and 9 months, lip closure supports movement of the bolus to the pharynx. Emerging lateralization of the tongue is noted for the preparation for more textured foods. Semisolid foods are introduced to initiate the chewing process and to stimulate the sensory and tactile systems. The caregiver should introduce textures and tastes slowly. Mixed textures should be avoided. Infant chewing resembles more of a munching quality rather than the rotary chewing of adults. At this time the infant is able to sit without support. From 9 to 12 months of age, finger foods and chopped solids are introduced. The ability to clear food from their lips is apparent, and they demonstrate a more controlled ability to bite as they gain gross motor movements integrated with feeding. Infants acquire more limb mobility, trunk stability, and head, neck, and shoulder stability. These motor milestones assist in the preparation for independent feeding. The normal feeding progression from birth to 24 months is summarized in Table 3-1. Developmental motor and communication milestones associated with feeding in older children are discussed in Chapter 4 (see Table 4-2).

TAKE HOME NOTES

1. It is important to understand and recognize the normal development of the fetus in relation to swallowing. Knowledge of the cardiac, pulmonary,

---

TABLE 3-1

Feeding Progression (Birth to 24 Months)

Age	Food	Oral Preparations and Oral Events	Feeding Utensil
Birth to 6 months	Milk, liquids	Suckling and then sucking	Breast or bottle
4-6 months	Cereals, puree	Initially sucking, then tongue to palate movement; may eject food from spoon involuntarily; gags on new textures	Spoon
6-9 months	Chunky puree, mashed food, soft finger foods	Emerging munching pattern, desensitization of gag reflex; lateralization of food to gums; deciduous teeth erupting	Spoon; drinking from cup (at 9 months)
9-12 months	Chopped food and finger food	Licking food off lips; biting of objects; controlled, sustained bite on hard food (e.g., biscuit/cracker)	Spoon, cup; self-feeds with fingers; weaning from breast/bottle as cup drinking increases
15-24 months	Full diet with some exclusionary items (e.g., nuts)	Licks food from lips, increased maturity of adult rotary chew pattern, and jaw stability in cup drinking; independence in self-feeding; straw drinking	Spoon, cup, fork; self-feeding predominates

From Cichero J, Murdoch B: *Dysphagia: foundation, theory, and practice*, Chichester, UK, 2006, John Wiley.

gastrointestinal, and neurologic control systems underlying swallowing are crucial. The NICU team assists the infant to continue to develop outside the uterus in a healthy manner for minimal future deficits.

2. It is important to remember the difference between nonnutritive sucking, nutritive suckling, and sucking. Each plays a significant role for the premature infant, helping to reduce stress and provide comfort. Nutritive suckling and sucking may be difficult and induce stress.

3. Breast milk for infants is universally accepted as the best food. It is highly encouraged for premature and term infants for at least the first 6 months of life. It is important for the NICU team to encourage the mother to start pumping her breasts (either by feeding her infant or with a breast pump) on the day of delivery and to continue every 2 to 3 hours until her milk supply is established. Some mothers may require electric breast pumps to establish milk flow.

4. Infants follow a progression of abilities from birth through 12 months to tolerate a variety of fluids and textured foods. These milestones are general guidelines for medical staff and parents to assess whether the infant is developing normally.

5. Providing protection of the auditory, visual, motor, taste, and smell development of the preterm infant is imperative to avoid permanent damage. The NICU medical teams and parents of the infant work together to ensure that the infant's systems are protected so that normal development can occur.

References

1. Moore KL, Persaud TVN: *The developing human, clinically oriented embryology,* ed 7, Philadelphia, 2003, Saunders.

2. Hall JW 3rd: Development of the ear and hearing, *J Perinatol* 20(8 Pt 2):S12, 2000.

3. Lickliter R: Atypical perinatal sensory stimulation and early perceptual development: insights from developmental psychobiology, *J Perinatol* 20:S45, 2000.

4. Shaker C: The early feeding skills assessment for preterm infants, *Neonatal Netw* 24:7, 2005.

5. Morris SE, Klein MD: *Pre-feeding skills,* ed 2, Austin, TX, 2000, ProEd.

6. Wolf LS, Glass RP: *Feeding and swallowing disorders in infancy,* Tucson, 1992, Therapy Skill Builders.

7. Arvedson JC, Brodsky L: *Pediatric swallowing and feeding: assessment and management,* ed 2, Albany, NY, 2002, Singular.

8. Hill A: The effects of nonnutritive sucking and oral support on the feeding efficiency of preterm infants, *Newborn Infant Nurs Rev* 5:133, 2005.

9. Cichero J, Murdoch B: *Dysphagia foundation, theory, and practice,* Chichester, UK, 2006, John Wiley.

10. Selley WG, Ellis RE, Flack FC et al: Coordination of sucking, swallowing and breathing in the newborn: its relationship to infant feeding and normal development, *Br J Disord Commun* 25:311, 1990.

11. Newman J, Pitman T: *The ultimate breastfeeding book of answers,* Roseville, CA, 2000, Prima.

Chapter **4**

Disorders in Infants and Children

JO PUNTIL-SHELTMAN AND HELENE TAYLOR

OBJECTIVES

1. Discuss the typical feeding disorders seen in infant and pediatric outpatient populations.
2. Understand the integration of developmental levels and feeding skills in the infant and pediatric outpatient populations.
3. Be able to discuss the impact of medical and developmental disorders on the development of feeding skills in the infant and pediatric outpatient population.

INFANT BACKGROUND

Feeding specialists should become familiar with common maternal and prenatal sequelae that occur during and after delivery when working in the neonatal intensive care unit (NICU) or on a well-baby unit. Not all these disorders or diseases affect an infant's swallowing and feeding, although special attention should be directed toward the infant's respiratory and cardiac systems because the coordination and endurance needed to feed successfully may be compromised as a result of poor cardiopulmonary development. There is a difference between a sick infant whose condition may decompensate because of an illness and a premature infant in stable condition. Feeding specialists should think beyond their comfort zone and provide an effective, holistic, and developmental approach to any evaluation and treatment process (see Chapters 11 and 13).

MATERNAL CONDITIONS

Many risk factors can result in early delivery or contribute to the problems infants encounter after birth. Contributing factors may include a mother's poor diet, multiparity (more than three living children), maternal weight (<100 lb or >200 lb), maternal age (<16 years or >35 years), smoking habits, and substance abuse such as excessive alcohol consumption. Preexisting medical conditions that may affect the fetus include diabetes mellitus or gestational diabetes, cardiac disease, preeclampsia and eclampsia (see below), and use of corticosteroids; anemia can contribute to early delivery or postdelivery problems. Maternal infections such as **toxoplasmosis**, rubella, and **cytomegalovirus**; herpes and sexually transmitted diseases; and group B streptococcus also may be contributing factors. **Intrapartum** risk factors include preterm labor, medications used during pregnancy and delivery, **abruptio placentae**, **placenta previa**, **umbilical cord prolapse**, breech delivery, shoulder **dystocia**, cesarean delivery, obstetric analgesia, and obstetric anesthesia.

Diabetes and Gestational Diabetes

Improved methods of prenatal care, ultrasound evaluations, and the ability to measure fetal lung maturity have reduced the risk associated with diabetes mellitus during pregnancy and the incidence of adverse perinatal outcomes of infants of diabetic mothers (IDMs). Strict glucose control is critical during the entire pregnancy. The most common complication of IDMs is congenital anomalies. Approximately 6% to 10% of pregnancies complicated by diabetes involve a structural abnormality directly related to glycemic control.[1] The most common fetal structural defects associated with maternal diabetes malformations are cardiac malformations, neural tube defects, **renal agenesis**, and skeletal malformations.[1] If the mother has hyperglycemia, it may result in fetal hyperglycemia and hyperinsulinemia that may lead to fetal overgrowth. These babies appear large at birth even when born prematurely. They are initially quiet and lethargic, rather than alert and robust. Poor feeding can be a major problem in IDMs. These babies feed slowly and may tire easily when beginning the feeding process.

Preeclampsia

Preeclampsia (or **toxemia**) is hypertension with edema preceding pregnancy or before 20 weeks' gestation with proteinuria (protein in the urine). Eclampsia is preeclampsia with seizure activity. Depending on the severity, the best treatment may be to induce labor. It is essential for the mother to monitor her blood pressure and stabilize it as much as possible. Infants born to mothers with preeclampsia may show evidence of intrauterine growth restriction (IUGR) and are frequently delivered prematurely. Some medications used either before or during birth may negatively affect the fetus. Short-term effects include hypotonia and respiratory depression.

Drugs

Perinatal substance abuse can affect the pregnancy, fetus, and neonate. Drugs such as tobacco, alcohol, stimulants, cannabinoids, narcotics and opioids, sedatives or hypnotics, and inhalants all may affect aspects of pregnancy, delivery, and the newborn's transition from uterine life to adaptation to extrauterine life. Common effects on the pregnancy include poor nutrition, spontaneous abortion, placenta previa, abruptio placentae, and preterm labor. The effects on the fetus include intrauterine growth restriction, congenital malformations and deformities, and perinatal death. The long-term effects on the neonate can include mental retardation, sudden infant death syndrome, and developmental delays, including cognitive integration disorders.

PREMATURITY

A preterm neonate is born before completing 37 weeks of gestation. Twelve percent of all U.S. births are premature, and approximately 2% occur at less than 32 weeks' gestation. Multiple-gestation births frequently occur with prematurity in 57% of twins and 93% of triplets.[2] A fetus is viable at 23 weeks. Problems that occur with prematurity may be respiratory, cardiovascular, neurologic, hematologic, nutritional, gastrointestinal, metabolic, renal, temperature regulatory, immunologic and/or ophthalmologic.

Normal birth weight is between 2500 and 3999 g, low birth weight is less than 2500 g, very low birth weight is less than 1500 g, and extremely low birth weight is less than 100 g. In general, the lower the birth weight the more likely the infant will be predisposed to medical complications that interfere with feeding.

Necrotizing Enterocolitis

A disorder of inflammation, tenderness, and pneumatosis (air in the bowel wall) of the intestine, necrotizing enterocolitis (NEC) usually is caused by an infection or decreased blood supply to the intestine. The seriousness of NEC varies. It may involve only the innermost lining or the entire thickness of the bowel. It is imperative that the physician diagnose this process as quickly as possible so that proper management is initiated. Causes of NEC are not well defined. NEC is a heterogeneous disease resulting from complex interactions ranging from mucosal injury caused by a variety of factors, including ischemia, infection, and poor host-protective mechanism(s) in response to injury.[3] Infants are restricted from oral feedings and receive total parenteral nutrition. Clinical characteristics of the infant may include respiratory distress, apnea and/or bradycardia, lethargy, temperature instability, irritability, poor feeding, hypotension, and **acidosis**. The infant can have abdominal signs such as bloody stools, emesis, abdominal distention, and decreased or absent bowel sounds. Long-term sequelae may include strictures, short-bowel syndrome, malabsorption, chronic diarrhea, and feeding disorders.

Gastroesophageal Reflux Disease

Gastroesophageal reflux (GER) is the flow of the stomach's contents back into the esophagus. GER is extremely common in premature infants and can be common in term infants. Gastroesophageal reflux disease (GERD) is pathologic reflux or reflux with complications. **Emesis** can be associated with the introduction or advancement of feedings in the premature infant, although in the absence of emesis, chronic GER may go undetected. The episodes of emesis and GER are most commonly related to intestinal dysmotility as a result of prematurity. Some infants respond negatively to this phenomenon, and some have no adverse effects. It is generally agreed that there are important interactions between GERD and a variety of disorders of the respiratory system.

Respiratory problems caused by gastrointestinal reflux include reactive airway disease, aspiration pneumonia, laryngospasm, stridor, chronic cough, and apnea. Infants with daily GER or regurgitation from birth through 12 months of age are more likely to have feeding difficulties during their second year of life even when regurgitation has apparently resolved. The NICU team can approach GER in several ways. The infant may be positioned either prone or left-side down during and after feedings. A tailored feeding schedule or pharmaceutical intervention may be the best for the infant. Pharmaceutical options can include acid suppressants, **proton pump inhibitors**, or **prokinetics**. At times, thickening feedings has reduced the amount and frequency of GER. Additional diagnostic testing may include an upper gastrointestinal series in radiology or 24-hour pH probe testing. The validity and usefulness of pH probe testing remains controversial. An infant's response to the treatment of GERD is paramount to successful feedings in both the NICU and after discharge.

Tracheoesophageal Fistula and Atresia

Tracheoesophageal fistula (TEF) and esophageal atresia (EA) occur early in the first trimester when the esophagus and trachea form abnormally. Pathologically, the trachea communicates directly with the esophagus through a small hole, and the esophagus ends in a blind pouch. There are five variants of TEF. Clinical signs of TEF may include choking, coughing, and cyanosis with feeding. The risk of aspiration is very high with accompanying respiratory distress. Abdominal distention may be noted because air cannot escape the stomach. The infant may show excessive salivation if EA is noted. A history of **polyhydramnios** in the mother may indicate a problem with the fetus being able to swallow amniotic fluid and should prompt suspicion of TEF or EA. After diagnosis, the infant is not fed orally and will require surgical intervention. These infants have difficulty eating orally postoperatively.

RESPIRATORY DISORDERS

Infants with prolonged respiratory illness may have difficulty with oral feedings. They must learn to coordinate the suck-swallow-breathe sequence (see Chapter 3) and have the endurance to safely complete an entire feeding. Infants supported by mechanical ventilation for lengthy periods can develop oral aversions as well as grooving on the palate from the endotracheal tube needed to support respiration. Consistent developmental care is encouraged during intubation and ventilation. Infants with tracheotomies and ventilation may be able to eat orally after a detailed evaluation of their swallowing.

Respiratory Distress Syndrome

Respiratory distress syndrome (RDS, also known as **hyaline membrane disease**) is the process of inadequate **surfactant** and a disease of prematurity. The incidence of RDS increases with decreasing gestational age. The pathophysiology of RDS includes surfactant deficiency, diffuse alveolar **atelectasis**, cell injury, and edema. Surfactant production depends on the maturity of the lung. Lack of surfactant causes a decrease in lung compliance because of collapse of the alveolar sacs. The initial signs of RDS appear shortly after birth. The infant will be **tachypneic** with worsening intercostal and sternal retractions, evidence of **paradoxic breathing**, **duskiness**, nasal flaring, apnea, and possible audible grunting. The key to management of these conditions is to prevent **hypoxemia** and acidosis, to stabilize fluid management and edema, reduce metabolic demands, and reduce lung injury. Current methods of treatment may include continuous positive airway pressure (CPAP) and positive end-expiratory pressure (PEEP) delivered mechanically. Surfactant replacement therapy, controlled delivery of oxygen, and varied methods of mechanical ventilation including high-frequency ventilation (HFV) are appropriate treatment interventions. The aim of mechanical ventilation is to reduce the risk of lung collapse, maintain alveolar inflation, and prevent or reduce lung injury. As the infant shows signs of improvement, the process of weaning from the ventilator occurs. A long-term complication from RDS is bronchopulmonary dysplasia. Infants with RDS are at risk for oral and pharyngeal abnormalities, including change in sensation from long-term devices such as orogastric tubes, nasogastric tubes, nasal cannulae, and endotracheal tubes. It is vital that they receive compassionate touch on the face and intraorally before oral feedings. A developmental approach before oral feedings will foster positive outcomes (see Chapter 13).

Transient Tachypnea of the Newborn

The cause of transient tachypnea of the newborn (TTN) is unknown but is most likely related to delayed clearance of the fetal lung fluid during the birth process. Most of the fluid is eliminated through the thoracic squeeze during the birth process. Other remaining fluid is drained through the lymphatic system. The fluid causes increased airway resistance and limited lung compliance. Infants with TTN breathe rapidly, usually at a rate greater than 80 breaths/min. They may show moderate respiratory distress and **cyanosis**, subcostal retractions, nasal flaring, and expiratory grunting. Management is supported by oxygen, although some infants need CPAP. Infants receiving CPAP are not fed orally. Infants receiving high respiratory support rates are often not fed orally or are fed with caution. TTN is usually temporary (24 to 72 hours) with a good prognosis.

Apnea

Apnea is the cessation of airflow. It is considered pathologic if it lasts for more than 20 seconds or is accompanied by bradycardia (heart rate <100 beats/min). Premature infants frequently have periodic respirations with apneic periods of 5 to 10 seconds followed by 5 to 10 seconds of rapid breathing. These apneic periods are abnormal if they last for more than 15 seconds and are accompanied by cyanosis, pallor, hypotonia, or bradycardia. As many as 25% of all premature infants who weigh less than 1800 g (about 34 weeks' gestational age) have at least one apneic episode. Usually, all infants at less than 28 weeks' gestational age also have apnea.[4] Apnea can be central nervous system mediated or caused by an obstruction. Mixed apnea, which is a combination of both causes, can also occur and usually starts with an obstruction that precipitates central apnea. One cause of apnea in the premature infant is immature **chemocontrol** of the respiratory drive. Apnea also can be caused by infections, metabolic disorder, impaired oxygenation, maternal drugs, intracranial lesions, poor temperature regulation, and GERD. Treatment of apnea includes continuous monitoring with gentle stimulation. Apnea of prematurity responds well to administration of theophylline and caffeine. These drugs stimulate the central nervous system to increase the infant's response to carbon dioxide levels. As the infant's respiratory control matures, the apneic periods decrease and usually disappear by weeks 34 to 35, although some infants experience apnea beyond this period.

Bronchopulmonary Dysplasia

Bronchopulmonary dysplasia (BPD) may develop in premature infants with severe respiratory failure in the first weeks of life. BPD results from an abnormal development of lung tissue. Immaturity, malnutrition, oxygen toxicity, and mechanical ventilation may contribute to BPD, which is characterized by inflammation and scarring in the lungs. *Broncho* refers to the airways or the bronchial tubes through which the oxygen is transported to the lungs. *Pulmonary* refers to the alveoli where oxygen and carbon dioxide are exchanged. *Dysplasia* means abnormal changes in the structure or organization of a group of cells. The cell changes in BPD take place in the smaller airways and lung alveoli, making breathing difficult and causing problems with lung function. Prolonged **hyperoxia** begins a sequence of lung injury that can lead to inflammation, diffuse alveolar damage, and pulmonary dysfunction. Infants with severe BPD may depend on oxygen or mechanical ventilation for months and may have symptoms of airway obstruction for years. Long-term consequences consist of pulmonary dysfunction in adolescents and young adults and potentially impaired growth and cognitive function.[5] The clinical presentation usually includes tachypnea and **rales** on auscultation. Infants with BPD have a difficult time learning to coordinate the timing of the suck-swallow-breathe sequence and often tire easily, especially when oral feedings are first introduced. With initial feeding of infants with BPD, they present with many sucks, then a swallow, and pauses for breathing. Often there is little rhythm to their feeding attempts.

Persistent Pulmonary Hypertension in the Newborn

The most common cause of persistent pulmonary hypertension of the newborn (PPHN) is a disruption of the fetal to neonatal circulatory transition and usually is caused by increased pulmonary vascular resistance (PVR). This condition can exacerbate into further **left-to-right shunting**, hypoxemia, and metabolic and respiratory acidosis. The infant in utero does not use the lungs as gas exchange organs. During fetal life pulmonary blood flow is low; less than 10% of the combined cardiac output is directed to the lungs. In fetal life numerous factors, including hypoxia, can maintain high PVR. After birth, PVR decreases and pulmonary blood flow increases dramatically as the lungs assume the function of gas exchange. The combination of rhythmic ventilation of the lung and increased alveolar oxygen tension stimulates these changes. In some newborns, the normal decrease in pulmonary vascular tone does not occur, and the result is PPHN. Treatment often includes mechanical ventilation. Because pain and anxiety may exacerbate the PPHN, the infant may need sedation and paralysis. Survivors of PPHN are at risk for possible chronic pulmonary disease, NEC, neurodevelopmental disabilities, intracranial hemorrhage or infarction, and hearing loss.

NEUROLOGIC DISORDERS

The human brain is extremely fragile and is constantly developing from the time of conception. If this process in interrupted, difficulties can develop, ranging from simple to significant disorders. Table 4-1

TABLE 4-1

Major Events in Human Brain Development and Peak Times of Occurrence

Major Developmental Event	Peak Time of Occurrence
Primary neutralization	3-4 weeks of gestation
Prosencephalic development	2-3 months of gestation
Neuronal proliferation	3-4 months of gestation
Neuronal migration	3-5 months of gestation
Organization	5 months of gestation to years after birth
Myelination	Birth to years after birth

From Volpe JJ: *Neurology of the newborn,* ed 4, Philadelphia, 2001, WB Saunders.

summarizes the major events in human brain development and the peak times of occurrence.

The following neurologic disorders are seen most frequently in the NICU.

Microcephaly

If the infant has a small brain or the occipitofrontal circumference (OFC) is more than 2 standard deviations below the mean for age and gender, he or she is considered microcephalic.[6] The risk factors for microcephaly include viral infection, metabolic conditions, medication or substance abuse, genetic conditions, and malnutrition. The fetal risk factors may be a prenatal or perinatal insult such as inflammation, hypoxia, and birth trauma. Microcephaly can be a **neuronal proliferation defect** that occurs between the third and fourth months of gestational age.

Hydrocephalus

Hydrocephalus results when there is an excess of cerebrospinal fluid (CSF) in the ventricles of the brain from a decrease in reabsorption or overproduction.[7] The clinical presentation is a large head with widened sutures. The infant may exhibit full and tense **fontanelles**, increasing OFC, **setting sun eyes**, vomiting, lethargy, and irritability. If an infant has hydrocephalus, a neurosurgical consult is warranted, and placement of a **ventriculoperitoneal shunt** for cerebral decompression may be considered. Deficits to the infant can be sensorimotor, cognitive, or both.

Intracranial Hemorrhage

Intracranial hemorrhages can be classified as subdural, subarachnoid, intracerebellar, periventricular, and intraventricular. Infants with any of these insults to the brain can demonstrate sudden deterioration, oxygen desaturation, bradycardia, metabolic acidosis, shock, hypotonia, hyperglycemia, seizure activity, recurrent apnea, respiratory distress, decreased level of consciousness, and asymmetry of motor function. Outcomes depend on the severity of hemorrhage. Frequent medical and developmental evaluations are warranted.

Seizures

Seizures are a symptom of neurologic dysfunction, not a disease. Seizures can be caused by metabolic conditions, infections, intracranial hemorrhage, intrapartum trauma, **kernicterus**, hypoxemia, intracerebral meningitis, withdrawal from drugs, or familial inheritance or may be **idiopathic**. The clinical presentation in newborns is often unique and variable. Symptoms include eye blinking or fluttering, deviation of the eyes, **pedaling** and other tonic-clonic movements, nonnutritive sucking, smacking of the lips, drooling, and periods of oxygen desaturation.

Periventricular Leukomalacia

Periventricular leukomalacia (PVL) is the result of ischemic or necrotic periventricular white matter changes. PVL may present as **multicystic encephalomalacia** with or without secondary hemorrhage.[8] PVL can be secondary to systemic hypotension severe enough to impair cerebral blood flow, a focal infarction or ischemia, and episodes of apnea and bradycardia. The clinical presentation may demonstrate frequent tremors or startles, irritability, and hypertonicity with or without an abnormal **Moro reflex**. The long-term outcomes can include spastic dysplegia, visual impairments, upper arm **paresthesias**, impaired intellectual development, and lower limb weakness. Outcome is based on the location and extent of the injury.

Birth Injuries

Some birth injuries may result in feeding disorders. Specific injuries can include **cephalohematoma**, **subgaleal hemorrhage,** skull fractures, **brachial nerve plexus** injuries, phrenic nerve paralysis, clavicle and humerus fractures, and traumatic facial nerve palsy.

CARDIOVASCULAR DISORDERS

Advances in fetal echocardiography have resulted in the prenatal diagnosis of many congenital heart defects, allowing parents time to make decisions about treatment before birth.[9] Although significant advancements have been made in the correction of cardiac disorders, there is now evidence of neurodevelopmental complications such as seizures and sen-sorimotor dysfunction after neonatal heart surgery.[10] Limperopoulos et al.[11] studied infants who underwent their first cardiac surgery before 12 months and surgery after 12 to 18 months. They found that 37% had moderate disability and another 6% showed severe disability. The disabilities were identified as motor and cognitive impairments, including 41% with neurologic abnormalities, 42% with gross and fine motor deficiencies, and 35% with behavioral problems.

Fetal cardiac development occurs rapidly from day 18 to 12 weeks after conception. This process includes development of the cardiac tube, **cardiac septation**, great vessel development, and circulatory development. Cardiac anomalies can include **patent ductus arteriosus**, ventricular septal defect, atrial septal defect (ASD), atrioventricular canal, **tetralogy of Fallot**, aortic stenosis, pulmonary stenosis, coarticulation of the aorta, tricuspid atresia, and **truncus arteriosus**. Management of these disorders includes hemodynamic and respiratory stabilization, cardiac catheterization, balloon dilatation, and extensive surgical repairs. Because of the serious nature of some of these defects and the surgical procedures required, **palliative** care may be necessary for the patient and family.

CONGENITAL ANOMALIES

Multiple congenital anomalies and syndromes result from chromosomal, environmental, multifactorial, or idiopathic causes. Some of the more common disorders include neural tube defects, structural abnormalities, and metabolic disorders. Some chromosomal anomalies include trisomy 21 (Down syndrome), trisomy 18 (Edwards syndrome), and trisomy 13 (Patau syndrome) defects. Multiple characteristics help define or accompany certain syndromes. Some of these characteristics may include abnormal facial features and musculoskeletal, cardiac, renal, gastrointestinal, and genital abnormalities. These syndromes are often accompanied by deficits in cognitive and motor impairments that may affect feeding. Numerous syndromes can affect the neurodevelopmental processes and common structural disorders may affect the head and neck. Common facial and head defects may include cleft lip and cleft palate and **amniotic band syndrome**.

Cleft Lip and Cleft Palate

A *cleft lip* results from failure of mesenchymal masses in the medial nasal and maxillary prominences to join.[12] The overall incidence of all types of clefts is approximately 1 in 700 live births. More boys than girls are affected, but more girls than boys have a cleft palate only. Infants can have a cleft of the lip alone, palate alone, or a combination of both, either unilateral or bilateral. Good outcome is noted with a variety of surgical corrections. These infants usually are fed with special bottles and nipples. They can breastfeed for short periods to continue the bonding process, although a bottle is usually necessary for appropriate hydration and nutrition (see Chapter 13).

The child with a unilateral or bilateral cleft lip and palate often presents a feeding challenge. However, when the cleft lip or palate is not part of another syndrome (see below), the management of the child is relatively simple. Babies with only a cleft lip usually are able to breastfeed or bottle feed. They require no further intervention for this difficulty. Children with cleft palate, however, almost always have difficulty achieving and maintaining an adequate suckling pattern; this is due to limited velar mechanics, which are needed for suction. Babies sometimes appear to be

suckling, and mothers often have been encouraged to breastfeed. These babies lose weight quickly and are at risk for dehydration. Babies with cleft palate rarely succeed at breastfeeding.[13]

Children with cleft lip and palate may have associated difficulties that affect feeding. Associated concerns may include cardiac anomalies such as in **DiGeorge** or **velocardiofacial syndrome**, developmental delay as in **Kabuki syndrome,** facial nerve palsy or paralysis (Möbius syndrome), hemifacial microsomia, airway maintenance concerns (as in **Pierre Robin sequence**), and sensory system dysfunction such as **CHARGE association**. Other oral and facial structural anomalies also may affect normal feeding, including **Beckwith-Wiedemann syndrome**, **Goldenhar's syndrome**, **Apert's syndrome**, **Treacher Collins syndrome**, and other syndromes that may affect muscle tone and movement patterns, such as **Freeman-Sheldon syndrome** and Down syndrome. Children who have had surgical procedures beyond closing of the cleft palate occasionally demonstrate feeding problems.[14] Children with syndromes that affect the airway, such as Pierre Robin sequence, may need a **tongue-lip adhesion**, mandibular advancement, or tracheostomy to address upper airway obstruction.

CLINICAL CORNER 4-1

A toddler was referred for a clinical feeding evaluation at age 20 months. His medical history includes maternal complications with prenatal alcohol and drug exposure and birth at 32 weeks' gestation. He is currently in the care of other family members who intend to adopt him. He stayed in the NICU for several months after birth. Current medical diagnoses include short-gut syndrome as a result of necrosis of the bowel. He has had numerous surgeries and visits to a variety of medical providers. His primary nutrition is by gastrostomy tube and total parenteral nutrition.

CRITICAL THINKING:

1. What are the medical and dietary restrictions that may be associated with short-gut syndrome?
2. What may be some of the developmental challenges associated with a child who was exposed to drugs during pregnancy?
3. What may be some of the developmental challenges associated with a child who was born at a gestational age of 32 weeks?
4. What may be some of the developmental challenges associated with a child who has experienced frequent hospitalizations?
5. Why is this information important in the development of the evaluation and therapy plan?

PEDIATRIC FEEDING DISORDERS

A pediatric feeding disorder is the inability of a child to consume sufficient calories for optimal growth and development. Sometimes, although not always, this inability is associated with swallowing dysfunction. The number of children identified with feeding and swallowing disorders has increased considerably over the past 20 years. Initially, many of the problems were attributed to the child's behavior or inappropriate parental feeding skills. It is now known that the origin of most childhood feeding disorders is the result of related medically based conditions, congenital anomalies, developmental delays, sensory processing disorders, and environmental factors.[15] The burden of care was historically on individual physicians; however, this has now moved to multidisciplinary care, and optimally the pediatric interdisciplinary feeding team.[16,17] The inclusion of the family in care planning has shown to considerably decrease the stress surrounding the child's feeding disorder.[18] The need for focused and coordinated treatment plans, which include family and caregiver education, has increased the content found in university curricula and available resources. There no longer appears to be a "general" population of children with feeding disorders. Twenty-five percent of all children are reported to present with feeding disorders, with that number increasing to 80% in the population of developmentally delayed children.[19] Feeding disorders are known to be associated with neurologic dysfunction, brain injury, prematurity, cardiac anomalies, liver function problems, gastrointestinal disorders, pulmonary disorders, metabolic disorders, autism, and a variety of other developmental syndromes discussed in the previous sections.[20] Feeding problems in the typically developing population include food refusal, disruptive mealtime behaviors, rigidity in the range of preferred foods, suboptimal growth, and failure to meet self-feeding milestones associated with the child's developmental level.[21] There has been an attempt to classify feeding disorders into organic problems and behavioral feeding problems. Beyond infancy, it becomes increasingly difficult to assign children with feeding problems to these specific categories. Toomey et al.[22] noted that "children with physical difficulties often develop 'behavioral' problems after their attempts to eat don't go well, and children with 'behavioral' eating difficulties develop physical disorders after having poor nutrition for a period of time." Signs and symptoms that may signal eating and feeding difficulty are summarized in Box 4-1.

BOX 4-1	**Signs of Problematic Eating**

- Poor weight gain
- Coughing, choking, or gagging during meals
- Problems with vomiting
- History of a traumatic choking incident
- History of eating and breathing coordination problems, with ongoing respiratory issues
- Inability to make the transition to baby food purees by 10 months
- Inability to accept table food solids by 12 months
- Inability to make the transition from breast to bottle to cup by 16 months
- Has not been weaned from baby foods by 16 months
- Aversion or avoidance of all foods of specific texture or food groups
- Food range of fewer than 20 foods, especially if foods are being dropped from the child's repertoire with no foods replacing those lost
- Crying or arching by the infant at most meals
- Family fighting about food and feeding
- Repeated parental reports that the child is difficult for everyone to feed
- Parental history of an eating disorder, with a child not meeting weight goals

TYPICAL DEVELOPMENT: INFANT TO CHILD

Understanding the typical developmental patterns of infants and children is essential in determining the presence or absence of any type of disorder. Regarding feeding, infants and toddlers must achieve specific milestones before the introduction of solids and the ability to progress to eating a higher food texture. Table 4-2 presents a summary of the milestones for typically developing children from birth to 2 years of age, including the relations among feeding skills, motor skills, respiration, and communication. The feeding specialist must have a clear understanding of the anatomic features of the mouth and pharynx as components of typical development. In the examination of the child and feeding skills, the feeding specialist examines the symmetry of the head and face, the structural integrity of the head and oral-facial structures, and the proportionality of the oral and facial structures. A difference in a single feature may or may not affect feeding. For example, a typically developing child with a high arch to the hard palate who has otherwise typical facial and oral characteristics likely will not exhibit a feeding problem. A child

with this same arch to the hard palate with very low muscle tone—and consequent limited lingual range of motion—may exhibit difficulty with bolus formation and propulsion, including packing of foods into the palatal arch.

Oral-facial changes occur as a process of development in all children, regardless of the presence or absence of a disorder. These changes occur at approximately 4 to 6 months of age. The lips are in a less everted position than in infancy; this allows the child to bring solid food into the mouth more easily. The tongue takes a lower position in the mouth and no longer takes up most of the oral space, allowing for management of formed solid foods. The uvula and the epiglottis are no longer in close proximity, and the body is now able to demonstrate more complete airway protection during eating and drinking. Similarly, the larynx has moved to a lower position in the airway. These changes are important, especially in children with developmental disorders such as cerebral palsy who initially demonstrate safe swallowing but may demonstrate more difficulty eating or signs and symptoms of dysfunctional swallowing as these developmental changes occur.

Text continued on page 65.

TABLE 4-2

Guidelines for Normal Feeding Development: Birth to 2 Years

Age	Oral Motor/Feeding Skills	Diet Recommendations	Self-Feeding	Motor Skills	Respiration	Communication Skills
Birth	Suckling pattern as tongue moves forward and backward (extension/retraction). Tongue moves with mandible. Jaw and tongue move within a narrow base. Mouth moves in a more closed position. Cheeks and lips are not active in sucking. Sucking pads within cheeks develop the last month before birth and provide stability for efficient sucking pattern of the newborn. Strong suckling response, rooting response, automatic phasic bite.	Breast milk or formula is the primary source of nutrition. Bottle introduction can begin at 3 weeks for breastfed infants.	Newborn moves mouth to attain hand. These activities assist the baby in organizing suck-swallow-breathe pattern.	**Gross motor:** Physiologic flexion provides stability for posture and random movements of arms and legs. Total body movements into flexion and extension (movements lack grading). Lack midline object orientation. **Fine motor:** Maintains object placed in hand with tight finger flexors. Grasp reflex with pressure into palm.	Rapid breathing. Belly breathing pattern. Upper respiratory structure is set up to protect the newborn during feeding. Obligatory nose breathers. (Development of neck extension as the baby matures increases breathing through the mouth.)	Sound production with body movements.
1 month	Suckling pattern predominates with sucking pattern emerging. Sequence 2 sucks before breath/swallow. Lacks good seal on nipple due to inactivity of lips and decreased flexion in the body. Rooting response and phasic bite continue.			**Gross motor:** Flexion decreasing. Move extremities in a wide arc. **Fine motor:** Grasp reflex present, reflexive scratching at objects/hands.	Sustained rhythmic belly breathing at rest and during quiet breathing. Crying in short duration due to poor respiratory control. Arrhythmic breathing with movements or when upset.	Listens to voices, cooing; expresses self with face, body tone, and increasing vocalizations.

Age					
2 months	Suckling pattern predominates with wide jaw movements, protrusion and retraction of tongue. Drooling increases with wide tongue and jaw movements.		**Gross motor:** Period of hypotonia due to decreasing physiologic flexion, which decreases structural stability. Raises head to 45 degrees in prone position. Holds head upright momentarily when trunk is supported. **Fine motor:** More purposeful movements of arms. Hands are more open with increased random movements.	Belly breathing.	Varied pitch with cooing. Smiles, squeals, coos when spoken to. Laughs, imitates several tones, quiets to music, cries if play is disrupted.
3 months	Long sequence of suck-swallow (20 or more). More closed position of the mouth. Improved organization of oral activity. Emerging sucking intermittently. Upper lip beginning to have discrete movement by itself. No lateral movement of tongue. Jaw stability is increasing. Rooting response and automatic phasic bite are diminishing. Strong gag continues.	Hand to mouth. Objects to mouth. May move hand to bottle as midline hand movement develops.	**Gross motor:** Functional head control in all positions. Postures of body are more symmetric. Sits upright for brief periods with upper trunk support. Head to 90 degrees in prone with extension in back and hips. **Fine motor:** Purposeful reach into a wider range, reaching with both hands but may not secure objects. Voluntary grasp of objects brought close to hands.	Deeper breaths with increased mobility in the ribs.	Increased variety of sounds. Cry is less nasal. Volume changes with movements. Strong cry before meals.

Continued

TABLE 4-2

Guidelines for Normal Feeding Development: Birth to 2 Years—cont'd

Age	Oral Motor/Feeding Skills	Diet Recommendations	Self-Feeding	Motor Skills	Respiration	Communication Skills
4 months	Small up-and-down jaw movements. Flattening and cupping of the tongue. Center of lips more active. Suckling predominates but true suck emerging with active jaw/cheek assistance. Sucking strength increases as tongue grasps nipple and up-and-down movement of tongue occurs, creating negative pressure. Tongue has more variability in movement and is able to flatten and cup. Easy coordination of suck-swallow-breathe sequence. Reduction of automatic phasic bite, gag continues, rooting absent except if breastfeeding.	Breast milk/formula are the primary source of nutrition. May begin iron-fortified cereal.	Explores objects by mouthing, which helps the gag move back. May begin spoon feedings. Child will do better with spoon feeding if fully supported in a semiupright position, such as a car seat or bouncy seat with additional support.	**Gross motor:** Period of symmetry. Prone play assists with bringing ribs down, elongating diaphragm, and increasing space between ribs. Rolls to side. Props on forearms in prone. Sits upright for longer periods with lower trunk support.	Thoracic expansion beginning as abdomen becomes more active and holds rib cage. Respiration during sleep is slow and rhythmic and shallower when awake.	Vocalizes in response to sound. Baby plays with sounds by changing breath, moving, or playing.

5 months	True suck on bottle. Attempts to disassociate or separate movements of tongue from jaw. Jaw becomes more stable with increased strength/stability of neck muscles. Tongue flattens and spreads as jaw opens and closes. Active lip movements. Child sucks and suckles food from spoon. Munching pattern. Unable to transfer food from center to sides.	Offer baby rice or oatmeal once a day.	Child attempts to assist with holding the bottle but may continue to feed better if bottle is held by caregiver.	**Gross motor:** Rolls prone to supine. **Fine motor:** Reach in prone on elbows. Visually directed reach. Unilateral reach emerging.	No longer an obligatory nose breather as oral structure changes. Decreased rate of breathing due to increased inhalation.	Quantity and variety of sounds increase. Pitch and rhythm of cry increase, allowing baby more expression.
6 months	Smaller jaw range. Rolling and shifting of tongue from side to side. Lower lip active. Active lip pressure on the spoon or cup. Upper lip closure around spoon. Suckle-suck pattern from cup with wide jaw movements. Liquid is lost during cup drinking. Child may choke or sputter with liquids from the cup because of inability to control the flow or speed of liquid. Vertical jaw movements with biting. Munching pattern with chewing. Rooting and automatic plasic bite are not present. Gag may occur with presentation of new tastes and textures through 10 months of age.	Spoon feeding usually more successful at this age, especially with a child who is able to sit independently for brief periods. Provide spoon foods (cereal mixed with plain fruit or plain vegetable twice daily).	Child able to hold his or her own bottle and cup. Does better with cup drinking if cup is held by an adult. Requires supportive position in high chair for efficient oral motor patterns with spoon feeding and cup drinking.	**Gross motor:** Head control is complete. Rolls supine to prone with rotation. Improved variety and complexity of movement. Sitting independently. Hands used intermittently for support in sitting. In prone, can sit and reach with control. **Fine motor:** Continues to reach primarily with both hands. Transfers objects from hand to hand. Beginning to use thumb to grasp.	Coordinates breathing with movements. Belly breathing with greater expansion and inhalation. Thoracic and abdominal breathing for more active abdominals.	Increased babbling and repetition of sounds. Produces vowel sounds and several consonant sounds (*d, b, l, m, n, sh, f*). Becomes excited during sound play. Expresses protest. Recognizes familiar objects.

Continued

TABLE 4-2

Guidelines for Normal Feeding Development: Birth to 2 Years—cont'd

Age	Oral Motor/Feeding Skills	Diet Recommendations	Self-Feeding	Motor Skills	Respiration	Communication Skills
7-9 months	Gag position now more similar to an adult. Bites toys, nipples, cup, spoon. Rolls tongue to both sides. Can take 2-3 swallows from cup. Increased awareness of jaw pressure with biting. Uses a munching pattern with chewing.	Eat spoon foods 3× per day. A cup of formula or breast milk should be provided at each meal. Offer thicker baby food cereals and stage 2 foods. Begin offering harder foods that can be held by the child to explore them in the mouth (e.g., zwiebac crackers, teething biscuits, raw large carrot sticks, strips of bagel). **8 months:** Offer soft mashed table foods and table food smooth purees of one texture. At 8-9 months a baby should be eating 4× per day. **9 months:** Meltable solids (e.g., town crackers, graham crackers) that can be held while a child explores the item in the mouth.	They can independently bottle feed at this age. They require support of surface to release so this makes placement of small objects into mouth difficult at this age. Upper lip is more active in spoon feeding. Improved coordination with cup drinking. Straw drinking has been observed at this age but is not typical.	**Gross motor:** Transition between sitting quadruped. Moves from sitting to prone. Sits on floor without arm support and can reach out farther in sitting to get toys and return to sitting. Rocks forward and back in quadruped or crawling position. Belly crawls in prone. **Fine motor:** Reaches out into the environment in sitting due to increased stability in this position.	Belly breathing with greater expansion and less rib flaring.	Babbling with inflections, pitch, and intonation. May begin having sounds for what he or she wants. Combining sounds. **8 months:** Can use sequences of a syllable strung together. Imitates mouth and jaw movements, coughs, tongue clicks, hisses. Express emotions. Begins to respond to words (no-no, bye). Will play games such as patty cake.

Continued

Age					Respiratory	Speech
10-11 months	More jaw control with mouthing and biting. Increased use of tongue tip elevation. Transfers food from center to side and side to center for chewing. May stick tongue under cup to gain stability. Active lip and cheek control with cup drinking. Lip closure over spoon. Biting is more controlled. Increased rotary control in chewing.	Meals 4× per day to be included along with bottles being offered every 3 hours during the day. Cup with formula or breast milk, soft mashed table food, and some type of finger food should be provided at each meal. Soft cubed foods can also be offered at this time. This includes foods like baby food fruits and vegetables, bananas, avocado, overcooked squash. May begin with smooth dairy products such as yogurt or mashed cottage cheese. **11 months:** May introduce soft foods such as fruit breads, fruit bars, muffins, soft small pasta, cubed lunch meat, thin deli meats in small rectangles.	Baby now has improved grasp patterns for picking up smaller objects and release is easier, so small finger foods can be introduced.	**Gross motor:** Dynamic sitting with weight shifts allowing for improved balance in sitting positions. Pulling to stand with improved leg or lower extremity control. Standing with less support. Cruising furniture. **Fine motor:** Grasps object with thumb and first two fingers. Pincer grasp with small objects. Uses mouth to reposition objects.	Abdominal thoracic breathing pattern developing.	Increased accuracy with imitation of inflection patterns. Uses 1-2 words. Begins to indicate wants by vocalizing. Understands whole-phrase grammatical pattern ("give it to daddy," "come to mama"). Demonstrates intense attention and response to speech over prolonged periods.
12 months	Jaw pressure controlled on soft foods. Both lips close around spoon. Stabilized cup by biting or by placing tongue under cup. Takes 4-5 swallows from cup. Transfers foods from center of mouth to both sides. Sufficient oral control to allow liquid needs to be attained primarily from cup. Lip closure over cup is complete.	Soft table foods. Provide a protein, starch, and fruit or vegetable at each meal and snack (a child this age should be sitting down for meals and snacks 5-6 times per day). One of these items should be some type of finger food. Add whole milk as primary source of nutrition.	Improved control with spoon but most of spoon feeding is still completed by caregiver. Provide the child with a spoon to hold to allow them a sense of independence with meals.	**Gross motor:** May take independent steps (norm for independent walking in the United States is 14-16 months). Standing alone. Feeding still most successful with a child of this age seated in high chair. **Fine motor:** Neat pincer (tip of finger and thumb). Bilateral coordination. Manipulates and explores objects.	Increased thoracic breathing. No longer asynchronous breathing even under stress.	Inflection and rhythm of vocalizations. More and more attempts to imitate words.

TABLE 4-2

Guidelines for Normal Feeding Development: Birth to 2 Years—cont'd

Age	Oral Motor/Feeding Skills	Diet Recommendations	Self-Feeding	Motor Skills	Respiration	Communication Skills
12-18 months	Increased awareness of mouth with tongue play. Licks lower lip and cleans lower lip by 15 months. Controlled bite on harder items developing at 16 months.	Child continues to receive the majority of calories and nutrition from whole milk through 24 months. Continue to provide a variety of soft table foods of protein, starch, and fruit or vegetables. Minimal to no juice is needed in a child's diet unless encouraged by the pediatrician. **16-18 months:** Harder foods can be provided such as Cheerios, pretzel sticks, saltine crackers, cookies, cereals.	Finger feeds many or most foods. Holds cup and drinks with some spilling. Uses spoon for scooping with some spilling by 18 months.	**Gross motor:** Walks well. Begins to pull items and walk backward. Good control with starting and stopping. Creeps up and backwards down stairs. Squats to play to pick up objects. Gets up to stand from the middle of the floor. **Fine motor:** Continues to improve quality and control of hand movements to enable them to interact more successfully with increased variety of toys. Improved grasp and release to allow the infant to dump and place objects into containers.	Fairly mature with increased endurance and thoracic expansion.	Expressive vocabulary expanding. Repeats new words. By 18 months is able to name familiar objects on request. Attempts to sing. Uses voice along with pointing. Begins to verbalize needs and desires. Initiates 2-word phrases. Makes a variety of sounds while babbling but often substitutes these sounds in words.
24 months	Controlled sustained bite on either side of mouth. Transfers food efficiently from side to side. Internal stabilization without biting cup.		Able to spoon-feed self with some mess. May begin using a fork (which is sometimes easier with tines pointed down).	Walking, running jumping. Lots of practicing of previously learned motor skills.		Expressive vocabulary of 50-300 words. Combining simple 2-word sentences. Uses and understands self-use of "no." Tries to use most sounds but will omit final sounds and some medial sounds. Uses some verbs. Retrieves object from another room when asked.

MEDICAL IMPACT ON FEEDING

The first section of this chapter discussed management of premature children in the NICU. However, the outpatient feeding specialist often sees many infants and young children who were born prematurely. Prematurity is defined as birth before 37 weeks' gestation. Infants who are born prematurely are at risk for significant medical conditions that may affect their feeding through the first year of their development or longer.

Premature infants have immature gastrointestinal systems (see Chapter 3). They do not have the same ability to digest breast milk and formula. They often receive formulas that are specifically designed for the less-mature digestive system. Breast milk is most easily tolerated, and mothers are encouraged to pump their breasts until their babies are able to breastfeed. Extreme prematurity can result in NEC, causing a

---

CLINICAL CORNER 4-2

A 12-month-old boy was referred for a clinical feeding evaluation. His medical history includes normal development, including feeding, through 11 months of age. He developed a high fever that led to seizures. These seizures were accompanied by vomiting and difficulty breathing. He was transferred to a medical facility by helicopter while in status epilepticus. The seizures were controllable by medication. He remained in the hospital for 17 days and returned home with a nasogastric feeding tube and developmental skills that had decreased to approximately a 4-month level. The nasogastric tube is causing vomiting and must be replaced several times per week. He has no allergies. He is taking several medications to address the seizures and altered muscle tone. Of significance, this family recently lost another child, age 4 years, to significant medical complications associated with extreme prematurity.

CRITICAL THINKING:

1. What motor and feeding skills may this child have developed before the onset of his seizures?
2. Given his described current level of motor functioning, what feeding skills may be expected?
3. How may you obtain information on this child's ideal weight and expected nutritional needs?
4. Which professionals may be involved in this child's care? What are their roles regarding care for this child?

---

section of the small intestine to die. NEC is the most common gastrointestinal gut syndrome, and long-term digestive problems will be present. Because their gastrointestinal systems are immature, infants who are born prematurely are also at higher risk for GER and gastric motility disorders. These also can be related to immature neurologic systems and related muscle tone disorders.

As previously discussed, infants who are born prematurely may have cardiac anomalies, cardiac function regulation (**tachycardia** and **bradycardia**) problems, respiratory problems, problems with metabolic regulation, immature or altered oral structures caused by extended periods of ventilation, and dysfunctional skills for sucking and swallowing. Each of these difficulties needs to be addressed with a view toward the individual component of the feeding disorder and in coordination with other aspects of the child's functional abilities.

Other problems noted in premature infants include difficulty coordinating the suckling process. Most studies show that success with nipple feeding begins to occur at 34 weeks' gestation; this occurs in coordination with increases in neurologic maturity. A "healthy" premature baby may be discharged from the NICU to home but still have trouble initiating and maintaining strong suckling patterns. Structured feeding intervention for the baby and education for the family will be of benefit until the infant is able to demonstrate more efficient feeding. When assessing and treating the infant or toddler who was born prematurely, it is important to consider the *corrected* age rather than the *chronologic* age until two chronologic years of life. For example, a baby who is at 12 months chronologic age and was born at 24 weeks' gestation is (in general) evaluated as a child who is 8 months of age. This is important because of the significant difference in the feeding skills of an 8-month-old child and a 12-month-old child.

Gastrointestinal Disorders

As previously discussed, GER is considered on a continuum from a normal event to a state of illness to a disease (GERD).[23] "Normal" reflux occurs in approximately 50% percent of otherwise healthy infants and is often noted as an infant "spitting up."[24] By 12 months the symptoms resolve in 80% of affected infants. In premature infants, however, studies have shown that significant GERD may occur in up to 100% of premature infants.[25] For children with pediatric reflux that is part of the continuum of illness or disease, clinical signs may be present in the oral and nasal cavity. Signs of pathologic reflux include bad- or sour-smelling breath, gagging during or after feedings, chronic ear infections, sinus infections, enamel erosion of the teeth, swallowing problems, throat clearing, chronic throat infections, chronic cough, bacterial pneumonia unrelated to dysfunctional swallowing, voice disorders with stridor, recurrent vomiting during or after meals, and **esophagitis**. Other clinical signs and symptoms include pain on swallowing, specific delay in developmental skills, sleep disturbance, limited quantities of ingestion, selectivity of food type, and anemia. Unresolved reflux in infants and young children almost always results in food preference restriction or food refusal.

Eosinophilic Esophagitis

Eosinophilic esophagitis (EE) is a gastroenterologic condition caused by an allergic response. The symptoms of EE include inflammation of the esophagus, unexplained oral feeding difficulty, failure to thrive, occasional swallowing dysfunction, pain similar to GERD, and a history of allergic disease including asthma and eczema.[26] The diagnosis of EE is made by endoscopy of the esophagus, stomach, and the first part of the small bowel. Biopsy samples are taken from these areas to test for the presence of **eosinophils**. EE is treated through a combination of medication and dietary modification. Therapeutic management is necessary for many children because they may have a learned aversion to feeding from long-term discomfort with eating. This conditioned response, noted with many gastroenterologic disorders, may continue well after the medical aspects of the EE are resolved. The feeding specialist needs to be aware of the strict dietary restrictions necessary for management of this disorder.

Celiac Disease

Celiac disease is a digestive disease that damages the small intestine and interferes with absorption of nutrients from food. People with celiac disease cannot tolerate the protein gluten, commonly found in wheat, rye, and barley. Gluten is found mainly in foods but also may be found in stamp and envelope adhesives, medicines, and vitamins. Celiac disease is classified as an autoimmune disorder. However, it is also classified as a disease of malabsorption because nutrients are not absorbed. Symptoms may include gas, recurring abdominal bloating and pain, chronic diarrhea, constipation, failure to thrive, fatigue, and irritability. A variety of tests are used by physicians, including measurements of specific antibodies. A biopsy of the small bowel also may be done. If celiac disease is confirmed, the only treatment is a gluten-free diet.

Other Disorders

The feeding specialist should be aware of other disorders of the gastrointestinal system because many directly affect feeding. These include functional gastrointestinal disorders and motility disorders. Examples of these disorders include **Hirschsprung's disease, cyclic vomiting syndrome, gastroparesis, intestinal pseudo-obstruction, irritable bowel syndrome, dyspepsia**, and constipation.

Cardiac and Respiratory Conditions

Children with cardiac and respiratory disorders are seen more often in the inpatient setting. However, once discharged, these children present with decreased endurance and high caloric needs. Field et al.[15] reported that more than 25% of 349 children with feeding disorders had cardiopulmonary complications. Special considerations in therapy must be made for feeding endurance and safety. Dietary requirements should be identified by a pediatric dietitian.

Disorders of the Head and Neck

One area that has not been extensively studied but is well known to many feeding specialists is the impact of frequent medical conditions involving the head

---

CLINICAL CORNER 4-3

John is a typically developing 4-year-old boy. He was referred for a clinical feeding evaluation due to decreased appetite and self-induced vomiting. His parents noted this approximately 6 months before the evaluation. He has had significant weight loss. He has a diagnosis of GER and is taking Prevacid and Reglan for this disorder. He has a history of anxiety. Other health history is unremarkable. The early history shows that he was born at term with no problems during pregnancy. He swallowed some amniotic fluid during birth and was kept in the hospital nursery for 2 extra days for respiratory difficulties. He also had jaundice and was treated with light therapy. He has no diagnosed food or environmental allergies.

CRITICAL THINKING:

1. What developmental and feeding skills are typical in a 4-year-old?
2. What are some of the (U.S.) cultural feeding challenges in children of this age?
3. What may be some of the social and personal concerns experienced by a family with a typically developing child with feeding difficulties?

and neck seen in childhood. These include chronic ear infections, chronic throat infections such as tonsillitis, and sinus infections. Chronic middle ear infections attributable to eustachian tube failure may cause uncomfortable or painful swallowing or increased ear pain when swallowing. Sinus infections may be painful and most often create difficulty in upper airway breathing patterns. The suck-swallow-breathe sequence may be interrupted in the infant as a result of disturbances in breathing patterns. For the older child, the ability to chew effectively may be affected by the child's difficulty in maintaining a closed mouth position. The drainage of fluid during the resolution phase of a sinus infection may also pose some difficulties with swallowing. Frequent coughing, choking, and gagging may be observed. As noted previously, children with chronic sinus infection may have underlying GERD as the primary source.

Children with enlarged tonsils (acute or chronic) often present with a variety of atypical feeding patterns. A child with very large tonsils may present to the feeding specialist as a child with tongue thrust as an effort to maintain an open airway. Because of the enlarged tonsils, the tongue does not have adequate space to move in a complete posterior fashion for swallowing. The mouth may also be held open as part of the child's effort to maintain an open airway. Some children also present with swallowing difficulty or limitations in accepted textures because of the structural impact of the tonsils on swallowing larger amounts of food.

Lymphatic malformations (LMs) are rare but may affect feeding and swallowing. LMs are congenital and are evident either at birth or are detected before 2 years of age. They are primarily related to malformation of the lymphatic channels, although they also may be in the form of a combined capillary-lymphatic malformation. The symptoms of LMs are related to the anatomic location of the malformation and the extent of involvement. LM presents in a variety of forms. The tongue may be affected, resulting in macroglossia and speech and feeding development disorders. The more severe forms of LM extensively involve the head and neck, producing deformities into the oral cavity, oropharynx, and preepiglottic space.[27] Therefore these children exhibit considerable feeding difficulties, including dysphagia, limitations in movement of the tongue, and breathing difficulties related to the coordination of the suck-swallow-breathe sequence. Some children with LMs require tracheotomy because of severe airway obstruction.

For most children, the impact of upper airway and middle ear conditions on feeding is transient; for other children the impact may be longer. A thorough history and prompt referral to the related physician is crucial in addressing and possibly resolving the feeding problem.

Allergies

It is estimated that between 2% and 2.5% of the U.S. population has food allergies. Eight foods account for 90% of all allergic reactions—peanuts, tree nuts, milk, eggs, wheat, soy, fish, and shellfish. Symptoms of food allergy include eczema, hives, breathing problems (including asthma), painful or uncomfortable gastro-enterologic responses, and **anaphylaxis**. The feeding specialist should obtain specific information regarding a child's food allergy. If there is a history of allergy in a family member, similar or identical responses are often seen in children. Objectives for management of allergies include understanding the characteristics of the child's allergy, ensuring dietary adequacy for the child, helping the family to understand the importance of label reading, and prompt referral to appropriate resources.

SENSORY IMPACT ON FEEDING

An individual's response to what is heard, felt, smelled, seen, and tasted has an effect on what is eaten. *Sensory processing* refers to the ability to receive information through our senses, organize that information, and make meaningful responses within the context of that information. Sensory experiences may have either a positive or negative impact on what a child eats. When a child begins to avoid or is reluctant to participate in certain experiences or shows specific preferences to seek a sensory experience (in other than a typical context), a sensory-processing disorder (SPD) may be suspected. SPD is a complex disorder of the brain that affects developing children and adults. People with SPD have abnormal interpretations of everyday sensory information. SPDs may include sensory defensiveness, **sensory modulation problems**, **sensory registration problems**, and sensory integration disorder. These disorders are not psychologically based, as in the case of an avoidance response related to a specific event such as a phobia. Rather, SPD is believed to be a neurologically based disorder that requires specific evaluation and treatment. Establishing the diagnosis of SPD requires careful evaluation by an occupational therapist specifically trained in this area. Similarly, the occupational therapist can suggest strategies for prefeeding preparation to maximize feeding therapy sessions and home programs.

Two specific categories of SPD often are noted during the case history portion of an evaluation or during the evaluation itself. SPD is evident in the child's eating experiences, although SPD often is not limited to eating alone. The two most common categories of impairment are sensory defensiveness (hypersensitivity) and registration problems (hyposensitivity).

Sensory defensiveness—hypersensitivity—usually appears as some type of avoidance of a specific food or entire groups of food. For example, the child with sensory defensiveness may avoid chewy foods, wet foods, or purees. The child may not like getting his or her hands wet or messy. The child may be unable to pick up certain foods but may accept the same food on a utensil. The child may gag easily in the presence of food smells, tastes, textures, or even seeing specific foods. This child may be termed a "picky eater."[28]

A second type of SPD is sensory underregistration—hyposensitivity. A child with this type of SPD usually has decreased awareness of messy hands or a messy face. The child frequently overfills the mouth and is unaware of items falling out of the mouth. Parents may term these children as "sloppy" or "messy" eaters. Some of these children have problems with drooling. They may have problems with coughing or choking on food due to incomplete oral management of certain food textures. Children with underregistration may enjoy chewing, licking, or eating nonfood objects. They almost always prefer savory, salty, or spicy foods over less flavorful foods. Similarly, these children prefer textured foods over pureed foods.[28]

General feeding treatment recommendations for children with sensory disorders include the use of preparatory strategies before the actual eating time. These strategies may include both non-food– and food-based activities. Activities should be linked to the foods and food types to be presented during the feeding therapy session. The child must be moved into optimal sensory functioning before introduction of any new or challenging task.[22] Children should be placed in seating positions that create postural stability. Visual and auditory distractions should be decreased. Clear visual and physical boundaries must be given for both seating and for tasks. For example, individualized containers, placemats, carpet squares, and name cards may be useful.

AUTISM SPECTRUM DISORDERS

Children with autism spectrum disorders (ASDs) may present with a variety of feeding problems. Field et al.[15] found that 62% of children with autism had food selectivity by type. Caregivers describe their child's diet as consisting of only a few foods, with starches as the most commonly accepted food type. Children with ASDs may present with GER(D) or chronic constipation, both of which adversely affect feeding. Other significant challenges present in children with ASDs include resistance to change and ritualistic behaviors surrounding mealtimes. Children with ASDs also present with sensory integrative dysfunction that affects a wide span of feeding areas, including visual characteristics, smell, touch (hands touching food), movement, feeling of food within the mouth, and the taste of foods. Language delays and disorders of learning and behavior also affect children's feeding skills and response to therapy. General treatment recommendations for children with ASD include attention to the sensory needs of the child, use of visual tools to establish the rules, and routines of eating time, such as timers, charts, **TEACCH** (Treatment and Education of Autistic and related Communication-handicapped Children) schedules (www.TEACCH.com), and **PECS** (Picture Exchange Communication System) (www.pecs-usa.com). Teaching communication strategies to facilitate the ability to make requests and strategies to improve pragmatics help to provide predictable routines. These routines often facilitate the eating circumstance. Children with ASDs should be assessed by an occupational therapist and SLP to ensure that the child's therapeutic needs are met.

CEREBRAL PALSY

Children with cerebral palsy (CP) are classified according to the location of neuromuscular involvement. With respect to the muscle movement patterns, these include spasticity, athetosis, and hypotonia. A child with CP may have diplegia (both lower extremities), quadriplegia (all four extremities), or hemiplegia (one side is more involved than the other). There may be a variety of severity levels within each of these classifications. CP is the most common cause of congenital neurogenic dysphagia. Typical feeding problems include poor growth, difficulty with lip closure for breastfeeding or bottle feeding, weak or inefficient sucking patterns, discoordinate tongue movement patterns, and increased risk of aspiration. Common oral phase eating problems include tongue thrusting patterns, a **tonic bite reflex**, and hypersensitivity in and around the mouth. A child's external muscular features are present within the gastrointestinal system because this system is primarily guided through muscle control. Therefore children with CP may show esophageal dysmotility, GER, and problems with constipation. An additional challenge for the feeding specialist and the family of children with CP is that children with spasticity and athetosis have higher energy expenditures that require more calories and other nutrients for growth. Studies have indicated that up to 90% of children with CP show evidence of undernutrition.[29] The challenge of undernutrition is noted in the presence of decreased oral efficiency and potentially atypical swallowing patterns. From a therapeutic perspective, children with CP should be assessed by physical therapy, occupational therapy, and the SLP so that all related needs can be coordinated for successful feeding.

BRAIN INJURY

Children with brain injury present a specific challenge to the feeding specialist. *Brain injury* may be classified as traumatic brain injury or acquired brain injury. The location and severity of the brain injury is significant with respect to the feeding challenges experienced by the child. Studies have indicated that between 30% and 60% of children with brain injury present with feeding difficulties.[15,30] The feeding specialist should obtain information on the previous feeding skills of the child to understand food preferences and skill areas to be addressed.

The most common feeding problems associated with brain injury include dysphagia, oral motor dysfunction, changes in appetite, and difficulties with self-feeding skills. Because frontal lobe injury occurs in many cases, children may display disinhibition during eating times, resulting in overeating and specific dysfunctional eating behaviors.[30] The neuropsychologist can be of assistance to the family and medical care team in developing an appropriate plan for the child's behaviors related to disinhibition.

A videofluoroscopic swallowing study should be completed in children with brain injury to determine swallowing safety. Children with dysphagia and oral motor dysfunction require a treatment plan that addresses swallowing dysfunction and oral motor difficulties. Such children often require a modified diet directed at safety and efficiency in eating. This may include pureed foods, soft solids, thickened liquids only, and other specific food limitations. Therapy activities may be directed at improving lip closure, tongue lateralization, biting and chewing patterns, and overall oral awareness. Some children may require supplemental tube feeding until their medical status and feeding skills allow for a transition to full oral feedings.

If the feeding specialist is not an occupational therapist, an occupational therapy evaluation should be requested for a child who was previously able to self-feed but who may not have the motor skills for successful performance. Optimizing independence is among the many goals for these children. A dietitian should be part of the clinical team for children with brain injury. Brain injury may alter the metabolic rate for some children who may require special dietary intervention and appetite enhancers. Instruction in dietary needs should be provided to both the family and the medical team. Multidisciplinary care optimizes the outcome for children with brain injury.

DOWN SYNDROME

Children with Down syndrome present with a variety of medical and developmental concerns that may affect the development of feeding skills. Approximately 80% of children with Down syndrome display feeding difficulties.[15] Accompanying cardiac and respiratory disorders may affect energy and endurance for eating. Children with Down syndrome are at a higher risk for complications from GER than typically developing children because of low muscle tone. Others may require supplemental oxygen, which can have effects on the coordination of breathing and swallowing. Low muscle tone may result in developmental delays in neck and head control, poor postural stability (including the ability to sit independently), and inadequate upper extremity skills for self-feeding. Specific feeding areas affected by low muscle tone include swallowing dysfunction and oral motor competency. Early feeding problems include weak sucking patterns and difficulties containing food in the oral cavity. Children with Down syndrome often have tongue thrusting patterns as a result of the low muscle tone and a small mouth in relation to the size of the child's tongue. Treatment techniques for children with Down syndrome include modification of diet, modification of feeding position, and support of the oral-facial structures.[31]

TAKE HOME NOTES

1. It is vital for the feeding specialist to understand the maternal conditions that can affect a fetus and how they may affect the overall development of the infant outside the uterus.
2. Infants with gastrointestinal issues such as NEC, prolonged and painful GERD, and tracheoesophageal fistula may have difficulty introducing and advancing oral feedings.
3. Infants with prolonged respiratory issues may have difficulty with initial feedings because of difficulty coordinating the suck-swallow-breathe bursts.
4. Infants with prolonged respiratory issues may have difficulty with the stages of feedings, especially the transitions from liquids to puree to textures.

5. Infants who require cardiac surgery may have neurodevelopmental complications after surgery.

6. The cause of feeding disorders in children may be specific or multidimensional. Rarely is only one specific cause responsible for their origin or longevity.

7. The evaluation and treatment of feeding disorders in the outpatient pediatric population is best accomplished by coordinating information with the family, medical care team, and the feeding specialist.

8. The developmental skills, more than chronologic age, determine the level of a child's feeding competency.

9. Each of the characteristic features of genetic syndromes must be understood in evaluating or treating a child with a feeding disorder.

10. Gastroesophageal reflux is one of the most common underlying features manifest in children with feeding disorders. It is important for the feeding specialist to recognize when to refer a child for evaluation and treatment of gastroesophageal reflux before feeding therapy.

References

1. Lee-Parritz A, Cloherty J: Maternal conditions that affect the fetus. In Cloherty JP, Eichenwald EC, Stark A, editors: *Manual of neonatal care*, ed 5, Philadelphia, 2004, Lippincott.

2. Cochran W, Lee K: Assessment of the newborn. In Cloherty JP, Eichenwald EC, Stark A, editors: *Manual of neonatal care*, ed 5, Philadelphia, 2004, Lippincott.

3. McAlmon KR: Necrotizing enterocolitis. In Cloherty JP, Eichenwald EC, Stark A, editors: *Manual of neonatal care*, ed 5, Philadelphia, 2004, Lippincott.

4. Stark A: Apnea. In Cloherty JP, Eichenwald EC, Stark A, editors: *Manual of neonatal care*, ed 5, Philadelphia, 2004, Lippincott.

5. Giacoia GP, Venkataraman PS, West-Wilson KI et al: Follow-up of school-age children with bronchopulmonary dysplasia, *J Pediatr* 130:400, 1997.

6. DeMyer W: Microcephaly, microcephaly, megacephaly and megalencephaly. In Swaiman KF, Ashwal S, editors: *Pediatric neurology: principles and practice*, St Louis, 1999, Mosby.

7. Ashwal S: Congenital structural defects. In Swaiman KF, Ashwal S, editors: *Pediatric neurology: principles and practice*, St Louis, 1999, Mosby.

8. DeVries SL, Rennie JM: *Textbook of neonatology*, ed 3, Edinburgh, 1999, Churchill Livingston.

9. Cuneo BF: Perinatal cardiology, *Newborn Infant Nurs Rev* 2:90, 2002.

10. Del Nido PJ: Developmental and neurologic outcomes late after neonatal corrective surgery, *J Thorac Cardiovasc Surg* 124:425, 2002.

11. Limperopoulos C, Majnemer A, Shevell M: Functional limitations in young children with congenital heart defects during the first day of life, *Pediatrics* 108:1325, 2001.

12. Moore LL, Persaud TVN, Shiota K: Congenital anomalies or birth defects. In Moore KL, Persaud TVN, Shiota K, editors: *Color atlas of clinical embryology*, ed 2, Philadelphia, 2000, Saunders.

13. Mohrbacher N, Stock J: *The breastfeeding answer book*, ed 3, Schaumburg, IL, 2003, La Leche League International.

14. Spring MA, Mount DL: Pediatric feeding disorder and growth decline following mandibular distraction osteogenesis, *Plast Reconstr Surg* 118:476, 2006.

15. Field D, Garland M, Williams K: Correlates of specific childhood feeding problems, *J Paediatr Child Health* 39:299, 2003.

16. Ayoob KT, Barresi I: Feeding disorders in children: taking an interdisciplinary approach, *Pediatr Ann* 36:478, 2007.

17. Martin C, Southall A, Shea E et al: The importance of a multifaceted approach in the assessment and treatment of childhood feeding disorders: a two-year old inpatient case study in the U.K. National Health Service. *Clin Case Stud* 7:79, 2008.

18. Greer, AJ, Gulotta CS, Mosler EA et al: Caregiver stress and outcomes of children with pediatric feeding disorders treated in an intensive interdisciplinary program, *J Pediatr Psychology* 33:612, 2008.

19. Manikam R, Perman JA: Pediatric feeding disorders, *J Clin Gastroenterol* 30:34, 2000.

20. Burklow KA, Phelps AN, Schults JR et al: Classifying complex pediatric feeding disorders, *J Pediatr Gastroenterol Nutr* 27:143, 1998.

21. Davies WH, Berlin KS, Sato AF et al: Reconceptualizing feeding disorders in interpersonal context: the case for a relational disorder, *J Fam Psychology* 20:400, 2006.

22. Toomey K, Kurtz M, Ross E: *When children won't eat: the SOS approach to feeding*, Denver, 2002, Toomey and Associates.

23. Pulsipher E: *The reflux book: a parent's guide to gastroesophageal reflux*, Garrett Park, MD, 2007, Intensive Care Parenting.

24. Vandenplus Y, Goyvaerts H, Helven R et al: Gastroesophageal reflux as measured by 24-hour pH monitoring in 509 healthy infants screened for risk of sudden infant death syndrome, *Pediatrics* 88;834, 1991.

25. Orenstein SR: Gastroesopohageal reflux, *Pediatr Rev* 20:24, 1997.

26. Pentiuk S, Miller CK, Kaul A et al: Eosinophilic esophagitis in infants and toddlers, *Dysphagia* 22:44, 2007.

27. McGill TJ: Vascular anomalies of the head and neck. In Wetmore RF, Munts HR, McGill TJ, editors: *Pediatric otolaryngology*, New York, 2000, Thieme.

28. Kranowitz CS: *The out-of-sync child: recognizing and coping with sensory integration dysfunction*, New York, 2005, Perigree.

29. Schwarz SM, Corredor J, Fisher-Medina J et al: Diagnosis and treatment of feeding disorders in children with developmental disabilities, *Pediatrics* 108:671, 2001.

30. Tomlin P, Clarke M, Robinson G et al: Rehabilitation in severe head injury in children: outcome and provision of care, *Devel Med Child Neurol* 44:828, 2002.

31. Wolf LS, Glass RP: *Feeding and swallowing disorders in infancy*, Tucson, 1992, Therapy Skill Builders.

Chapter 5

Adult Neurologic Disorders

MICHAEL A. CRARY

CHAPTER OUTLINE

OBJECTIVES

1. Explain why is it important to possess a basic understanding of the nervous system to clinically manage swallowing disorders resulting from neurologic disease.
2. Name some of the sensorimotor characteristics associated with impairments at different levels of the nervous system.
3. Identify some of the dysphagia characteristics that might be seen in diseases affecting various levels of the nervous system.
4. Describe some of the dysphagia-related problems that might be seen in patients with neurologic disease.
5. Describe some aspects of change in dysphagia over time in neurologic diseases.
6. Identify some of the more common treatment issues, decisions, options, and/or practices in different forms of neurogenic dysphagia.

PRELIMINARY CONSIDERATIONS: SWALLOWING SYMPTOMS AND NEUROLOGIC DEFICITS

Swallowing disorders are symptoms of underlying disease processes. One implication of this perspective is that swallowing disorders in patients with neurologic disorders should manifest the characteristics of damage to different areas of the nervous system. This premise has long been accepted in the arena of motor speech disorders (**dysarthria**).[1] For example, spastic dysarthria results from damage to the **upper motor neuron** system governing speech production. Upper motor neuron damage results in specific patterns of neuromotor impairment, including spasticity, slowed movement, exaggerated reflexes, and reduced range of movement. The characteristics of spastic dysarthria are believed to be the direct result of spasticity in the corticobulbar system governing speech production. Patients with spastic dysarthria demonstrate a slow rate of speech, limited movement of the speech articulators, equalized stress patterns, and other characteristics reflecting the underlying neuromotor characteristics of spastic weakness.

A similar framework helps clinical specialists evaluate and plan treatment for patients with swallowing disorders resulting from neurologic deficit. Patients with damage to upper motor neuron systems characteristically demonstrate spastic weakness with resultant slowness and reduced range of movement. This may translate to reduced speed of swallowing (i.e., a delay in initiating one or more components of the swallow) and/or reduced range of movement in the swallowing mechanism (i.e., reduced transport of the bolus contributing to post-swallow residue). To understand better the potential clinical applications of such a framework, clinical specialists must be famil-

iar with neuroanatomy, neurologic functions and dysfunctions of various nervous system components, and sensorimotor components of swallowing at different stages of the swallow. Chapter 2 describes the basic anatomy and neuroanatomy of swallowing functions. A summary of some common neurologic functions associated with various levels within the central nervous system follows.

Brief Overview of Functional Neuroanatomy Relative to Swallowing Functions

Motor and sensory systems work together to produce movement, including movement associated with swallowing. However, in clinical practice motor and sensory functions frequently are described separately as they may relate to impaired swallowing physiology. To facilitate a clinical perspective, a top-down approach to the nervous system is followed in which sensory and motor components are described at each level. Figure 5-1 is a simplified schematic depicting each "level" of the nervous system. Table 5-1 summarizes neurobehavioral and sensorimotor functions associated with each level.

CORTICAL FUNCTIONS

Functional control of sensorimotor behaviors in the human cortex frequently is described in reference to various areas or regions. The frontal lobe cortex is deemed responsible for multiple aspects of motor control, ranging from intent and initiation of movement to coordinating a movement in time and space to executing the movement in an organized and timely fashion. In general, parietal lobe regions are responsible for recognizing and interpreting sensory functions. These functions might include identifying the presence of a sensory stimulus or the interpretation of a sensory stimulus in reference to

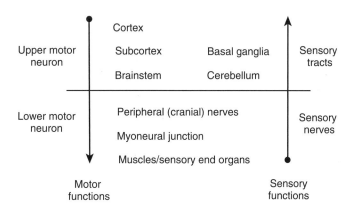

FIGURE 5-1. Simplified schematic of various levels of the nervous system.

TABLE 5-1

Basic Sensorimotor Functions Associated With Different Levels of the Nervous System

Level	Motor	Sensory
Cortical	Intent Initiation Programming Execution	Recognition Awareness Motor tuning
Subcortical (basal ganglia)	Initiation Refinement Inhibition	Motor tuning Awareness Sensory conduit

Brainstem	Junction box:
	    upper motor
	      neuron/
	      lower motor
	      neuron
	Motor/sensory
	    "centers":
	      Swallow
	      Respiration
	      Heart
		Reflexes
		Sensory conduit

Cerebellum	Refinement Inhibition	Refinement
Peripheral nerves	Lower motor neuron Drive movement	Sensory conduit
Muscles and sensory receptors	Effect movement	Sensation reception

an appropriate motor response. Sensorimotor impairments resulting from cortical damage may vary in response to the location of neurologic deficit, extent of the deficit (larger areas of damage are believed to result in more severe or widespread behavioral impairments), and whether the neurologic damage is unilateral or bilateral.

Other important functions housed within the cortex are those of human communication and cognition. Damage to primarily the left side of the brain may result in a number of difficulties in the ability to communicate. Focal attention is frequently afforded to the area of the inferior frontal lobe and superior temporal lobe, although damage to these areas often is accompanied by damage to adjacent motor control areas of the frontal lobe and/or sensory control areas of the parietal lobe. Cognitive deficits associated with cortical dysfunction may present in various forms with different levels of severity and different clinical courses depending on the location of damage and the nature of the underlying disease process.

Arriving to and leaving from the cortex are the major sensory and motor tracts within the central nervous system. Damage to the sensory tracts arriving in the primary sensory strip of the anterior parietal lobe results in loss of recognition of sensory stimuli

in the corresponding body area. Damage to the motor tracts leaving the primary motor strip in the posterior frontal lobe (upper motor neurons) results in paresis or paralysis of the corresponding body area. Sensory or motor deficits are similar regardless of the location of the damage along the tracts. For example, cortical level damage to the upper motor neuron system results in the same type of motor weakness as subcortical or brainstem upper motor neuron damage.

Cortical Functions and Swallowing Impairment

If motor functions of the cortex range from intent to execution, then swallowing deficits resulting from cortical damage may range from no observable swallow activity to poorly coordinated execution of the act of swallowing. In considering these possibilities, frequent cortical pathologic conditions such as stroke, dementia, and traumatic brain injury should be reviewed.

Before reviewing dysphagia characteristics in various cortical pathologies, a worthwhile question to ask is "Where is swallowing function represented in the human cortex?" Given the complexity of motor control involved in oropharyngeal swallowing, it is logical to implicate the frontal cortex, specifically areas involved in various components of motor control. In fact, results of both animal and human studies using lesion or cortical stimulation techniques implicate the importance of the lateral frontal cortex, the inferior frontal lobule, and the insula in various motor acts associated with feeding and swallowing. Recent studies using functional magnetic resonance imaging (**fMRI**) implicate a wide range of cortical, subcortical, and brainstem structures involved in swallowing performed by healthy volunteers.[2] Not surprisingly, the primary motor and sensory cortical areas consistently participated in swallowing function. In a comparison of ischemic stroke patients with dysphagia and stroke patients without dysphagia, the internal capsule emerged as the only brain region significantly associated with dysphagia. However, other areas of the sensorimotor cortex and the basal ganglia also were frequently associated with the presence of dysphagia in stroke patients.[3]

Although findings from many studies implicate a dysphagia based in poor motor control resulting from damage to the anterolateral and precentral frontal cortex, no consensus exists concerning the specific characteristics of these dysphagias. Still, hemispheric damage to frontal areas underpinning motor control resulting in direct movement deficits should raise significant clinical concern for the presence of dysphagia.

What about cortical or hemisphere lesions that impair sensory function? These sensory areas of the hemisphere may be important in understanding swallowing functions and impairments. In fact, some studies report that many stroke patients with dysphagia have damage to the parietal lobe with associated sensory deficits.[4] Primary sensory areas of the cortex have extensive interconnections with the motor areas of the cortex. Sensory function is deemed important in the control of voluntary movement. Beyond direct sensory loss, we should consider conditions in which the patient cannot interpret sensory information, for example, **neglect**. Patients with neglect may not respond to a stimulus in the swallowing tract (food or liquid bolus), not because of direct sensory loss, but because of a cortical deficit in processing and interpreting sensory information. In at least one study, hemispatial neglect was related to nonoral intake of food and liquid, but not severity of dysphagia, in patients evaluated 3 days after hospital admission for stroke.[5] Unfortunately, these investigators did not interpret the association between neglect and nonoral intake. As a result, the presence of neglect may be related to feeding limitations rather than swallowing deficits leading to nonoral intake.

More recently, increased systematic attention has been afforded sensory functions in swallowing and swallowing impairment.[6-8] Continued emerging information and clinical observations suggest that impaired sensory functions may have a direct influence on swallowing functions. A better understanding of the role of sensory systems on swallowing function and impairment may lead to improved sensory-based interventions for dysphagia.

Issues of Unilateral Versus Bilateral Hemispheric Lesions

The issues previously raised regarding hemispheric contribution to swallowing control also raise the question of whether such control is unilateral or bilateral. A traditional perspective is that patients with bilateral lesions often demonstrate the most severe and persistent dysphagia characteristics.[9] Still, patients with unilateral hemisphere lesions may demonstrate dysphagia to varying degrees. Recent research using the technique of transcranial magnetic stimulation has suggested an interesting point of view on the hemispheric representation of swallowing function. Transcranial magnetic stimulation involves sending a magnetic current across the cranium over discrete hemisphere regions. These magnetic currents stimulate motor activity that is measured in various muscles by **electromyography**. This interesting work on the

---

CLINICAL CORNER 5-1

Sensory deficits may be observed in many neurologic (and nonneurologic) diseases and disorders. They may range from a direct loss of sensory input (e.g., numbness, blindness) up to and including the inability to interpret an intact sensory signal (e.g., agnosia, cortical blindness). Depending on the nature of the sensory deficit, patients may have reduced (and at times insufficient) oral intake of food and liquid. However, this deficit level of oral intake of food and liquid may not represent a dysphagia (here meaning specific difficulty swallowing food). Rather, certain sensory deficits may contribute to feeding limitations that reduce oral intake of food and liquid. Clinical specialists in the area of dysphagia need to be able to differentiate various sensory deficits and interpret their impact on feeding versus swallowing impairments.

CRITICAL THINKING

1. What types of sensory problems might occur within the swallowing mechanism—specifically the oral and pharyngeal components of the mechanism? Consider various diseases and/or disorders that might contribute to these sensory deficits. Be sure to consider direct sensory loss versus deficit interpretation of sensory input.
2. How would you evaluate sensory functions within the swallow mechanism from direct sensory loss up to poor interpretation of sensory information?
3. What practical impact might sensory deficits have on the oral intake of food and liquid? Consider specific clinical examples.

---

hemispheric control of swallowing function can be summarized as follows:

1. Swallowing motor functions are bilaterally represented in the hemispheres.
2. If the dominant hemisphere is impaired, a contralateral "backup" area may be available to facilitate recovery.
3. A form of **cortical plasticity** may occur over time, increasing the utility of the intact, nondominant hemisphere to control swallowing motor functions.
4. Bilateral strokes would result in the most tenacious dysphagias.[10-13]

In some respects, this perspective is consistent with traditional clinical observations; bilateral strokes produce the most severe dysphagias, and many patients with unilateral strokes often recover the ability to swallow after a period of dysphagia.

SWALLOWING DEFICITS IN HEMISPHERIC STROKE SYNDROMES

Several issues must be addressed when considering dysphagia secondary to hemispheric strokes. These issues may be simplified into two general considerations: location of damage and functional consequences of the damage. These considerations are not mutually exclusive. Location of the damage may be important in understanding sensory and/or motor impairments and in understanding the severity and potential for recovery based on unilateral versus bilateral lesions. In clinical practice, information on lesion location often is not available at the time of the dysphagia evaluation. Therefore a strong reliance on the clinical examination of functional impairment after stroke may provide the best "road map" to understanding and perhaps predicting dysphagia characteristics. Table 5-1 provides a basic orientation to some of the functional impairments that may be clinically observed after impairment to various levels of the nervous system. At the hemisphere level, intent to swallow may be an important consideration. If the patient indicates such intent, a subsequent consideration would be motor initiation of the swallow. Patients with damage to premotor areas (e.g., supplemental motor cortex) may have generalized difficulty with motor initiation. The clinical picture may be that of a patient who holds a bolus in the mouth for an abnormally long period with associated movements that indicate the intent to swallow but without initiating a swallow.

Patients with sensory deficits may demonstrate a variety of dysphagia characteristics, including retention of a portion of a bolus in the mouth, oropharynx, or hypopharynx with no attempt to clear the residue. These patients also may be more susceptible to aspiration of material into the upper airway as a result of the sensory deficit. Another category of sensory deficit may be seen in the patient with neglect. Such patients may not recognize material presented to one side of the swallowing tract. These patients may hold material in the mouth with no apparent intent to swallow, but in fact they are unaware of the material in the mouth.

Finally, patients with hemispheric stroke may have significant communication deficits or cognitive deficits that reduce their ability to relate to the clinical examiner the nature of the dysphagia complaints. Patients who are asleep, lethargic, have waxing and waning alertness, or difficulty participating in the

swallowing evaluation because of cognitive deficits present significant challenges to a valid evaluation of swallowing abilities. Also, the inability to describe swallowing difficulties may delay or hinder clinical evaluation and/or implementation of rehabilitation strategies. Figure 5-2 depicts general hemisphere areas

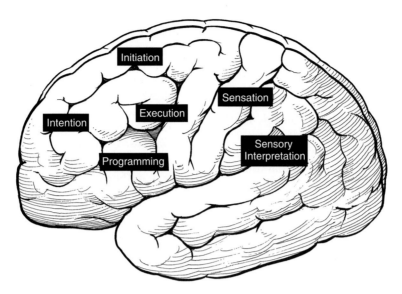

FIGURE 5-2. Various hemisphere areas that may be associated with sensorimotor functions supporting swallowing function.

BOX 5-I	General Sensorimotor Considerations for Various Swallowing Deficits in Hemisphere Stroke

- Volitional motor control
  - Initiation difficulties
- Paresis/paralysis
  - Transport difficulties
- Sensory recognition
  - Residue
  - Aspiration
- Communication deficits
  - Inability to describe difficulties

that may be associated with various sensorimotor functions associated with swallowing. The left hemisphere is shown for descriptive purposes only. Box 5-1 presents various swallowing characteristics that may be associated with sensorimotor deficits after hemispheric stroke.

A variety of swallowing deficits have been reported after hemispheric stroke. In general, hemispheric lesions (including both cortical and subcortical damage) contribute to many swallowing deficits (Box 5-2), including (1) poor initiation of saliva swallows (sometimes termed the *dry swallow*); (2) delay in initiation of the pharyngeal component of the swallow; (3) incoordination of the oral components of swallowing; (4) increased pharyngeal transit time and reduced pharyngeal constriction and clearing; (5) aspiration; (6) dysfunction of the pharyngoesophageal segment (cricopharyngeal muscle); and

Practice Note 5-2

Acute stroke patients may present a variety of clinical signs and certainly are at risk for a variety of morbidities. One issue that seems obvious but may not be apparent to all health care providers is the level of alertness presented by the patient. Some stroke patients may be generally lethargic, whereas others may demonstrate a waxing and waning level of alertness.

A few years ago, I was working on the inpatient service in our hospital when I received a request for a consultation from a neurologist whom I knew well. The consult was to "evaluate and treat" dysphagia in a patient who had survived a recent stroke. On entering the patient's room I found her asleep. I tried to gently awaken her by speaking close to her ear, then by speaking louder, then by washing her face and hands with a cloth rinsed in cold water. Nothing worked. I entered a note in the chart that the patient could not be aroused and that the service should reconsult when her status improved. The next day I received another consultation request from the same neurologist. I visited the patient at a different time during the day with the same result. In fact, I went back at different times on the same day with the same result. I called the neurologist and arranged to be with him when he next saw this patient. Together we agreed that this patient could not realistically participate in a swallowing examination and we would wait and watch. In another few days she "woke up" and we evaluated her swallow and began small amounts of oral intake.

(7) poor relaxation of the lower esophageal sphincter. These collective observations indicate that hemispheric stroke can impair swallowing functions from the mouth to the stomach. Furthermore, a wide spectrum of swallowing deficits has been noted, ranging from impaired initiation of the swallow to poor transport of the bolus to aspiration into the airway. To date no report has emerged comparing specific sensorimotor stroke sequelae with specific swallowing impairments. However, the above list suggests that the array of potential swallowing deficits after stroke is extensive and may relate to the spectrum of poststroke sensorimotor impairments.

BOX 5-2	Swallowing Deficits in Patients After Hemisphere Stroke

- Reduced ability to initiate a saliva swallow
- Delayed triggering of pharyngeal swallow
- Incoordination of oral movements in swallow
- Increased pharyngeal transit time
- Reduced pharyngeal constriction
- Aspiration
- Pharyngoesophageal segment dysfunction
- Impaired lower esophageal sphincter relaxation

Practice Note 5-3

Recently I saw two patients within a short time frame who had similar histories and clinical presentations. Both patients were stroke survivors and at least 6 months past the stroke event. Both were deemed medically stable. Both were dependent on nonoral percutaneous esophageal gastrostomy (PEG) feedings. And both had difficulty managing their oral secretions; they drooled and carried a towel to "mop up the problem." Finally, neither patient had functional speaking ability, but both could vocalize and phonate simple vowels. These patients were referred for evaluation and treatment of pharyngeal dysphagia.

On the surface, this clinical presentation may make sense. However, the basic problem for both patients was not pharyngeal dysphagia, but rather *oral apraxia*. Admittedly, oral apraxia was quite severe in both patients. Both presented with a persistent open-mouth posture but in the absence of overt weakness within the facial or oral musculature. Both could close the mouth in response to intraoral sensory stimuli and both spontaneously swallowed, though infrequently. A key feature of the clinical examination in both cases was the absence of overt cranial nerve deficits. Also, each patient had the ability to close the mouth, but this was context dependent (e.g., they did not close the mouth on command, but when liquid was placed in the posterior mouth they did close and a spontaneous swallow was observed). As part of the clinical swallow examination, liquid was placed in the oropharyngeal area with a straw as a pipette. As this liquid trickled into the hypopharynx, we occasionally observed a swallow. Under endoscopic inspection we delivered additional liquid to the oropharynx in this fashion. I also learned that both patients protected their airway and that no residue remained after these volume-dependent swallows.

Based on these clinical and endoscopic findings I did not enroll these patients in therapy for pharyngeal dysphagia. The dysphagia was primarily the result of a severe oral apraxia that limited oral motor control for voluntary tasks, including swallowing.

I did make simple recommendations that I hoped would improve oral functions for feeding and oral control for swallowing. Because I observed intermittent spontaneous swallows when liquid was placed in the posterior part of the mouth, I recommended this technique in an attempt to stimulate improved oral swallow initiation. I suggested to the local therapist that if the frequency of spontaneous swallowing improved, she should vary the type and amount of material used in this fashion and gradually place the material more forward within the mouth. Later I heard from one of the local therapists that her patient had increased the frequency of spontaneous swallowing and was taking more oral intake. Sometimes success comes in small steps.

Refer to Videos 5-2, *A* and *B* on the Evolve site for endoscopic and fluoroscopic examples of a single patient who demonstrated significant oral apraxia in the presence of preserved pharyngeal swallowing function.

Dysphagia is highly prevalent in acute stroke, with estimates that well over 50% of all patients are affected. However, the majority of acute stroke patients recover functional swallowing ability within the first 1 to 6 months after stroke, whereas swallowing problems develop in a small percentage of patients during the postacute period.[14-16] These observations emphasize the importance of accurate identification and management of swallowing deficits in acute stroke patients. Furthermore, it is important to understand the factors that might predict persistent swallowing problems beyond the acute recovery period. The importance of this perspective is highlighted by the observation that acute and chronic swallowing problems in stroke patients are associated with many complications, including dehydration, malnutrition, aspiration, chest infections and, in some cases, death. Furthermore, dysphagia during acute stroke is associated with poor long-term outcome, including death and an increased rate of institutionalization.[17]

Treatment Considerations

Perhaps the most obvious statement about dysphagia in stroke is that it changes over time. From that perspective, dysphagia intervention strategies should also change over time. Table 5-2 presents clinical considerations and decisions that may affect treatment planning over time. Early in the course of a stroke, focus should be given to basic decisions such as the safety of oral feeding versus the need for nonoral feeding routes, the presence of **comorbid conditions** such as pneumonia, malnutrition, or dehydration, and the overall medical condition of the patient.

TABLE 5-2	
Treatment Considerations and Decisions for Dysphagia After Stroke*	
Considerations	**Decisions**
Acute (0-1 Month)	
Most comorbid conditions	How to avoid or minimize complications
Resolving dysphagia	Need and readiness for therapy
Malnutrition	How to maintain and improve nutrition
Improving (1-6 Months)	
Patient more stable with better endurance	Need and readiness for therapy
Comorbid conditions often under medical control	Type of therapy
Feeding routes established for most	
Malnutrition may still be a factor	
Chronic (After 6 Months)	
Feeding routes more established	Therapy or no therapy (prognosis?)
Patients eating orally may have impaired swallow	Type of therapy
Compensations that interfere with swallow	
Impact of prior therapy	

*Changing issues with time after onset.

The acute stroke patient is at greatest risk for dysphagia and morbidities associated with dysphagia. During the acute phase of stroke, patients are likely to demonstrate significant weakness contributing to reduced stamina and perhaps reduced mental status, including alertness and attention. These factors significantly limit any meaningful clinical (or other) evaluation of swallowing ability. Thus a conservative strategy would be to observe the patient's status and postpone any in-depth assessment or intervention until the patient is more alert and has better endurance. Acute stroke patients also are at risk for respiratory abnormalities. Respiratory abnormalities range from basic weakness in expiratory muscles that might reduce cough effectiveness,[18] to increased episodes of oxygen desaturation,[19,20] to deviations in the respiratory rate,[21] to alterations in the coordination between respiration and swallowing.[22,23] Collectively, these respiratory deviations noted in acute stroke patients suggest an increased risk of aspiration of swallowed materials and pooled secretions and potential limitations in clearing aspirated secretions as a result of reduced cough efficiency. Given these potential risks, respiratory functions in the acute stroke patient should be evaluated as part of the comprehensive swallowing examination.

Pneumonia is commonly noted in acute stroke patients. Pneumonia is a significant morbidity because it is related to both an increased number of hospital readmissions[24] and short-term and long-term mortality.[25] Causes of pneumonia in the poststroke patient are multifactorial; however, dysphagia, especially dysphagia accompanied by aspiration, is significantly related to the presence of pneumonia.[16] In fact, dysphagia screening leading to early identification and treatment of swallowing deficits in acute stroke patients has been associated with a reduction in pneumonia rates.[26]

The presence of dysphagia after stroke may contribute to pneumonia in various ways. Although the focus is often on aspiration of orally ingested food and liquid, aspiration of pooled pharyngeal secretions also may contribute to chest infection. Aspiration of secretions may be especially problematic in the acute stroke population because oral bacteria colonization is prominent in these patients.[27] Patients dependent on tube feeding, specifically nasogastric tube feeding, may have a higher degree of bacterial colonization than patients who feed orally.[28] In fact, at least one study has reported that stroke patients who were completely dependent on nonoral feeding (e.g., nothing by mouth) demonstrated higher rates of respiratory infections than did stroke survivors who were feeding orally.[29] One implication of these findings is that reduced frequency of swallowing contributes to an increased risk of aspirating pharyngeal secretions in the presence of higher rates of bacterial colonization within the swallowing mechanism. This premise is supported by treatment studies demonstrating that swallowing therapy[30] and strategies to improve oral hygiene[31] reduce the incidence of pneumonia in stroke patients. Thus the dysphagia clinician should consider more than aspiration of food and liquid when providing swallowing interventions to patients after acute stroke.

Nutritional deficits are prevalent among stroke patients on admission and may worsen during hospitalization. On admission, the prevalence of such deficits has been estimated at approximately 16%; this figure increases to 22% to 26% through discharge from acute care.[32-34]

Nutritional decline continues beyond acute care. The prevalence of nutritional deficits in stroke patients at admission to rehabilitation approximates 50%.[35] At approximately 1 month after stroke, nutritional status begins to improve and continues to improve up to 4 months after stroke. In the acute stroke patient nutritional deficits are not overtly linked to dysphagia.[33,36] However, later during the rehabilitation period and thereafter, swallowing and/or feeding difficulties may contribute to the maintenance or increase in poor nutritional status.[37] Still, some suggest that poor nutrition during the acute phase of stroke contributes to poor longer term functional outcomes.[38] Nutritional evaluation and intervention are outside the scope of practice for most dysphagia clinicians. However, all dysphagia clinicians should be aware of the potential impact of swallowing and feeding abilities on nutritional status and participate in multidisciplinary health care teams, including nutritional specialists.

As the patient's condition improves and more active rehabilitation is initiated (usually well within the first month after stroke), dysphagia treatment strategies also may change. One consideration is spontaneous resolution of dysphagia as the patient recovers from the effects of acute stroke. Although many stroke patients have some degree of recovery in swallowing ability, estimates of persisting dysphagia range from 11% to 50% at 6 months after stroke.[14,39] During this period of improvement the patient with persistent dysphagia is likely to be engaged in active swallowing rehabilitation. By this time a decision about oral or nonoral feeding has already been established and comorbid conditions are often under medical control. Of importance to active dysphagia rehabilitation are various patient issues and the nature of the swallowing deficit. If the patient is able to participate in active rehabilitation and is motivated, direct and intense swallowing therapy is expected to produce significant benefit. Benefits from swallowing therapy extend beyond improved swallowing abilities to include reduced pneumonia rates and improved nutritional status.[29,40-42] Decisions about therapy technique(s) selection depend in large part on the specific dysphagia characteristics demonstrated by individual patients (see Chapter 14).

Chronic dysphagia is reported in some stroke survivors, although no study has documented the prevalence of dysphagia in stroke patients beyond 6 months after stroke. Typically, if the swallowing deficit persists beyond 6 months, it is considered chronic. Available reports indicate that stroke patients with chronic dysphagia can benefit from intense therapy.[43-45] Such therapies are typically active and directed at changing specific physiologic features of the swallowing deficit.

In summary, dysphagia is highly prevalent after stroke and may be related to pneumonia, nutritional deficits, and other health complications. Dysphagia does resolve to varying degrees in the poststroke period, but the few estimates available suggest that up to 50% of stroke patients demonstrate some degree of persistent dysphagia. Dysphagia therapy has been shown to improve swallowing ability, reduce pneumonia rates, and improve nutritional status in stroke patients. Even stroke survivors with chronic dysphagia can experience functional benefit from intensive swallowing therapy.

SWALLOWING DEFICITS IN DEMENTIA

Another form of cortical impairment that can affect swallowing ability is the category of progressive diseases known as *dementia*. Several types of dementias have been described; the most frequent is Alzheimer's disease. Other forms of dementia include dementia caused by cerebrovascular disease, Lewy body dementia, frontotemporal dementia, alcoholic dementia, and metabolic and/or nutritional dementia.[46] The hallmark of all dementias is a progressive deterioration in cognitive abilities, including memory, judgment, abstract reasoning, and personality changes. Other cortical disturbances such as **apraxia** and/or **aphasia** might be noted.

Swallowing deficits are well documented in advanced dementia.[47-50] Persistent weight loss may be the first indication that patients with dementia have a significant swallowing problem; however, weight loss may not be directly related to feeding or swallowing difficulties.[49,51] As a result, such individuals are at significant risk for nutritional deficits that may further compromise their health status. Pneumonia is a common cause of death in patients with dementia.[50] Although dysphagia, including aspiration, is associated with pneumonia in this population,[51] it is not the only contributing factor and may not be the critical contributing factor.[49,50,52]

General characteristics of swallowing deficits in dementia are listed in Box 5-3. Prominent on this list is the presence of oral-stage dysfunction. It has been suggested that certain oral aspects of swallowing are under volitional motor control. The generalized cognitive impairments in dementia may contribute to deficits in volitional motor control and hence oral aspects of dysphagia. These may be characterized by lack of initiation of the swallow in which the patient holds food in the mouth, has incoordinated oral control of food and liquid, and/or delayed initiation of the oral component of the swallow, thus prolonging mealtimes.

Although the majority of dysphagia information in dementia is derived from studies of patients in advanced stages of the disease, patients with mild-stage dementia also demonstrate feeding and swallowing deficits.[53] Box 5-4 summarizes the salient findings regarding feeding and swallowing abilities in mild-stage dementia. These impairments are similar to, though not as severe as, those reported in more advanced stages of the disease. Specifically, patients with dementia demonstrate an overall slowing of the swallowing process from the oral aspects of food manipulation through the response of the pharynx accepting the bolus. This slowing of the swallowing process can have direct consequences for longer mealtimes and hence increase the risk of declining nutritional status. In addition, slowing of the pharyngeal response in swallowing may reduce airway protection, resulting in an increase of coughing and choking behaviors during mealtimes.

In addition to overall slowness in the swallowing process, individuals with dementia frequently demonstrate self-feeding difficulties. Self-feeding difficulties may relate to numerous factors, including cognitive impairment, motor deficits such as weakness or apraxia, loss of appetite, and food avoidance. Consequences of self-feeding difficulties can include weight loss and associated nutritional decline as well as dependency for feeding. Dependency for feeding can contribute to dysphagia-related health problems, including pneumonia.[54-56] Self-feeding difficulties may be noticed in the mild stages of the disease and become more pronounced as the disease progresses. For patients with self-feeding difficulties, clinicians or caregivers may need to offer increased verbal or environmental cues or provide direct assistance. Refer to Video 5-3 on the companion Evolve site of this text for an example of feeding difficulties in a single patient with primary progressive aphasia (PPA). PPA is a form of dementia in which language and communication abilities deteriorate and are initially followed by deterioration of other functions. This patient appeared to have a specific form of apraxia that influenced her use of eating utensils.

At the beginning of this chapter the premise was offered that different neurologic deficits contribute to different clinical presentations of swallowing deficits. At least one study has evaluated differences in feeding and swallowing abilities in patients with Alzheimer's disease compared with patients with frontotemporal dementia.[57] As the name implies, frontotemporal dementia is often characterized by frontal lobe signs, including loss of insight, disinhibition, impulsivity, poor self-care, stereotypic behavior, and more. Conversely, Alzheimer's disease is characterized by progressive memory deficits that may affect many tasks of daily life because of forgetfulness, disorientation, or impaired **executive functions**. Ikeda et al.[57] used caregiver questionnaires to evaluate eating behaviors in patients with frontotem-

---

BOX 5-3	**Swallowing Deficits Seen in Patients with Cognitive Decline (Dementia)**

- Unexplained weight loss*
- Oral-stage dysfunction*
- Pharyngeal-stage dysfunction
- Combined oral and pharyngeal dysfunction
  - Minor aspiration
  - Major aspiration
- Feeding limitations

*More commonly observed characteristics.

BOX 5-4	**Examples of Swallowing and Feeding Deviations in Mild-Stage Dementia**

SWALLOWING DEVIATIONS
- Slow oral movement
- Slow or delayed pharyngeal response
- Overall slow swallowing duration

FEEDING DEVIATIONS
- Increased self-feeding cues (specifically related to food preparation or utensil use)
- Direct assistance with utensil use for food preparation or convenience
- Imitation of feeding behavior from the meal partner

Practice Note 5-4*

Successful oral care and swallowing for the patient with advanced Alzheimer's disease is very much in the hands of the caregiver. I learned this firsthand by caring for my mother, who had Alzheimer's disease. As speech-language pathologists, we are often in a position to offer insight into the process of these two activities by combining our knowledge of swallowing with our knowledge of dementia. The following anecdotal examples illustrate this point.

First, how may the sensory input of taste trigger an oral behavior? Good oral hygiene is critical, but what do you do when it is no longer feasible to use regular toothpaste, since it often mismanaged and swallowed? Toddler toothpaste (designed to be safe if swallowed) is an option and a popular flavor is bubble gum. There were occasions when the desired swish and spit was accomplished after the predictable brushing action. However, months later, when giving her liquid Tylenol (also in bubble gum flavor) she *remembered* to successfully swish and spit.

Second, and this may be very case specific, we encountered the dilemma of trying to cue chewing and swallowing during a meal. Although the process was slow and laborious, it seemed sensible that this should be done slowly with verbal and tactile cues with each step and a pause between each bite to check for residual food in the oral cavity. However, I stunned the nursing assistant by trying to follow a successful swallow with another bite without pausing. For a time this was a successful strategy. Why did I try this? One of the four "A's" of Alzheimer's disease is *apraxia*. I recalled that it is at the point of transition that motor planning seems to break down. Therefore if we minimized the pause between successful swallows, an almost "automatic" second swallow of food followed.

---

*AUTHOR'S NOTE: This practice note was provided by my former student and good friend, Dr. Nancy J. Haak, who cared for her mother with Alzheimer's dementia in her home. In multiple conversations with Nancy, I learned much about the practical management of dysphagia in patients with dementia and felt it appropriate to share at least one example in this text.—M.A.C.

poral dementia versus Alzheimer's disease. They evaluated five categories: swallowing problems, appetite change, food preferences, eating habits (including table manners and stereotype behaviors), and other oral behaviors. In general, swallowing problems occurred less frequently than other limitations and the frequency of dysphagia did not differ among the types of dementia. However, swallowing problems tended to occur earlier in the course of disease progression in the patients with Alzheimer's disease. Patients with frontotemporal dementia demonstrated more frequent changes in appetite. These patients were more likely to demonstrate increased appetite compared with reduced appetite in patients with Alzheimer's disease. In addition, patients with frontotemporal dementia demonstrated more food preferences than patients in the Alzheimer's group. Still, more than 20% of the patients with Alzheimer's disease demonstrated increased preference for sweets and other taste-related changes. As might be expected from the basic profile, patients with frontotemporal dementia demonstrated more deviations in eating behaviors. Patients in the Alzheimer's disease group did demonstrate longer meal durations, decline in table manners such as eating with hands, and a tendency to prefer eating at the same time each day. Finally, the category of "other oral behaviors" included observations such as overstuffing the mouth, eating nonedible objects, snatching any food item within reach, or vomiting, including self-induced vomiting. In general, patients with Alzheimer's disease scored low on these behaviors with the exception of overfilling the mouth when eating. This is an interesting study in many ways. First, it details caregivers' observations of eating and swallowing behaviors in different groups of patients with dementia. Second, it supports the basic premise that the characteristics of the underlying neurologic disease affect the clinical presentation of dysphagia. Finally, it provides at least an initial description of feeding and swallowing behaviors that may be used by dysphagia clinicians in evaluating swallowing and related behaviors in patients with dementia.

Treatment Considerations

Dementia is a progressive disease with no known cure. Dysphagia intervention for patients with any form of dementia should keep that focus and incorporate basic principles of quality of life, dignity, and comfort.[58,59] Dysphagia treatment options for patients with dementia may range from simple environmental adjustments to the use of nonoral feeding sources. Depending on specific problems in individual patients, some potential treatment avenues may include special food preparations, diet restriction, enhanced taste and flavor, changing the mealtime environment, increased mealtime supervision and cueing, or a variety of other behavioral or environmental changes to facilitate increased food and liquid intake. Direct behavioral therapy to change swallowing mechanics also may be indicated (see Chapter 14).

Feeding tubes are frequently recommended for patients with advanced dementia as a mechanism to maintain nutritional support and avoid dysphagia-related comorbid conditions. However, the available evidence on the benefit of feeding tubes for this population suggests that they do not reduce the risks of aspiration pneumonia, may not prevent further decline in nutritional status, may not prolong survival, and seem to have no impact on overall functional status.[60] A recent survey of national databases (Minimum Data Set and Medicare Claims Files) indicated that most feeding tubes were placed in nursing home residents with dementia during acute hospitalization.[61] The most common reasons for these hospitalizations included pneumonia, dehydration, and dysphagia. The 1-year mortality rate was 64%, with median survival of 56 days after tube placement. Patients with feeding tubes also had a significantly higher rate of health care use after tube insertion. These observations are nearly opposite the results of a survey completed by speech-language pathologists working in the area of dysphagia.[62] In that survey, many respondents believed that percutaneous endoscopic gastrostomy (PEG) improves nutritional status and increases survival, and nearly 40% believed that PEG was the standard of care for patients with advanced dementia. However, the majority of respondents did not believe that tube feeding improved quality of life or functional status for these patients. These misperceptions and lack of knowledge are not confined to speech-language pathologists. Pelletier[63] evaluated dysphagia and feeding knowledge of certified nursing assistants working in nursing homes. Even though these professionals were actively participating in patient feeding activities, their knowledge of dysphagia and feeding was greatly limited. The results of this study and others suggest that focused education is vital in managing dysphagia and feeding limitations in patients with dementia. In fact, at least one study has demonstrated that educational programs for medical and allied health staff on end-of-life care and feeding management in patients with dementia resulted in a reduction in feeding tube placement in these patients.[64] An additional study indicated that trained feeding assistance focusing on patients' self-feeding ability, social stimulation during meals or snack periods, and increased availability of choices for foods and liquids increased the daily intake of food and liquid in 90% of nursing home residents. Both feeding assistance and the availability of between-meal snacks resulted in increased oral intake.[65] Col-

lectively, the available information suggests that (1) feeding tubes do not produce significant benefit to most patients with dementia, (2) they do not promote quality of life or compassionate care, (3) alternatives are available, and (4) education on the problems and intervention strategies can benefit patients. See Chapter 15 for more information on the use of feeding tubes.

SWALLOWING DEFICITS IN TRAUMATIC BRAIN INJURY

Traumatic brain injury (TBI) typically results in diffuse neurologic deficits that affect several aspects of behavioral control. Various studies have indicated the prevalence of dysphagia in acute or subacute TBI ranges from 60% to more than 90%.[66-68] Oral-phase difficulties and pharyngeal-phase deficits are roughly evenly distributed within this population.[67] The primary factor related to the presence of dysphagia in these patients is the severity of neurotrauma assessed by clinical scales such as the **Glasgow Coma Scale (GCS)**, the **Rancho Los Amigos Scale (RLAS)**, or the **Functional Independence Measure (FIM)**.[66-68] At least one study has suggested that the level of functional oral intake at admission to subacute rehabilitation as measured by the Functional Oral Intake Scale (FOIS; see Chapter 9) is one predictive component of return to total oral feeding in patients with TBI.[68] Another study reported that a level IV on the RLAS was required to initiate oral feeding and that a level VI on this scale was needed for return to total oral feeding.[66] Recovery of swallowing function in TBI is good; most patients regain some degree of functional swallowing within the first 3 to 6 months after injury.[68-70] The severity of the initial injury emerges as a strong predictor of both the presence of swallowing deficits and time to recovery of functional swallowing ability.

Pneumonia is frequently seen in patients with TBI, especially early in the posttraumatic course of treatment.[71,72] Hansen et al.[72] reported that 27% of patients admitted with a brain injury for early rehabilitation were being actively treated for pneumonia and that pneumonia developed in an additional 12% during rehabilitation. Clinical factors associated with the presence of pneumonia included severity of neurotrauma (GCS, RLAS), no oral intake on admission, and presence of tracheostomy tube and/or feeding tube. Woratyla et al.[71] added prolonged intubation time and field intubation versus in-hospital intubation as risk factors for pneumonia. Thus level of consciousness and tracheostomy tube or feeding tube plus type of intubation appear to related to the development of early pneumonia in patients with TBI.

In addition to the effects of neurotrauma on swallowing ability in patients with TBI, swallowing may be affected by factors such as the need for **tracheostomy** and/or **ventilator** support, the presence of communicative and cognitive deficits, and the presence of physical deficits that may interfere with self-feeding ability. Tracheostomy tubes indicate some degree of compromise in the respiratory system, which is integral in the swallowing process. Also, these tubes may have a mechanical impact on swallowing physiology. However, at least one study has reported that the presence of tracheostomy tubes was not associated with increased rates of dysphagia or aspiration in trauma patients.[73] Patients with communicative and/or cognitive deficits present additional challenges to clinicians in the design of swallowing assessments or rehabilitation strategies because of patients' reduced understanding and/or interaction. Finally, physical deficits impose a degree of dependency for activities such as self-feeding.[74]

Treatment Considerations

In as much as the deficits observed in TBI are multifactorial, the potential treatment strategies and techniques are also multifactorial. Cherney and Halper[75] provide a brief but excellent review of the roles of interdisciplinary team members that may be required in the management of dysphagia in patients with TBI. Standard intervention approaches included diet modifications, postural adjustments, feeding adaptations, and behavioral maneuvers and compensations (see Chapter 14).[76] In cases of severe injury with widespread comorbid conditions, alternate feeding routes may be indicated, especially in the early postinjury course. The good news is that many patients with dysphagia after TBI do regain the ability to eat by mouth with appropriate clinical intervention.

SUBCORTICAL FUNCTIONS

The basal ganglia are a group of cell bodies in the subcortical brain hemispheres that influence the quality of movement. Basal ganglia functions regulate tone (resting tension level of muscles) and steadiness of movement, among other functions. Impairment to basal ganglia functions may create excessive tone and/or extra, unintended movements. Excessive tone may create delays in the initiation of movement, slowed movements, and/or a reduced amount of movement. Extra, unintended movements disrupt the smooth, coordinated nature of voluntary movement attempts. Movement disruptions may be seen as

BOX 5-5	General Dysphagia Consideration in Patients with Basal Ganglia Deficits

- Poor bolus control: involuntary movements
  - Oral
  - Oropharyngeal
- Residue from inefficient swallow
  - Oral
  - Oropharyngeal
  - Pharyngeal
- Difference among swallow types
  - Automatic versus intentional movements
- Severity dependent

tremor, regular **clonic movements**, slow sustained postural interruptions (**dystonias**), or other unintentional movements superimposed on the normal resting state of muscle groups or during intended movements. Box 5-5 lists general swallowing problems that may be associated with various characteristics of basal ganglia deficits.

SUBCORTICAL FUNCTIONS AND SWALLOWING IMPAIRMENT: PARKINSON'S DISEASE

Parkinson's disease (PD) is a slowly progressive disease of the basal ganglia. The key problem is an impairment in the execution of voluntary movement. The classic features of PD include **resting tremor**, **bradykinesia**, and **rigidity**. The cause of this disease is essentially unknown, but the immediate cause for the motor changes is the depletion of the neurochemical dopamine, which results in impaired basal ganglia functioning during voluntary movements. These changes may also result from long-term use of certain medications and/or be part of more encompassing degenerative diseases that can influence basal ganglia performance.[77-79]

Patients with PD may present with a variety of interrelated clinical signs. They may demonstrate slowness in cognitive tasks and in some cases a form of dementia. As the disease progresses, they may show a masklike face that appears expressionless. They often demonstrate a characteristic dysarthria, impaired writing (**micrographia**), changes in body posture and gait, and other potential changes associated with reduced movement ability or instability. The progression of PD varies among patients, and no cure currently exists for PD. Medical management consists primarily of medications, although recent efforts have described surgical approaches to management.

Swallowing deficits in patients with PD are common and reflect the underlying motor impairments, the extent of the disease progression, and potentially the effects of medications. Miller et al.[80] identified dysphagia in 84% of a sample of 137 adults with PD; 23% demonstrated severe dysphagia and could not complete a 150-mL water swallowing task. These prevalence data may be lower than the true clinical picture because patients, especially those in the earlier, milder stages of the disease, do not reliably report swallowing difficulties.[80,81] In general, oropharyngeal swallowing deficits may result from poor bolus control caused by involuntary movements or from residue or misdirection of the bolus from an inefficient, possibly weakened swallow. In addition, an overall slowness characterizes swallowing deficits in patients with PD that may reflect the degree of underlying bradykinesia.[82] Box 5-6 lists some of the oropharyngeal swallowing-related deficits in patients with PD.

Drooling, in some contexts termed **sialorrhea**, is a common problem for patients with PD and may be related to the presence and severity of dysphagia.[83] Results from preliminary studies have suggested that patients with **diurnal** sialorrhea are at increased risk for silent aspiration,[84] which may, in turn, increase their risk for respiratory infections and subsequent death.[85] These risks are higher in later stages of the disease and in patients with severe sialorrhea.

Swallowing deficits in PD extend beyond the oral and pharyngeal components of the swallowing mechanism. Gross et al.[86] describe impaired coordination between swallowing and respiration that may contribute to reduced airway protection during swallowing. Moreover, various esophageal abnormalities have been reported, including delayed transport through the esophagus, esophageal stasis, abnormal contractions, and lower esophageal abnormalities.[81] Patients with PD have been reported to demonstrate problems farther along the digestive tract—**gastroparesis** and various defecatory dysfunctions.[87] Again, these irregularities may be related to the movement disorder and/or the influence to some of the medications used to treat the disease. Still, dysphagia clinicians should at least discuss the entire spectrum of gastrointestinal functions in evaluating dysphagia in patients with PD.

It is important to remember that patients with PD must cope with a widespread assortment of daily problems resulting from the disease and, at times, from the treatments for the disease. These deficits extend beyond the swallowing mechanism and may affect related acts such as food shopping, preparation of meals, and self-feeding activities.[88] Thus dysphagia in patients with PD and associated daily activities may contribute to increased patient and caregiver burden.[89] In the absence of appropriate support systems, these dysphagia-related impairments could have a direct, and potentially negative, influence on the nutritional and health status of individual patients.

Treatment Considerations

Clinical research on the effectiveness of dysphagia therapy for patients with PD is limited. In fact, a systematic review by Baijens and Speyer[90] identified only 16 articles describing rehabilitative, surgical, pharmacologic, or other therapies for swallow difficulties in PD. Not surprisingly, each article reported some degree of positive benefit from its particular intervention(s). In fact, it is conceivable that a variety of interventions may improve some aspects of swallow function in patients with PD. For example, Felix et al.[91] reported improved swallowing of water and to a lesser extent biscuits after a 2-week period of performing the effortful swallow technique with adjunctive biofeedback. El Sharkawi et al.[92] reported that some swallowing variables improved after 1 month of Lee Silverman Voice Treatment (LSVT). LSVT is a well-known therapy for speech and voice improvement in patients with PD. This study examined the **cross-system effect** of LSVT on swallowing performance. Finally, Pitts et al.[93] reported that 4 weeks of expiratory muscle strength training improved both voluntary cough and some swallowing parameters. Collectively, these studies represent a wide range of

BOX 5-6	**Oropharyngeal Swallowing Deficits in Patients with Basal Ganglia Deficits (Parkinson's Disease)**

ORAL STAGE
- Lingual tremor
- Repetitive tongue pumping*
- Prolonged ramplike posture
- Piecemeal deglutition
- Velar tremor
- Buccal retention*

PHARYNGEAL STAGE
- Vallecular retention*
- Piriform sinus retention
- Impaired laryngeal elevation*
- Airway (supraglottic) penetration
- Aspiration
- Pharyngoesophageal segment dysfunction

*More commonly observed characteristics.

behavioral interventions both in terms of the focus and outcomes of therapy. However, each intervention may be appropriate and helpful to select individual patients with dysphagia attributable to PD. In addition, dysphagia clinicians are advised to remember that medical and surgical interventions may be appropriate for certain patients. From an evidence-based perspective, the available literature reflects small numbers of patients with generally weaker study designs. As the clinical sciences mature, the expectation is that clinicians and patients will benefit from more rigorous knowledge on the effectiveness of various dysphagia interventions for patients with PD.

As with all dysphagias, treatment planning interacts with an understanding of the underlying mechanisms contributing to the dysphagia. In addition, because PD is a progressive disease, intervention strategies are expected to change. Finally, some evidence suggests that medications may have a positive effect on swallowing function in patients with PD[94]; however, this benefit may not extend to all patients or to some aspects of swallow function.[95] Because medications tend to work in time cycles, it may be important to time meals in relation to the maximum beneficial effect of medications. Finally, Table 5-3 summarizes intervention strategies recommended by Yorkston et al.[96] that may be appropriate for patients with PD. Although clinicians should not limit treatment options to those listed in the table, the recommendations do reflect the changing nature of dysphagia in PD over time and represent a range of potential interventions from patient counseling and education to modifying swallowing activity to adjusting diets. As such, this information may serve as a general guide to dysphagia clinicians with common sense suggestions at various severity levels of PD.

BRAINSTEM FUNCTIONS

The brainstem is much like a junction box. Here the major ascending sensory tracts receive input from the head and neck region by way of the cranial nerves. The head and neck musculature also receives motor innervation from the upper motor neurons of the corticobulbar system. These upper motor neurons synapse with the motor components of the individual cranial nerves, which function as **lower motor neurons**. Thus damage to the brainstem typically results in sensory deficits to the head and neck region in addition to motor deficits associated with both upper and lower motor neuron damage. The first of these is characterized by spastic weakness and associated movement impairments, whereas the second is characterized by flaccid weakness and associated movement impairments.

TABLE 5-3

Summary of Swallowing Interventions in Parkinson's Disease

	Normal Swallow	Early Swallowing Problems	Moderate Swallowing Disability	Severe Swallowing Disability
Presenting features	No observable changes	Reduction in pharyngeal peristalsis	Pharyngeal peristalsis worsens	Aspiration both during and after swallow
		Repetitive rocking motion of the tongue	Delay in swallowing reflex	
			Cricopharyngeal dysfunction	
			Laryngeal closure during swallowing may be inadequate	
Intervention	Monitor weight	Provide counseling to bring swallowing under voluntary control	Introduce aids and devices to promote independence	Teach chin-tuck swallowing
	Answer questions	Monitor weight	Increase sensory input	Switch to soft diet
		Coordinate eating with drug cycle	Teach double swallow	
			Recommend small, frequent, highly nutritious meals	

From Yorkston KM, Miller RM, Strand EA: *Management of speech and swallowing in degenerative diseases*, Tucson, AZ, 1995, Communication Skills Builders.

Years ago I saw a patient with PD for whom a feeding tube was being considered. I do not recall the stage of the disease, but he was nonambulatory outside his home, had some obvious degree of rigidity, and presented with a significant dysarthria (likely a 4 or 5 on the Hoehn and Yahr functional rating scale). I do remember that his wife was pleading with me and the radiologist to recommend that this patient could continue oral feeding, even if a feeding tube had to be placed for nutritional support. He had already had one episode of pneumonia, which prompted his referral for swallowing evaluation. Furthermore, the wife insisted that her husband could drink milkshakes at home with no difficulty.

Initially, the fluorographic swallow evaluation incorporated small volumes (5 mL or less) of thin liquid, thickened liquid, and pudding material provided to the patient by spoon. As expected, we noted poor oral control with material entering the pharynx before the airway was closed. We also noticed residue that increased in amount as the thickness of swallowed material increased. Given the wife's report of successful milkshake drinking at home, we provided the patient with a cup of nectar-thickened liquid and a straw. To our surprise, his swallow improved dramatically under this condition. We observed no aspiration and only a small amount of residue once the sequence of multiple swallows was completed. This patient continued to take oral nutrition oral supplements by mouth that were adequate for a short period. Even after a feeding tube was placed, he was able to continue drinking milkshakes by straw.

CRITICAL THINKING

1. How would you explain the difference in swallowing performance based on straw drinking versus small volumes taken by spoon provided by the examiner? Consider neurologic, swallow mechanics, and context variables in your discussion.

2. Do you think this distinction may be specific to patients with PD or might other patients respond in a similar manner?

3. When do you think it is appropriate to evaluate swallowing abilities in patients diagnosed with PD?

 Refer to Video 5-4 on the Evolve site for an example of how different swallowing strategies and different bolus volumes may affect swallow function in a patient with PD. The initial swallow is a thick liquid presented by the clinician from a spoon. Subsequent swallows are taken sequentially by the patient with a straw.

The brainstem also is believed to be home to a "swallowing center" located in the rostral brainstem.[97,98] This group of nuclei (often focusing on the nucleus tractus solitarius) is believed to facilitate coordination among the various components of the swallowing mechanism (oral, pharyngeal, esophageal) and coordinate swallowing functions with respiration. Individuals with damage to this area of the brainstem usually demonstrate a severe dysphagia in addition to the basic sensory and motor signs associated with brainstem deficits.

Brainstem Functions and Swallowing Impairment

Swallowing deficits subsequent to brainstem stroke provide a good example of the relation between neurologic deficits and dysphagia. In general, dysphagia in brainstem stroke involves two aspects: incoordination presumably related to disruption of the "swallowing center" and weakness resulting from damage to the corticobulbar system (sensory deficits also may be present). The collective effects of these deficits often are manifest clinically as incoordination among "stages" of swallowing and between swallowing and respiration, as well as weakness in one or more of the muscle groups innervated by the corticobulbar system (velum, pharynx, larynx, pharyngoesophageal segment). The resulting swallow has been described as the *incomplete swallow*.[43,99] Although *incomplete swallow* is not a specific term, it does offer an overt description of the impairment in swallow physiology observed in these patients. Box 5-7 summarizes features of the incomplete swallow often seen in patients with dysphagia subsequent to brainstem stroke. Videos 5-5, *A* and *B* on the companion Evolve site show endoscopic and fluoroscopic examples of the swallow incoordination typically seen after brainstem impairment. In this specific case, the patient had a tumor in the medulla. The author saw him nearly 3

BOX 5-7	Pharyngeal Swallowing Deficits in Patients After Brainstem Stroke

- Absent or delayed pharyngeal response
- Reduced hyolaryngeal elevation
- Reduced oropharyngeal constriction
- Reduced pharyngeal constriction
- Reduced laryngeal closure
- Reduced pharyngoesophageal segment opening
- Brief swallow event
- Generalized incoordination (including respiration)

years after medical treatment. He presented with deficits to cranial nerves X and XII on the left and was dependent on a feeding tube. Two months before the evaluation he had a thyroplasty to medialize a paralyzed left vocal fold.

Treatment Considerations

Similar to hemispheric stroke patients, patients with brainstem stroke recover some degree of swallow function over time.[100] Likewise, the clinical presentation of dysphagia and comorbid conditions varies considerably. Given these perspectives, treatment approaches to dysphagia in the patient who has survived a brainstem stroke are symptomatic and change over time.

A careful assessment of the components of dysphagia and related deficits is mandatory in this group of patients. For example, the patient requiring tracheostomy for respiratory support presents a different clinical profile than does the patient who does not require tracheostomy. The patient with minimal cranial nerve deficits may have better physiologic support for rehabilitative efforts than the patient with multiple cranial nerve deficits. And the nonambulatory patient presents different challenges than the patient who can walk assisted or unassisted.

In the acute poststroke phase, intervention tends to be more cautious with a prophylactic component. At this point the patient may be at greatest risk for pulmonary complications from inappropriate oral intake. Depending on the severity of neurologic impairment and the overall health status of the patient, treatment strategies at this stage may range from nothing (monitoring recovery) to passive sensorimotor activities (oral hygiene and/or movement exercises) to more active swallowing efforts involving compensatory maneuvers (postural adjustments, changes in the swallow behavior, etc.).

Because recovery facilitates an overall improvement in the patient's health status, dysphagia intervention may be more direct and aggressive. At some point the need for continuation of tracheostomy tubes should be addressed. Direct and intensive swallowing rehabilitation has been effective in facilitating return to oral feeding in chronic patients.[43-45] Although limited, clinical research has suggested that therapy approaches focused on increasing strength and coordination of swallowing are likely to improve swallow function (see Chapter 14 for examples of therapy approaches). The key for the dysphagia specialist is interaction with medical and other rehabilitative specialists to understand the patient's larger health status picture and selection of treatment strategies consistent with the patient's global needs and still provide the potential for improved swallowing function.

The Role of the Cerebellum in Swallowing

The *cerebellum* is adjacent to the brainstem and is located posterior and slightly superior to most brainstem structures. The role of the cerebellum in the control of swallowing is poorly understood. This structure does appear to play a role in swallow activity; several functional imaging studies have demonstrated activation, often bilateral activation, in the cerebellum on volitional swallowing.[101-103] From a clinical perspective, cerebellar damage results in unsteadiness (**ataxia**), **intention tremor** (tremor that is exaggerated at the initiation of movement), and **hypotonia** (low muscular tone). When present in the swallowing mechanism, these movement deficits are expected to impair coordinated swallowing functions. Motor unsteadiness and weakness resulting from cerebellar damage may contribute to difficulty in controlling a bolus, directing that bolus in a timely fashion, and residue from reduced swallowing effort. Video 5-6 on the companion Evolve site presents an endoscopic swallowing examination of a patient with cerebellar deficit who demonstrates tremor that contributes to poor oral control of a liquid bolus with subsequent aspiration.

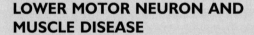

LOWER MOTOR NEURON AND MUSCLE DISEASE

Lower motor neurons proceed through the body and connect with muscles at the **myoneural junction**. Deficits to the peripheral nerves or the myoneural junction produce flaccid weakness. However, myoneural junction deficits demonstrate significant deterioration of motor function with use but recovery with extended rest.

The end points in the sensorimotor chain of events are the muscle and sensory end organs. Motor impairments at the muscle level are termed **myopathies**. These are characterized by a severe flaccid weakness within the affected muscle groups. Sensory loss may come in many forms, resulting from both neurologic and nonneurologic processes. Reduction or loss of tactile sensation is considered particularly important in swallowing problems because it may lead to unawareness of residual food along the swallowing mechanism or it may contribute directly to aspiration of food and liquid materials into the airway.

Lower Motor Neuron Functions and Swallowing Impairment

Amyotrophic lateral sclerosis (ALS) is one disease that reflects the relation between lower motor neuron impairment and dysphagia. ALS, sometimes referred to as Lou Gehrig's disease or motor neuron disease, is a progressive degenerative disease of unknown cause. The clinical presentation is progressive weakness; approximately 30% of patients show the initial effects of this disease in the corticobulbar musculature.[104] When present, corticobulbar deficits contribute to a significant and progressive dysphagia.

Neurologic deficits in ALS are not confined to the lower motor neurons of the peripheral nervous system. Central nervous system structures also are involved. As a result, the motor deficits in ALS are mixed—incorporating both flaccid (lower motor neuron) and spastic (upper motor neuron) weakness. The mixture of flaccid and spastic weakness may be seen in the musculature of the swallowing mechanism, in the respiratory musculature, and throughout the remainder of the body. ALS is progressive and terminal, and although many patients survive for longer than 5 years, the majority do not.[104] Substantial variability in progression rates exists among individuals. Respiratory failure is a common cause of death. Available research suggests that the different subtypes of ALS do not progress differentially.[105]

In addition to dysphagia, individuals with ALS experience movement difficulties with the arms and legs, dysarthria, respiratory decline from chest muscle weakness and, in some cases (though rare), cognitive changes (including **emotional lability** and dementia). Obviously the impact of this disease on all aspects of daily functions is severe. These factors certainly are considered in planning any rehabilitative efforts, including swallowing rehabilitation.

Swallowing deficits are progressive and widespread. As might be expected, they reflect a weakness across the muscle groups used to prepare and transport a bolus. Early in the course of the disease, dysphagia may be characterized by oral limitations resulting from lingual weakness.[106] In addition to poor oral transport of a bolus, patients with ALS, even those with no bulbar symptoms, demonstrate pharyngeal residue.[107] However, pharyngeal esophageal segment opening and laryngeal elevation may demonstrate relative maintenance even in advanced dysphagia.[107] As might be expected, respiratory aspects of swallowing are negatively affected in ALS. Nozaki et al.[108] reported that swallow apnea, or **hypopnea**, was

increased in patients with ALS and that patients with severe respiratory limitations or presence of aspiration on fluoroscopic swallow examination presented the longest apnea durations. General considerations for dysphagia are listed in Box 5-8, and specific dysphagia characteristics are presented in Box 5-9. In general, these deficits reflect limitations in oral bolus control, reduced ability to transport the bolus with resulting residue, and reduced airway protection. Because lingual weakness is an early aspect of dysphagia in ALS, it is not surprising that speech production also is affected. In fact, speech and swallow functions in ALS tend to show a highly related course of deterioration.

BOX 5-8   **General Dysphagia Considerations in Patients with ALS and Associated Sensorimotor Deficits**

- Oral control of bolus
  - Perioral weakness
  - Lingual weakness
- Reduced transport
  - Velar leak
  - Reduced tongue pump
  - Reduced pharyngeal contraction
- Residue
- Airway protection
  - Bradykinesia
  - Residue

BOX 5-9   **Oropharyngeal Swallowing Deficits Seen in Patients with ALS**

ORAL STAGE
- Leakage
- Mastication
- Bolus formation
- Bolus transport
- Residual pooling

PHARYNGEAL STAGE
- Nasopharyngeal regurgitation
- Valleculae pooling
- Piriform sinus pooling
- Airway spillage
- Ineffective airway clearance
- Shortness of breath

Early in the disease course, no significant dysphagia may be reported. As weakness in the swallowing mechanism progresses, patients may have difficulty chewing solid food, loss of food or liquid from the lips, and food-specific difficulties. This may cause patients to begin to reject specific foods or to alter their diet or chewing or swallowing mechanics. As the disease progresses further, patients need more extensive diet modifications and risk rapid weight loss, leading to nutritional decline. This situation, perhaps combined with the loss of a positive social environment surrounding mealtimes, may lead to the decision to use an alternate feeding source (see Chapter 15). Initially, patients may be able to continue some oral feeding, but at some point total reliance on alternate feeding sources may occur. Table 5-4 summarizes a variety of intervention strategies suggested by Yorkston et al.[96] across various stages of severity in ALS.

Muscle Diseases and Swallowing Impairment

A variety of pathologic conditions may have a negative influence on muscles related to swallowing function. These diseases typically result in weakness in muscle groups that contribute to dysphagia. Examples of disease processes that might impair peripheral muscle function (in some cases including the peripheral nerve) include polyneuropathy, myasthenia gravis, polymyositis, scleroderma, systemic lupus erythematosus, and dystrophy. Unless working as part of a specialized health care team, the typical dysphagia specialist does not encounter large numbers of patients with these disorders or diseases. However, it is important to recognize the potential impact of each condition on swallowing function and to be able to differentiate other causes of dysphagia from these clinical conditions. From that perspective, each of these muscle diseases with the potential to affect swallowing function is discussed briefly in relation to dysphagia characteristics.

Polyneuropathy

Literally meaning "pathology to many nerves," polyneuropathies may result from many sources. Systemic diseases such as diabetes can result in polyneuropathies, as can other processes that affect peripheral nerves. Perhaps most common to dysphagia, and often forgotten, is the peripheral nerve damage that can result from radiotherapy in the treatment of head/neck cancer. These patients have fibrosis in tissue as well as nerve deficits in the affected areas (see Chapter 6). Weakness in peripheral nerves innervat-

Practice Note 5-5

A woman in her late 50s was referred for speech and swallow evaluation by her neurologist. Roughly 18 months before the evaluation she began to have speech difficulties. These were progressive, and roughly 5 months before the evaluation she noticed increased difficulty swallowing.

At the time of the clinical evaluation she was able to take all foods orally but she was avoiding "heavier" foods such as certain meats. She also engaged in swallow compensations, including cutting any masticated food into small pieces and using liquids to "wash" heavier food down when she ate them. She also reported difficulty with controlling oral secretions, with resultant drooling day and night.

On clinical examination this woman demonstrated a mixed dysarthria. The tongue presented with bilateral fasciculations but other cranial nerves were grossly intact. Her score on the Mann Assessment of Swallowing Ability (MASA; see Chapter 9) was 166 of 200, indicating moderate dysphagia. Her score on the speech scale of the ALS Severity Scale was 6, indicating the need to repeat some messages, and her score on the swallowing subscale was 7, reflecting her diet changes.

Endoscopic and fluoroscopic swallowing examinations are presented in Videos 5-7, *A* and *B* on the Evolve site. On endoscopic examination this patient demonstrates basic single and simple movement but impairment on rapid and/or sequential movements. Still, her swallow abilities seemed functional. On fluoroscopic examination, she demonstrated a pattern of slowness with possible weakness, but she again gave the impression of a functional swallow.

I saw her again 2 months later. At this point she demonstrated little clinical change, although her MASA score had lowered to 154 with noted changes in tongue function and increased coughing during meals. The patient was having obvious difficulty coping with the apparent diagnosis and indicated a desire for no further clinical follow-up. These wishes were respected and she has not returned for additional evaluation or clinical assistance or advice.

ing the swallowing musculature contributes directly to weakness in the muscles used for chewing and swallowing. Polyneuropathies also may result in sensory deficits with resulting impact on the ability to safely ingest food and liquid. Guillain-Barré syndrome is one example of a neurogenic polyneuropa-

TABLE 5-4				
Summary of Swallowing Interventions in ALS				
	Early Swallowing Problems	**Dietary Consistency Changes**	**Unable to Meet Needs Orally**	**Salivary Problems**
Presenting features	Solid foods difficult to eat	Weight loss	Decline in calorie intake	Complaints of too much saliva
	Longer mealtimes	Chronic dehydration	Decline in fluid intake	Complaints of drooling
	Need for smaller bites	Loss of enjoyment	Food spillage from mouth	
			Respiratory fatigue	
Intervention	Use chin-tuck position	Change to soft diet	Insert PEG or insert nasogastric tube or insert intermittent orogastric tube	Maintain adequate hydration
	Maintain liquid intake	Maintain liquid intake		Use aspirator
	Try using a straw	Eat calorie-dense foods		Use medication
	Eliminate caffeine	Increase taste, temperature (colder), and texture sensations of liquids		Surgically relocate salivary ducts
	Use double swallow			
	Learn choking first aid			
	Avoid washing foods down with liquids			

PEG, Percutaneous endoscopic gastrostomy.
From Yorkston KM, Miller RM, Strand EA: *Management of speech and swallowing in degenerative diseases*, Tucson, AZ, 1995, Communication Skill Builders.

thy in adults. Nearly all patients with Guillain-Barré syndrome have some degree of dysphagia. According to Chen et al.,[109] the majority of patients present with moderate to severe pharyngeal dysphagia, but nearly half of the patients they studied also had oral-phase swallowing deficits. Most patients recovered swallowing functions to varying degrees, but those with more severe dysphagia later in the disease tended to have persistent complaints.

Myasthenia Gravis

Myasthenia gravis (MG) is a disease process in which the neurotransmitter substance between motor nerves and muscles is depleted with use. In this regard, initial movements (such as chewing) are often intact or at least at their strongest at the beginning of movement (such as a meal). With repeated use the muscles fatigue into a flaccid weakness. Thus any swallowing activity that requires sustained and/or repeated movement (i.e., most of them) results in fatigue and reduced function. Colton-Hudson et al.[110] described dysphagia characteristics in 20 adults with MG. These investigators reported oral and pharyngeal deficits in all patients, and approximately 30% demonstrated aspiration. In addition, Linke et al.[111] reported that esophageal transit often is compromised in MG. Thus patients with MG may present with dysphagia characteristics reflecting weakness along the entire

course of the upper swallowing mechanism. Finally, Warnecke et al.[112] used a fiberoptic examination of swallowing (FEES) examination (see Chapter 10) to evaluate the immediate impact of the Tensilon test. Injection of Tensilon into a symptomatic patient with MG reduced symptoms within a short time. These authors reported that the combination of the FEES examination and the Tensilon test represents a clinical tool useful in the early diagnosis of MG-related dysphagia.

Polymyositis, Scleroderma, and Systemic Lupus Erythematosus

Polymyositis, scleroderma, and systemic lupus erythematosus are inflammatory muscle diseases more generally classified as *connective tissue diseases*. A brief but informative summary of dysphagia in these diseases is provided by Sheehan.[113] *Polymyositis (dermatomyositis)* is an inflammation of striated muscle. It often is initially seen in proximal muscle groups, and when present in the head and neck musculature can contribute to oropharyngeal dysphagia. In these instances clinical characteristics may include nasopharyngeal regurgitation, residue in the pharynx, and airway compromise by food and/or liquid. Deficits of the cervical esophagus are also frequently reported.

Scleroderma (progressive systemic sclerosis) is an inflammation of smooth muscle tissue. In this respect dysphagia is often esophageal in nature, primarily resulting from dysfunction in the distal third of the esophagus. At some point in the disease process many patients with scleroderma experience solid food dysphagia as a result of esophageal dysfunction. However, oropharyngeal dysphagia also may be seen with this disease.

Systemic lupus erythematosus is a disease process that affects women more frequently than men. The clinical presentation may vary because the disease may involve many organ systems. The time course is also variable. Patients may demonstrate proximal muscle weakness (including head and neck musculature), cranial nerve abnormalities, or deficits in the central nervous system. Often the presentation is of acute deterioration with slow recovery between exacerbations. Many patients report esophageal-based dysphagias.

Other diseases in the category of connective tissue or systemic rheumatic diseases can contribute to dysphagia. The general presentation is fatigue, malaise, pain, reduced appetite, and often dysphagia. Dysphagia may present as oropharyngeal or esophageal or both. Often the determining factor is which muscle groups are involved.

Muscular Dystrophy

Muscular dystrophy is another muscle disease that can affect various muscle groups. One type of dystrophy that may directly contribute to dysphagia is *oculopharyngeal muscular dystrophy* (OPMD).[114,115] OPMD is a slowly progressive disorder characterized by dysphagia, dysarthria, **ptosis**, and face and trunk weakness. As the name implies, pharyngeal muscles are likely to be weakened and thus contribute to dysphagia. Depending on the stage of the disease, dysphagia may be mild or severe.

Treatment Considerations

Many diseases that affect lower motor neurons and/or peripheral muscle groups are progressive and thus present special challenges to the patient and the clinician. As with other neurogenic dysphagias, swallowing interventions often are symptomatic, reacting to the specific set of clinical circumstances presented at any given time. Various strategies may be used; these range from behavioral compensations to diet modifications. The use of strengthening exercises or related strategies may be questionable in some situations. Exercise fatigues muscle groups. If the underlying disease creates weakness in muscles required for swallowing, attempts to overexercise these same muscle groups may exaggerate the underlying weakness rather than ameliorate it. Thus it is important to understand the impact of the underlying neurologic condition on sensorimotor capability of the individual patient.

Clinicians attempting to improve swallowing function also must remember that these patients are receiving ongoing medical care. They often take multiple medications that may be changed from time to time. It is important for the dysphagia specialist to maintain good communication with other members of the health care team to understand better the impact of various medications and make optimum decisions about changes in the dysphagia management plan. Remember, many of these diseases are progressive, necessitating changes in dysphagia management strategies over time. Hillel and Miller[116] provide an excellent perspective on the team approach to management of dysphagia and other bulbar symptoms in patients with ALS. Much of their sage clinical advice is applicable to management of dysphagia in patients with other progressive neuromuscular diseases.

IDIOPATHIC OR IATROGENIC DISORDERS OF SWALLOWING THAT RESEMBLE NEUROGENIC DYSPHAGIA

A variety of contributing factors may create a neurogenic dysphagia in the absence of overt neurologic disease. These factors include undetected vascular

CLINICAL CORNER 5-3

A 75-year-old man was referred for evaluation of dysphonia and dysphagia after knee replacement surgery. His endoscopic swallow examination is presented in Video 5-8 on the Evolve site. Note the nonmoving left true vocal fold, weakness in the left hemipharynx, and pooled secretions.

CRITICAL THINKING

1. What factors might contribute to both dysphonia and dysphagia in this specific patient?

2. Speculate about the relation between knee surgery and dysphonia and dysphagia in this patient.

3. What is the clinical significance of the hemipharyngeal weakness "on top" of the nonmoving left true vocal fold? How might this affect treatment planning for this patient?

deficits (ministrokes), decompensation with advancing age, decompensation in complex medical conditions, medication-induced changes, initial symptoms of a progressive disease, and postsurgical changes.[117,118] When dysphagia appears to result from neurologic dysfunction in the absence of overt neurologic disease or damage, these factors should be considered. A good rule of thumb is to treat a suspected neurogenic dysphagia as the result of a neurologic process until proven otherwise.

TAKE HOME NOTES

1. Dysphagia resulting from neurologic disorders reflects the underlying sensorimotor characteristics of the neurologic deficit.
2. Treatment of neurogenic dysphagias is often symptomatic but relies heavily on a strong understanding of the underlying neurologic process. In many cases behavioral treatment interacts significantly with medical treatment.
3. Many neurogenic dysphagias change over time, necessitating different intervention strategies. Change may occur both toward recovery or deterioration of function depending on the specific neurologic disease or disorder.
4. Medical treatments (including surgery) for various neurologic diseases and disorders also contribute to dysphagia.
5. In the absence of overt neurologic disease, dysphagia that appears to be neurogenic should be considered reflective of an underlying neurologic cause until proven otherwise.

CLINICAL CASE EXAMPLE 5-1

A 69-year-old man had a brainstem stroke 7 months before seeking rehabilitation for dysphagia. The patient takes no food or liquid by mouth and is receiving all nutrition by PEG. He expectorates saliva into a cup except at nighttime. Within the past month he has tasted food but not attempted to swallow. His anxiety level is high about the possibility of aspiration but he is highly motivated to initiate oral feeding. He has experienced no chest infections or other complications since discharge from acute rehabilitation. Clinical examination revealed a left facial weakness but he was able to make a strong lip seal. He demonstrated right body weakness greater in the arm than the leg, and he was able to walk with a quad cane. Endoscopic evaluation revealed slight paresis of the left vocal fold and in the left hemipharynx. Fluoroscopic examination of swallowing function revealed incomplete swallow attempts with limited hyolaryngeal excursion, limited opening of the PES (a small amount of material entered the esophagus), post-swallow residue for thicker materials, and a small amount of aspiration with thin liquid. He demonstrated a strong reactive cough to the aspiration and the ability to clear residue back into the mouth, where it was expectorated.

INTERPRETATION

This patient would be considered in the chronic poststroke phase because more than 6 months have elapsed since his stroke. He has had no swallowing experience during that period, but the observation that he does not expectorate at night (and does not complain of a "soggy" pillow in the morning) possibly suggests that he is swallowing saliva while asleep. The fact that he has tasted food supports his motivation to undertake aggressive therapy. His anxiety about aspiration is understandable and may be a factor to consider once therapy begins. The fact that he has had no chest infections and no history of tracheostomy are positive indications for the respiratory system. Ambulatory status is considered a positive sign because active patients are believed to be less susceptible to respiratory infections than are bedridden patients. The alternating hemiplegia (left face, pharynx, and vocal fold versus right side of the body) is characteristic of brainstem stroke. The incomplete swallow is characterized by incoordination and limited excursion of movement of the hyolaryngeal complex with reduced PES opening. Material entering the esophagus is a positive finding, as is the strong reactive cough and the ability to clear residue.

This patient is a good candidate for direct, intensive swallowing therapy. An appropriate therapy program for this individual would address airway protection (either by choice of material to be swallowed or compensatory maneuver), hyolaryngeal excursion (increase upward and forward movement), and swallow coordination (in some cases, slowing the speed of the swallow with prolonged maneuvers may accomplish this outcome). If successful, the functional outcome should be increased oral intake of food and liquid.

CLINICAL CASE EXAMPLE 5-2

A 72-year-old woman presented to the clinic with a diagnosis of primary progressive aphasia. The primary complaint was weight loss and unfinished meals. The patient lived independently and attended an adult day-care facility where she reportedly was observed to cough during lunch. Her brother had a history of esophageal disease and a concern was expressed by the family. The patient was ambulatory and presented no overt physical impairments. She was limited in her ability to communicatively interact. Her expressive communication was limited to head nods and a few vocalizations but no meaningful words were produced. She was able to respond appropriately to many basic commands and requests and participated interactively with a dysphagia examination. Oral mechanism examination was unremarkable with no overt signs of corticobulbar deficit. Videofluorographic examination of swallowing was completed. The only mild abnormality was the observation that the patient tilted her head upward as she initiated a swallow and that oral initiation and transit were prolonged. Subsequently, a feeding examination was completed in which the patient was provided a tray of food and liquid (regular-grade diet) and requested to eat. She surveyed the tray of food and promptly began to eat using her fingers. She was handed a fork and used this appropriately until she faced a situation in which she had to cut her food. She was handed a knife and proceeded to use it as a fork. Despite multiple cues she persisted to use the knife as a fork and could not be encouraged to use two tools (knife and fork) simultaneously.

INTERPRETATION

This specific case contains features commonly associated with dementias (weight loss, reduce food intake, poor communicative interaction) in addition to a more rare and specific finding. *Primary progressive aphasia* is a form of dementia in which language skills are impaired early in the course of the dementia, rendering the initial symptoms to those of a progressive aphasia. The observations of utensil use by this patient suggest a form of apraxia that seemed specific to mealtime and self-feeding. Because at her age and in her situation these social functions were central to her life and her well-being, this form of apraxia

had a significant functional impact on her life. The immediate therapy for this individual was environmental. The family was instructed to prepare meals that could be eaten with a single utensil (i.e., fork or spoon). The patient was quite successful with this strategy. Also, it is important to take into consideration the progressive, deteriorating nature of dementia. Although the mealtime adjustment of a single utensil was effective in the short term, as this disease progresses, this patient would require additional strategies to ensure adequate nutrition and hydration. In this respect, her treatment plan must contain periodic and regular monitoring of the success of any adaptation used to maintain oral food and liquid intake and the nutritional consequences of that intake (see Video 5-3 on the accompanying Evolve site).

References

1. Duffy JR: *Motor speech disorders: substrates, differential diagnosis, and management*, ed 2, St Louis, 2005, Elsevier Mosby.

2. Humbert IA, Robins J: Normal swallowing and functional magnetic resonance imaging: a systematic review, *Dysphagia* 22:266, 2007.

3. Gonzalez-Fernandez M, Kleinman JT, Ky P et al: Supratentorial regions of acute ischemia associated with clinical important swallowing disorders: a pilot study, *Stroke* 39:3022, 2008.

4. Gordon C, Hewer RL, Wade DT: Dysphagia in acute stroke, *Br Med J (Clin Res Ed)* 295:411, 1987.

5. Schroeder MF, Daniels SK, McClain M et al: Clinical and cognitive predictors of swallowing recovery in stroke, *J Rehabil Res Devel* 43:301, 2006.

6. Hays NP, Robers SB: The anorexia of aging in humans, *Physiol Behav* 30:257, 2006.

7. Perlman PW, Cohen MA, Setzen M et al: The risk of aspiration of pureed food as determined by flexible endoscopic evaluation of swallowing with sensory testing, *Otolaryngol Head Neck Surg* 130:80, 2004.

8. Setzen M, Cohen MA, Mattucci KF et al: Laryngopharyngeal sensory deficits as a predictor of aspiration, *Otolaryngol Head Neck Surg* 124:622, 2001.

9. Ickenstein GW, Kelly PJ, Furie KL et al: Predictors of feeding gastrostomy removal in stroke patients with dysphagia, *J Stroke Cerebrovasc Dis* 12:169, 2003.

10. Michou E, Hamdy S: Cortical input in control of swallowing, *Curr Opin Otolaryngol Head Neck Surg* 17:166, 2009.

11. Hamdy S, Rothwell JC, Aziz Q et al: Organization and reorganization of human swallowing motor cortex: implications for recovery after stroke, *Clin Sci (Lond)* 99:151, 2000.

12. Hamdy S, Aziz Q, Rothwell JC et al: Recovery of swallowing after dysphagic stroke relates to functional reorganization in the intact motor cortex, *Gastroenterology* 115:1104, 1998.

13. Hamdy S, Aziz Q, Rothwell JC et al: The cortical topography of human swallowing musculature in health and disease, *Nat Med* 2:1217, 1996.

14. Mann G, Hankey GL, Cameron D: Swallow function after stroke: prognosis and prognostic factors at 6 months, *Stroke* 30:744, 1999.

15. Smithard DG, O'Neill PA, England RE et al: The natural history of dysphagia following stroke, *Dysphagia* 12:188, 1997.

16. Martino R, Foley N, Bhogal S et al: Dysphagia after stroke: incidence, diagnosis, and pulmonary complications, *Stroke* 36:2756, 2005.

17. Smithard DG, Smeeton NC, Wolfe CD: Long-term outcome after stroke: does dysphagia matter? *Age Ageing* 36:90, 2007.

18. Harraf F, Ward K, Man W et al: Transcranial magnetic stimulation study of expiratory muscle weakness in acute ischemic stroke, *Neurology* 71:2000, 2008.

19. Sulter G, Elting JW, Stewart R et al: Continuous pulse oximetry in acute hemiparetic stroke, *J Neurol Sci* 179:65, 2000.

20. Ali K, Cheek E, Sills S et al: Day-night differences in oxygen saturation and the frequency of desaturations in the first 24 hours in patients with acute stroke, *J Stroke Cerebrovasc Dis* 16:239, 2007.

21. Leslie P, Drinnan MJ, Ford GA et al: Resting respiration in dysphagic patients following acute stroke, *Dysphagia* 17:208, 2000.

22. Leslie P, Drinnan MJ, Ford GA et al: Swallow respiration patterns in dysphagic patients following acute stroke, *Dysphagia* 17:202, 2002.

23. Butler SG, Stuart A, Pressman H et al: Preliminary investigation of swallowing apnea duration and swallow/respiratory phase relationships in individuals with cerebral vascular accident, *Dysphagia* 22:215, 2007.

24. Bravata DM, Ho SY, Meehan TP et al: Readmission and death after hospitalization for acute ischemic stroke, *Stroke* 38:1899, 2007.

25. Saposnik G, Hill MD, O'Donnell M et al: Variables associated with 7-day, 30-day, and 1-year fatality after ischemic stroke, *Stroke* 39:2318, 2008.

26. Hinchey JA, Shephard T, Furie K et al: Formal dysphagia screening protocols prevent pneumonia, *Stroke* 36:1972, 2005.

27. Millns B, Gosney M, Jack CIA et al: Acute stroke predisposes to oral gram-negative bacilli—a cause of aspiration pneumonia? *Gerontology* 49:173, 2003.

28. Leibovitz A, Dan M, Zinger J et al: *Pseudomonas aeruginosa* and the oropharyngeal ecosystem of tube-fed patients, *Emerg Infect Dis* 9:956, 2003.

29. Langdon PC, Lee AH, Binns CW: High incidence of respiratory infections in "nil by mouth" tube-fed acute ischemic stroke patients, *Neuroepidemiology* 32:107, 2009.

30. Carnaby G, Hankey GJ, Pizzi J: Behavioural intervention for dysphagia in acute stroke: a randomized controlled trial, *Lancet Neurol* 5:31, 2006.

31. Kikiwada M, Iwamoto T, Takasaki M: Aspiration and infection in the elderly, *Drugs Aging* 22:115, 2005.

32. Axelsson K, Asplund K, Norberg A et al: Nutritional status in patients with acute stroke, *Acta Med Scand* 224:217, 1988.

33. Davalos A, Ricart W, Gonzalez-Huix F et al: Effect of malnutrition after acute stroke on clinical outcome, *Stroke* 27:1028, 1996.

34. Gariballa SE, Parker SG, Taub N et al: Influence of nutritional status on clinical outcome after acute stroke, *Am J Clin Nutr* 68:275, 1998.

35. Finestone HM, Greene-Finestone LS, Wilson ES et al: Malnutrition in stroke patients on the rehabilitation service and at follow-up: prevalence and predictors, *Arch Phys Med Rehabil* 76:310, 1995.

36. Crary MA, Carnaby-Mann GD, Miller L et al: Dysphagia and nutritional status at the time of hospital admission for ischemic stroke, *J Stroke Cerebrovasc Dis* 15:164, 2006.

37. Poels BJ, Brinkman-Zijiker HG, Dijkstra PU et al: Malnutrition, eating difficulties and feeding dependence in a stroke rehabilitation centre, *Disabil Rehabil* 28:637, 2006.

38. Yoo SH, Kim JS, Kwon SU et al: Undernutrition as a predictor of poor clinical outcomes in acute ischemic stroke patients, *Arch Neurol* 65:39, 2008.

39. Smithard DG, O'Neill PA, Park C et al: Complications and outcome following acute: does dysphagia matter? *Stroke* 27:1200, 1996.

40. Neumann S, Bartolome G, Buchholz D et al: Swallowing therapy of neurologic patients: correlation of outcome with pretreatment variables and therapeutic methods, *Dysphagia* 10:1, 1995.

41. Elmståhl S, Bülow M, Ekberg O et al: Treatment of dysphagia improves nutritional conditions in stroke patients, *Dysphagia* 14:61, 1999.

42. Foley N, Teasell R, Salter K et al: Dysphagia treatment post stroke: a systematic review or randomized controlled trials, *Age Ageing* 37:258, 2008.

43. Crary MA: A direct intervention program for chronic neurogenic dysphagia secondary to brainstem stroke, *Dysphagia* 10:6, 1995.

44. Huckabee ML, Cannito MP: Outcomes of swallowing rehabilitation in chronic brainstem dysphagia: a retrospective evaluation, *Dysphagia* 14:93, 1999.

45. Crary MA, Carnaby-Mann GD, Groher ME et al: Functional benefits of dysphagia using adjunctive sEMG biofeedback, *Dysphagia* 19:160, 2004.

46. Focht A: Differential diagnosis of dementia, *Geriatrics* 64:20, 2009.

47. Easterling C, Robbins J: Dementia and dysphagia, *Geriatr Nurs* 29:275, 2008.

48. Langmore SE, Olney RK, Lomen-Hoerth C et al: Dysphagia in patients with frontotemporal lobar dementia, *Arch Neurol* 64:58, 2007.

49. Kalia M: Dysphagia and aspiration pneumonia in patients with Alzheimer's disease, *Metabolism* 52:36, 2003.

50. Chouinard J: Dysphagia in Alzheimer disease: a review, *J Nutr Health Aging* 4:214, 2000.

51. Chouinard J, Lavigne E, Villeneuve C: Weight loss, dysphagia, and outcome in advanced dementia, *Dysphagia* 13:151, 1998.

52. Knol W, van Marum RJ, Jansen PA et al: Antipsychotic drug use and the risk of pneumonia in elderly people, *J Am Geriatr Soc* 56:661, 2008.

53. Priefer BA, Robbins J: Eating changes in mild-stage Alzheimer's disease: a pilot study, *Dysphagia* 12:212, 1997.

54. Rothan-Tondeur M, Meaume S, Girard L et al: Risk factors for nosocomial pneumonia in a geriatric hospital: a control-case one-center study, *J Am Geriatr Soc* 51:997, 2003.

55. Langmore SE, Skarupski KA, Park PS et al: Predictors of aspiration pneumonia in nursing home residents, *Dysphagia* 17:298, 2002.

56. Wada H, Nakajoh K, Satoh-Nakagawa T et al: Risk factors for aspiration pneumonia in Alzheimer's disease patients, *Gerontology* 47:271, 2001.

57. Ikeda M, Brown J, Holland AJ et al: Changes in appetite, food preference, and eating habits in frontotemporal dementia and Alzheimer's disease, *J Neurol Neurosurg Psychiatry* 73:371, 2002.

58. Volicer L: Goals of care in advanced dementia: quality of life, dignity, and comfort, *J Nutr Health Aging* 1:481, 2007.

59. Amella EJ: Feeding and hydration issues for older adults with dementia, *Nurs Clin North Am* 39:607, 2004.

60. Finucane TE, Christmas C, Travis K: Tube feeding in patients with advanced dementia, *JAMA* 282:1365, 1999.

61. Kuo S, Rhodes RL, Mitchell SL et al: Natural history of feeding-tube use in nursing home residents with advanced dementia, *J Am Med Dir Assoc* 10:264, 2009.

62. Sharp HM, Shega JW: Feeding tube placement in patients with advanced dementia: the beliefs and practice patterns of speech-language pathologists, *Am J Speech Lang Pathol* 2008 Dec 23 [Epub ahead of print].

63. Pelletier C: What do certified nurse assistants actually know about dysphagia and feeding nursing home residents? *Am J Speech Lang Pathol* 13:99, 2004.

64. Monteleoni C, Clark E: Using rapid-cycle quality improvement methodology to reduce feeding tubes in patients with advanced dementia: before and after study, *BMJ* 329:491, 2004.

65. Simmons SF, Schnelle JF: Individualized feeding assistance care for nursing home residents: staffing requirement to implement two interventions, *J Gerontol A Biol Sci Med Sci* 59:M966, 2004.

66. Mackay LE, Morgan AS, Bernstein BA: Swallowing disorders in severe brain injury: risk factors affecting return to oral intake, *Arch Phys Med Rehabil* 80:365, 1999.

67. Terré R, Mearin F: Prospective evaluation of oropharyngeal dysphagia after severe traumatic brain injury, *Brain Inj* 21:1411, 2007.

68. Hansen TS, Engberg AW, Larsen K: Functional oral intake and time to reach unrestricted dieting for patients with traumatic brain injury, *Arch Phys Med Rehabil* 89:1556, 2008.

69. Ward EC, Green K, Morton AL: Patterns and predictors of swallowing resolution following adult traumatic brain injury, *J Head Trauma Rehabil* 22:184, 2007.

70. Terré R, Mearin F: Evolution of tracheal aspiration in severe traumatic brain injury-related oropharyngeal dysphagia: 1-year longitudinal follow-up study, *Neurogastroenterol Motil* 21:361, 2009.

71. Woratyla SP, Morgan AS, Mackay L et al: Factors associated with early onset pneumonia in the severely brain-injured patient, *Conn Med* 59:643, 1995.

72. Hansen TS, Larsen K, Engberg AW: The association of functional oral intake and pneumonia in patients with severe traumatic brain injury, *Arch Phys Med Rehabil* 89:2114, 2008.

73. Sharma OP, Oswanski MR, Singer D et al: Swallowing disorders in trauma patients: impact of tracheostomy, *Am Surg* 73:1117, 2007.

74. Duong TT, Englander J, Wright J et al: Relationship between strength, balance, and swallowing deficits and outcomes after traumatic brain injury: a multicenter analysis, *Arch Phys Med Rehabil* 85:1291, 2004.

75. Cherney LR, Halper AS: Swallowing problems in adults with traumatic brain injury, *Semin Neurol* 16:349, 1996.

76. Schurr MJ, Ebner KA, Maser AL et al: Formal swallowing evaluation and therapy after traumatic brain injury improves dysphagia outcomes, *J Trauma* 46:817, 1999.

77. Harris MK, Shneyder N, Borazanci A et al: Movement disorders, *Med Clin North Am* 93:371, 2009.

78. Jankovic J: Parkinson's disease: clinical features and diagnosis, *J Neurol Neurosurg Psychiatry* 79:368, 2008.

79. Alverez MV, Evidente VG, Driver-Dunckley ED: Differentiating Parkinson's disease from other parkinsonian disorders, *Semin Neurol* 27:356, 2007.

80. Miller N, Allcock LM, Hildreth T et al: Swallowing problems in Parkinson's disease: frequency and clinical correlates, *J Neurol Neurosurg Psychiatry* 2008 Nov 21 [Epub ahead of print].

81. Potulska A, Friedman A, Królicki L et al: Swallowing disorders in Parkinson's disease, *Parkinsonism Relat Disord* 9:349, 2003.

82. Nagaya M, Kachi T, Yamada T et al: Videofluorographic study of swallowing in Parkinson's disease, *Dysphagia* 13:95, 1998.

83. Nóbrega AC, Rogrigues B, Torres AC et al: Is drooling secondary to a swallowing disorder in patients with Parkinson's disease? *Parkinsonism Relat Disord* 14:243, 2008.

84. Nóbrega AC, Rodrigues B, Melo A: Silent aspiration in Parkinson's disease patients with diurnal sialorrhea, *Clin Neurol Neurosurg* 110:117, 2008.

85. Nóbrega AC, Rodrigues B, Melo A: Is silent aspiration a risk factor for respiratory infection in Parkinson's disease patients? *Parkinsonism Relat Disord* 14:646, 2008.

86. Gross RD, Atwood CW, Ross SB et al: The coordination of breathing and swallowing in Parkinson's disease, *Dysphagia* 23:136, 2008.

87. Pfeiffer RF: Gastrointestinal dysfunction in Parkinson's disease, *Lancet Neurol* 2:107, 2003.

88. Andersson I, Sidenvall B: Case studies of food shopping, cooking and eating habits in older women with Parkinson's disease, *J Adv Nurs* 35:69, 2001.

89. Miller N, Noble E, Jones D et al: Hard to swallow: dysphagia in Parkinson's disease. *Age Ageing* 35:614, 2006.

90. Baijens LW, Speyer R: Effects of therapy for dysphagia in Parkinson's disease: systematic review, *Dysphagia* 24:91, 2009.

91. Felix VN, Corréa SM, Soares RJ: A therapeutic maneuver for oropharyngeal dysphagia in patients with Parkinson's disease, *Clinics* 63:661, 2008.

92. El Sharkawi A, Ramig L, Logemann JA et al: Swallowing and voice effects of Lee Silverman Voice Treatment (LSVT): a pilot study, *J Neurol Neurosurg Psychiatry* 72:31, 2002.

93. Pitts T, Bolser D, Rosenbek J et al: Impact of expiratory muscle strength training on voluntary cough and swallow function in Parkinson disease, *Chest* 135:1301, 2009.

94. Monte FS, da Silva-Júnior FR, Braga-Neto P et al: Swallowing abnormalities and dyskinesia in Parkinson's disease, *Mov Disord* 20:457, 2005.

95. Lim A, Leow L, Huckabee ML et al: A pilot study of respiration and swallowing integration in Parkinson's disease: "on" and "off" levodopa, *Dysphagia* 23:76, 2008.

96. Yorkston KM, Miller RM, Strand EA: *Management of speech and swallowing in degenerative diseases*, Tucson, AZ, 1995, Communication Skill Builders.

97. Miller AJ: *The neuroscientific principles of swallowing and dysphagia*, San Diego, 1999, Singular.

98. Lang IM: Brain stem control of the phases of swallowing, *Dysphagia* 2009 Apr 28 [Epub ahead of print].

99. Crary MA, Baldwin BO: Surface electromyographic characteristics of swallowing in dysphagia secondary to brainstem stroke, *Dysphagia* 12:180, 1997.

100. Chua KS, Kong KH: Functional outcome in brain stem stroke patients after rehabilitation, *Arch Phys Med Rehabil* 77:194, 1996.

101. Malandraki GA, Sutton BP, Perlman AL et al: Neural activation of swallowing and swallowing-related tasks in healthy young adults: an attempt to separate the components of deglutition, *Hum Brain Mapp* 2009 Feb 26 [Epub ahead of print].

102. Harris ML, Julyan P, Kulkarni B et al: Mapping metabolic brain activation during human volitional swallowing: a positron emission tomography using [18F] fluorodeoxyglucose, *J Cereb Blood Flow Metab* 25:520, 2005.

103. Suzuki M, Asada Y, Ito J et al: Activation of cerebellum and basal ganglia on volitional swallowing detected by functional magnetic resonance imaging, *Dysphagia* 18:71, 2003.

104. Wijesekera LC, Leigh PN: Amyotrophic lateral sclerosis, *Orphanet J Rare Dis* 2009 Feb3;4:3 [Epub ahead of print].

105. Magnus T, Beck M, Giess R et al: Disease progression in amyotrophic lateral sclerosis: predictors of survival, *Muscle Nerv* 25:709, 2002.

106. Kawai S, Tsukuda M, Mochimatsu I et al: A study of the early stage of dysphagia in amyotrophic lateral sclerosis, *Dysphagia* 18:1, 2003.

107. Higo R, Tayama N, Nito T: Longitudinal analysis of progression of dysphagia in amyotrophic lateral sclerosis, *Auris Nasus Larynx* 31:247, 2004.

108. Nozaki S, Sugishita S, Saito T et al: Prolonged apnea/hypopnea during water swallowing in patients with amyotrophic lateral sclerosis, *Rinsho Shinkeigaku* 48:634, 2008.

109. Chen MY, Donofrio PD, Frederick MG et al: Videofluoroscopic evaluation of patients with Guillain-Barré syndrome, *Dysphagia* 11:11, 1996.

110. Colton-Hudson A, Koopan WJ et al: A prospective assessment of the characteristics of dysphagia in myasthenia gravis, *Dysphagia* 17:147, 2002.

111. Linke R, Witt TN, Tatsch K: Assessment of esophageal function in patients with myasthenia gravis, *J Neurol* 250:601, 2003.

112. Warnecke T, Teismann I, Zimmerman J et al: Fiberoptic endoscopic evaluation of swallowing with simultaneous Tensilon application in diagnosis and therapy of myasthenia gravis, *J Neurol* 255:224, 2008.

113. Sheehan NJ: Dysphagia and other manifestations of oesophageal involvement in the musculoskeletal diseases, *Rheumatology (Oxford)* 47:746, 2008.

114. Rüegg S, Lehky Hagen M, Hohl U et al: Oculopharyngeal muscular dystrophy—an under-diagnosed disorder? *Swiss Med Wkly* 135:574, 2005.

115. Brais B, Rouleau GA, Bouchard JP et al: Oculopharyngeal muscular dystrophy, *Semin Neurol* 19:59, 1999.

116. Hillel AD, Miller RM: Management of bulbar symptoms in amyotrophic lateral sclerosis, *Adv Exp Med Biol* 209:201, 1987.

117. Buchholz DW: Neurogenic dysphagia: what is the cause when the cause is not obvious? *Dysphagia* 9:242, 1994.

118. Buchholz DW: Oropharyngeal dysphagia due to iatrogenic neurological dysfunction, *Dysphagia* 10:248, 1995.

Chapter 6

Dysphagia and Head/Neck Cancer

MICHAEL A. CRARY

OBJECTIVES

1. Define cancer and describe its potential impact on the individual patient.
2. Describe the various treatments for head/neck cancer and their side effects.
3. Describe factors that contribute to dysphagia in patients being treated for head/neck cancer.
4. Describe the dysphagia characteristics that might be associated with head/neck cancer treated with different modalities.
5. Elaborate on dysphagia-related complications seen in patients treated for head/neck cancer.
6. Discuss the when, what, and why aspects of dysphagia intervention for patients being treated for head/neck cancer. What are the anticipated outcomes for the various dysphagia interventions?

CANCER AS A DISEASE

Cancer is currently the second leading cause of death in the United States. An estimated half of all men and one third of all women will have some form of cancer. Millions of people are either living with cancer or have had cancer. These facts clearly indicate that prevention, early detection, and treatment of cancer, as well as appropriate rehabilitation for the cancer survivor, are among today's primary health concerns.

What Is Cancer?

Cancer is the result of cell growth that is out of control. In simple terms, cells become abnormal and grow rapidly, forming extra, unwanted, and potentially destructive tissue. This proliferation of cell growth is called **hyperplasia**. The abnormality that causes cancer cells results from damaged DNA within cells. This damaged DNA may be inherited or it may result from exposure to an environmental cause such as smoking. In fact, the primary risk factors for head and neck cancer (with the exception of nasopharyngeal cancer) have been identified as tobacco (including smokeless tobacco), heavy alcohol use, poor oral hygiene, and mechanical irritation.[1] One potential problem caused by these abnormal cancer cells is that they can travel to various places in the body, begin to grow and proliferate, and replace normal body cells. This traveling of cells is referred to as **metastasis**. Metastasis may occur when cancer cells enter the bloodstream or the **lymph** system and travel to a different part of the body.

Cancer usually forms as a *tumor,* which technically means a swelling or enlargement, although not all cancers form tumors and not all tumors are cancerous. Some tumors are **benign** rather than **malignant**. Different types of cancers grow at different rates, create different problems, and respond to different treatments. One way to conceptualize cancer is as a group of diseases with different symptoms and signs. *Symptoms* are noticed by a patient and taken as an indication that something is not right in the body. *Signs* are also indicative of health problems but are more definitive of disease as observed by a physician or other health care professional. Symptoms and signs of cancer may change as the disease changes over time. The specific symptoms and signs depend on the location of the cancer; the size of the tumor; direct impact on any surrounding organs, blood vessels, or nerves; and any metastasis of the cancer. Both general and specific symptoms have been associated as warning signs of cancer. These are summarized in Box 6-1.

BOX 6-1	General and Specific Signs Associated with Cancer (Not Specific to Head/Neck Cancer)

GENERAL CANCER WARNING SIGNS
- Unexplained weight loss
- Fever
- Fatigue
- Pain

SPECIFIC CANCER WARNING SIGNS
- Change in bowel or bladder function
- Sores that do not heal
- Unusual bleeding or discharge
- Thickening or a lump in any part of the body
- Indigestion or difficulty swallowing
- Recent change in a wart or mole
- Nagging cough or hoarseness

BOX 6-2	Salient Characteristics of Cancer-Related Fatigue

- Feeling tired, weary, or exhausted even after sleep
- Lacking energy to do regular daily activities
- Trouble concentrating, thinking clearly, or remembering
- Negative feelings, irritability, impatience, lack of motivation
- Lack of interest in day-to-day activities
- Less attention to daily appearance
- Spending more time lying in bed or sleeping

Different problems may be encountered depending on the type and location of a cancer. The symptoms listed in Box 6-1 provide general categories of problems that may be encountered. Pain is perhaps the most feared of cancer-related problems. Pain does not result from all cancers, but when it does occur it may be the result of tumor growth or result from the treatments used to eradicate the cancer. Another common problem is fatigue. Like pain, fatigue may result either directly from the cancer or as a side effect of cancer treatment. Box 6-2 summarizes some of the salient characteristics that may be associated with cancer-related fatigue.

Cancers may also contribute to significant weight loss and impaired immune function. These problems are not mutually exclusive because malnutrition also contributes to impaired immune function. Impaired immune function contributes to increased complications, poor wound healing, and opportunistic infections. Together, poor nutrition and impaired immune function may contribute to a less-optimistic outcome for patients with cancer. An estimated 30% to 50% of patients with head/neck cancer demonstrate some degree of malnutrition.[2] Up to half of patients with head/neck cancer reveal some degree of weight loss when cancer is first diagnosed.[3,4] Average weight loss has been estimated between 5% and 10% of baseline body weight.[4,5] Weight loss may result from reduced ingestion or digestion of food and/or impaired absorption or utilization of nutrients by the body in the presence of adequate food and liquid intake. This latter situation may be complicated by the need for increased caloric intake resulting from increased energy expenditure in some patients with cancer. Thus some patients have a biologic need for more caloric intake, but as a result of poor food and liquid intake, absorption, or utilization they actually have a significantly reduced caloric reservoir. This can become a vicious cycle leading to **cachexia**. Weight loss may be accompanied by **anorexia**, nausea and/or constipation, and fatigue. Box 6-3 summarizes some of the more general consequences of malnutrition in patients with head/neck cancer.

Early detection and timely treatment for cancers of the head/neck often are associated with improved outcomes. From that perspective, it is important to facilitate early recognition of the symptoms and signs of cancer and obtain appropriate medical diagnosis early in the course of the disease.

Diagnosis of Cancer

As noted, the initial indications of cancer are often symptoms identified by the patient. These should not be ignored because early detection and prompt treatment lead to a better outcome. Depending on the type and location of cancer, various diagnostic tests may be used. These tests are used to identify the specifics of the cancer and help plan the best possible treatment.

BOX 6-3	General Consequences of Malnutrition

- Increased susceptibility to infection
- Reduced immune functions
- Respiratory failure
- Poor wound healing
- Skin breakdown
- Death

Patients with head/neck cancer require careful examination by a multidisciplinary team of health care providers. Such teams may vary but a common core membership might include a head/neck surgeon, radiation oncologist, medical oncologist, dentist, social workers, and rehabilitation specialists. The goal of the team evaluation is to characterize the cancer and develop the best comprehensive treatment approach (including rehabilitation when indicated). The team may use a variety of diagnostic procedures, including radiography, computed tomographic and/or magnetic resonance imaging, endoscopy (including both laryngoscopy and esophagoscopy), biopsy and **histopathologic** confirmation, and physical examination.

Staging

A common procedure involved in evaluating cancer is *staging*. In simple terms, staging is the process of determining how far the cancer has spread. This process is important in determining the best treatment options, estimating complications or comorbid conditions, and formulating a prognosis. Although

CLINICAL CORNER 6-1

Some cancers are identified early, which is believed to lead to earlier treatment and better outcomes. In my practice, I typically ask patients what the initial signs were that "something was wrong." The answers vary greatly. Some men report that they felt a small lump (size of a pea) in their neck when shaving. Others have told me that their dentist found a growth during routine dental examination. Still others have reported sore throat, persistent dysphonia, or swallowing difficulties. However, the most unusual report was from an elderly man who indicated that he had trouble keeping his dentures in place. This man has a diagnosis of nasopharyngeal carcinoma (NPC). When I looked into his mouth, the reason for the ill-fitting dentures was obvious (see Figure 6-1, *A*). Subsequently on endoscopic examination the complete tumor was clearly seen (see Figure 6-1, *B*). Despite the size and location of this growth, this man reported no difficulties with either nasal breathing or the sense of smell.

Remember that NPC often has no early signs and these tumors may grow large before any overt signs are noted by the patient.

CRITICAL THINKING

1. What other head/neck cancer shares this dubious distinction?
2. How might NPC affect swallowing function?

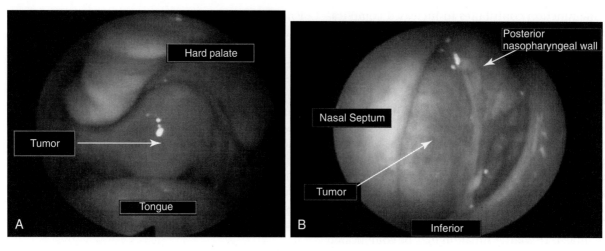

FIGURE 6-1. Photograph of a nasopharyngeal tumor protruding into oral cavity (**A**) and viewed with transnasal endoscopy (**B**).

more than one system is available for cancer staging, the TNM system is used most often.[6] *T* (tumor) describes the size of the tumor and extension into any neighboring tissues. *N* (nodes) describes any spread of the cancer into nearby lymph nodes. *M* (metastasis) describes spread of the cancer to other organ systems within the body. A number or additional letter after each letter is assigned to provide more detail. In general, lower numbers mean smaller, more localized cancers. Higher numbers mean larger, spreading cancers. Therefore a T1N0M0 tumor is small, has not invaded neighboring lymph nodes, and has not spread to other body organ systems. Conversely, a T4N2M1 tumor is large, has invaded neighboring lymph nodes, and has metastasized to other body organ systems. Box 6-4 lists TNM definitions for oropharyngeal cancer. Similar, but not identical, definitions are used for hypopharyngeal and laryngeal cancers. One difference is the inclusion of anatomic subsites for these latter areas.

After TNM description, cancers may be grouped together into stage classifications. In general, five stages are used (stage 0 through 4). Stage 4 has three subdivisions (A, B, and C). A lower stage classification indicates a smaller, nonmetastasized cancer. A higher stage classification indicates a more serious, widespread cancer. Box 6-5 shows the staging system based on TNM descriptions.

TREATMENTS FOR HEAD/NECK CANCERS

Many cancers of the head/neck region can be cured if they are found early. Choice of treatment and outcome

---

BOX 6-4	TNM Definitions for Oropharyngeal Cancer

PRIMARY TUMOR (T)

TX:	Primary tumor cannot be assessed
T0:	No evidence of primary tumor
Tis:	Carcinoma in situ
T1:	Tumor 2 cm or less in greatest dimension
T2:	Tumor more than 2 cm but not more than 4 cm in greatest dimension
T3:	Tumor more than 4 cm in greatest dimension
T4:	Tumor invades adjacent structures

REGIONAL LYMPH NODES (N)

NX:	Regional lymph nodes cannot be assessed
N0:	No regional lymph node metastasis
N1:	Metastasis in a single ipsilateral lymph node, 3 cm or less in greatest dimension
N2:	Metastasis in a single ipsilateral lymph node, more than 3 cm but not more than 6 cm in greatest dimension (N2a); or in multiple ipsilateral lymph nodes, none more than 6 cm in greatest dimension (N2b); or in bilateral or contralateral lymph nodes, none more than 6 cm in greatest dimension (N2c)
N3:	Metastasis in lymph node more than 6 cm in greatest dimension

DISTANT METASTASIS (M)

MX:	Distant metastasis cannot be assessed
M0:	No distant metastasis
M1:	Distant metastasis

frequently depend on many factors, including location and stage of the cancer, the patient's age and general health status, the experience of the medical team treating the patient, and available facilities. Although curing the cancer is a primary goal, the patient's posttreatment function and quality of life are also important considerations in choosing the type of treatment because each treatment has potential side effects and sequelae. Another aspect to consider is whether the treatment is intended to be **palliative** or curative. Three primary options are frequently used in the treatment of head/neck cancers: surgery, radiation, and chemotherapy. These may be used in isolation or in various combinations depending on the type of cancer and the goals of treatment. Surgery and radiation therapy are considered the only curative therapies for cancer in the head/neck region.

Chemotherapy is used in the **neoadjuvant** or **adjuvant** setting but is not considered a curative therapy.[7]

Surgery

Surgery refers to removal of the cancerous tumor and some of the surrounding healthy tissue, referred to as the *margin*. Surgery is intended to remove as much of the primary tumor as possible and leave no trace of cancer cells in the margin. However, this is not always possible, and surgery often is combined with radiation therapy and/or chemotherapy. In some cases, more than a single surgery may be required to remove the cancer or restore the anatomic or functional deficit caused by the primary surgery. For example, if the cancer has spread to the lymph nodes in the neck, the lymph nodes will be removed. This is called a *lymph node dissection* or a *neck dissection*. In other situations reconstruction may be required. This involves moving tissue from another part of the body to fill a gap created by the cancer **resection**. A variety of procedures have been described to relocate tissue to the head/neck region. Generally referred to as *flaps,* these are often named for the location from which the replacement tissue is taken. Therefore a pectoralis major flap would be constructed from tissue obtained from the pectoralis major muscle. Other flaps might include a lateral thigh flap, a radial forearm flap, or similar procedures. Figure 6-2 depicts a pectoralis major flap on the left side. Figure 6-3 shows a flap reconstruction of the floor of the mouth and tongue. In some situations bone tissue may be relocated to reconstruct bony deficits in the mandible, or if a majority of the mandible is removed an implant may be used to replace the missing bone (Figure 6-4). If surgical reconstruction is not feasible, a **prosthodontist** may be consulted to construct

BOX 6-5	Staging System for Oropharyngeal Cancer Based on TNM Descriptions
Stage 0:	Tis, N0, M0
Stage I:	T1, N0, M0
Stage II:	T2, N0, M0
Stage III:	T3, N0, M0
	T1, N1, M0
	T2, N1, M0
	T3, N1, M0
Stage IVA:	T4, N0, M0
	T4, N1, M0
	Any T, N2, M0
Stage IVB:	Any T, N3, M0
Stage IVC:	Any T, Any N, M1

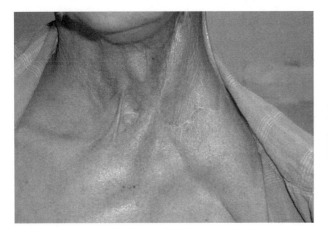

FIGURE 6-2. Photograph of a pectoralis major flap on the left side of the neck.

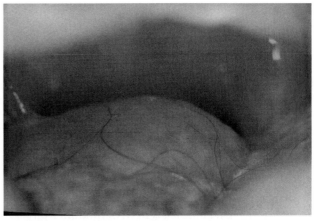

FIGURE 6-3. Photograph of a flap reconstruction of the tongue and floor of the mouth.

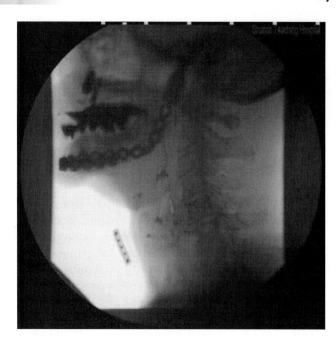

FIGURE 6-4. Example of mandibular reconstruction with an implant.

artificial dental or facial parts to fill a space created by the initial surgery. If the primary tumor surgery creates a risk to breathing, a **tracheotomy** may be performed. If severe swallowing problems are anticipated, a **gastrostomy** may be performed. Either or both of these procedures may be performed at the time of the primary cancer surgery if the surgical team anticipates airway or swallowing problems as a direct result of the surgery.

Surgery is a primary treatment consideration for all small cancers. Contraindications to surgical removal of a small tumor are the possibility of significant deficits to function (speaking, chewing, swallowing) or cosmetic defects. Advanced cancers often require a combination of surgery and/or radiation or chemotherapy. Various surgical approaches may be used depending on the location and size of the cancerous tumor. Box 6-6 lists some of the more common surgeries associated with head/neck cancer treatment.

Surgery, like other cancer treatments, has a number of side effects that can be problematic for patients. Side effects typically depend on the location and type of surgery. Some of these are temporary and others are more permanent. All side effects have an impact on the patient's quality of life. Box 6-7 lists some of the more frequent side effects from cancer surgery in the head/neck region. The length of time after surgery was performed is an indicator of the prominent side effects. For example, edema will be pronounced in the

| BOX 6-6 | Common Surgeries Associated with Head and Neck Cancer Treatment |

Primary tumor surgery: removal of tumor and surrounding tissue

Mandibulectomy: removal of a piece of the jawbone

Mandibulotomy: splitting the mandible to gain access to a tumor

Maxillectomy: removing all or part of the hard palate

Mohs surgery: removal of a tumor in thin slices, evaluating each slice under a microscope for cancer cells until all cancer cells are gone

Laser surgery: using a narrow, intense beam of light to remove cancer

Laryngectomy: removal of the entire larynx

Partial laryngectomy: removal of part of the larynx: supraglottic, hemilaryngectomy, supracricoid, vocal cord

Laryngopharyngectomy: removal of larynx and pharynx

Tracheostomy: establishing a hole in the anterior neck (stoma) into the trachea to establish an airway

Gastrostomy: creating a fistula into the stomach by way of the abdominal wall; often used to place a feeding tube

Neck dissection: removal of lymph nodes and other tissue in the neck considered at risk for metastatic disease; radical neck dissection involves more tissue removal than modified neck dissection

Reconstructive surgery: any surgery that attempts to replace missing anatomy to improve function and/or appearance

| BOX 6-7 | Potential Side Effects of Surgery to Treat Head/Neck Cancer |

- Swelling of the mouth and/or throat, resulting in difficulty breathing
- Impaired speech and/or voice
- Difficulty chewing and swallowing
- Facial disfigurement
- Numbness in the face, neck, or throat
- Reduced mobility in the neck and shoulder area
- Decreased function of the thyroid gland

acute postoperative period. Edema may be accompanied by pain. As the primary surgical site heals, scarring may reduce movement of anatomic structures spared and in the vicinity of the surgery. In addition, if cranial nerves are damaged during the primary surgery or as a result of postoperative scarring, the patient may sustain motor or sensory deficits from nerve damage.

Radiation Therapy

Radiation therapy uses high-energy x-rays to kill cancer cells. Death of the cancer cells leads to shrinkage of the tumor. Radiation therapy may be used as the primary treatment for small tumors, after surgery to destroy residual small pockets of cancer cells, or before surgery to shrink tumors in the hope of more successful surgical removal with fewer residual deficits. Radiation may be administered in two ways: external-beam radiation and internal radiation. *External-beam radiation* involves aiming a high-energy radiation beam at the tumor and surrounding tissues. External-beam radiation may be applied on a conventional, once-daily schedule or on an altered fractionation schedule. The latter form of radiation therapy may increase acute toxicity, but late effects are similar between these two techniques.[7] A newer form of external-beam radiation is known as *intensity-modulated radiation therapy*. This procedure allows more effective doses of radiation to be delivered to the tumor while hitting less healthy tissue around the tumor. This method is intended to result in fewer side effects. Other recent advances in radiotherapy include *radiosensitization* (using drugs to make cancer cells more sensitive to radiation) and *hyperfractionation* (giving radiation in small doses several times per day). In general, treatment strategies leading to a lower dose of radiotherapy or radiotherapy to more confined anatomic regions results in less-severe and more transient dysphagia.[8-10]

Internal radiation therapy, often referred to as **brachytherapy,** involves implanting small pellets or rods containing radioactive material into the cancer or near the cancer site. Patients remain hospitalized during this procedure while the implants remain in place.

Side effects from radiation therapy are common both during treatment (acute toxicity) and after treatment (late effects or late toxicity). Some of these effects are transient and others are persistent. In addition, certain side effects may be latent—that is, they may not appear for a substantial period (in some cases years) after the completion of radiation therapy. Many side effects of radiation therapy to the head/neck region contribute directly to dysphagia and resulting decline in nutritional status. If these occur during treatment, patients may experience interruptions in therapy. Box 6-8 lists several side effects that may occur from radiation therapy to the head/neck region.

BOX 6-8	Potential Side Effects of Radiation Therapy to Treat Head/Neck Cancer

- Redness and skin irritation in area treated
- Permanent change to salivary glands leading to persistent dry mouth or thickened saliva
- Bone pain
- Nausea and vomiting
- Fatigue
- Mouth sores and/or sore throat
- Dental problems
- Painful swallowing
- Loss of appetite
- Reduced sense of taste (and sometimes smell)
- Earaches resulting from hardening of ear wax
- Hypothyroidism
- Fibrosis leading to reduced movement
- Peripheral neuropathy
- Bone, cartilage, soft tissue necrosis

Before the initiation of radiation therapy, all patients should undergo a complete dental examination. Damaged or decayed teeth may need to be removed because radiation can cause tooth decay. Also, patients who receive radiation to the anterior neck region are at risk for damage to the thyroid gland, contributing to **hypothyroidism**. This condition may worsen any feelings of fatigue already experienced by the patient. For these patients, thyroid gland function should be monitored on a regular basis.

Chemotherapy

Chemotherapy refers to the use of drugs to kill cancer cells. These agents are typically very powerful drugs that can cause several unpleasant side effects. Chemotherapy may be administered by mouth, intravenously, by injection into a muscle or under the skin, or by injection directly into the tumor. Chemotherapy may be used to palliate symptoms in patients with incurable disease or as an adjuvant to radiation therapy, surgery, or both. Chemotherapy may be used before or after surgery (and/or radiation therapy). Chemotherapy has been used in combination with radiation therapy to treat certain laryngeal cancers in an attempt to preserve the larynx (avoid a total laryngectomy) and subsequent voice functions. As previously mentioned, certain drugs may be used in combination with radiation therapy as a form of

BOX 6-9	Potential Side Effects from Chemotherapy to Treat Head/Neck Cancer

- Fatigue
- Nausea and vomiting
- Hair loss
- Dry mouth
- Loss of appetite
- Reduced sense of taste
- Weakened immune system
- Diarrhea and/or constipation
- Open sores in the mouth potentially leading to infection

radiosensitization. Although these approaches are promising, many combined therapies are still considered experimental. One negative aspect of combined therapies is the risk of increased severity or a wider range of side effects. For example, large clinical studies reported increased acute toxicity in patients receiving concomitant chemoradiation therapy.[11] However, at least one review has concluded that posttreatment swallowing dysfunctions noted in patients receiving concomitant chemoradiation therapy were similar to those seen in patients receiving only radiation therapy.[12] Box 6-9 lists several possible side effects from chemotherapy in the treatment of head/neck cancer. Each patient should be evaluated for the presence of one or more of these possible side effects resulting from primary cancer treatments that may affect swallowing function.

DYSPHAGIA IN PATIENTS WITH HEAD/NECK CANCER

Many—in fact, a majority—of patients treated for head/neck cancer have some degree of swallowing difficulty. Some dysphagia symptoms result directly from the cancer and thus may be present before medical treatment, whereas others are the result of various treatments for the cancer. In general, patients receiving radiation therapy (alone or in combination with surgery) are at greater risk for swallowing difficulties than are patients receiving surgical treatments without radiation.[13-15] Dysphagia subsequent to cancer treatments may be described as resulting from reduced swallowing efficiency, which may be complicated by anatomic changes within the swallow mechanism. Reduced swallow efficiency is characterized by reduced

movement of structures within the swallowing mechanism, leading to prolonged duration of various aspects of the swallow and reduced opening of the pharyngoesophageal segment.[16,17] The reduction of movement during swallowing contributes to postswallow residue along the swallowing mechanism and poor clearance of saliva.[12,18] Food and saliva residue may build up over time, increasing the risk of aspiration or necessitating frequent expectoration by the patient.

Dysphagia from Surgical Intervention

Surgery for head/neck cancer results in the loss, rearrangement, or reconstruction of structures that are important for swallowing function. A traditional rule for predicting dysphagia after surgery for head/neck cancer is the "50% rule."[19,20] This "rule," which seems to result from experiences with oral cancers, suggests that removal of less than 50% of a structure will not result in a significant and permanent swallowing problem. However, this rule has been challenged with the introduction of surgical reconstruction techniques as clinicians report good postoperative swallowing function after surgical flap reconstruction.[21,22] Thus individual patient characteristics should be carefully examined both before and after surgery to identify and manage any resulting swallowing impairments.[23] A general guideline is that the more tissue removed or relocated, the higher the probability for postsurgical dysphagia. Of course, this guideline requires modification when combined modalities are used (radiation therapy and/or chemotherapy in addition to surgery). The following text provides a brief overview of certain dysphagia characteristics that may result from surgery involving various aspects of the swallowing mechanism. Table 6-1 presents a summary of certain surgeries with the associated physiologic impact and anticipated swallow deficit.

Surgery for Oral Cancers

Generally speaking, the oral cavity involves the anterior aspect of the tongue, floor of the mouth, submental structures, the mandible, and the maxilla. Oral surgeries often involve more than a single structure. For example, a **mandibulotomy** may be required to gain adequate surgical access to tumors in the floor of the mouth or other areas of the oral cavity. In general, surgeries for oral cancers may limit mastication, bolus formulation and containment, and bolus transport from the front to the back of the mouth. Surgeries restricted to the tongue often result in transient dysphagia with good functional outcome; however, this may depend on the extent of the tissue removed and

TABLE 6-1		
Common Swallowing Disorders Resulting from Various Surgeries to Treat Head/Neck Cancer		
Resection	**Physiologic Effect**	**Swallowing**
Partial glossectomy	Removes <50% of tongue Anterior tissue removal ↑ difficulties	Difficulty holding and preparing a bolus for swallowing
Total glossectomy	Removal >50% of tongue Flap technique influences result	Difficulty moving materials from the oral cavity Reduced tongue driving force May show reduced pharyngeal clearance
Tonsil/base of tongue	Reduced anterior tongue range	Reduced tongue driving force Difficulty moving materials through the oropharynx
Palatal resection	Removal of >50% of soft palate Incomplete velar seal	Velar leak results in retrograde movement of materials into the nasopharynx
Anterior/lateral floor of mouth	Reduced anterior tongue range; unable to lateralize tongue Reduced ability to elevate hyoid/larynx Reduced opening of upper esophageal sphincter	Reduced control of oral bolus Reduced tongue driving force Difficulty moving material through the oropharynx Delayed triggering of pharyngeal swallow Reduced clearance of bolus from pharynx
Partial pharyngeal resection	Reduced pharyngeal wall constriction Reduced elevation of hyoid/larynx	Difficulty clearing materials from the pharynx Delay triggering swallow
Hemilaryngectomy	Unilateral resection Partial airway closure	Unilateral pharyngeal weakness Reduced airway protection
Supraglottic laryngectomy	Incomplete posterior tongue movement, restricted arytenoids motion, partial airway closure	Delay in bolus propulsion Difficulty with elevation of structures for swallow Reduced airway protection
Total laryngectomy	Removal of vibratory source Alternative source surgically developed	Issues with reduced negative pressure, bolus transit Anatomic or physiologic stenosis of PES possible

PES, Pharyngeal esophageal segment.

the shape of the reconstructed tongue if flap reconstruction is completed.[24,25] When present, swallowing problems resulting from limited tongue resections involve bolus control and transport difficulties and may be transient.

With more extensive resections involving the tongue and floor of mouth with or without flap reconstruction, dysphagia may be expected for varying periods. Such dysphagia typically involves problems with mastication, bolus control, transport to the posterior oral cavity and, in some cases, airway protection as a result of loss of control of the bolus within the oral cavity.[26-28] In addition, pain may result from alterations to the temporomandibular joint. In cases of dramatic resection and reconstruction of the mandible, limitations in the pharyngoesophageal segment may result from reduced upward pull from the hyolaryngeal complex that attaches to the mandible. Conversely, some patients with resection limited to oral structures will have functional pharyngeal aspects in swallowing and will do well if compensations can be used for oral deficits. Video 6-1 on the Evolve site demonstrates functional pharyngeal aspects of swallowing in a patient with significant tongue reconstruction. Contrast liquid is delivered to the pharynx by a small straw connected to a syringe to compensate for limited oral control. Note the increase in residue resulting from thicker materials. Also note the patient's spontaneous compensations to adjust for limited tongue movement.

Surgery for Oropharyngeal Cancers

The oropharynx begins where the oral cavity stops, extending superiorly from the hard palate to the hyoid bone inferiorly. This area includes the tongue base, faucial arches, tonsils and tonsillar fossa, **retromolar trigone**, soft palate, and the pharyngeal walls of the superior and lateral pharynx. General aspects of dysphagia resulting from surgery in the oropharynx include nasal regurgitation (sometimes called *nasopharyngeal reflux*), decreased bolus transit, aspiration, and pharyngoesophageal segment (PES) dysfunction. Surgery in this area often involves multiple structures, thus increasing the extent of swallowing deficit.

Surgery limited to the tongue base may result in a reduced force applied by the tongue to move the bolus into the pharynx, which could result in

Practice Note 6-1

Many devices have been suggested to compensate for reduced oral transit in patients with limited tongue movement as a result of resection or paralysis. Glossectomy spoons have been described but are not always accepted by patients. We treated a patient who had floor of mouth and lingual resection and repair with a microvascular flap. As a result of these surgeries, the patient had reduced lingual movement, impaired ability to contain a liquid bolus in the mouth, and impaired ability to transit a pudding or thicker bolus posteriorly in the mouth. We were able to increase oral intake by placing a "cocktail straw" (small straw) on a syringe so that the patient could place liquid (thin and thick) in the posterior mouth where she could control delivery to the pharynx and swallow without complication. View Video 6-1 on the Evolve site for this text for an example of these types of deficits.

post-swallow residue in the area of the tongue base/valleculae. Surgery in this region also can result in reduced upward pull on the pharyngoesophageal segment, contributing to reduced opening of this region and post-swallow residue in the piriform recesses. In general, surgery limited to the tongue or limited surgery to the tongue base has a favorable outcome regarding the ability to ingest food and/or liquid by mouth.[14,29,30] A related consideration is the use of reconstructive procedures in this region. Newer microvascular reconstruction techniques have shown promise for improved swallow function after surgery in the oropharynx.[31]

Patients undergoing surgery involving more than one structure in the oropharynx tend to have more severe and persistent dysphagia.[32] For example, if the tongue and palate are both resected, the patient may have difficulty propelling a bolus into the pharynx, poor bolus control, and nasal regurgitation. Patients who have extensive reconstruction with flaps may have swallowing difficulties related to both the ablative surgery and the flap reconstruction. Flaps used in reconstruction may contribute to swallowing problems related to altered sensation, poor movement, or bulk added to the oropharynx. Each of these factors should be clinically evaluated in patients with flap reconstruction in the swallowing mechanism.

Surgery for Hypopharyngeal Cancers

The pharynx is a tubelike structure extending from behind the nose to the entrance of the esophagus.

The portion referred to as the *hypopharynx* is the section of the tube beginning at the hyoid bone and extending to below the cricoid cartilage of the larynx. The hypopharynx includes the piriform recesses, postcricoid area, and pharyngeal walls. The larynx rests within the hypopharynx but is not technically part of this structure. The most common site for hypopharyngeal cancer is the piriform recess. The hypopharynx has extensive lymph drainage into the cervical neck region, and metastasis to the cervical neck lymph nodes is frequent with hypopharyngeal cancer.[7] Thus neck dissection commonly is performed in combination with any surgery to the hypopharynx. Also, hypopharyngeal tumors often do not create overt symptoms early in the course of the disease. For this reason, hypopharyngeal tumors are often advanced and require extensive surgery that may involve both the larynx and the neck.[33] Such patients may have concurrent therapies, including extensive surgeries such as **laryngopharyngectomy**, along with a neck dissection. In some cases, only a partial removal of the larynx is required and vocal functions may be somewhat preserved. In advanced cancers in this region, reconstruction with a **gastric pull-up** or **jejunal transfer** may be used to retain as much swallowing function as possible. Given the location of hypopharyngeal cancers and the frequent spread of these cancers to adjacent structures (larynx, neck), dysphagia resulting from surgeries to treat these cancers is severe. However, newer surgical approaches using transoral laser microsurgery offer promise for good control of the cancer with lower rates of treatment-related morbidity.[34]

Surgery for Laryngeal Cancers

The larynx can be subdivided into three regions: the supraglottic region, glottic region, and subglottic region. Subglottic cancers are rare compared with cancers in the other regions, and when identified often involve the vocal folds (glottic region). Supraglottic cancers have a higher rate of spread to the lymph system of the neck than isolated vocal fold tumors and thus may require neck dissection.[7] Supraglottic and glottic tumors both contribute to early overt changes in voice and/or swallowing and thus may be identified and treated early in the course of the disease. These small tumors may be successfully treated with limited surgeries, including laser surgery.[35-37] As the size of the tumor and/or metastasis to adjacent structures increases, the need for more extensive surgical resection is indicated; these may be considered as a partial laryngectomy or a total laryngectomy.

Partial laryngectomy procedures may include a cordectomy, in which only a true vocal fold (vocal cord) is removed; a hemilaryngectomy, in which one half (right or left) of the larynx is removed; or a supraglottic or supracricoid laryngectomy, in which the structures above the glottis are removed. Figure 6-5 depicts the larynx of a patient after right cordectomy. Each partial laryngectomy procedure may contribute to a reduction in airway protection during swallowing by compromising either the glottis or the supraglottic mechanisms that contribute to airway closure. The extent of the surgery and the functional aspects of any reconstruction may be predictive of the presence and severity of any postoperative dysphagia. Recent reports suggest that partial laryngectomy, specifically supracricoid laryngectomy, has a good prognosis for return of functional swallowing, but airway protection is a persistent concern in the period after surgery.[38-40]

Patients with total laryngectomy typically do not present with risk of airway compromise because the airway and the swallowing tract are separated. In these patients a new airway opening is established by way of a stoma in the anterior neck. By removing transnasal airflow and redirecting it to the neck stoma, these patients also have a diminished sense of smell, which may further contribute to reduced food intake. The more common dysphagia problem faced by patients with total laryngectomy is **stenosis** in the **neopharynx** created after surgical removal of the larynx. The terms *anatomic stenosis* and *physiologic stenosis* may be applied as simple descriptors of whether this narrowing results from structural (anatomic) or muscle (physiologic) irregularities. Typically, this narrowing of the swallowing mechanism limits the ability of the patient to ingest solids foods, whereas liquids may be swallowed more easily. In cases of severe stenosis, patients may report difficulty swallowing both solids and liquids. Other problems faced by the patient after total laryngectomy may include tissue breakdown, leading to fistulas and/or surgical scarring. One variant of a postsurgical scar deficit in the neopharynx is the presence of a pseudoepiglottis, or pull-apart pouch. On lateral radiograph this "structure" may give the impression of an epiglottis in a patient who has none. Video segments 6-2 and 6-3 on the Evolve site provide endoscopic and fluoroscopic studies of a pseudoepiglottis. Video 6-4 is a fluoroscopic study showing a stricture in the neopharynx of a patient after total laryngectomy. Video segment 6-5 is an endoscopic view of a patient who received a supraglottic laryngectomy.

Dysphagia from Radiation Therapy

Radiation therapy in the treatment of head/neck cancer may be used in isolation or in combination with surgery and/or chemotherapy. Radiation therapy may be used as the treatment of choice for small tumors to preserve tissue function (as in the larynx) or for advanced tumors that are not resectable. A general impression is that swallowing problems after radiation therapy either in isolation or in combina-

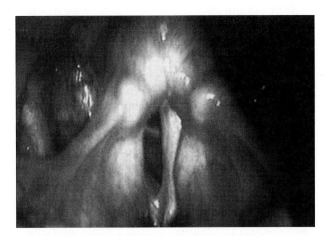

FIGURE 6-5. Photograph of a larynx after right true vocal cord removal by laser (laser cordectomy). The larynx is in the fully adducted (closed) position as indicated by approximation of the arytenoid cartilages. Note the large glottal opening resulting from the surgical procedure.

Practice Note 6-2

Although patients with total laryngectomy are at minimal risk for aspiration during eating and drinking, some patients aspirate in an unusual way. A few years ago, I saw a patient who reported chronic coughing when he drank any liquids. We had been seeing him for minor adjustment with his tracheoesophageal speaking valve and wondered if he might be "leaking" around the valve. Clinically we did not see any visible signs of leaking around the valve, so we completed a fluoroscopic evaluation of swallowing. To our surprise, this patient had a long but narrow pharyngocutaneous fistula that opened in the anterior midline of the neck approximately 1 inch above the stoma. After a few sips of liquid barium he began coughing. The barium tracked along the fistula and dripped into his trachea through the stoma. A simple bandage reduced this unusual source of aspiration and the fistula was brought to the attention of our head and neck surgical team.

tion with surgery are worse than those after surgery alone.[41,42]

Radiation therapy contributes to a variety of mucosal and muscle tissue changes that can complicate any existing swallowing difficulties and create new problems. Box 6-10 lists several complications resulting from radiation therapy to the head/neck region that may contribute to dysphagia. One or more of these complications occur in almost every patient who receives radiation therapy for the treatment of head/neck cancer. These changes may occur to both mucosal tissue and muscle/nerve tissue. Clinical experience with this population suggests that in the early stages of treatment pain and dryness, as a result of mucositis and xerostomia, and edema of structures in the swallowing mechanism directly contribute to reduced frequency and efficiency of swallowing ability. Swallowing difficulties that persist or develop after radiation treatment often are linked to fibrosis, muscle weakness from disuse atrophy, and/or peripheral nerve deficits. The time course of these tissue changes and resulting dysphagia are variable across patients and are related to many different factors. In general, an intense mucosal tissue response is noted within the first 3 to 4 weeks after the initiation of radiation therapy. Shortly thereafter the patient may be at greatest risk for development of new and severe dysphagia symptoms. If candidiasis (fungal infection) occurs, pain from mucositis may be increased and contribute further to dysphagia complaints. Finally, the impact of radiation therapy on dentition must be considered. Often, especially if the patient has poor dentition, a dentist will be consulted for corrective action before the initiation of radiation therapy. Even with this preventive action, the remaining teeth will be affected to some extent by radiation therapy. Figure 6-6 depicts various postradiation effects that can occur in the swallowing mechanism. Video 6-6 on the Evolve site is an endoscopic study of a patient revealing significant postradiation mucosal changes, including edema in the larynx, pharyngeal stenosis, and thickened secretions.

Dysphagia Characteristics after Radiation Therapy

General characteristics of dysphagia encountered by patients treated with radiation therapy for head/neck cancer are listed in Box 6-11. The listed percentages are from a single published report and thus should be considered only as estimates.[43] This list contains both contributing factors (dry mouth, pain) and dysphagia characteristics (small amounts, multiple swallows). Only general characteristics are listed. In many, but not all, cases of dysphagia during or after radiation therapy pain, dryness, and edema contribute to reduced frequency of swallowing, misdirection of a

BOX 6-10	**Potential Complications and Side Effects of Radiation Therapy That May Contribute Directly to Dysphagia**

- Mucositis
- Xerostomia
- Sensory changes in taste and smell
- Fibrosis (including trismus)
- Neuropathy
- Changed anatomy (e.g., stricture)
- Odynophagia (painful swallowing)
- Loss of appetite
- Edema
- Infection (fungal, bacterial)
- Dental changes

CLINICAL CORNER 6-2

A 48-year-old man was treated with a concomitant chemotherapy/radiation therapy regimen for cancer at the base of his tongue. During his therapy a PEG tube was placed for primary nutrition and hydration. He attempted to maintain some oral intake, but this steadily declined and he eventually was limited to sips of water. At the time of our initial evaluation I reported the presence of an anatomic stenosis (stricture) beginning at the top region of the PES and continuing into the proximal esophagus. The entire length of this stenosis was estimated to be greater than 20 mm. The patient was referred to the gastroenterology service for dilatation. Several weeks after this procedure the patient returned for repeat fluoroscopic evaluation and reported increased oral intake but prolonged meal time. The report from the gastroenterology service indicated that the stricture was dilated to 48 Fr (approximately 16 mm). During the fluoroscopic study we again noted a severe stricture in the same area and the patient was unable to ingest more than a small sip of liquid without significant aspiration.

CRITICAL THINKING

1. How do you reconcile the radiographic findings of a stricture with the gastroenterology report of a successful dilatation?
2. What next steps would you consider for this patient?

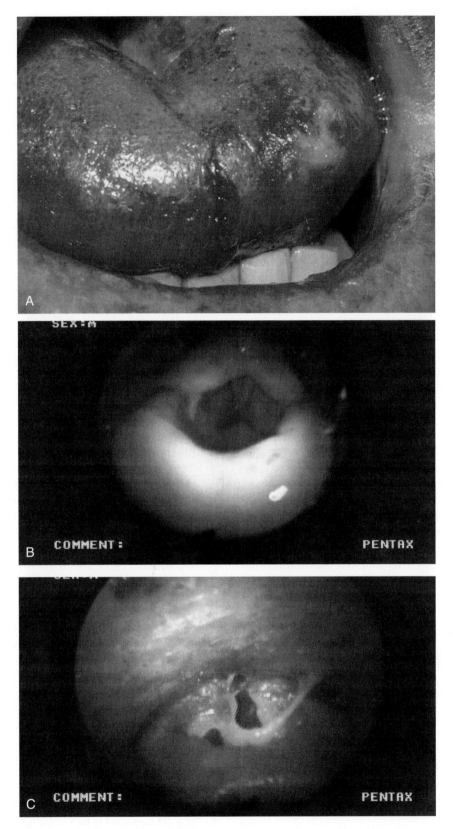

FIGURE 6-6. Postradiation changes to the swallowing mechanism. **A,** Mucositis of the tongue.
B, Edema of the larynx, including epiglottis. **C,** Persistent and adhering mucus.

bolus leading to aspiration, inefficient swallow leading to post-swallow residue, the need for multiple swallows, and prolonged mealtimes.

Pain from mucositis is a significant problem for patients early in the radiotherapy period and may last well beyond the initial treatment period. Oral mucositis also may result from chemotherapy and is enhanced in combined treatment protocols. The consequences of oral pain from mucositis extend beyond speech and swallowing functions and include potential interruption in the cancer treatment regimen[44] and economic consequences for the patient and family.[45] In general, oral mucositis is related to patient report of oral dysfunction and distress in patients receiving cancer therapy.[46]

Dry mouth, or *xerostomia,* is perhaps the most clinically significant and long-lasting difficulty faced by patients who undergo radiation therapy in the treatment of head and neck cancer. Patient surveys report associated xerostomia with significant negative emotional impact, in addition to difficulty talking and eating.[47] Interestingly, xerostomia may not be directly related to swallowing physiology. That is, the physiologic movement of a bolus through the swallowing mechanism is not significantly affected by xerostomia. Rather, xerostomia seems to have a negative impact on patients' perception of swallowing as a result of altered sensory processes.[48,49]

Many patients describe reduced or altered senses of taste and smell that limit eating enjoyment.[50] Taste impairments may relate to reduction in the number of taste buds during radiotherapy, but in some instances taste buds return after cessation of radiotherapy and thus the sense of taste improves.[51] In fact, one recent study reported that the four basic tastes returned to baseline levels by 6 months after radiotherapy in patients who received either conventional or hyperfractionated radiotherapy for primary tumors of the oropharynx.[52] Note that these chemosensory impairments are not limited to diminished senses of taste and smell; some patients report abnormal and adverse tastes and smells that contribute to eating avoidance. Another perspective on taste aversions in patients with cancer is that they are learned through negative sensory experiences during radiotherapy and chemotherapy.[53] Thus primary sensory deficit or the learned negative reaction to it may contribute to reduced overall intake of food and liquid, resulting in threats to what may be an already compromised nutritional state.

Poor dentition may further complicate any existing dysphagia by limiting the patient's ability to masticate solid foods. Reduced mouth opening from trismus also may limit the variety and/or amount of food or liquid that a patient may consume by mouth and have negative implications for oral care. One group has tried to operationally define the degree of reduced mouth opening that may contribute to a functional cutoff point for trismus. By comparing vertical mouth opening with a mandibular function impairment questionnaire, this group identified a mouth opening of 35 mm or less as a functional cutoff for trismus in patients with head/neck cancer.[54]

BOX 6-11	General Characteristics of Dysphagia Associated with Radiation Therapy for Head/Neck Cancer*

- Bolus control deficits (63%)
- Small amounts per bolus and multiple swallow attempts
- Increased meal times
- Reduced frequency of swallowing
- Dry mouth (92%)
- Pain (58%)
- Altered taste (75%)

*Percentages are estimates.

Practice Note 6-3

Sensory changes in patients treated with radiation therapy can have a profound impact on oral intake. On multiple occasions we have encountered patients who refuse to take any material beyond liquids by mouth. One reason is that more solid foods cause them to gag; often to the point of vomiting. In conjunction with an otolaryngologist several years ago, we decided to "numb" the tongue of one patient with this complaint. We painted 4% lidocaine gel on the tongue dorsum and gave this patient the exact material on which he had gagged just minutes before. He was able to swallow this material without difficulty. The physician gave him a bottle of lidocaine to take home. On return to the clinic in 1 month, the patient had greatly increased the variety and amount of soft foods taken by mouth. Although this strategy has not always worked, we have since used it successfully for many patients. Whether gagging in these individuals was physiologic or psychological, altering the status quo sensory system by topical application of lidocaine seemed to help these patients move forward in oral intake.

ASSESSMENT STRATEGIES FOR DYSPHAGIA IN HEAD/NECK CANCER

Chapters 9 and 10 provide detailed information on the clinical and instrumental evaluation of dysphagia in adult patients. This section reviews certain assessment strategies of specific importance to the evaluation of swallow function in patients who are treated for head and neck cancer. Because of the diversity in clinical presentation of head/neck cancers (e.g., some cancers may contribute to pretreatment swallowing deficits, whereas others have minimal impact), the nature of their treatments, and the changing time course of the clinical signs and symptoms during and after treatment, patients who have been treated for head/neck cancer often present a unique clinical challenge to the dysphagia clinician. The basics of dysphagia assessment described in Chapters 9 and 10 are appropriate for these patients, but at least two additional factors should be considered: the timetable of evaluations and the assessment of impact factors.

Timing of Swallow Evaluations

Many patients demonstrate some degree of swallow deviation before any medical treatment as a result of the cancer or other factors. Interestingly, slightly more than half of these patients actually report swallow difficulty, and a majority demonstrate functional swallowing ability.[16] On the basis of these estimates, more than half of patients in whom head/neck cancer is diagnosed are not evaluated for swallow ability before cancer treatment. This approach may not provide the best patient care because pretreatment deficits may be neglected that may have an impact on posttreatment dysphagia status and rehabilitation. In addition, a pretreatment evaluation provides the patient an additional opportunity to discuss potential difficulties that may occur during radiotherapy or posttreatment deficits that may occur after surgery or radiotherapy.[23]

Timing of the postsurgical evaluation of swallowing function should be determined between the speech-language pathologist (SLP) and the surgeon. In the early postsurgery period the patient may have significant edema that limits swallowing ability and the extent of any evaluation. Still, early evaluations may be helpful in determining the extent of dysphagia, identifying factors that contribute to any dysphagia, and establishing a time course for more intensive rehabilitation. In patients who demonstrate some functional swallow ability in the early postsurgery period, early evaluation may be critical to identify strategies that will facilitate safe "swallowing" with the potential to limit dysphagia-related complications during the hospital stay.

Patients treated with radiation therapy protocols should be evaluated before treatment as well as during treatment for acute toxicity side effects that will have a negative impact on swallow function. Also, these patients should have follow-up for the emergence of late-occurring effects of radiotherapy that may impair swallow function.[55]

Assessing Impact Factors

Impact factors are patient characteristics that directly or indirectly have a negative impact on swallowing functions. In patients with head/neck cancer, frequent impact factors include pain, xerostomia, taste and smell deviation, fibrosis, nutritional status, and psychological status.

Pain may be present after surgery or during or after radiation therapy. Alterations in swallowing related to painful swallowing (**odynophagia**) should be differentiated from dysphagia, in which movement of the swallowing mechanism is impaired because the course of treatment differs between these two clinical entities. Pain is typically managed medically with a variety of analgesic medications. If pain medications—particular narcotic class medications—are used for a prolonged period, the dysphagia clinician must also consider gastroparesis in the profile of potential swallowing deficits.[56] As a minimal attempt to differentiate odynophagia from other forms of swallowing difficulty, clinicians should ask patients to identify, localize, and rate the severity of any pain within the swallowing mechanism. When pain is related to oral mucositis as a result of radiation therapy, oncologists and/or oncology nurses often use a standard rating scale to grade oral mucositis. Among these scales is the World Health Organization Grading Scale,[57] which relies heavily on the patient's ability to eat by mouth in determining the severity of oral mucositis (Table 6-2). Clinicians should become familiar with the rating scale used in their facilities and the functional interpretation of that scale as it may pertain to a patient's swallowing ability. In addition, clinicians should be aware that pain within the swallowing mechanism can result from fungal infections or peripheral nerve injury. A basic understanding of the source of pain within the swallow mechanism allows the dysphagia clinician to interact with the rest of the cancer rehabilitation team to best meet the patient's comprehensive needs. As pain diminishes with appropriate medical treatment, patients with reduced oral intake caused by odynophagia should increase both

TABLE 6-2	

World Health Organization Scale for Grading Oral Mucositis

Grade	Clinical Findings
0	No symptoms
1	Sore mouth, no ulcers
2	Sore mouth with ulcers, but able to eat normally
3	Liquid diet only
4	Unable to eat or drink

BOX 6-12	University of Michigan Xerostomia Questionnaire*

1. Rate your difficulty in talking because of dryness.
2. Rate your difficulty in chewing because of dryness.
3. Rate your difficulty in swallowing solid food because of dryness.
4. Rate the frequency of your sleeping problems because of dryness.
5. Rate your mouth or throat dryness when eating food.
6. Rate your mouth or throat dryness while not eating.
7. Rate the frequency of sipping liquids to aid swallowing food.
8. Rate the frequency of sipping liquids for oral comfort when not eating.

*Patients rate each item on a scale from 0 to 10. Higher scores indicate worse xerostomia.

the amount and variety of foods and liquids taken by mouth.

Xerostomia is a common side effect of radiotherapy. As previously described, xerostomia may affect swallowing by altering the normal sensory function within the oral cavity and thus change the patient's perception of his or her swallowing ability. Regardless of the specific impact of xerostomia on swallowing ability, it is a pervasive and long-lasting impairment in most patients treated with radiation therapy. The ability to rate the severity of xerostomia adds an objective dimension to the clinical evaluation of the patient with head/neck cancer. Researchers at the University of Michigan developed and validated a patient report scale for xerostomia that is widely used as a clinical scale.[58] The scale items from this xerostomia questionnaire are listed in Box 6-12. Patients rate each item from 0 to 10 (higher scores denote worse xerostomia). Clinicians should also discuss with the patient his or her perception of the impact of xerostomia on swallowing and other oral functions. Beyond the patient's report, clinicians should note the presence, type (thin and watery, thick, etc.), and amount of secretions on the tongue dorsum and in the anterior sublingual vault.

The senses of taste and smell are critical to the enjoyment of eating. Both radiotherapy and chemotherapy can have a negative impact on these senses. Taste is mediated by the tongue, with only five basic tastes identified (sweet, sour, bitter, salty, and **umami**). Many lingual tissue changes from radiotherapy and/or chemotherapy can diminish or alter the sense of taste. Flavor is mediated through olfaction. Often the sense of smell is not impaired or perhaps is only temporarily diminished in the patient with head/neck cancer. Diminished senses of taste and smell can reduce a patient's enjoyment of eating and may negatively affect food choices and overall intake. Altered senses of taste and smell can have a direct, negative impact on oral intake because patients will avoid foods that are perceived as aversive. Although standard protocols exist for the systematic evaluation of taste and smell function, patient report is typically sufficient to document the presence of these sensory deficits and their impact on oral intake of food and liquid. If impaired senses of taste or smell are determined to be a primary factor on reduced oral intake, patients should be referred to an appropriate oral health professional for more extensive evaluation and potential treatment.

Radiotherapy can damage skin and muscle along with devascularization and damage to peripheral nerves. Soft tissue of the skin and muscle can become fibrosed, which reduces movement in the swallowing mechanism and in the head and neck region in general. Dysphagia clinicians should attempt to differentiate the underlying cause of reduced movement primarily between muscle weakness and tissue fibrosis. Even passive movement will be restricted because of fibrosis. The patient with soft tissue fibrosis demonstrates hard, or "woody," presentation of a region that has been irradiated such as the anterior aspect of the neck. Simply grasping both sides of the larynx and trying to move this structure from side to side gives some indication of the degree of movement and hence fibrosis. Subsequently, the clinician can attempt to feel laryngeal movement during a volitional swallow. The combination of reduced passive and volitional movement suggests that fibrosis may be a

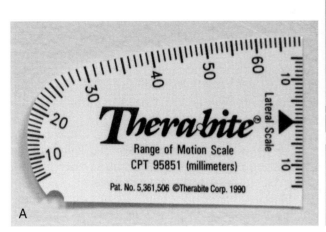 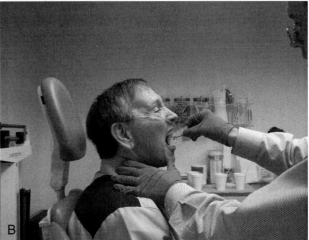

FIGURE 6-7. Measuring mouth opening. **A,** TheraBite mouth opening ruler. **B,** Use of the ruler in a patient to measure vertical mouth opening.

limiting factor. If possible, endoscopic inspection of the larynx and pharynx helps determine whether the effects of fibrosis are limited to the superficial skin and muscles or if deeper structures are involved. More details of this evaluation are provided in Chapter 10, but the key feature is to evaluate movement within the larynx, pharyngeal walls, and the base of the tongue.

Fibrosis may also alter other structures within the swallow mechanism. The upper esophageal sphincter (also termed *pharyngoesophageal segment*) may become fibrotic and stenosed as a result of radiation therapy. Strictures in this segment reduce the sphincter opening and limit the amount of food the patient is able to swallow. This impairment should be considered in patients with head/neck cancer who report difficulty swallowing solid foods. Finally, a common and potentially debilitating form of fibrosis can lead to reduced mouth opening, or **trismus**. Trismus may result from reduced flexibility of the masseter and temporalis muscles, which are the primary muscles of jaw closure. If these muscles become fibrotic, they pose a substantial force against the muscles of jaw opening and limit the degree of vertical opening of the mouth. This situation can negatively affect mastication, swallowing, speech, and general oral care. As previously mentioned, a vertical mouth opening of less than 35 mm may be considered reduced and indicative of trismus. TheraBite (Atos Medical AB, West Allis, Wis.) is a therapeutic device for the treatment of trismus; a simple cardboard "ruler" is available from the manufacturer of this device for the systematic measurement of mouth

opening. Measurement of mouth opening is recommended for all patients who have been treated for head/neck cancer, but especially those who have been treated with a radiotherapy protocol. Figure 6-7 depicts the TheraBite mouth opening ruler and its use.

Malnutrition in cancer patients is multifactorial and can lead to poor quality of life, reduced survival, and treatment-related morbidity. As previously mentioned, between 30% and 50% of patients with head/neck cancer demonstrate a degree of malnutrition before, during, or after treatment. Reasons for malnutrition may include dysphagia, odynophagia, taste deviations, poor appetite (which in itself may be multifactorial), increased caloric needs, or other metabolic, physical, or psychological factors. Nutritional status may be evaluated by a variety of methods. Weight change is a general guideline for nutritional change, and unintentional weight loss is often used as a clinical sign of potential nutritional risk. The body mass index (BMI) is an extension of weight change reflected in a ratio between weight and height. BMI calculators are common and easily accessed on the Internet. Beyond these simple clinical tools, if significant nutritional deficit is suspected, the referring physician should always be notified and a consultation sought with a qualified nutritional specialist.

Psychological status may affect rehabilitation efforts. Cancer patients often cope with pain, fatigue, disfigurement, communication difficulties, dysphagia, and various gastric complaints, including nausea and vomiting. These conditions are chronic in many cases and may contribute to distress and depression. Psychological consultation is helpful in identifying potential factors and suggesting direction to minimize their impact on rehabilitative efforts.

THERAPY STRATEGIES FOR DYSPHAGIA IN HEAD/NECK CANCER

Chapters 12 and 14 provide more extensive detail on developing therapy plans for adult patients and a variety of therapeutic interventions. However, the patient who has been treated for head/neck cancer often represents a specific set of clinical challenges for dysphagia therapy resulting from both the cancer and its treatment. Most reports of therapy efforts in patients with head/neck cancer are based on small numbers of patients. For these reasons, much remains to be learned about the best therapy for such patients. Many patients, especially those with more advanced cancers, are treated with a combination of surgery and radiation therapy. In this situation, the effects of both treatments must be considered in therapy planning.

Timing of Swallowing Therapy

One important consideration for dysphagia therapy in patients treated for head/neck cancer is when to provide therapy. Many studies suggest that the sooner therapy is initiated after cancer treatment, the better the eventual outcome.[59-61] To the author's knowledge, no study suggests waiting for a prolonged period before initiating dysphagia therapy. Unfortunately, no consensus has emerged regarding the optimal time after cancer treatment to begin dysphagia therapy. As a general guideline, therapy should begin as soon as possible. It is advisable to consult with the head and neck surgeon regarding readiness of patients to initiate different therapeutic activities after surgery. Moreover, some patients who have only minor problems or those who substantially recover swallowing function after treatment develop new dysphagia symptoms or notice deterioration in swallowing function months or years after primary cancer treatment. Still, published clinical research does offer hope even for patients with chronic dysphagia after treatment of head/neck cancer.[62,63]

A different approach considers intervention strategies before or during cancer treatment that may prevent or reduce the severity of dysphagia after cancer treatment. This paradigm has been applied recently, primarily to patients being treated with radiotherapy with or without chemotherapy. Results from a single cancer treatment center indicate benefit to patient quality of life[64] and in certain aspects of swallow function[65] after radiation therapy (with or without chemotherapy) when patients completed swallowing-related exercises 2 weeks before cancer treatment. The exercises were commonly reported exercises (detailed in Chapter 14) and included tongue resistance, tongue hold, head lift, effortful swallow, and the Mendelsohn maneuver.

In at least one small, randomized clinical trial, active exercise-based therapy provided daily during radiotherapy treatment reduced the severity of dysphagia after cancer treatment with the benefits lasting up to 6 months of follow-up.[66] Results of this study included preservation of muscle structure and functional maintenance of swallowing ability in patients who received intensive exercise-based therapy versus a sham therapy versus usual care involving no active intervention during cancer treatment. Exercises used in this study were simple and focused on tongue, larynx, pharynx, and jaw movement. They included tongue resistance activities, effortful swallow, falsetto, and jaw stretch against mild resistance. Secondary findings from this study implicated preservation of salivary flow and smell sensation in the active exercise group. Both of these variables are considered contributory to dysphagia in this population. These initial findings are encouraging for patients and strongly suggest that engaging in active swallow exercises during (or before) radiation therapy may have widespread benefit for patients treated with this modality for head/neck cancer.

Dysphagia characteristics may develop in patients receiving radiation therapy during the course of treatment. A percutaneous endoscopic gastrostomy (PEG) tube may be used to maintain nutrition and hydration during and after treatment until oral food and liquid intake can be reestablished. In such situations, it is important to maintain contact with the patient during and after treatment to either initiate swallowing therapy or reevaluate for oral feeding possibilities. At the very least, patients should be given exercises focusing on both strength and flexibility of the swallowing mechanism to limit or eliminate weakness and restricted movement that may contribute to dysphagia after treatment. Although some patients do require long-term use of alternative feeding sources after treatment for head/neck cancer, many centers report only temporary use of these strategies (often between 2 and 4 months).[67] In these situations, the dysphagia specialist plays an important role in the patient's transition from nonoral to oral feeding.[68]

Given the variation in size and location of head/neck cancers and the resulting diversity in the medical and surgical treatments, no single approach to dysphagia therapy in this patient group is all-encompassing. In addition, the timing of dysphagia therapy after cancer treatment results in different clinical presentations within and across patients treated with the same medical and surgical strategies. Thus in an attempt to simplify what may be a complicated clinical issue, bolus transport and airway protection problems after head/neck cancer treatment are the focus of this section. In addition, an overview of interventions that may be indicated to address mucosal and muscle changes resulting from radiation therapy is provided.

Therapy for Bolus Transport Problems

In designing therapy for bolus transport problems, the first step is to identify the changes in the swallowing mechanism that are contributing to the transport problems. These changes may result from either surgical intervention or radiation therapy. The common attribute is reduced movement of the structures comprising the swallowing mechanism. Surgical treatment may remove structures that are important to bolus movement. If structures have been removed, a maxillofacial prosthodontist is a valuable resource. In combination with a speech-language pathologist (SLP), this professional can fabricate palatal lifts, obturators, maxillary-shaping devices, or other intraoral prostheses that can contribute to improved swallowing function.[69] A *palatal lift* is helpful to lift the existing soft palate into a raised position, thus creating improved velopharyngeal closure. An *obturator* is a device that fills a gap created by surgical resection. If the soft palate is removed (or, for that matter, part of the hard palate), an obturator can be used to facilitate separation of the oral and nasal cavities. A *maxillary-shaping device* is a prosthesis that fits over the hard palate (much like an upper denture). This device may be thickened or shaped to facilitate maximal contact with a weakened or partially resected tongue. Increased lingual-palatal contact should facilitate improved oral bolus transport. However, at least one study has cast doubt on the overall benefit of these prostheses in patients who have been surgically treated for oropharyngeal cancer.[70] Video 6-7 on the Evolve site accompanying this text is an endoscopic study revealing a "gap" in the left aspect of the velopharyngeal sphincter. The SLP and the maxillofacial prosthodontist agreed that an obturator may provide benefit to both speech and swallowing functions in this patient. Videos 6-8, *A* and *B*, show an endoscopic evaluation that (a) depicts a complete and symmetrical incompetence of the velopharynx and (b) a fluoroscopic evaluation showing sufficient soft palate tissue that may produce benefit from a palatal lift.

When structures are restricted in movement (from either surgery or radiation), changes in head posture, use of feeding devices, and/or dietary changes may be indicated. Range of motion (i.e., stretching) exercises also may be helpful in some instances. Patients who have limited tongue movement may benefit from elevating the chin to allow gravity to transport a bolus to the back of the mouth or even into the pharynx. In these cases, good airway protection is an important part of the clinical picture. The risk of aspiration is increased if the patient cannot protect the airway and propels a bolus into the pharynx by gravity. Another consideration is that elevating the chin may increase the pressure within the PES.[71] If patients have existing problems opening the PES, this technique may be contraindicated. Logic dictates that use of this postural technique requires a bolus that is amenable to movement by gravity. This may limit the oral diet to liquids or very soft and liquefied foods.

Feeding devices have been described that allow patients to place a more solid bolus in the posterior oral cavity.[72] These so-called glossectomy spoons have been used to place soft foods in the posterior mouth in patients who have lingual paralysis or otherwise restricted lingual movement. In cases of severe movement restriction, patients may use syringes or even soft catheters to place food into the posterior oral cavity, the pharynx, or in some cases directly into the upper esophagus (some patients can learn to pass an orogastric tube themselves).

Stretching exercises may be helpful, especially if performed before scarring or fibrosis is so severe that any movement is severely restricted. Positive results have been shown specifically in increasing mouth opening for patients with trismus. Two primary methods for stretching have been recommended. Active and passive stretching with physical therapy exercises has been suggested to be beneficial by some authors,[73] but this benefit has been questioned by other investigators.[74] Various devices also have been proposed to aid in passive stretching of the jaw in the treatment of trismus. Traditionally, tongue blades were used by stacking the tongue blades, placing them between the incisor teeth (or gums in edentulous patients), and adding blades to increase the degree of stretch. More recent devices include the Therabite and the Dynasplint Trismus System (Dynasplint Systems, Inc., Severna Park, Md.). All three "systems" have shown benefit in the treatment of trismus after irradiation in the treatment of head/neck cancer.[75,76] Among the three techniques, the Therabite device appears to have been studied most extensively in clinical research.[75] Improved mouth opening in patients with trismus has also been demonstrated in limited studies with microcurrent electrotherapy and use of the drug pentoxifylline, which is used to increase peripheral blood flow.[75]

Other maneuvers and compensations such as the effortful swallow or the Mendelsohn maneuver may also be useful in improving bolus transport in response to specific dysphagia characteristics. (See Chapter 14 for a more complete review of various maneuvers and compensations and their impact on swallowing physiology and function.)

Therapy for Airway Protection Problems

Airway protection deficits result from compromise of the laryngeal valve or from incoordination of the swallow event. Laryngeal changes may result either from surgical or radiation therapies that either impair the anatomy of the larynx or the movement of laryngeal structures. From this perspective, therapeutic endeavors to protect the airway will focus on improved laryngeal closure and/or improved coordination of the swallow focusing on airway protection.

In some instances, surgical correction of reduced glottal closure is indicated. Two frequently used techniques are medialization of a nonmoving vocal fold by a technique termed *thyroplasty* or injection of an acceptable biosubstance into a vocal fold. The determining factors in the selection of the specific technique may be the degree of glottal incompetence, the experience of the surgeon with the respective techniques, and factors regarding the patient's overall medical condition. Figure 6-8 shows the same larynx

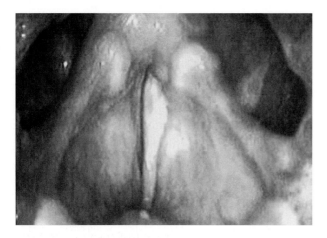

FIGURE 6-8. Photograph of the same larynx shown in Figure 6-4 after medialization of the right true vocal cord remnant by thyroplasty. Note the improved glottal closure by comparing the two photographs.

depicted in Figure 6-4 but after medialization by thyroplasty on the right side of the larynx. Note the improved glottal closure. Injection of biomaterials into one or both vocal folds has also been shown to be effective in improving glottal closure.[77-79] Although different techniques are available to surgeons to inject the vocal folds, recent techniques have focused on in-office procedures that allow patients to avoid general anesthesia in the operating room. One such technique incorporates an injection through the thyrohyoid membrane and injecting the vocal fold with endoscopic visualization.[80]

Various behavioral therapy techniques have been shown to reduce aspiration during swallowing. These techniques may be appropriate in cases of altered laryngeal anatomy but should be considered when incoordination of the swallowing event contributes to aspiration of swallowed materials. These compensatory techniques include the chin-down position, the head-turn posture, the supraglottic swallow, and the super-supraglottic swallow. Each of these techniques is discussed in greater detail in Chapter 14. Video segments depicting these techniques are also described in Chapter 14. The chin-down position may be helpful when a patient demonstrates a delay in the pharyngeal component of the swallow. This head position narrows the oropharyngeal opening and causes the patient to swallow "uphill" over the tongue. The head-turn posture helps to both direct a bolus to one side (hopefully the more intact side) of the pharynx and to lower the intrasphincter pressure on the contralateral side of the PES. This postural adjustment during the swallow may help direct a bolus away from the airway and to reduce the amount of post-swallow residue that may be aspirated after the swallow event. Both supraglottic swallow maneuvers focus on closing the airway before the swallow occurs and coughing lightly to clear any residue in the larynx immediately after the swallow. The difference between these two maneuvers is that the "super" variation includes effort during the breath-hold phase in an attempt to ensure and/or increase the degree of laryngeal closure. One additional swallow maneuver, the Mendelsohn maneuver, may indirectly facilitate improved airway protection by improving swallowing coordination. Video series 6-9 depicts changes in a patient's ability to perform the Mendelsohn maneuver with progressing therapy over a 6-week span. Each video segment was obtained at 2-week intervals. The patient was a cancer survivor with a severe dysphagia and difficulty protecting his airway during swallowing. He was taught the maneuver during the initial fluoroscopic study (Video 6-9, *A*) and with therapy he was able to learn the Mendelsohn maneuver and improved airway protection that led to increased oral intake. Note that even though this patient demonstrated increased skill with this maneuver, intermittent aspiration was still noted for some materials. This case raises a question on what clinicians should expect as a result of any given technique or maneuver. A summary of this patient's history and progress in treatment follows.

CLINICAL CASE EXAMPLE 6-1

A 66-year-old man had left neck dissection and radiation therapy (RT) for cancer of the left tonsillar fossa (T2N2A). The patient completed radiation therapy 4 months before his first visit to the outpatient dysphagia clinic. A left neck dissection was planned after RT; however, at the completion of RT he presented with pneumonia that was presumed to be related to aspiration and was hospitalized for treatment. A PEG tube was placed during that hospital stay. During that hospitalization a fluorographic swallowing evaluation revealed no aspiration. Two months later (2 months before presentation to the dysphagia clinic), a left neck dissection was completed. Three weeks after this surgery, a repeat fluorographic study did show aspiration and the patient was recommended to take only thickened liquids. Four weeks later he presented to our outpatient dysphagia clinic. Endoscopic assessment of swallowing functions identified no aspiration of thin liquids. Penetration of thick liquids was noted and these were effectively cleared with a cough. He showed moderate post-RT changes in the pharynx, including reduced movement of the pharyngeal wall during falsetto, adhering mucus in the pharynx, and post-swallow residue that increased as the viscosity of the bolus increased. Subsequent fluorographic study indicated better swallowing performance (no aspiration, less residue) with thin liquids than with thicker materials. Swallow movements were deemed adequate to support functional swallowing but reduced in degree of movement (reduced hyolaryngeal excursion, reduced pharyngeal constriction, reduced PES opening). The recommendation at that time was to initiate oral intake of thin liquids and gradually increase viscosity as tolerated up to a soft food consistency. He was to be followed up by his local physician and SLP.

Ten months later this patient was again hospitalized with right lower lobe pneumonia. Fluo-rographic study at that time indicated aspiration with a recommendation for the patient to cease all oral intake of food or liquid. Two months later he again presented to the dysphagia clinic. Fluorographic study at that time indicated aspiration when attempting to swallow 10 mL of thick liquid but not with thin liquid or smaller volumes of thick liquid (5 mL). Both a supraglottic swallow and a Mendelsohn maneuver were taught and both were successful in reducing or eliminating aspiration during larger bolus swallows. At this point, intensive swallowing therapy was recommended with a focus on airway protection and increasing hyolaryngeal excursion, pharyngeal constriction, and PES opening during swallowing. The Mendelsohn maneuver with increasing effort was emphasized and a progression of materials beginning with thin liquid and progressing to thick liquids and pureed foods was introduced. Surface electromyographic (sEMG) biofeedback was used to teach the maneuver and monitor increased swallowing effort. Post-swallow airway clearance was monitored with cervical auscultation.

After 2 weeks of daily therapy sessions, the patient demonstrated increased base of tongue contact to the posterior pharyngeal wall, increased extent and duration of pharyngeal constriction, and increased hyolaryngeal excursion. He was able to take larger volumes of thin liquid without aspiration (cup drinking) and demonstrated less residue with swallows of thick liquid. After 2 additional weeks of daily therapy this patient was able to ingest thickened liquids without aspiration and minimal residue and able to ingest "moist puree" foods with only minimal residue and no signs of aspiration. At this point, he met with our team dietitian to discuss strategies for increasing to total oral feeding while reducing tube feedings. Subsequently, the PEG tube was removed and he returned to total oral intake of food and liquid. His diet was restricted to liquids and soft foods but he reported that this was indeed better for him than tube feedings.

This patient represents a case of moderate reduction of movement within the swallowing mechanism as a result of RT. His case was complicated by pneumonia after completion of RT and by the inconsistent findings of aspiration across instrumental examinations. This inconsistency might result from variability within the patient over time or from variability in how these examinations were completed. One consistent finding was that he swallowed thin liquid better than thicker materials. This may result from less force applied to a bolus as a result of reduced movement of structures within the swallowing tract or perhaps from xerostomia, which would create more adherence between oral mucosa and thicker materials. The initial approach to increase oral intake for this patient was to start with material deemed safe based on instrumental study and allow him to progress at his own pace under supervision of his physician and local therapist. This was somewhat successful, but the level of intensity of his attempts and his compliance with a routine were unknown with this approach. The subsequent therapy program for this patient focused on attempting to increase movement of oropharyngeal structures during swallowing attempts while taking precaution to reduce the risk of aspiration of material into the airway. In this case, he improved even though it was more than a year after RT. Possibly because he was continuing to swallow during this period some flexibility in the mechanism was retained or at least not further compromised. This case presents many interesting questions, not all of which can be answered directly. Still, this case does demonstrate that swallowing rehabilitation can be successful and safe even in patients with chronic conditions and those who are at risk for airway compromise.

Therapies for Mucosal and Muscle Changes Resulting from Radiation Therapy

When radiation therapy creates mucosal and muscle tissue changes that interfere with swallowing, it is in the patient's best interest for the therapy plan to incorporate activities directed at minimizing the impact of those tissue changes. Box 6-13 summarizes some of the more common interventions for both mucosal and muscle tissue changes created by RT in the treatment of head/neck cancer.

Xerostomia (dry mouth) can contribute to swallowing difficulties as a result of reduced watery saliva that mixes with food to assist in bolus transport. At least two studies have suggested that oral xerostomia after radiation therapy affects the sensory aspects more than the motor aspects.[48,49] Another function of

---

BOX 6-13	Common Interventions for Mucosal and Muscle Changes Resulting from Radiation Therapy for Head/Neck Cancer

MUCOSAL CHANGES
Salivary supplements
Water
Analgesics
Ice chips
Mouthwash
Gels
Prescription medications
Mechanical cleansing

MUSCLE CHANGES
Cold (including ice chips)
Stretching activities
Various exercises

---

saliva is to promote improved oral and dental health. Reduced salivary flow can contribute to impaired oral and dental health.[81,82]

Unfortunately, xerostomia can be long lasting or even permanent after radiation therapy. Various interventions have been introduced, but none has been completely effective across the wide array of patients with this disabling clinical problem.[82,83] For some patients, especially those with some preservation of salivary flow, chewing gum may increase salivary output. Flavored gum may be superior in this regard because saliva flows in response to taste (particularly sour and bitter). In this regard, some patients may benefit from gums or lozenges (sugar free!) that have the potential to increase salivary flow by mechanical and chemosensory stimulation. Synthetic saliva or other moisturizing agents are commercially available as a replacement or compensation for lost natural saliva. These agents come in various forms, including mouthwash, sprays, and gels. When saliva substitutes are used, it is important to instruct the patient to coat the entire oral mucosa and to place a small pool of the liquid under the anterior aspect of the tongue. Some patients will benefit from use of these materials and others reject them. In general, any obtained benefit typically is temporary; therefore if xerostomia is a factor in dysphagia, patients should be instructed to apply these agents before eating. Many patients report using a water spritzer bottle as needed for dry mouth. These patients also use liquids frequently during meals to help transport food through the swallowing mechanism and to remove post-swallow residue with this liquid wash. Of course, this strategy requires adequate airway protection to minimize or eliminate risk of aspiration.

Physicians may prescribe medication to increase salivary flow. These agents tend to require extended use and the cost may be prohibitive for some patients. These medications also increase fluid secretion from many glands in addition to salivary glands. Some patients report profuse sweating when taking these medications. In reality, many patients who have xerostomia experiment with different approaches to improving oral lubrication. Clinicians can help this process by providing a wide range of options and information. One consideration for patients with xerostomia is oral hygiene. Reduction of saliva can compromise oral and dental health. Clinicians should counsel patients to engage in a routine of frequent oral hygiene activities consistent with the condition of the oral cavity.

Oral pain from mucositis can be a significant problem resulting from acute toxicity in the patient treated with RT protocols (also with chemotherapy). In severe cases, this pain can be excruciating and cause the individual to reduce the frequency of swallowing or cease oral intake of food and liquid altogether. Few proven strategies are available to combat this situation. Simple techniques that do not require medical support include mechanical cleansing with saline solution and use of ice chips.[84] Foam "toothettes" are not recommended for mechanical cleansing because they tend to disintegrate on the dry mucosa. Instead, patients are encouraged to use a very soft toothbrush in light salt water and to brush the oral mucosa to remove any debris. Ice chips use both cold, which can provide temporary relief from oral pain in some cases, and water, which can help lubricate the oral mucosa. Some patients report using oral analgesic gels similar to those used for babies who are teething. For severe pain, physicians may prescribe analgesic patches of strong pain-suppressing medication. In milder cases, an over-the-counter liquid medication to suppress pain may be adequate.

A series of Cochrane reviews has been completed to evaluate the effectiveness of interventions for oral mucositis.[85] The most recent review concluded that only weak, unreliable evidence was available to support the use of allopurinol mouthwash or other medical approaches. However, despite this absence of proven interventions in the treatment of oral mucositis, at least two positive views should be mentioned. Oral mucositis is a side effect of acute toxicity and thus is often a temporary condition. When it is well managed, the duration and impact of oral

mucositis in the irradiated area can be contained to various degrees. Second, clinicians and researchers continue to investigate new and perhaps unusual methods to help patients with this disabling condition. Some novel approaches include the topical application of pure honey[86] and the use of low-level laser therapy.[87]

Changes in muscle tissue occur in the direction of restricted movement of structures resulting from fibrosis or neuropathy in muscles that have been irradiated. Also, disuse atrophy leading to weakness should be considered in patients who are not taking food and liquid by mouth. No single therapy has been shown to be a panacea for all patients. Consultation with a physical therapist may be valuable to identify strategies to increase movement in fibrotic muscles, especially when fibrosis restricts functional head and/or neck movement. One general strategy is to stretch the restricted structure and thereby the fibrotic muscles. As previously described, repetitive stretching has improved movement, especially in the jaw. If movement is reduced from muscle weakness, exercise approaches to muscle rehabilitation should be investigated. This applies to the swallowing mechanism as well as the general head and neck region.

In severe cases of radiation changes in mucosa and/or muscle tissue, patients are not able to maintain any oral intake of food or liquid. In these cases, the physician providing the cancer treatment may opt for nonoral feeding strategies. Available evidence supports the use of a PEG tube over a nasogastric tube.[88] PEG feedings have been shown to be superior to nasogastric feeding in regard to less mechanical failure, better nutritional outcomes, and fewer associated chest infections in this patient population. The decision to pursue nonoral feeding strategies is typically based on individual patient circumstances and is often done in consultation with a dietitian and an SLP. As noted, it is important to monitor these patients over time to determine whether oral feeding may be reestablished or if swallowing therapy may be beneficial. In addition, it is important for these patients to follow a prophylactic exercise regimen to limit the potential atrophic effects of muscle disuse within the swallowing mechanism while the patient relies on a nonoral feeding source for nutrition and hydration.

TAKE HOME NOTES

1. Cancer within the swallowing mechanism and the treatments for cancer contribute to dysphagia and other life-altering changes. The primary treatments

for cancer are surgery and radiation therapy. These may be used alone or in combination. Chemotherapy may be used in combination with one of these primary approaches.

2. Dysphagia characteristics resulting from treatments for head/neck cancer vary depending on the type and extent of the treatment. One common feature is reduced movement within the swallowing mechanism. This contributes to reduced swallowing efficiency, which may be observed in many ways. Knowledge of the nature and extent of the cancer treatment is helpful in understanding and developing therapeutic strategies for resulting dysphagia.

3. Patients who receive radiation therapy in isolation or in combination with surgery may have dysphagia related to reduced movement of structures within the swallowing mechanism and/or from pain and dryness in the oropharyngeal structures. If present, these treatment complications may require direct intervention to facilitate improved swallowing function.

4. In evaluating swallowing function in the patient who has been treated for head/neck cancer, it is important to evaluate dysphagia-related conditions, including nutritional status, senses of taste and smell, endurance, and oral pain.

5. Therapy for dysphagia in patients with head/neck cancer often focuses on bolus transport issues and airway protection issues. A variety of surgical and behavioral therapy strategies are available to improve swallowing function. Recent research has suggested that the earlier therapy is initiated, the better the expected outcome.

References

1. National Cancer Institute Factsheet: *Head and neck cancer: Questions and answers*: http://www.cancer.gov/cancertopics/factsheet/Sites-Types/head-and-neck. Accessed March 28, 2008.

2. van Bokhorst-de van der Schuer MA, van Leeuwen PA, Kuik DJ et al: The impact of nutritional status on the prognoses of patients with advanced head and neck cancer, *Cancer* 86:519, 1999.

3. Fietkau R: Principles of feeding cancer patients via enteral or parenteral nutrition during radiotherapy, *Strahlenther Onkol* 174(Suppl 3):47, 1998.

4. Lees J: Incidence of weight loss in head and neck cancer patients on commencing radiotherapy at a regional oncology centre, *Eur J Cancer Care (Engl)* 8:133, 1999.

5. Johnston CA, Kean TJ, Prudo SM: Weight loss in patients receiving radical radiation therapy for head and neck cancer: a prospective study, *J Parenter Enteral Nutr* 6:399, 1982.

6. American Joint Committee on Cancer: *AJCC cancer staging manual*, ed 6, New York, 2002, Springer.

7. Mendenhall WM, Riggs CE, Cassisi NJ: Treatment of head and neck cancers. In DeVita VT, Hellman S, Rosenberg SA, editors: *Cancer: principles and practice of oncology*, Philadelphia, 2005, Lippincott Williams & Wilkins.

8. Smith RV, Goldman Y, Beitler JJ et al: Decreased short- and long-term swallowing problems with altered radiotherapy dosing used in an organ-sparing protocol for advanced pharyngeal carcinoma, *Arch Otolaryngol Head Neck Surg* 30:831, 2004.

9. Levendag PC, Teguh DN, Voet P et al: Dysphagia disorders in patients with cancer of the oropharynx are significantly affected by the radiation therapy dose to the superior and middle constrictor muscle: a dose-effect relationship, *Radiother Oncol* 85:64, 2007.

10. Jensen K, Overgaard M, Grau C: Morbidity after ipsilateral radiotherapy for oropharyngeal cancer, *Radiother Oncol* 85:90, 2007.

11. Adelstein DJ, Li Y, Adams GI et al: An intergroup phase III comparison of standard radiation therapy and two schedules of concurrent chemoradiotherapy in patients with unresectable squamous cell head and neck cancer, *J Clin Oncol* 21:21, 2003.

12. Mittal BB, Pauloski BR, Harah DJ et al: Swallowing dysfunction—preventive and rehabilitation strategies in patients with head-and-neck cancers treated with surgery, radiotherapy, and chemotherapy: a critical review, *Int J Radiation Oncology Biol Phys* 57:1219, 2003.

13. Logemann JA, Pauloski BR, Rademaker AW et al: Swallowing disorders in the first year after radiation and chemoradiation, *Head Neck* 30:148, 2008.

14. Zuydam AC, Lowe D, Brown JS et al: Predictors of speech and swallowing function following primary surgery for oral and oropharyngeal cancer, *Clin Otolaryngol* 30:428, 2005.

15. Pauloski BR, Rademaker AW, Logemann JA et al: Speech and swallowing in irradiated and nonirradiated postsurgical oral cancer patients, *Otolaryngol Head Neck Surg* 118:616, 1998.

16. Pauloski BR, Rademaker AW, Logemann J et al: Pretreatment swallowing function in patients with head and neck cancer, *Head Neck* 22:474, 2000.

17. Kendall K, McKenzie S, Leonard R et al: Timing of swallowing events after single-modality treatment of head and neck carcinomas with radiotherapy, *Head Neck* 20:720, 1998.

18. Kotz T, Abraham S, Beitler JJ et al: Pharyngeal transport dysfunction consequent to an organ-sparing protocol, *Arch Otolaryngol Head Neck Surg* 125:410, 1999.

19. Conley JJ: Swallowing dysfunctions associated with radical surgery of the head and neck, *Arch Surg* 80:602, 1960.

20. Summers GW: Physiologic problems following ablative surgery of the head and neck, *Otolaryngol Clin North Am* 7:217, 1974.

21. Hsiao HT, Leu YS, Lin CC: Tongue reconstruction with free radial foreman flap after hemiglossectomy: a functional assessment, *J Reconstr Microsurg* 19:137, 2003.

22. Seikaly H, Rieger J, Wolfaardt J et al: Functional outcomes after primary oropharyngeal cancer resection and reconstruction with the radial forearm flap, *Laryngoscopy* 113:897, 2003.

23. Crary MA, Carnaby-Mann GD: Rehabilitation after treatment for head and neck cancer. In DeVita VT, Hellman S, Rosenberg SA, editors: *Cancer: principles and practice of oncology*, ed 7, Philadelphia, 2005, Lippincott Williams & Wilkins.

24. Frazell EL, Lucas JC: Cancer of the tongue: report of the management of 1,554 patients, *Cancer* 15:1085, 1962.

25. Kimata YSM, Hishinuma S, Ebihara S et al: Analysis of the relations between the shape of the reconstructed tongue and postoperative functions after subtotal or total glossectomy, *Laryngoscope* 113:905, 2003.

26. Hirano M, Kuriowa Y, Tanaka S: Dysphagia following various degrees of surgical resection for oral cancer, *Ann Otol Rhinol Laryngol* 101:138, 1992.

27. McConnell FMS, Logemann JA: Diagnosis and treatment of swallowing disorders. In Cummings CW, editor: *Otolaryngology, head and neck surgery (update II)*, St Louis, 1990, Mosby.

28. Khariwala SS, Vivek PP, Lorenz RR et al: Swallowing outcomes after microvascular head and neck reconstruction: a prospective review of 191 cases, *Laryngoscopy* 117:1359, 2007.

29. Tei K, Maekawa K, Kitada H et al: Recovery from postsurgical swallowing dysfunction in patients with oral cancer, *J Oral Maxillofac Surg* 65:1077, 2007.

30. Pauloski BR, Rademaker AW, Logemann J et al: Surgical variables affecting swallowing in patients treated for oral/oropharyngeal cancer, *Head Neck* 26:625, 2004.

31. Reiger JM, Zalmanowitz JG, Sytsanko A et al: Functional outcomes after surgical reconstruction of the base of tongue using the radial forearm flap in patients with oropharyngeal carcinoma, *Head Neck* 29:1024, 2007.

32. Borggreven PA, Verdonck-de Leeuw I, Rinkel RN et al: Swallowing after major surgery of the oral cavity or oropharynx: a prospective and longitudinal assessment of patients treated by microvascular soft tissue reconstruction, *Head Neck* 29:638, 2007.

33. Wycliffe ND, Grover RS, Kim PD et al: Hypopharyngeal cancer, *Top Magn Reson Imaging* 18:243, 2007.

34. Martin A, Jackel MC, Christiansen H et al: Organ preserving transoral laser microsurgery for cancer of the hypopharynx, *Laryngoscope* 118:398, 2008.

35. Preuss SF, Cramer K, Klussmann JP et al: Transoral laser surgery for laryngeal cancer: outcome, complications and prognostic factors in 275 patients, *Eur J Surg Oncol* 35:235, 2009.

36. Hinni ML, Salassa JR, Grant DG et al: Transoral laser microsurgery for advanced laryngeal cancer, *Arch Otolaryngol Head Neck Surg* 133:1198, 2007.

37. Hartl DM, de Mones E, Hans S et al: Treatment of early-stage glottic cancer by transoral laser resection, *Ann Otol Rhinol Laryngol* 116:832, 2007.

38. Lewin JS, Hutcheson KA, Barringer DA et al: Functional analysis of swallowing outcomes after supracricoid partial laryngectomy, *Head Neck* 30:559, 2008.

39. Pellini R, Pichi B, Ruscito P et al: Supracricoid partial laryngectomies after radiation failure: a multi-institutional series, *Head Neck* 30:372, 2008.

40. León X, López M, García J et al: Supracricoid laryngectomy as salvage surgery after failure of radiation therapy, *Eur Arch Otorhinolaryngol* 264:809, 2007.

41. Pauloski BR, Rademaker AW, Logemann J et al: Speech and swallowing in irradiated and nonirradiated postsurgical oral cancer patients, *Otolaryngol Head Neck Surg* 118:616, 1998.

42. Pauloski BR, Logemann J, Rademaker AW et al: Speech and swallowing function after oral and oropharyngeal resections: one-year followup, *Head Neck* 16:313, 1994.

43. Epstein JB, Emerton S, Kolbinson DA et al: Quality of life and oral function following radiotherapy for head and neck cancer, *Head Neck* 21:1, 1999.

44. Rosenthal DI: Consequences of mucositis-induced treatment breaks and dose reductions on head and neck cancer treatment options, *J Support Oncol* 5:23, 2007.

45. Murphy BA: Clinical and economic consequences of mucositis induced by chemotherapy and/or radiation therapy, *J Support Oncol* 5:13, 2007.

46. Cheng KK: Oral mucositis, dysfunction, and distress in patients undergoing cancer therapy, *J Clin Nurs* 16:2114, 2007.

47. Dirix P, Nuyts S, Vander Poorten V et al: The influence of xerostomia after radiotherapy on quality of life: results of a questionnaire in head and neck cancer, *Support Care Cancer* 16:171, 2008.

48. Logemann J, Smith CH, Pauloski BR et al: Effects of xerostomia on perception of performance of swallow function, *Head Neck* 23:317, 2001.

49. Logemann J, Pauloski BR, Rademaker AW et al: Xerostomia: 12-month changes in saliva production and its relationship to the perception and performance of swallow function, oral intake, and diet after chemoradiation, *Head Neck* 25:432, 2003.

50. Mirza N, Machtay M, Devine PA et al: Gustatory impairment in patients undergoing head and neck irradiation, *Laryngoscope* 118:24, 2008.

51. Yamashita H, Nakagawa K, Tago M et al: Taste dysfunction in patients receiving radiotherapy, *Head Neck* 28:508, 2006.

52. Sandow PL, Hejrat-Yazdi M, Heft MW: Taste loss and recovery following radiation therapy, *J Dent Res* 85:608, 2006.

53. Schiffman SS: Critical illness and changes in sensory perception, *Proc Nutr Soc* 66:331, 2007.

54. Dijkstra PU, Huisman PM, Roodenburg JL: Criteria for trismus in head and neck oncology, *Int J Oral Maxillofac Surg* 35:337, 2006.

55. Zackrisson PMC, Strander H, Wennerberg J et al: A systematic overview of radiation therapy effects in head and neck cancer, *Acta Oncol* 42:443, 2003.

56. Levin AA, Levine MS, Rubesin SE et al: An 8-year review of barium studies in the diagnosis of gastroparesis, *Clin Radiol* 63:407, 2008.

57. World Health Organization: *Handbook for reporting results of cancer treatment*, Geneva, 1997, World Health Organization.

58. Meirovitz A, Murdoch-Kinch CA, Schipper M et al: Grading xerostomia by physicians or by patients after intensity-modulated radiotherapy of head-and-neck cancer, *Int J Radiation Oncology Biol Phys* 66:445, 2006.

59. Denk DM, Kaider A: Videoendoscopic biofeedback: a simple method to improve the efficacy of swallowing rehabilitation of patients after head and neck surgery, *Otorhinolaryngol* 59:100, 1997.

60. Denk DM, Swoboda H, Schima W et al: Prognostic factors for swallowing rehabilitation following head and neck cancer surgery, *Acta Otolaryngol* 117:769, 1997.

61. Zuydam A, Rogers S, Brown J et al: Swallowing rehabilitation after oro-pharyngeal resection for squamous cell carcinoma, *Br J Oral Maxillofac Surg* 38:513, 2000.

62. Crary, MA, Mann, GD, Groher ME et al: Functional outcomes of dysphagia therapy with adjunctive sEMG biofeedback, *Dysphagia* 19:160, 2004.

63. Carnaby-Mann GD, Crary MA: Adjunctive neuromuscular electrical stimulation in the treatment of chronic pharyngeal dysphagia, *Ann Otol Rhino Laryngol* 117:279, 2008.

64. Kulbersh BD, Rosenthal EL, McGrew BM et al: Pretreatment, preoperative swallowing exercises may improve dysphagia quality of life, *Laryngoscope* 116:883, 2006.

65. Carrol WR, Locher JL, Canon CL et al: Pretreatment swallowing exercises improve swallow function after chemoradiation, *Laryngoscope* 118:39, 2008.

66. Carnaby-Mann GD, Crary MA, Amdur R et al: Preventative exercise for dysphagia following head/neck cancer [abstract], *Dysphagia* 22:381, 2007.

67. Al-Othman MO, Amdur RJ, Morris CG et al: Does feeding tube placement predict for long-term swallowing disability after radiotherapy for head and neck cancer? *Head Neck* 25:741, 2003.

68. Crary MA, Groher ME: Reinstituting oral feeding in tube fed patients with dysphagia, *Nutr Clin Pract* 21:576, 2006.

69. Light J: A review of oral and oropharyngeal prostheses to facilitate speech and swallowing, *Am J Speech Lang Pathol* 4:15, 1995.

70. Pauloski BR, Logemann JA, Colangelo LA et al: Effect of intraoral prostheses on swallowing function in postsurgical oral and oropharyngeal cancer patients, *Am J Speech Lang Pathol* 5:31, 1996.

71. Castell JA, Castell DO, Shultz A et al: Effect of head position on the dynamics of the upper esophageal sphincter and pharynx, *Dysphagia* 8:1, 1993.

72. Fleming SM: Treatment of mechanical swallowing disorders. In Groher M, editor: *Dysphagia: diagnosis and management,* ed 3, Boston, 1997, Butterworth-Heinemann.

73. Grandi G, Silva ML, Streit C et al: A mobilization regimen to prevent mandibular hypomobility in irradiated patients: an analysis and comparison of two techniques, *Med Oral Pathol Oral Cir Bucal* 12:E105, 2007.

74. Dijkstra PU, Sterken MW, Pater R et al: Exercise therapy for trismus in head and neck cancer, *Oral Oncol* 43:389, 2007.

75. Dijkstra PU, Kalk WW, Roodenburg JL: Trismus in head and neck oncology: a systematic review, *Oral Oncol* 40:879, 2004.

76. Shulman DH, Shipman B, Willis FB: Treating trismus with dynamic splinting: a cohort, case series, *Adv Ther* 25:9, 2008.

77. Umeno H, Chitose S, Sato K et al: Efficacy of additional injection laryngoplasty after framework surgery, *Ann Otol Rhinol Laryngol* 117:5, 2008.

78. Dursun G, Boynukalin S, Bagis Ozgursoy O et al: Long-term results of different treatment modalities for glottic insufficiency, *Am J Otolaryngol* 29:7, 2008.

79. Morgan JE, Zraick RI, Griffin AW et al: Injection versus medialization laryngoplasty for the treatment of unilateral vocal fold paralysis, *Laryngoscope* 117:2068, 2007.

80. Amin MR: Thyrohyoid approach for vocal fold augmentation, *Ann Otol Rhinol Laryngol* 115:699, 2006.

81. Scully C: The role of saliva in oral health problems, *Practitioner* 245:841, 2001.

82. Cassolato SF, Turnbull RS: Xerostomia: clinical aspects and treatment, *Gerodontology* 20:64, 2003.

83. Fox PC: Salivary enhancement therapies, *Caries Res* 38:241, 2004.

84. Symonds RP: Treatment-induced mucositis: an old problem with new remedies, *Br J Cancer* 77:1689, 1998.

85. Worthington HV, Clarkson JE, Eden OB: Interventions for treating oral mucositis for patients with cancer receiving treatment, *Cochrane Database Syst Rev* (2):CD001973, 2007; (2):CD001973, 2004; (1):CD001973, 2002.

86. Motallebnejad M, Akram S, Moghadamina A et al: The effect of topical application of pure honey on radi-ation-induced mucositis: a randomized clinical trial, *J Contemp Dent Pract* 9:40, 2008.

87. Arora H, Pai KM, Maiya A et al: Efficacy of He-Ne laser in the prevention and treatment of radiotherapy-induced oral mucositis in oral cancer patients, *Oral Surg Oral Med Oral Pathol Oral Radiol Endod* 105:180, 2008.

88. Magné N, Marcy PY, Foa C et al: Comparison between nasogastric tube feeding and percutaneous fluoroscopic gastrostomy in advanced head and neck cancer patients, *Eur Arch Otorhinolaryngol* 258:89, 2001.

Esophageal Disorders

MICHAEL E. GROHER

OBJECTIVES

1. Discuss the structural disorders of the esophagus that affect swallowing.
2. Discuss the motor disorders of the esophagus that affect swallowing.
3. Detail disorders of the pharyngoesophageal segment.
4. Show how disorders of esophageal origin might affect other aspects of the swallowing chain.
5. Discuss possible treatment approaches for swallowing disorders of esophageal and pharyngoesophageal origin.

ROLE OF THE SPEECH-LANGUAGE PATHOLOGIST

It is not the role of the speech-language pathologist (SLP) to diagnose and treat dysphagia of esophageal origin. In most cases this is done by the gastroenterologist. However, because of the interdependency of the oral, pharyngeal, and esophageal stages of swallowing it is important for the speech pathologist to be aware of how esophageal-based dysphagia might affect other compartments involved in swallowing. It also is important for the SLP to be aware of the types of swallowing problems that should be referred to the gastroenterologist and what types of treatments they might recommend. Sometimes treatments (e.g., medications) might affect other parts of the swallowing chain, and patients might need certain instructions about taking their medications reinforced by other health care providers. One example is patients who take medication to control their gastroesophageal reflux disease (GERD). On careful questioning, it is revealed that they only take their medicine when they perceive they might be eating a meal that would cause an increase in reflux events. In most cases patients should be taking their medication on a daily basis, so reinforcing this point or reviewing proper dietary restrictions may be needed to avoid an increase in reflux events. In these circumstances knowledge of other professional roles and methods of evaluation and treatment can be beneficial to improve patient compliance and answer any questions patients might have about their dysphagia.

It is becoming more common for the SLP to include a screening of the esophagus in patients who are able to stand during the modified barium swallow study. The screenings are useful because they might detect a disorder that helps explain the patient's oropharyngeal symptoms. It is the role of the radiologist—rather than the SLP—to document and comment on these abnormalities. If further tests are warranted the SLP might include them in his or her progress note but with the approval of the radiologist.

STRUCTURAL DISORDERS

Esophageal dysphagia can be caused by a change in the ability of the esophagus to fully open during swallowing, resulting in a blockage of bolus passage. A change in the structure of the esophagus may be caused by a luminal stenosis or narrowing or by a luminal deformity such as another structure compressing it, thereby limiting its ability to open.

Esophageal Stenosis

Esophageal stenosis is conceptually the easiest mechanism of dysphagia to understand. When the lumen narrows, solid food may be too large to pass through it. Esophageal stenosis typically causes dysphagia for solid food. In addition, the *type* of solid material ingested often is important for symptom production. For instance, dysphagia of esophageal origin is more likely when solids are tough or fibrous. Softer, more easily chewed foods are much less likely to cause symptoms of esophageal dysphagia. An exception to this tough food–soft food dichotomy is that many patients also have particular trouble with soft, absorbent foods such as bread or pasta, which swell when mixed with saliva during mastication. Once bolus impaction occurs, the patient may have difficulty with liquids as well, obscuring the characteristic solids-only nature of esophageal stenosis. However, a careful history usually reveals that liquid dysphagia begins with ingestion of solids (see differential diagnosis later in this chapter).

Clinicians often rely too much on the patient's sensation of where food is sticking. The common wisdom that patients accurately localize symptoms to the site of obstruction is often inaccurate. In fact, approximately one third of patients with obstructing lesions of the distal esophagus point to the neck as the site of obstruction.[1] Conversely, one third of patients with dysphagia localized to

---

CLINICAL CORNER 7-1

A 57-year-old man came to the clinic because of solid and liquid dysphagia. He felt that food was sticking in the back of his throat. He had a long history of GERD but could not afford his medication. His oral peripheral examination was normal, and a modified barium swallow with liquids and solids was performed. Because he was an outpatient and was able to stand, the bolus was followed by the radiologist from the mouth to the region of the stomach. The radiologist commented that it appeared that the bolus flow through the PES was normal but was delayed with solid food boluses in the midesophageal region. For this reason he recommended a full examination of the esophagus with the patient in the supine position to more fully investigate this impression.

CRITICAL THINKING

1. Why is it necessary to study the esophagus with the patient in the supine or side-lying position?
2. How could GERD cause a swallowing problem?

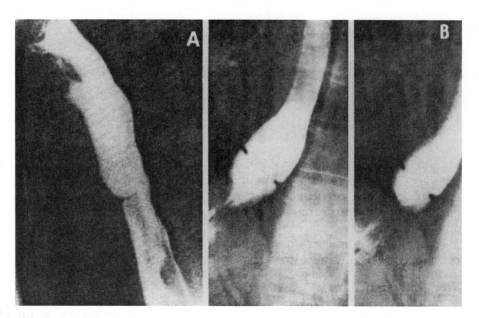

FIGURE 7-1. Thin, bandlike stenotic lesions are generally referred to as *rings* when located at or near the esophagogastric junction and *webs* when located elsewhere in the esophagus. **A,** A web is located at the pharyngoesophageal segment. **B,** Schatzki's ring located at the esophagogastric junction. The webs are seen as *darkened lines (slits)* on the white barium column. (Courtesy Bronwyn Jones, MD.)

the pharynx have an isolated abnormality of the esophagus.[2]

It is surprising how well some patients fare despite dramatic stenosis. Based on radiographic observations in patients with Schatzki's rings, it is often stated that patients with luminal diameters of more than 18 to 20 mm are never symptomatic, whereas those with diameters less than 10 to 12 mm are always symptomatic.[3] When the radiologist examines the esophagus for suspected stenosis, a **radiopaque** pill that is 13 mm in diameter is used to detect a stenosis. Between these extremes (20 and 10 mm), symptoms vary both in frequency and severity depending on the presence of associated motor dysfunction and the choice and preparation of food. Stenosis is treated by opening or removing the narrowed segment, depending on the specific cause. This is usually accomplished with **Maloney (bougie) dilators** or with **balloon dilatation**.

Common intrinsic structural abnormalities that narrow the esophagus include mucosal rings, benign strictures, and malignant tumors.

Rings and Webs

The esophagus may be narrowed by a band of tissue composed of mucosa and submucosa. By tradition, this type of lesion is called a *ring* when located at the esophagogastric junction and a *web* when located elsewhere in the esophagus or hypopharynx.

Although classically described in patients with iron-deficiency anemia *(sideropenic dysphagia),* the majority of esophageal webs are not associated with iron deficiency. Webs of the pharyngoesophageal segment or cervical esophagus are frequently asymmetric, most often impinging on the esophageal lumen from the anterior wall (Figure 7-1, *A*). A suspected web at the cervical level also can be seen in Video 7-1 on the Evolve site accompanying this text.

Schatzki's rings are the most common bandlike constriction of the esophagus. This lesion is typically symmetric and located at the esophagogastric junction (Figure 7-1, *B*). Asymptomatic Schatzki's rings are detected in approximately 10% of the population.[4] The ring is always noted in the presence of a **hiatal hernia**. However, most hiatal hernias are not associated with Schatzki's rings. The etiology of a Schatzki's ring is unknown. Because they are rarely seen in childhood and generally are first noticed in middle age, it is unlikely that a Schatzki's ring represents a congenital abnormality. A video image of a Schatzki's ring can be seen in Video 7-2 as a narrowing of the esophageal lumen in the distal esophagus during swallowing of a thicker bolus.

Webs and rings typically produce dysphagia for solids only. Patients often report that symptoms are intermittent and less likely if they select their food wisely and chew carefully (see the section on differential diagnosis). Conversely, symptoms are more likely if the patient eats away from home or carries on a conversation while eating; in these situations the choice of food is more restricted and proper preparation of food before swallowing is more difficult. The patient often must end the episode by inducing regurgitation. Once the food is dislodged, the patient often can return to the meal without further difficulty.

The extent to which attention to the mechanics of cutting and chewing controls symptoms is limited. When the lumen is severely compromised, the patient may find it impossible to maintain the level of attention required to remain symptom free without avoiding solids entirely. The patient may describe symptoms without any apparent progression in frequency or severity that date back for many years. Progression, when it does occur, usually is slow.

Radiographically, rings and webs appear as thin (2 to 4 mm) bands that form shelflike constrictions anywhere along the esophagus. Although radiologists occasionally refer to thicker lesions as webs or rings, these are probably short strictures or abnormal muscular contractions.

Treatment of webs or rings involves dilatation or rupture of the ring by any one of a variety of esophageal dilator systems. The ring is thin, nonfibrotic, and easy to dilate. Complete, or nearly complete, symptomatic relief can be anticipated. Failure to respond is unusual. Dilatation may provide permanent relief, although a large proportion of patients need periodic redilatation at variable intervals.[5]

Benign Stricture

Strictures are rarely seen in children, although congenital strictures do occur. The majority of benign esophageal strictures are acquired in adulthood as a consequence of esophagitis. In a circular structure such as the esophagus, edema resulting from ongoing inflammation and **fibrosis** as part of the healing process occurs at the expense of luminal diameter.

As with webs and rings, dysphagia is generally for solids only. However, dysphagia is progressive, with episodes becoming more frequent and severe over a period of months or years. As luminal narrowing increases, the patient reports trouble swallowing food that previously caused no difficulty. Stenosis occasionally can become so severe that even thick liquids cause dysphagia. Even then, however, dysphagia is virtually always greater for solids than liquids.

Benign strictures are usually secondary to reflux-induced esophagitis, although most patients with gastroesophageal reflux disease (GERD) do not have esophagitis. *Esophagitis* refers to inflammation of the lining of the esophagus. Esophagitis may vary in severity from microscopic inflammation to mucosal

BOX 7-1	Differential Diagnosis of Esophagitis

1. Gastroesophageal reflux
2. Infections (*Candida*, viral)
3. Trauma (prolonged nasogastric intubation)
4. Acute chemical ingestion (lye, industrial acids)
5. Drug-induced esophagitis (tetracycline, iron, potassium, quinidine, nonsteroidal antiinflammatory drugs)
6. Radiation
7. Skin conditions (pemphigus, cicatricial pemphigoid, epidermolysis bullosa dystrophica, lichen planus, toxic epidermal necrolysis, Stevens-Johnson syndrome)
8. Others (Crohn's disease, Behçet's syndrome)

edema to erosion, ulcerations, and stricture. Patients usually describe a history of heartburn or chest pain and may report the frequent use of antacids or other ulcer medications. In some patients the esophagus appears to be relatively insensitive to acid exposure. These individuals never experience significant reflux symptoms despite severe esophagitis and progression to stricture formation. Although most benign esophageal strictures are a result of reflux esophagitis, any source of esophagitis can cause stricture formation (Box 7-1).

Drug-induced or pill esophagitis can be seen in young or elderly patients. Typically, commonly administered medications that are larger in size (tetracycline, potassium, quinidine) become lodged at the level of the aortic arch and dissolve, causing inflammation and stricture. Symptoms of chest pain, odynophagia, heartburn, and dysphagia may be present, usually more acutely in younger patients.[6]

Radiographically, a benign stricture is seen as a narrowed segment of esophageal lumen that may range from 1 cm to many centimeters long (Figure 7-2). The stricture usually is smooth and gradually tapering, with a symmetric lumen that follows the anticipated path of the normal esophagus. Ongoing inflammation may produce an eroded appearance along its course. A lateral and anteroposterior (AP) video image of a midesophageal stricture caused by GERD can be seen in Video 7-3 on the Evolve site. In the AP view barium flow is interrupted, with barium building up above the stricture. The lateral view shows a long, tapered appearance of a stricture in the esophagus.

Proper management requires both treatment of the underlying inflammation and dilation of the stricture. Treatment of the cause of esophagitis requires accu-

Practice Note 7-1

One day my neighbor, aware of my background with swallowing disorders, came to tell me that her 18-year-old son suddenly could not swallow. Because sudden onset of a swallowing disorder is rare in younger persons, the only potential cause that came to mind was pill-induced esophagitis. When I asked whether he was taking medication, she reported that he had just started taking tetracycline for his acne and the day before he had forgotten to take his medication at home using the normal amount of water. Instead he took his dose in the classroom without water. Undoubtedly, the pill did not reach the stomach before it dissolved, which created an inflammatory reaction with subsequent stenosis. I speculated that he had temporary dysphagia from pill-induced esophagitis. His symptoms spontaneously resolved within 2 days.

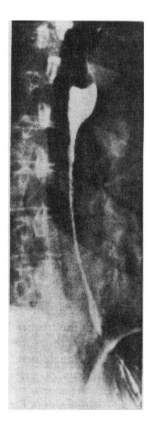

FIGURE 7-2. Long and symmetric benign stricture with a lumen that tapers gradually. The lumen follows the anticipated line of the normal esophagus. The barium within the narrowed lumen has a somewhat irregular appearance because of the erosions. (Courtesy Bronwyn Jones, MD.)

rate diagnosis. Although reflux is the most common cause of esophagitis, other possibilities must be considered, especially in patients with atypical histories, an unusual distribution of inflammation, or failure to respond to reflux treatment.

Dilatation often can be performed by using the same techniques available for a Schatzki's ring. However, the stricture may be relatively unyielding and require stiffer dilator systems. Effective dilatation usually improves symptoms, although edema from inflammation may result in less-complete symptomatic relief than with a Schatzki's ring and in relatively rapid restenosis. Frequent dilatations are more often required in benign strictures than with Schatzki's rings. Even when ongoing inflammation completely ceases, periodic dilatation may be necessary, especially during the first year after initial treatment, when maturation of the fibrotic reaction continues at the expense of luminal diameter.

Malignant Stricture

Although benign tumors may arise from the esophagus, the majority of clinically significant tumors of the esophagus are malignant. In the past, most esophageal malignancies were **squamous cell carcinomas**, although recent studies suggest a dramatic increase in **adenocarcinoma** of the distal esophagus. Most esophageal adenocarcinomas appear to arise from Barrett's esophagus, a premalignant condition in which columnar cells replace the usual squamous epithelium covering the lower end of the esophagus as a result of severe GER.

As with other types of stenotic lesions, dysphagia initially occurs for solids only. However, it usually progresses rapidly, with dysphagia for soft foods and even liquids developing within a few months of the onset of symptoms.

Radiographically, esophageal malignancies appear as strictures of variable length. By the time of presentation, the cancerous tumor or area is usually many centimeters long and involves the entire circumference of the esophageal lumen, producing a stricture. The typical malignant stricture is characterized by its shelflike proximal margins and irregular channel, which may diverge substantially from the anticipated course of the esophageal lumen (Figure 7-3). However, not all esophageal cancers are obviously malignant on barium radiography, and occasional malignant-looking strictures may be benign.[6] For this reason, endoscopy with tissue sampling by biopsy with or without **cytologic brushing** is essential to differentiate benign and malignant strictures.

Curative treatment is primarily surgical, although apparent cures by radiotherapy have been reported.

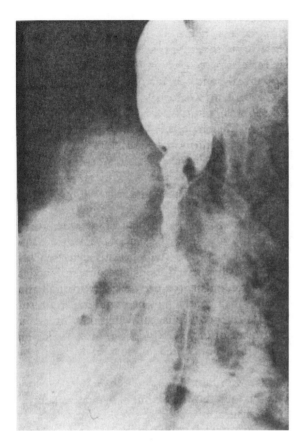

FIGURE 7-3. Malignant circumferential stricture. Characteristics distinguishing it from a benign stricture include the sharp, shelflike proximal margin and the more irregular configuration of the stenotic segment. Unlike some malignant strictures, this stricture follows the anticipated path of the esophageal lumen. Compare the appearance with the benign stricture shown in Figure 7-2. (Courtesy Bronwyn Jones, MD.)

Unfortunately, by the time symptoms develop, the cancer is usually very advanced and incurable. The overall 5-year survival rate for esophageal cancer is only approximately 5%.[1] Even among those in whom resection for apparent cure is possible, the 5-year survival rate is only approximately 15%.[7] Recent studies suggested that the 5-year survival rate could be doubled with a combination of preoperative radiotherapy and chemotherapy.[8] Surprisingly, almost 25% of patients had no evidence of cancer by gross or histologic examination. Among these patients, survival was improved fourfold over rates reported for surgery alone and twofold over those with evidence of residual tumor at surgical resection.

For patients in whom curative resection is not possible, palliative resection often is still feasible

and provides good symptomatic relief. In the past, a high perioperative mortality rate of approximately 29% combined with the infrequency of cure made surgery unattractive.[9] However, with better nutrition provided by preoperative and perioperative hyperalimentation the risk of palliative surgery has declined.[10]

Alternative approaches include dilatation, tumor ablation (thermal treatment to destroy tumor obstructing the esophagus) by laser or bipolar electrocautery, and **stent** placement. Each of these approaches is directed at opening the esophageal lumen to permit eating, in recognition that the major cause of early death in patients with esophageal cancer is malnutrition and aspiration pneumonia.

Dilatation generally provides limited and short-lived relief but is useful in preparing for other forms of therapy. The choice between other modalities depends on specific features of the tumor and local technical expertise and resources. Endoscopic laser therapy and bipolar electrocautery can be used to destroy tumor tissue that blocks the esophageal lumen; this may provide a number of months of relief, allowing continuing oral intake. Treatment can be repeated if obstruction recurs.

An esophageal stent is a tube with a large channel that can be placed through the strictured segment to maintain luminal patency. The stent permits ingestion of a modified diet, concentrating on soft, easily chewed foods and purees. The use of stents for palliation has decreased dramatically since the development of thermal methods of treatment. However, stents continue to be useful in certain situations, especially in the presence of a **tracheoesophageal fistula** that often complicates the natural history or treatment of esophageal cancer. In this situation, a properly placed stent can maintain the esophageal lumen while covering the opening to the airway. The recent introduction of expandable metal stents has made insertion easier and provides a larger internal luminal diameter, allowing patients to eat a less-restrictive diet.

Although endoscopic treatment with laser, bipolar electrocautery, or stent placement may be highly successful in reestablishing luminal patency, a substantial proportion of patients with esophageal cancer have poor appetites and are unable to gain weight. The early use of endoscopically placed or fluoroscopically guided gastrostomies should be considered in patients who do not eat once the lumen is reestablished or who are scheduled to undergo chemotherapy or radiotherapy, treatments that may produce or exacerbate anorexia. (See Chapter 8 for a discussion of transhiatal esophagectomy.)

Luminal Deformities

Extrinsic Compression

Some degree of luminal deformity caused by extrinsic compression by normal **mediastinal** structures (the aortic knob, the left mainstem bronchus, and the left atrium of the heart) is normally seen on barium studies and rarely, if ever, causes symptoms. More pronounced compression can occur with mediastinal conditions, such as aortic aneurysm, **cardiomegaly**, congenital abnormalities of the large mediastinal arteries (e.g., aberrant subclavian artery), enlarged mediastinal lymph nodes, and lung cancer. Video 7-4 on the Evolve site shows a patient with cardiomegaly and reduced bolus flow. The enlarged heart is seen as a large shadow (note heartbeat) in the middle of the video image. The elasticity of the contralateral esophageal wall usually tends to minimize symptoms until compression is far advanced. Dilatation is usually ineffective because the force of dilatation is absorbed by the elastic, uninvolved wall. Effective treatment, when necessary, requires shrinking or removing the mass producing the compression. Unfortunately, this is often not practical in patients in whom compression produces significant symptoms.

Esophageal Diverticulum

Compared with **diverticula** of the hypopharynx, esophageal diverticula are rare and usually asymptomatic, even when they are relatively large. When symptoms do occur, they include dysphagia for liquids and solids, regurgitation of previously swallowed food back into the mouth, or both. Regurgitation without dysphagia is not uncommon.

Most often, esophageal diverticula are a consequence of obstruction distal to the region of bolus collection. Increased pressure in the esophagus results in bulging at a point of relative weakness. Less commonly, diverticula can result from periesophageal inflammation, which causes traction on the esophageal wall (traction diverticulum). Although most traction diverticula occur in the midesophagus, most midesophageal diverticula, like their distal esophageal counterparts, are caused by **pulsion**. Video 7-5 shows a diverticulum that fills and causes a momentary obstruction to bolus flow.

Treatment of pulsion-type diverticula is necessary only if a diverticulum is symptomatic. Because they frequently give rise to motor or structural disorders, it is important to look for pulsion-type abnormalities as causes for the development of the diverticulum. It may be difficult to distinguish between the underlying obstructive disorder and the diverticulum as a cause of symptoms. It is appropriate to attempt to treat the underlying cause of increased pressure with dilatation in the case of structural obstruction or with drugs for dysmotility. In some patients symptoms initially believed to be a consequence of the diverticulum improve significantly or resolve entirely with such conservative therapy.

Surgical removal of the diverticulum is required if medical management fails. Surgery limited to diverticulectomy, however, is associated with a high incidence of early **anastomotic leakage** or late recurrence, probably because it fails to deal with the underlying cause of increased intraesophageal pressure and creates an area of relative esophageal wall weakness. Therefore diverticulectomy should be combined with treatment of the underlying disorder—motor (with a surgical **myotomy**) or structural (with dilatation).

ESOPHAGEAL MOTILITY DISORDERS

An orderly, progressive peristaltic wave is not uniformly present after every swallow, even in individuals without dysphagia. The dividing line between normal and pathologic degrees of dysmotility is poorly defined. The incidence of abnormal contractions changes with bolus type (it is increased with dry swallows), although not with age.

A variety of schemes have been proposed to classify esophageal dysmotility. In abnormalities of esophageal peristalsis, contraction amplitude may be too high or low, contraction duration prolonged, or the orderly progression of the contractile wave down the length of the esophagus uncoordinated. In abnormalities of lower esophageal sphincter (LES) function, the pressure may be too high or too low and relaxation may be incomplete. Finally, the esophageal body and LES can misbehave separately or together. The individual characteristics of commonly described motility disorders are not necessarily unique. In many ways the separation between entities is somewhat arbitrary.

Disorders of Peristalsis

Motor dysfunction of the body of the esophagus may cause symptoms of dysphagia, chest pain, or regurgitation. Dysphagia is usually for liquids as well as solids, although not necessarily in equal measure. Chest pain may mimic that of cardiac disease and cause considerable concern on the part of both patient and physician. Although pain initiated or exacerbated by swallowing strongly implicates the esophagus as the site of origin, a clear relation to eating is often

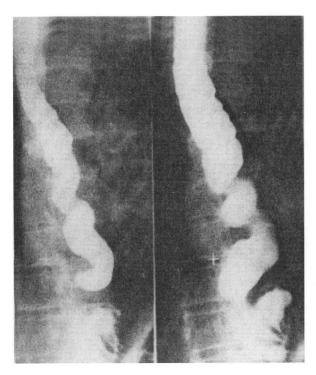

FIGURE 7-4. Radiographic appearance of esophageal dysmotility. A variety of patterns of abnormal peristalsis may be seen on barium radiography. In spot film, the silhouette of the barium column in the upper portion of the esophagus has a serrated appearance, whereas in the lower portion there is a corkscrewlike configuration. In addition, there is a hiatal hernia. (Courtesy Bronwyn Jones, MD.)

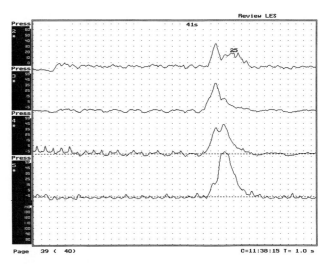

FIGURE 7-5. Manometric appearance of esophageal spasm. The manometric findings in esophageal dysmotility are characterized by various combinations of simultaneous, multiphasic, high-amplitude, and prolonged contractions. The more severe forms are designated *diffuse esophageal spasm,* although the boundaries between this diagnosis and lesser degrees of dysmotility are not well established. In addition, occasional abnormal contractions may be seen in normal individuals. In the manometric study shown, the four tracings are from pressure sensors spaced at 2-cm intervals in the distal esophagus (the distance of the distal sensor from the nares and timing of swallow are indicated by number and letter at the top). The initial upstroke in all leads is simultaneous. In addition, each demonstrates a secondary upstroke that also begins simultaneously. The amplitude and duration of contraction are within normal limits. The dashed lines represent intraesophageal resting pressure. (Vertical axis scale, 1 increment = 10 mm Hg; horizontal scale, 1 increment = 1 second.)

absent. Similarly, the presence of other symptoms implicating the swallowing mechanism supports the possibility that the esophagus is the cause of chest pain. However, cardiac disease is sufficiently common, especially in older patients, to justify a cardiology evaluation.

Diffuse Esophageal Spasm

Esophageal spasm is a graphic term with an imprecise meaning. The diagnosis of esophageal spasm is used quite freely among physicians, including gastroenterologists. All too often esophageal spasm is diagnosed on the basis of minor degrees of dysmotility seen radiographically (Figure 7-4) or manometrically (Figure 7-5), or even on the basis of consistent symptoms in the absence of radiographic or manometric confirmation. Esophageal spasm constitutes the end of a spectrum of nonspecific esophageal dysmotility. At one end of the range are the abnormal contractions seen occasionally in normal individuals. At the other are repeated high-amplitude, prolonged, simultaneous, or multiphasic contractions or some combination of these in the absence of any normal peristaltic

activity (Figures 7-5 and 7-6). Although few would argue against calling the latter *spasm,* little agreement exists on where less-severe abnormalities of esophageal peristalsis end and spasm begins.

An interesting feature of these criteria is the inclusion of high LES pressures and incomplete relaxation as an associated finding. LES dysfunction in diffuse esophageal spasm is well recognized, with failure of complete relaxation noted in one third of patients.[11] The presence of LES dysfunction in diffuse esophageal spasm and of spastic contractions in a variant of achalasia ("vigorous achalasia") obscures the distinction between the two (see achalasia below).

Nutcracker Esophagus

Brand et al.[12] described a group of patients with chest pain or dysphagia that occurred in association with manometric findings of high amplitude but with normally progressive peristaltic waves. This syndrome,

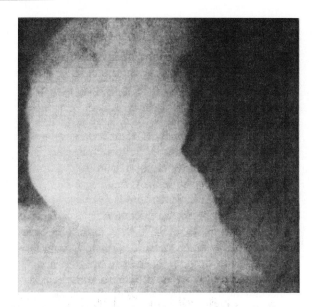

FIGURE 7-6. Radiographic appearance of achalasia. A barium esophagram with the patient in an upright position demonstrates the typical features of achalasia: a dilated esophagus and a smooth, tapering narrowing at the esophagogastric junction ("parrot-beaked deformity") holding up a column of barium mixed with retained food. In more extreme cases, the esophagus may take on a tortuous appearance (sigmoid esophagus). (Courtesy Bronwyn Jones, MD.)

often called *the nutcracker esophagus,* is considered by some authorities to be the most commonly detected disorder of esophageal motility.

A number of questions surround the manometric pattern of the nutcracker esophagus. First, the criterion for diagnosis has changed. Originally described as a mean pressure of more than 120 mm Hg, recent studies of healthy individuals indicate that this value is too low, especially for the older population. Castell[13] has suggested that to avoid overdiagnosis the term *nutcracker esophagus* should be restricted to patients with mean pressures higher than 180 mm Hg.[13]

Second, the pressures measured during serial motility studies performed in the same individual may change substantially, resulting in the manometric interpretations changing from abnormal (i.e., nutcracker) to normal on different recordings in the same patient.[14] Interestingly, the pressures tend to be highest at the initial recording, suggesting that anxiety associated with the procedure may play a role in this manometric pattern.

Third, why nutcracker esophagus produces symptoms is not clear. Barium esophagrams demonstrate normal stripping function. Although increased pressure could conceivably cause discomfort, most patients with high-amplitude contractions during motility do

not have pain at the time of the examination, and it is often difficult to appreciate differences between contraction amplitude and appearance during spontaneous episodes of pain that are witnessed manometrically.[15] Nutcracker esophagus may represent a marker of patients with intermittent diffuse esophageal spasm.

Nonspecific Motility Disorders

Disagreement about the criteria for esophageal spasm aside, a large number of patients referred to the esophageal function laboratory have abnormalities of esophageal motility in which the degree and type of motility abnormalities detected are not sufficient to be labeled esophageal spasm or nutcracker esophagus.[15] These lesser patterns of dysmotility are called *nonspecific esophageal motor disorders.* Their clinical significance remains unclear. On the one hand, it is difficult to ignore the potential significance of disordered peristalsis in patients with dysphagia. On the other hand, similar degrees of abnormality are so common in normal volunteers that their mere presence cannot be considered proof of causality.

Treatment of Motility Disorders

The medical therapy for esophageal dysmotility is often of limited benefit. A variety of smooth muscle–relaxant drugs (nitrates, hydralazine, calcium channel blockers) have been used in an attempt to decrease esophageal contractile amplitude and repetitive contractions. Although some patients experience a dramatic response, many do not. Controlled clinical trials thus far have failed to demonstrate a convincing beneficial effect of these drugs on symptoms.[16] The symptomatic response to these drugs is quite variable and often incomplete. Potential side effects related to the **hypotensive** effects of the drugs severely limit their use.

The most common mistake in the treatment of esophageal dysmotility is to assume that the patient has a primary disorder of esophageal motility. Esophageal dysmotility is like anemia; it is a laboratory finding that requires further evaluation. As for anemia, there is a differential diagnosis of esophageal dysmotility. The most common cause of dysmotility is esophageal irritation, most commonly by GER. Disordered esophageal peristalsis also may result from esophageal obstruction, ganglion degeneration (i.e., vigorous achalasia), autonomic neuropathies (e.g., caused by diabetes or alcohol abuse), or collagen vascular diseases (especially scleroderma and mixed connective tissue disease). Only patients with esophageal dysmotility in the absence of an underlying cause are considered to have a primary (or **idiopathic**) esophageal dysmotility.

Reflux-induced dysmotility is probably the most common cause of esophageal dysmotility and is more easily treated than idiopathic dysmotility. Because heartburn is not always present, reflux should be considered in any patient with symptoms of esophageal spasm. Ironically, the drugs used to treat idiopathic dysmotility may make reflux worse by further impairing LES pressure. Esophageal stenosis, another cause of esophageal dysmotility, may be missed occasionally by barium studies and endoscopy. Dilatation should be considered if there is any question of a structural obstruction.

LOWER ESOPHAGEAL SPHINCTER ABNORMALITIES

Achalasia

Achalasia is a condition in which a nonrelaxing or incompletely relaxing LES prevents the passage of swallowed material into the stomach. Patients usually present with dysphagia for both liquids and solids. Regurgitation is common and characteristically results in regurgitation of recognizable food hours after it was eaten. Late regurgitation of undigested food is a feature seen in only a few cases of dysphagia, primarily achalasia and hypopharyngeal (Zenker's) or esophageal diverticulum. During barium swallow, with the patient in the upright position, the esophagus is generally dilatated and a column of barium of variable height is maintained above a tight esophagogastric junction (see Figure 7-6). The possibility that this appearance could represent a tight esophageal stricture is ruled out at endoscopy when the endoscope passes into the stomach with mild to moderate resistance.[15]

Although the impairment of LES response to swallow is key to the functional obstruction of the flow of food into the stomach, the motor abnormalities of achalasia include the complete loss of progressive peristalsis (Figure 7-7). In the more common variant of achalasia (classic achalasia), low-amplitude, aperistaltic contractions in the body of the esophagus are combined with a high or high-normal, nonrelaxing sphincter. The simultaneous low-amplitude increases in pressure with swallow are often attributed to pharyngeal pressure, transmitted into the dilated esophagus, rather than to true esophageal contractile activity.[15]

A variant of achalasia, called *vigorous achalasia*, has been recognized. In this condition, the typical LES findings of achalasia are associated with higher amplitude, prolonged, multiphasic contractions, indicating

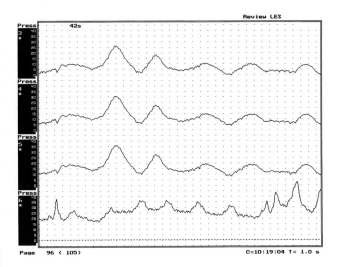

FIGURE 7-7. Radiographic appearance of achalasia. A barium esophagram with the patient upright shows a markedly dilated esophagus with a narrowing at the tip of the column *(lower right)* similar in shape to a bird's beak. The lower esophageal sphincter has failed to relax, allowing material to back up above the level of the blockage. (Courtesy Bronwyn Jones, MD.)

that intrinsic esophageal motor response to swallowing, however deranged, is still present.

The manometric features of achalasia include an LES with a high or high-normal resting pressure that fails to relax appropriately with swallow. In addition, a complete loss of progressive peristalsis occurs. Occasional patients with identical manometric findings as a result of tumor infiltration of the esophagogastric junction have been described; their condition is labeled *secondary achalasia* or *pseudoachalasia*.[17] Pseudoachalasia also has been described in a few nonmalignant conditions. Features that should raise suspicion of secondary achalasia include older age of onset, shorter duration of symptoms, modest dilation of the esophagus, and rapid and profound weight loss.

Compared with other primary esophageal motor disorders, identification and treatment of achalasia usually is successful. Although achalasia involves motor abnormalities of both the esophageal body and LES, the LES dysfunction is largely responsible for obstruction with resultant symptoms. Most patients are sufficiently affected by their symptoms at presentation to warrant therapy. The major absolute indication for treatment is nighttime regurgitation, which puts the patient at risk for aspiration during sleep. Treatment also is warranted if the obstruction is severe, nutrition is impaired, or the esophagus progressively dilates over time.

A number of treatment choices are available for achalasia, including smooth muscle–relaxant drugs, balloon dilatation, botulinum injections, and surgery. The treatment goal of all these choices is to decrease LES pressure, thereby diminishing the resistance to the flow of food and liquid. None has a clinically significant effect on abnormal motor function in the esophageal body.

Calcium channel blockers and long-acting nitrites do lower LES pressure significantly and have been used for achalasia, although complete relief of symptoms may not be achieved. Patients then may undergo either dilatation or surgery. Typically, if a trial of dilatation fails, a surgical myotomy is performed.

The endoscopic injection of a potent neurotoxin (botulinum toxin [Botox]) directly into the sphincter segment has been successful in treating achalasia. A placebo-controlled study has demonstrated a symptomatic response similar to that with dilatation.[18] This approach is technically simple and the risks appear to be confined to those associated with endoscopy alone. The effect of a successful injection lasts on average for 1 to 4 years. Those who respond initially often respond to repeated injection.

Isolated Abnormalities of the Lower Esophageal Sphincter

LES dysfunction is not limited to patients with achalasia. As previously mentioned, incomplete relaxation of the LES occurs in perhaps one third of patients with other evidence of severe esophageal dysmotility. In addition, occasional patients referred for esophageal manometry have isolated abnormalities of LES function, either hypertensive LES pressure or incomplete relaxation in response to swallow. Few of these patients have any radiographically detectable impairment of function. They may represent a preclinical stage in the evolution of achalasia, abnormalities related to esophageal spasm during periods of otherwise normal peristaltic activity, or a secondary reaction to intragastric phenomenon in which the LES reaction is directed at preventing GER. In most patients the explanation and clinical significance of isolated abnormalities of LES function cannot be determined.

Motor Weakness

Intermittent impairment of contraction amplitude or peristalsis is relatively common. Radiologists frequently mislabel weakness as spasm when they see the escape of barium above the peristaltic wave.[15] This distinction is important because medication directed toward esophageal spasm, which generally decreases contractile amplitude, would be inappropriate if the problem actually is weakness. In practice, the esophagus can empty by gravity, and many patients with esophageal paresis are asymptomatic. Although some

medications can increase esophageal contractility, their effect in patients with severe paresis usually is limited.

Severe esophageal weakness is relatively rare. It is most characteristically found in patients with collagen vascular disease, such as scleroderma and mixed connective tissue disease. The esophagus is the second most common organ involved in scleroderma.[19] Esophageal involvement varies from mild to nonspecific to the complete absence of a contractile response to swallow. The loss of esophageal motility can be appreciated on barium swallow studies. The patient in Video 7-6 initially had the diagnosis of rheumatoid arthritis and later reported solid food dysphagia. Eventually a diagnosis of overlap syndrome that included scleroderma was made. Many of these patients have low LES pressure on manometry. The resulting severe GER with poor esophageal clearance makes them particularly susceptible to esophageal inflammation and strictures.

GASTROESOPHAGEAL REFLUX DISEASE

GER is the normal movement of gastric contents into the esophagus. Because of constantly changing pressure relations between the stomach and esophagus during normal activity, this movement of contents is considered normal (physiologic reflux) and usually is not accompanied by dysphagia or heartburn. The relaxation of the LES is brief and the stomach contents that enter the distal esophagus typically are immediately cleared back into the stomach. Therefore all events of reflux are not pathologic. GER is a common physiologic event. Many apparently normal individuals describe heartburn on a regular basis. A study of healthy hospital employees indicates that approximately 33%, 14%, and 7% reported they had heartburn on a monthly, weekly, and daily basis, respectively.[20] Therefore it appears that reflux is a feature of normal life and does not necessarily reflect a pathologic condition.

However, when gastric contents (usually acid, pepsin, and bile) entering the esophagus are not immediately cleared or when the transient relaxations are frequent, typical symptoms—such as heartburn, regurgitation, odynophagia, and dysphagia—may develop. GER is not necessarily related to the levels of acid or pepsin but to the barriers that allow it to be pathologic. When symptoms become overt, it is referred to as gastroesophageal reflux *disease* (GERD). Despite its name, heartburn (or the sensation of burning in the chest) is generally of esophageal origin, although when severe it may be confused with cardiac disease. Heartburn is the archetypical symptom of GERD, although it may occasionally represent a nonspecific response to other types of esophageal dysmotility. Atypical symptoms, such as chest pain, recurrent sinusitis, chronic cough, hoarseness, asthma, laryngitis, globus sensation, and middle ear infections, also may be associated with GERD.[21] The negative effects on quality of life resulting from GERD are well known.[22] Detection and confirmation of typical and atypical GERD symptoms often can be done with a thorough history.[23] When the offending refluxate reaches the pharynx, it is called *laryngopharyngeal reflux* (LPR). Patients with LPR may represent a different diagnostic entity from those with classic GERD symptomatology (see section on laryngopharyngeal reflux later in this chapter).

Mechanisms of Reflux

Dysphagia associated with GER may be attributable to a variety of mechanisms. GER, with or without esophagitis, is a common cause of esophageal dysmotility. Patients with GERD that does not result in esophagitis but who may have symptoms of heartburn and dysphagia are classified as patients with nonerosive gastroesophageal reflux disease (NERD). The differential diagnosis between these two groups of patients is important because the management strategies (medication regimens) for controlling their symptoms may differ.[24] Although not definitely proven, it is conceivable that constant acid and pepsin irritation of the esophageal lumen results in edema that secondarily precipitates dysmotility with symptoms of heartburn and dysphagia, but not esophagitis. A subgroup of patients with NERD are those with functional heartburn. These patients report heartburn symptoms but have normal **24-hour pH** study findings, unlike some of those with NERD. Finally, chronic inflammation in the esophagus of any type can cause strictures and dysphagia.

A compete understanding of the pathophysiology of GER has progressed substantially over the past decade but still remains incomplete. The major components of the "antireflux barrier" are the LES acting in combination with the anatomic configuration of the esophagogastric junction. In particular, the diaphragmatic crura act as a sphincter during inspiration through their contraction at the level of the esophagogastric junction, whereas the fibers of the LES are more active on expiration (Figure 7-8).

Together these structures maintain an equilibrium of pressure between the stomach and esophagus. Reflux was initially believed to be more likely when the tone in the LES was low; however, it is now known that abrupt periods of relaxation during nonswallow events with normal LES tone are the explanatory

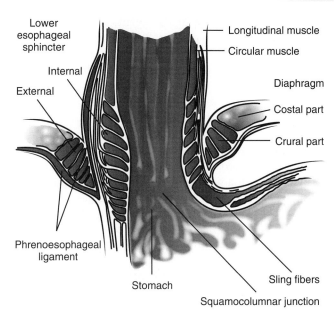

FIGURE 7-8. The distal esophagus pierces the diaphragmatic hiatus as it joins the stomach. On inspiration the crural diaphragmatic ligaments contract, pinching on the esophagus to maintain a pressure equilibrium between the stomach and esophagus. The longitudinal and circular fibers of the lower esophageal sphincter form the esophageal sphincter where the stomach and esophagus join. Together, this combination of muscular and ligamentous arrangement participates in the control of reflux.

mechanism.[25] These abrupt periods of relaxation are called *transient lower esophageal sphincter relaxations* (tSLERs). Patients with symptomatic GERD tend to have more tSLERs than those without symptoms, although mucosal injury may depend more on the ability of the esophagus to clear refluxed contents and the mucosal defense system in the wall of the distal esophagus.[26] Some evidence suggests that the frequency of tSLERs may be related to high **postprandial** pressures accompanied by slow gastric emptying.[26] In addition, the LES protective barrier is compromised in patients with hiatal hernia, in which the stomach herniation pushes the LES into the chest cavity, effectively eliminating the protective mechanisms of the LES and crural diaphragm.

Measuring Reflux

Continuous (24-hour) pH monitoring allows the objective evaluation for reflux under near-physiologic conditions. In most studies of esophageal acidification, a pH of 4.0 or less is considered abnormal. The patient performs the activities of normal daily living, including eating, working, and sleeping. A catheter is placed through the nose into the esophagus and is connected to a device measurement device the patient wears at the waist. When the patient experiences heartburn symptoms, he or she depresses a button that records the time of the event. Continuous pH monitoring provides quantitative information on the presence and severity of acid reflux. The incidence and duration of reflux events can be calculated and analyzed for the entire recording period and for segments of particular interest. The severity of reflux detected by pH monitoring correlates fairly well with the probability of esophageal inflammation and Barrett's esophagus.[27] Continuous pH monitoring is currently considered the best single test for the diagnosis of GERD, with a sensitivity and specificity of approximately 90%.[28] Barium (radiographic) studies, although important in evaluating patients with dysphagia, confirm the presence of reflux in only the minority of patients with symptomatic reflux disease.

Treatment of Gastroesophageal Reflux Disease

Treatment of GERD is directed at enhancing the strength of the antireflux barrier, improving esophageal clearance and gastric emptying, and decreasing the noxiousness of gastric contents. Antireflux therapy has three components: alteration in lifestyle, drugs, and surgery.

For many patients, reflux is provoked by dietary indiscretion and physical activity. Decreasing or eliminating foods that decrease LES pressure (e.g., fat, chocolate) or stimulate gastric acid production (e.g., coffee, tea) is important, especially in patients who ingest large amounts or note the association of symptoms with ingestion of these substances. In some patients with reflux, dietary modification is enough to control symptoms. Smoking and alcohol intake also impair esophageal function and should be eliminated. In addition, patients are instructed to elevate the head of the bed on 6-inch blocks and avoid lying down within 3 hours of eating. These measures allow gravity to assist in reflux prevention and enhance esophageal clearance.

Self-medication with antacids is common in patients with heartburn. Unfortunately, antacids alone are rarely sufficient to control esophagitis in patients with atypical symptoms. Antacids are primarily used for symptomatic relief of intermittent, infrequent heartburn. Most patients with severe symptoms or esophagitis require more potent acid-lowering agents. Prescribed most often are proton-pump inhibitors (PPIs) such as lansoprazole, rabeprazole, pantoprazole, or omeprazole. They are most effective in combination with lifestyle changes related to weight control and dietary modifications. Histamine antagonists, or H_2-blockers (e.g., cimetidine, ranitidine, nizatidine, famotidine), although less effective in curing esophagitis, are available in over-the-counter preparations. The control of typical and atypical manifesta-

tions in GERD is most effective with PPI therapy. Interestingly, control of symptoms in some patients does not always correlate with intraesophageal or intragastric acid suppression.[29] Because all patients in whom GERD is suspected respond uniformly to either H_2-blockers or PPI therapy, various algorithms that address success and failure, including dosage option and options other than medications, have been developed.[30]

Prokinetic drugs such as mosapride, tegaserod, urecholine, and metoclopramide have been used to improve gastric emptying to reduce intragastric pressure and events of reflux. Although these drugs have potential beneficial effects on upper gastrointestinal motor function, results have generally been disappointing when they are used as single agents. The use of metoclopramide has been further limited by the frequent occurrence of neuropsychiatric side effects, including agitation, insomnia, and lethargy. Prokinetic agents are occasionally used as adjunctive agents in combination with H_2-blockers and PPIs in patients with more severe disease.

Reflux can be controlled in the majority of patients the judicious use of medication. Surgical intervention is generally reserved for occasional patients whose disease is **refractory** to medical management. A number of operations have been described; most involve reestablishing the intra-abdominal location of the esophagogastric junction (hiatal hernia repair) in combination with wrapping a portion of the stomach around part or the whole circumference of the lower esophagus (fundoplication). **Laparoscopic** approaches to antireflux surgery have been developed and appear to be as effective as traditional surgical approaches with a more rapid recovery. Surgery is effective in controlling reflux in approximately 80% to 90% of patients in whom it is used.[15]

Newer nonsurgical, endoscopic approaches used to control GERD include suturing of the LES and radiofrequency ablation (Stretta procedure). Radiofrequency ablation attempts to place lesions in the wall of the stomach to reduce the frequency of tSLERs. Although no randomized trials have compared the Stretta procedure to other surgically based procedures, early data suggest a trend toward a reduction of PPI use and an increase in quality-of-life scores.[31] Specific subject selection for these procedures and efficacy data still need to be established.

LARYNGOPHARYNGEAL REFLUX

Laryngopharyngeal reflux (LPR) occurs when stomach contents reach the laryngeal level, frequently resulting in odynophagia, hoarseness, sore throat, a **globus sensation**, and chronic throat clearing. Painful

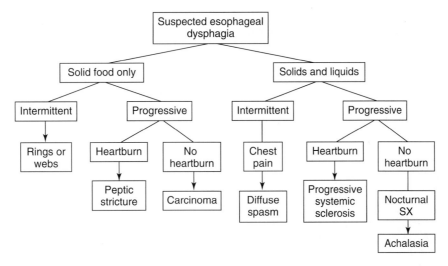

FIGURE 7-9. The distal esophagus pierces the diaphragmatic hiatus as it joins the stomach. On inspiration the crural diaphragmatic ligaments contract, pinching on the esophagus to maintain a pressure equilibrium between the stomach and esophagus. The longitudinal and circular fibers of the lower esophageal sphincter form the esophageal sphincter, where the stomach and esophagus join. Together, this combination of muscular and ligamentous arrangement participates in the control of reflux. *SX*, Symptoms.

swallow and a feeling that something is sticking in the cervical region frequently give rise to reports of dysphagia. The mechanism by which refluxate reaches the level of the posterior larynx is unknown. Endoscopic evaluation of the upper airway shows mucosal abnormalities on the posterior pharyngeal wall, marked edema on the arytenoid cartilages, and generalized **erythema** in the laryngeal aditus. Patients with LPR differ from those with classic GERD in the following ways: (1) most events occur during the day without nighttime episodes, (2) higher doses of medication are needed for longer periods to achieve adequate control, and (3) esophageal motility and acid clearance mechanisms are normal. Patients with LPR and GERD are similar in the following ways: (1) results of 24-hour pH or radiographic studies may not always be positive, (2) the pharyngeal esophageal segment (PES) and LES often are normal, and (3) heartburn may be described.

DIFFERENTIAL DIAGNOSIS

Unlike disorders that affect oropharyngeal function, clues to the cause of esophageal disorders often can be determined with a thorough history. Because the disorders can be conveniently divided into structural and motor, and because of the importance of asking the question of whether solids, liquids, or both is important to the diagnosis, the use of a decision tree can be useful in guiding the clinician in the decision of what tests to order and what signs and symptoms to evaluate. Donner and Castell[32] suggest the use of a

decision tree to guide differential diagnosis (Figure 7-9). The decision tree is normally used when the patient denies events of coughing and choking during meals (highly correlated with oropharyngeal dysphagia) and most likely has more complaints about solid food than liquids.

DISORDERS OF THE PHARYNGOESOPHAGEAL SEGMENT

The differential diagnosis of disorders from failed PES mechanics include disorders from poor traction (hyoid bone deficits); disorders of relaxation (neurogenic); disorders within the cricopharyngeal muscle, such as fibrosis, webs, **myositis**, and dystrophy; and disorders from failure of the cricopharyngeal muscle to relax or contract. Radiographic studies typically show a restriction of bolus flow through the region, particularly for solid food and often on multiple, consecutive attempts with fluids. When the diagnosis is confirmed as a PES abnormality, patients often initially report food sticking at the level of the cervical esophagus. However, most patients who describe solid food sticking at the level of the cervical esophagus often have disorders of esophageal origin (see the section on pharyngoesophageal relations in this chapter).[33]

Cricopharyngeal Bar

The radiographic appearance of a "bar" at the level of the cricopharyngeal muscle (C6-C7) is believed to be the result of failure of the muscle to fully distend (Figure 7-10). In most cases manometric relaxation is

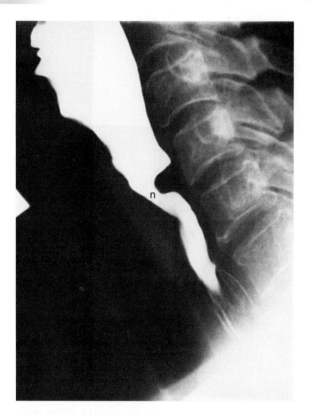

FIGURE 7-10. The cricopharyngeal muscle has pushed into the barium column, causing a narrowing (n) of the barium column. This creates the visual impression of a bar.

CLINICAL CASE EXAMPLE 7-1

An 81-year-old man reported a progressive history of solid food dysphagia. He was referred to a gastroenterologist who ordered a barium esophagram, the results of which were normal. On closer questioning the man reported that he thought food was sticking in the upper part of his neck, so he was referred for a modified barium swallow study. The results of the study can be seen in Video 7-7. On multiple swallows of thin liquid, a small indentation at the level of the PES was visualized, with no obvious restriction of bolus flow into the esophagus. However, when the patient was given a larger, solid bolus a cricopharyngeal bar at the C6 level was apparent. The patient was referred to the otolaryngologist, who chose dilatation of the PES as the treatment of choice. Myotomy was not considered because of the patient's age and history of cardiac disease, both of which constituted a surgical risk. The patient's solid food complaints resolved after two dilatations, and he continued to be symptom free for 10 months, after which he was lost to follow-up.

found to be normal.[34] Failure of distention may range from mild to severe. In the severe forms, restriction of bolus flow may cause retrograde propulsion with spillage into the airway. Cricopharyngeal bars may be seen in 30% of older adults with no symptoms of dysphagia,[35] even though the intrusion of the muscle into the bolus pathway may be small or transitory. Some studies have suggested that the failure of the cricopharyngeal muscle to distend adequately is related to muscle hypertrophy rather than failed PES mechanics and is more common in older adults. These findings on autopsy suggest a change in muscle fiber composition with aging and the potential for decreased cricopharyngeal muscle performance.[36,37] One theory for the formation of cricopharyngeal bars is that they result from increased tone (higher PES pressures) in the cervical esophagus as a result of the failure of the LES to relax.[38] This suggests that patients with cricopharyngeal bars should have a complete evaluation of the esophagus, including manometric and radiographic swallowing studies. Treatment for symptomatic cricopharyngeal bars includes dilatation[39] and cricopharyngeal myotomy.[40]

The formation of so-called pharyngeal pouches (diverticula) may be related to the pathophysiology of cricopharyngeal bars, although they may not always coexist. *Pharyngeal pouches* are lateral protrusions on the pharyngeal wall seen at the level of the thyrohyoid membrane. When they are large, these pouches collect swallowed material, delay bolus flow, and may cause dysphagic symptoms. Pouches that empty after the swallow may result in piriform sinus accumulation with the possibility of post-swallow aspiration.[41] Similar to cricopharyngeal bars, they may be the result of an unyielding PES with a subsequent increase in hypopharyngeal pressures that causes pouch formation above the level of the obstruction. Video 7-8 shows a patient with lateral pharyngeal pouches.

Zenker's Diverticulum

The name *Zenker's diverticulum* is reserved for a diverticulum that develops on the posterior pharyngeal wall in the region of the PES. Most often it represents a protrusion of the hypopharyngeal mucosa at the boundary of the transverse fibers of the cricopharyngeal muscle and the oblique fibers of the inferior constrictor muscle (Killian's dehiscence). These diverticula may be small and remain confined to the hypopharyngeal region. When larger, they may extend into

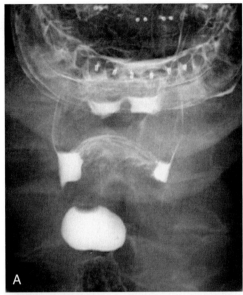
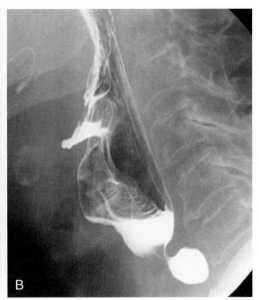
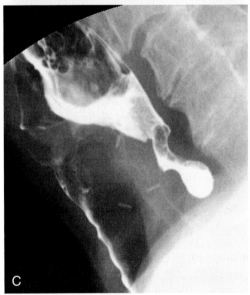

FIGURE 7-11. **A** and **B** show the frontal and lateral views, respectively, centered on the hypopharynx of a barium-filled diverticulum extending posteriorly near the junction with the cervical esophagus. **A,** The diverticulum is seen at the inferior portion of the image. Above the diverticulum the piriform and vallecular spaces also are filled with barium. **B,** In the lateral view the narrowing of the pharyngeal esophageal segment can be seen with the barium column in the piriform sinus above it. **C,** Another patient (lateral view) with a diverticulum seen inferiorly with a considerable collection of barium in the pharynx that has spilled into the trachea; this is seen as a *line* of barium on the *left side* of the image. (From Pickhardt PJ, Arluk GM: *Atlas of gastrointestinal imaging: radiologic-endoscopic correlation,* 2007, Saunders Elsevier.)

the cervical esophagus. They often are associated with reduced flow through the PES and may cause post-swallow aspiration. Figure 7-11, *C*, is representative of the radiographic appearance of a Zenker's diverticulum with tracheal aspiration. An example of a Zenker's diverticulum can also be seen in Video 7-9.

The origin of the development of a Zenker's diverticulum is controversial. Some have suggested that the pouch develops from high intrabolus pressure created by a resistance to flow through the PES, possibly either from failure of the cricopharyngeus muscle to relax or from premature closure.[34] Over time, the continued high pressures cause the hypopharyngeal mucosa to herniate through Killian's dehiscence, resulting in the

formation of a diverticulum. Cook et al.[42] studied 14 patients with Zenker's diverticulum using videofluoroscopy and manometry. They concluded that the diverticulum was not responsible for the poor flow through the PES. They suggested that because mechanical traction and relaxation parameters were normal, the resistance to flow with subsequent development of a diverticulum must be from a lack of compliance (fibrosis or **myopathy**) within the cricopharyngeal muscle body, resulting in a higher than normal resting tone. Other investigators have found a relation between premature closure of the PES caused by GERD, perhaps as a compensation for keeping any offending refluxate from entering the upper airway.[43]

Sasaki et al.[44] have proposed the esophageal shortening theory and GERD as a possible explanation of the development of Zenker's diverticulum. During normal swallowing the esophagus shortens to propel the bolus to the stomach. In patients with chronic GERD, the inflammatory response to acid results in abnormal shortening capability of the esophageal longitudinal muscle. Therefore when the esophagus contracts abnormally, it pulls the hypopharyngeal musculature distally away from its caudal attachments, allowing the pouch to form.

PHARYNGOESOPHAGEAL RELATIONS

As detailed in Chapter 2, the stages of swallowing are interdependent. Primary disease in one stage may affect other stages. Examples of this concept may be common in patients who describe dysphagia localized to the neck but who may have a primary disorder of the esophagus as the cause of their symptoms. In fact, a select group of patients does appear to have abnormal PES function with dysphagic symptomatology; however, it is likely to be the result of a disorder of esophageal origin.

For instance, numerous investigators have found both manometric and radiologic abnormalities in the PES caused by achalasia.[38,45-47] One possible theory is that resistance to flow in the LES causes pressure changes in the esophagus above the level of obstruction perceived by the patient at the level of the PES. Interestingly, there is evidence that successful dilatation of the LES relieves the dysphagic symptoms localized to the neck in patients with achalasia.[47] There also is some evidence that patients with GERD may have dysphagia localized to the level of the PES, possibly as a response to esophageal acidification resulting in a esophageal-PES hypercontractility[48] or because chronic GERD may result in pharyngeal-based compensations that change the mechanics of the PES.[49,50] A change in pharyngeal biomechanics is subsequently perceived by the patient as dysphagia. The relation between GERD and PES symptoms has not been proven, and there is no evidence that controlling GERD reduces symptoms localized to the cervical esophagus. Nonetheless, patients who report cervical dysphagia without abnormal findings after modified barium swallow studies might be candidates for an evaluation of GERD, even in the absence of the traditional symptoms of heartburn and regurgitation.

Zenker's diverticulum is treated either by surgical reduction to include cricopharyngeal myotomy[51] or by endoscopic stapling.[52]

CLINICAL CASE EXAMPLE 7-2

A 64-year-old woman told her primary care physician that over the past 6 months she felt food was sticking in her throat. She was referred to the SLP for a modified barium swallow study. The evaluation of her oropharyngeal mechanism was normal, and she denied any history of esophageal-related disease. The modified barium swallow study was done with thin and thick barium while the patient was standing. The study showed normal flow through the region of the PES in the lateral view. In the frontal view, a restriction of flow was seen at the level of the LES as a mild indentation of the barium column (Video 7-10). A follow-up esophagram revealed a suspected Schatzki's ring that was confirmed on endoscopy by a gastroenterologist. The patient underwent dilatation and the cervical dysphagic symptoms resolved.

CLINICAL CASE EXAMPLE 7-3

A 40-year-old man came to the clinic and stated that over the past year he felt that solid food was sticking in his throat. He reported that he had a significant history of GERD and was taking PPIs irregularly. He noted that he had lost 10 pounds in the past 3 months. A videofluorographic swallowing study revealed a hypertrophic cricopharyngeal muscle that caused a reduction of solid food through the region of the PES. However, the solid food bolus did enter the esophagus and did not spill into the airway. Because the obstruction to solid food was not judged as severe and the patient had a past history of GERD that had not been reevaluated, a standard barium esophagram was ordered. This study revealed a marked narrowing in the region of the LES with abnormal esophageal motility and a dilated esophagus. It was suggested that the patient be referred to a gastroenterologist for esophageal endoscopy. Endoscopy revealed marked esophageal stenosis at the junction of the esophagus and stomach.

In this case, the patient's report of solid food sticking in the neck was verified by the videofluorographic swallowing study. However, the history suggested that the patient had lost a significant amount of weight. The amount of weight loss seemed disproportionate to the degree of PES narrowing. In addition, the patient had a history of GERD that probably was not well controlled. Because of this, he was susceptible to primary esophageal disease, and tests confirmed this suspicion. The abnormality seen in the PES probably was a result of excessive pressure changes on the PES from a lack of esophageal motility. Alternate hypotheses for PES dysfunction include direct acid contact that resulted in cricopharyngeal hypertrophy, or an irritation of cranial nerve X that resulted in poor PES opening and closing mechanics. Treatment in this case would be aimed at dilatation of the LES stricture and medication to control the GERD.

TAKE HOME NOTES

1. The esophagus has two sphincters, the upper esophageal sphincter and the lower esophageal sphincter. The upper esophageal sphincter shares physiologic functions with the hypopharyngeal musculature. Physiologically this region is best described as the pharyngoesophageal segment (PES).
2. Structural disorders such as a stricture as a result of gastroesophageal reflux disease affect the lumen of the esophagus, causing a reduction of bolus flow and dysphagia.
3. External compression of the esophagus, such as from an enlarged heart, could narrow the lumen of the esophagus with resultant dysphagia.
4. Motor (motility) disorders affect the movement or peristalsis of the esophagus. Diffuse esophageal spasm and achalasia are examples of motor disorders.
5. Disorders of the PES may have numerous causes that result in either reduced relaxation or opening of the PES. These include oral and pharyngeal weakness that may cause disorders of traction (opening), neurologic disease (loss of relaxation), disorders within the PES musculature such as myositis and fibrosis, and disorders of esophageal motility that secondarily affect PES function.
6. Disorders specific to the region of the PES include cricopharyngeal bars, lateral pharyngeal pouches, and Zenker's diverticulum.
7. Patients who report solid food dysphagia with food sticking in the cervical region may be susceptible to disorders of the esophagus and not disease affecting the hypopharyngeal or cervical region.

References

1. Edwards DAW: Diagnostic procedures: history and symptoms of esophageal disease. In Vantrappen G, Hellemans J, editors: *Diseases of the esophagus*, New York, 1974, Springer-Verlag.
2. Jones B, Ravich WJ, Kramer SS et al: Pharyngoesophageal interrelationships: observations and working concepts, *Gastrointest Radiol* 10:225, 1985.
3. Schatzki R: The lower esophageal ring: long term follow-up of symptomatic and asymptomatic rings, *Am J Roentgenol Radium Ther Nucl Med* 90:805, 1963.
4. Goyal RK, Bauer JL, Spiro HM: The nature and location of the lower esophageal ring, *N Engl J Med* 284:1175, 1971.
5. Groskreutz JL, Kim CH: Schatzki's ring: long-term results following dilatation, *Gastrointest Endosc* 36:479, 1990.
6. Ravich WJ, Kashima H, Donner MW: Drug-induced esophagitis simulating esophageal cancer, *Dysphagia* 1:13, 1986.
7. Earlam R, Cunha-Melo JR: Oesphageal squamous cell carcinoma: a critical review of surgery, *Br J Surg* 67:381, 1980.
8. Forastiere AA, Orringer MB, Perez-Tamayo C et al: Preoperative chemoradiation followed by transhiatal esophagectomy for carcinoma of the esophagus, *J Clin Oncol* 11:1118, 1993.
9. Parker EF, Moertel CF: Is there a role for surgery in esophageal carcinoma? *Am J Dig Dis* 23:730, 1978.
10. Kinoshita Y, Endo M, Nakayama K et al: Evaluation of ten-year survival after operation for upper- and midthoracic esophageal cancer. *Int Adv Surg Oncol* 1:173, 1978.
11. Dimarino AT, Cohen S: Characteristics of lower esophageal sphincter function in symptomatic diffuse esophageal spasm, *Gastroenterology* 66:1, 1974.
12. Brand Dl, Martin D, Pope CE: Esophageal manometrics in patients with anginal type chest pain, *Am J Dig Dis* 23:300, 1977.
13. Castell DO: The nutcracker esophagus and other primary esophageal motility disorders. In Castell DO, Richter JE, Dalton CB, editors: *Esophageal motility testing*, New York, 1987, Elsevier.
14. Dalton CB, Castell DO, Richter JE: The changing faces of the nutcracker esophagus, *Am J Gastroenterol* 83:623, 1988.
15. Ravich WJ: Esophageal dysphagia. In Groher ME, editor: *Dysphagia: diagnosis and management*, Boston, 1997, Butterworth-Heinemann.
16. Davis HA, Lewis MJ, Rhodes J et al: Trial of nifedipine for prevention of esophageal spasm, *Digestion* 36:81, 1987.

17. Kahrilas PJ, Kishk SM, Helm JF et al: Comparison of pseudoachalasia and achalasia, *Am J Med* 82:439, 1987.

18. Pasricha PJ, Ravich WJ, Hendrix TR et al: Intrasphincteric botulinum toxin for the treatment of achalasia. *N Engl J Med* 332:774, 1995.

19. D'Angelo WA, Fries JF, Masi AT et al: Pathologic observations in systemic sclerosis (scleroderma): a study of 58 autopsy cases and 58 matched controls, *Am J Med* 46:28, 1969.

20. Castell DO, Johnston BT: Gastrointestinal reflux disease. Current strategies for patient management, *Arch Fam Med* 5:221, 1996.

21. Napierkowski J, Wong R: Extraesophageal manifestations of GERD, *Am J Med Sci* 326:279, 2003.

23. Liker H, Hungin P, Wiklund I: Managing gastroesophageal reflux disease in primary care: the patient perspective, *J Am Board Fam Pract* 18:393, 2005.

23. Manterola C, Munoz S, Grande L et al: Initial validation of a questionnaire for detecting gastroesophageal reflux disease in epidemiological settings, *J Clin Epidemiol* 55:1041, 2002.

24. Dickman R, Bautista JM, Wong WM et al: Comparison of esophageal acid exposure distribution along the esophagus among the different gastroesophageal reflux disease (GERD) groups, *Am J Gastroenterol* 101:2463, 2006.

25. Dent J: Patterns of lower esophageal sphincter function associated with gastroesophageal reflux, *Am J Med* 103:29S, 1997.

26. Richter JE, Castell DO: Drugs, foods and other substances in the cause and treatment of reflux esophagitis, *Med Clin North Am* 65:1223, 1981.

27. Iascone C, DeMeester TR, Little AG: Barrett's esophagus: functional assessment, proposed pathogenesis, and surgical therapy, *Arch Surg* 118:543, 1983.

28. Richter JE, Castell DO: Gastroesophageal reflux disease: pathogenesis, diagnosis, and therapy. In Castell DO, Johnson LF, editors: *Esophageal function in health and disease*, New York, 1983, Elsevier.

29. Milkes D, Gerson LB, Triadafilopoulos G: Complete elimination of reflux symptoms does not guarantee normalization of intraesophageal and intragastric pH in patients with gastroesophageal reflux disease (GERD), *Am J Gastroenterol* 99:991, 2004.

30. Tytgat GN, McColl J, Tack J et al: New algorithm for the treatment of gastro-oesophageal reflux disease, *Aliment Pharmacol Ther* 27:249, 2008.

31. Reymunde A, Santiago N: Long term results of radiofrequency energy delivery for the treatment of GERD: sustained improvements in symptoms, quality of life, and drug use at 4 year follow-up, *Gastrointest Endosc* 65:361, 2007.

32. Donner MW, Castell DO: Evaluation of dysphagia: a careful history is crucial, *Dysphagia* 2:65, 1987.

33. Roeder BE, Murray JA, Dierkhising A: Patient localization of esophageal dysphagia, *Dig Dis Sci* 49:697, 2004.

34. Goyal RK: Disorders of the cricopharyngeus muscle, *Otolaryngol Clin North Am* 49:115, 1984.

35. Leonard R, Kendall K, McKenzie S: UES opening and cricopharyngeal bar in nondysphagic elderly and nonelderly adults, *Dysphagia* 19:182, 2004.

36. Torres WE, Clements JL, Austin GE et al: Cricopharyngeal muscle hypertrophy: radiologic-anatomic correlation, *AJR Am J Roentgenol* 142:927, 1984.

37. Xu S, Tu L, Wang Q et al: Is the anatomical protrusion on the posterior hypopharyngeal wall associated with cadavers of only the elderly? *Dysphagia* 21:163, 2006.

38. Zhang ZG, Diamant NE: Repetitive contractions of the upper esophageal body and sphincter in achalasia, *Dysphagia* 9:12, 1994.

39. Wang AY, Kadkade R, Kahrilas PJ et al: Effectiveness of esophageal dilation for symptomatic cricopharyngeal bar, *Gastrointest Endosc* 61:148, 2005.

40. Bonavina L, Khan AN, DeMeester TR: Pharyngoesophageal dysfunctions: the role of cricopharyngeal myotomy, *Arch Surg* 120:541, 1985.

41. Jones B, Donner MW: *Normal and abnormal swallowing: imaging in diagnosis and therapy*, New York, 1990, Springer-Verlag.

42. Cook IJ, Gabb M, Panagopoulos V et al: Pharyngeal (Zenker's) diverticulum is a disorder of upper esophageal sphincter opening, *Gastroenterology* 103:1229, 1992.

43. Brady AP, Stevenson GW, Somers S et al: Premature contraction of the cricopharyngeus: a new sign of gastroesophageal reflux disease, *Abdom Imaging* 20:225, 1995.

44. Sasaki CT, Ross DA, Hundal J: Association between Zenker diverticulum and gastroesophageal reflux disease: development of a working hypothesis, *Am J Med* 115:1695, 2003.

45. Jones B, Donner MW, Rubesin SE et al: Pharyngeal findings in 21 patients with achalasia of the esophagus, *Dysphagia* 2:87, 1987.

46. DeVault KR: Incomplete upper esophageal sphincter relaxation: association with achalasia but not other esophageal motility disorders, *Dysphagia* 12:157, 1997.

47. Yoneyama F, Miyachi M, Nimura Y: Manometric findings of the upper esophageal sphincter in esophageal achalasia, *World J Surg* 22:1043, 1998.

48. Torrico S, Kern M, Aslam M et al: Upper esophageal sphincter function during gastroesophageal reflux events revisited, *Am J Physiol Gastrointest Liver Physiol* 279:G262, 2000.

49. Sivit CJ, Curtis DJ, Crain M et al: Pharyngeal swallow in gastroesophageal reflux disease, *Dysphagia* 2:151, 1988.

50. Mendell DA, Logemann JA: A retrospective analysis of the pharyngeal swallow in patients with a clinical diagnosis of GERD compared with normal controls, *Dysphagia* 17:220, 2002.

51. Sen P, Lowe DA, Farnan T: Surgical interventions for pharyngeal pouch, *Cochrane Database Syst Rev* 3:CD004449, 2005.

52. Casso C, Lalam M, Ghosh S et al: Endoscopic stapling diverticulotomy: an audit of difficulties, outcome, and patient satisfaction, *Otolaryngol Head Neck Surg* 134:288, 2006.

Chapter 8

Respiratory and Iatrogenic Disorders

MICHAEL E. GROHER

OBJECTIVES

1. Detail how disorders of respiration might affect swallowing performance.
2. Discuss common medical and surgical complications that lead to or exacerbate dysphagia.
3. Review how artificial supports for respiration might interfere with swallowing.

BACKGROUND

As detailed in Chapter 2, the interactions between breathing and swallowing are well known. Swallow coordination and subsequent upper airway protection depend on the normal interaction between these two related phenomena. It follows that disorders of breathing might either be the cause of dysphagia or could exacerbate it—such as after stroke.[1] Some patients enter the acute hospital setting with primary respiratory tract disease, such as congestive obstructive pulmonary disease with or without accompanying dysphagia. Others enter the acute care setting for medical reasons not related to their cardiopulmonary status but have cardiopulmonary complications, such as patients who undergo cardiac bypass surgery requiring **intubation**, support by respirator, and/or tracheotomy. Medical and/or surgical complications that result in dysphagic complications can be classified as *iatrogenic*. The side effects of radiation therapy on swallowing after treatment of cancer are classified as iatrogenic but are discussed in detail in Chapter 6.

ARTIFICIAL AIRWAYS

Patients with compromised respiratory status may require special interventions to support basic life functions. These supports include endotracheal or tracheostomy tubes that may or may not be connected to a mechanical respirator and oxygen delivered either by facial mask or through a nasal cannula. A potential side effect of oxygen use is xerostomia with its attendant negative impact on swallowing.

Endotracheal Tubes

Endotracheal tubes are long plastic, flexible tubes that are inserted through the mouth, through the vocal folds, and into the trachea to aid the patient in respiratory distress. They are designed to be connected to a respirator to help the patient breath. At the end of the tube is a cuff that is inflated to prevent oral secretions from entering the lungs by sealing the tracheal lumen and to keep air from escaping from the lungs past the tube (Figure 8-1). Keeping the desired respiratory volumes within the lungs is important to restore respiratory competence. Respirator settings are determined by the medical team and are implemented by the respiratory therapist. Placement of an endotracheal tube is considered a temporary measure (7 to 12 days) to establish respiratory competence. Longer periods of intubation may cause permanent laryngeal and lung injury because of local irritation to the mucosa. **Granulomas** and **hematomas** on the vocal folds and pharyngeal ulceration and edema may

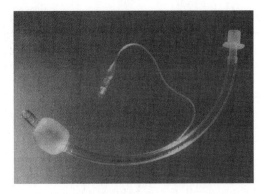

FIGURE 8-1. The endotracheal tube is designed to go through the mouth and below the level of the vocal folds into the trachea. This example shows the cuff on the end in the inflated position. The cuff is inflated by the small catheter in the middle of the photograph. (Photo courtesy Smiths Medical.)

give rise to voice and swallowing complications. In some cases vocal fold paralysis or weakness may develop. Settings (inhalation and exhalation cycles) on the respirator are progressively adjusted to allow the patient to regain independent breathing. The endotracheal tube is removed as normal breathing patterns are achieved. Removal of the endotracheal tube does not guarantee that the patient will not experience further respiratory distress requiring reintubation. Multiple reintubations suggest that the patient's respiratory status is tenuous and may lead to a longer term approach to airway maintenance—tracheotomy.

Bypassing the functions of the upper airway with an endotracheal tube precludes the patient from eating and swallowing because the vocal folds and oral cavity and pharynx are not available for swallowing activity because of the presence of the tube. If successful **extubation** is achieved, the physician may request a swallowing evaluation before the patient starts oral feeding. Because the traditional method of breathing has been altered for some time, these patients may have difficulty speaking and swallowing immediately after the removal of the endotracheal tube. Partik et al.[2] studied 21 patients with videofluoroscopy who were intubated for a mean of 24.6 days. They found that 86% of this group showed signs of aspiration after intubation. The majority of aspiration occurred before the swallow response, suggesting oral-stage weakness and subsequent poor laryngeal elevation. deLariminat et al.[3] were interested in whether difficulty with postextubation swallowing was acute or chronic. Using swallow response times as the measurement of function, they found swallow delay on all bolus volumes on day 1; shorter, but abnormal latencies on day 2; and normal response times by day 7. These results imply that interruptions in normal respiratory function may inhibit normal swallow response time but that, over time, they will recover without specific treatment.

Tracheotomy Tubes

Patients for whom weaning from endotracheal intubation is not possible may require the surgical placement of a tracheotomy tube. A vertical incision typically is made between the second and third tracheal rings so that the tube is below the level of the vocal folds to allow the medical team access to the lungs for suctioning. Other advantages over endotracheal intubation include the possibility for swallowing and speaking, less trauma to the vocal folds, and patient comfort. Tracheotomy tubes are available in various sizes, usually determined by the inner diameter of the lumen. Commonly used sizes are 8, 6, and 4 mm. The larger the tube size, generally the more difficult it is to get air around the tube up to the level of the vocal fold for phonation (Figure 8-2).

Decreasing the tube size (from 8 to 6 mm) is commonly done to reinvolve the upper airway for speech and swallowing and eventually for total decannulation. However, there are no prospective, empirical data studying the role of tracheotomy downsizing and its effect on speech and swallow. Figure 8-3 shows a patient who underwent a tracheostomy with a close-up view of the tube in place. Complications of a tracheotomy tube include decreased sense of smell and taste because the direction of airflow is not through the nose and mouth, infection at the tracheotomy site, and increased secretions from the body's response to a foreign object. *Tracheomalacia,* or a breakdown of tissue on the posterior pharyngeal wall as a result of constant irritation, is rare. When severe, such tissue breakdown may create a tracheoesophageal fistula with resultant aspiration of food or secretions.

Tracheotomy tubes are either cuffed or noncuffed. The *cuff* refers to a portion on the end of the tube that can be inflated with air externally by using a syringe (Figure 8-4). When the cuff is inflated it theoretically seals off the entrance to the lungs in an effort to prevent aspiration of secretions or food. If the patient is also receiving ventilation from a respirator, the cuff ensures that the volume of air being delivered does

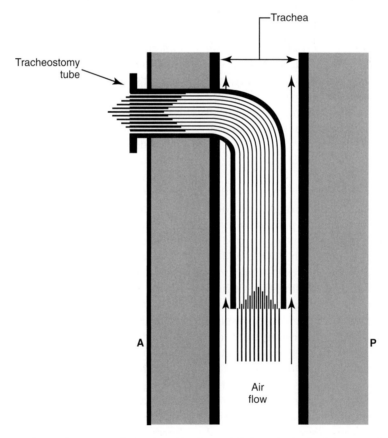

FIGURE 8-2. The tracheotomy tube is placed in the neck below the level of the vocal folds. The larger the diameter of the tube in the trachea, the more difficult it is to get air past the tube up to the vocal folds. Most of the pulmonary air for speaking would be directed through the tube. The smaller the tube lumen, the easier it is to get air up to the vocal folds. *A,* Anterior neck; *P,* posterior neck.

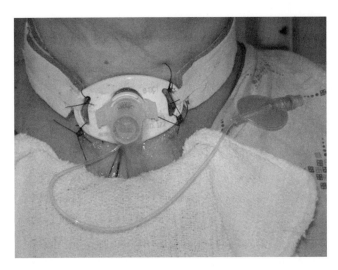

FIGURE 8-3. Close-up view of a tracheostomy tube. The tube is initially anchored by sutures and held in place around the neck by ties. The inner diameter of the tube can be read as 8 mm on the upper right section of the flange. The outer diameter is marked as 12.7 mm. The patient's secretions coughed from the lungs can be seen in and around the tube.

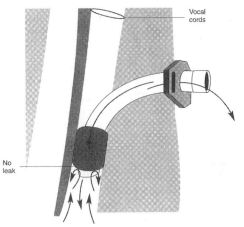

FIGURE 8-5. The inflated cuff protects the lung from secretions entering the airway above the level of inflation and keeps air from entering the upper airway. In addition, because the cuff is inflated, the laryngeal framework is anchored, potentially restricting laryngeal elevation during swallowing. (From Dikeman KJ, Kazandjian MS: *Communication and swallowing management of tracheostomized and ventilator-dependent adults,* 2nd edition, Belmont, CA, 2003, Cengage Learning.)

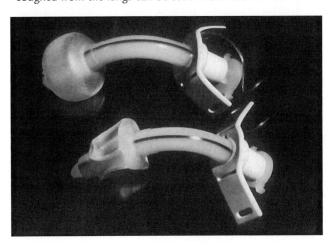

FIGURE 8-4. An example of a cuffed tracheotomy tube inflated *(top)* and deflated.

CLINICAL CORNER 8-1

A 76-year-old man had cardiac bypass surgery and was doing well until the second postoperative day, when he had a respiratory arrest. An endotracheal tube was immediately placed and connected to a respirator. Eventually a cuffed tracheotomy tube had to be placed. The speech-language pathologist was consulted for a swallowing evaluation. As part of the evaluation he wanted to check the patient's voice.

CRITICAL THINKING:

1. Why would an evaluation of the patient's voice be important?
2. To start the evaluation of voice, what would the speech-language pathologist want to ask the physician or nurse?

not leak into the upper airway. The cuff may be advantageous in protecting the lungs, but its presence restricts voice and limits swallow by anchoring the larynx (Figure 8-5). In a retrospective review of videofluoroscopic evaluations of patients swallowing with the cuff inflated and deflated, Ding and Logemann[4] found a higher prevalence of silent aspiration and changes in laryngeal biomechanics in the group with the cuff inflated.

Reexamination of Figure 8-3 shows the external catheter line to the internal cuff on the patient's chest. The balloon on the end of the catheter line is flat, indicating that the cuff on the end of the tracheotomy tube is deflated. When the balloon on the patient's chest is inflated, the cuff on the end of the tracheotomy tube can be assumed to be inflated.

In addition to the cuff versus no-cuff option, tracheotomy tubes may be fenestrated or nonfenestrated. A *fenestration* is a hole placed in the top of the tracheotomy tube to allow increased airflow to the upper airway, primarily for speaking (Figure 8-6).

SWALLOWING AND TRACHEOSTOMY

Numerous studies from critical care medicine have noted a higher prevalence of aspiration events in patients with tracheotomy compared with those without tracheotomy.[5-7] Factors that may place patients with a tracheotomy at greater risk for aspiration include loss of subglottic air pressure,[8] poor

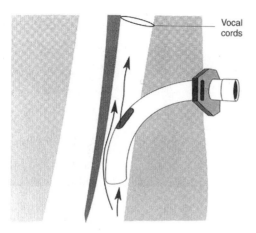

Vocal cords

FIGURE 8-6. The fenestration in the top of the tracheotomy tube allows additional pulmonary air to flow to the vocal folds. (From Dikeman KJ, Kazandjian MS: *Communication and swallowing management of tracheostomized and ventilator-dependent adults,* 2nd edition, Belmont, CA, 2003, Cengage Learning.)

CLINICAL CORNER 8-2

A 37-year-old woman had acute kidney and liver failure and eventually required a tracheotomy and underwent multiple, failed intubations. Her respiratory status was not stable, but the patient wanted to eat so the speech-language pathologist was consulted. She noted that with the No. 8 tracheotomy cuff down the patient was unable to phonate and suggested that if possible the medical staff consider either downsizing the tracheotomy tube or placing a No. 8 fenestrated tube. A No. 8 fenestrated tube was placed the next day and the speech-language pathologist went back for another evaluation. At this time, the patient was unable to phonate again.

CRITICAL THINKING:

1. What might explain why the patient still could not phonate?
2. Could the speech-language pathologist still check the patient's swallow even if she did not hear voicing?

laryngeal elevation related to the mechanical presence of the tube,[5] loss of upper airway sensitivity because of airway bypass, loss of the normal laryngeal closure reflex during swallow,[9] and the fact that patients requiring tracheotomy are acutely ill and may not be able to coordinate a normal swallow because of muscle weakness and/or mental status fluctuations.

Laryngeal Elevation

Although there are many anecdotes that tracheotomy tethers the larynx to the neck to reduce laryngeal elevation with subsequent aspiration, only one study has measured its effects on elevation. Terk et al.[10] studied seven patients with tracheotomy tubes without known dysphagia and concluded that elevation with the tracheotomy tube in place compared with when it was not in place showed no significant changes in laryngeal elevation measurements. However, factors of age, extent of respiratory illness, and prior medical history all must be considered before concluding that a tracheotomy tube does not affect laryngeal elevation.

Restoring Subglottic Pressure

Occlusion of the stoma at the tracheotomy site theoretically should help restore subglottic air pressure and improve swallow performance. Various methods of stoma occlusion have been studied, including digital occlusion, occlusion with a one-way valve such as a **Passy-Muir valve**, and occlusion from a cap placed at the stoma on the tracheotomy tube.

Digital occlusion in eight patients with head/neck cancer showed mixed results.[11] In general, aspiration events were either reduced or eliminated. Some patients benefited with some bolus types, whereas others did not. All biomechanical measures, however, were normalized. The investigators concluded that the response to digital occlusion should be evaluated on a patient-by-patient basis. In a similar group of 16 postsurgical patients, Leder et al.[12] found no difference in the prevalence of aspiration with or without finger occlusion. The use of one-way speaking valves and their effect on swallowing have been evaluated by numerous investigators with mixed findings.[13-16] Comparisons of studies are difficult because of subject selection variance, type of instrumentation to measure the effects on swallowing, swallowing outcome of interest, and length of time the valve was in place before the studies were conducted to assess swallowing status. All agree, however, that the placement of a valve improves speech and reduces upper airway secretions, restores olfaction, and improves patient ability to cough and clear secretions. In a mixed group of patients with chronic respiratory disease, Leder et al.[17] did not find any change in swallow-generated pharyngeal and cervical esophageal pressures with occlusion, either in those who aspirated or those who did not. Using endoscopy to study aspiration, Donzelli et al.[18] studied 37 patients—first with the tracheotomy in place and then with it removed with light digital occlusion over the tracheotomy site. Although some patients showed differences in aspiration and penetration patterns, for the majority there were no significant differences.

Practice Note 8-1

Digital occlusion of a tracheotomy tube always is done with a gloved finger to prevent any contamination of the open airway. The examiner typically occludes the trachea at the moment of swallow. Digital occlusion is easiest with the thumb. Firm pressure is needed to achieve an adequate seal. Some patients can be taught self-occlusion and often benefit from a mirror to learn the process. Occlusion may assist in swallow performance and help the patient regain his or her speaking voice.

CLINICAL CASE EXAMPLE 8-1

A 67-year-old man entered the hospital for knee replacement surgery. During the procedure he had a cardiac arrest and was resuscitated. After resuscitation he was intubated. Intubation includes insertion of an endotracheal tube and placement on a ventilator. A tracheotomy tube was inserted on the tenth postoperative day. The man's pulmonary status improved to the point where his physicians were considering decannulation. Before this point he was fed by nasogastric tube, and a modified barium swallow study was ordered to evaluate his ability to eat orally. Video 8-1 on the Evolve site shows the patient's modified barium swallow study, first with the tracheotomy tube unoccluded. On thin liquid swallows there is obvious aspiration with cough that cleared some, but not all, of the aspirated contents. The chin-down position did facilitate airway protection. Thicker boluses showed penetration of the airway. After the study, the results were shared with the physician, who believed the feeding tube should remain in place. The physician was anxious to move toward decannulation and ordered that the patient's tube be capped as the first step. After tolerating the capped tube for 24 hours without difficulty, the patient was rescheduled for a modified barium swallow study before beginning oral feeding. Video 8-2 shows that with the tube capped (visible at the bottom of the image), the patient was able to protect his airway on all bolus types and volumes. A soft mechanical diet was ordered. After the patient successfully swallowed three meals, the tracheotomy tube was removed. The marked difference in swallowing safety demonstrated by this patient should not be generalized to all patients. Success or failure after tracheotomy occlusion should be put into the context of a patient's medical history and current medical status.

Practice Note 8-2

Decannulation, or removal of a tracheotomy tube, while in the patient's best interest, may be one of the most disorganized and consequently lengthy processes in the medical center. Although some criteria for tube removal do exist—such as tolerances for breathing without supports and maintenance of adequate blood gases—rarely does one medical service or individual take responsibility for making the decision for removal. This is partly because of a lack of consensus on removal criteria and partly because of the physician's uncertainty that the patient will not incur any negative medical consequences once the tube is removed and possibly require reintubation.

POSTSURGICAL CAUSES OF DYSPHAGIA

Some surgical procedures, particularly those in the neck, predispose patients to postoperative dysphagia. Dysphagia results from (1) edema that restricts movement of swallowing structures such as the pharynx; (2) interference to the peripheral nerve supply to the muscles of swallowing, such as in endarterectomy, thyroidectomy, and cervical spinal fusion; (3) loss of central nervous system (brainstem) innervation, such as from posterior fossa or skull base surgery; or (4) replacement of swallowing structures that also may interfere with peripheral cranial nerves, such as in transhiatal esophagectomy. In surgical procedures that involve the neck region, it is difficult to identify the fibers of the pharyngeal plexus that innervate the pharyngeal constrictor muscles. This surgery may result in postoperative bilateral pharyngeal weakness that cannot be explained by isolated injury to the recurrent laryngeal nerve.[19]

Thyroidectomy

Surgical resection of all or part of the thyroid gland potentially can involve some disruption of motor and sensory branches of cranial nerve (CN) X. Unilateral vocal fold paralysis as a surgical complication compromises both voice and swallow. After follow-up of 39 patients for voice and swallow for 3 months after total thyroidectomy, Lombardi et al.[20] found persistent mild symptoms of voice and swallow abnormalities. In a series of 33 patients with thyroidectomy, Wasserman et al.[21] reported that 49% had preoperative swallowing difficulty, whereas 73% reported acute postoperative difficulty. They speculated that the prevalence of swallowing complaints was the result of injury to the extrinsic perithyroidal neural plexus innervating the pharyngeal and laryngeal structures. In a follow-up study of 60 patients, Pereira et al.[22] found that 15% of their patients had what they termed "nonspecific upper aerodigestive" complaints, including neck strangling, voice changes, and dysphagia. None of these studies provided objective, instrumental swallowing data on the type or severity of the swallowing disorder.

Carotid Endarterectomy

Ekberg et al.[23] studied the swallowing ability of 12 patients before and after carotid **endarterectomy**. Findings for all swallowing studies were normal before surgery, but five patients had pharyngeal dysfunction and dysphagia after surgery. At 1 month after surgery, only two had swallowing complaints. These investigators speculated that the dysfunction was either attributable to peripheral nerve injury (vagus) or cerebrovascular damage during the procedure. Monini et al.[24] acknowledged the potential for cranial nerve involvement after carotid endarterectomy. Their follow-up of patients included serial examinations of voice and swallow for 60 days after surgery. Although most patients had only transient difficulty, 17.5% continued to have symptoms. Of those, only 9% required rehabilitation. In a related prospective study of 19 patients after endarterectomy, swallow endoscopies were done at 5 and 90 days after surgery. During the first evaluation, 15 of the 19 patients had dysphagia. Within 1 month, 10 patients returned to their regular diet, and an additional six did so by 90 days. The investigators suggested that the swallowing skills of patients after endarterectomy be closely monitored and rehabilitation strategies implemented if difficulties persisted.[25]

Cervical Spine Procedures

Surgical stabilization of the cervical spine after trauma or surgery to eliminate pain and sensory/motor weakness from spinal nerve compression may secondarily result in oropharyngeal dysphagia. Surgical approaches to the cervical spine usually are through the anterior muscles of the neck. In some cases, a posterior approach or a combination of both may be used. Frequently, stabilization plates with screws are placed for long-term support of the cervical spine. Figure 8-7 shows a patient with an extensive posterior and ante-

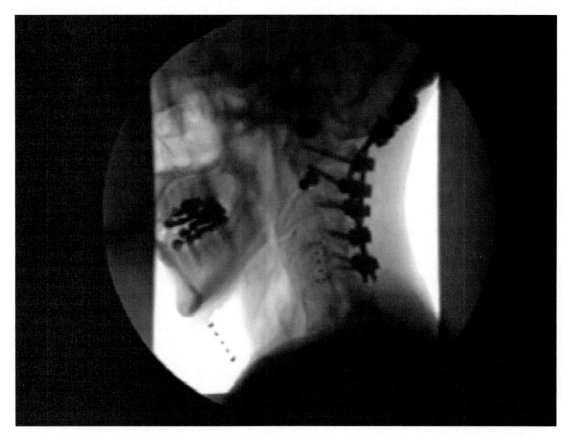

FIGURE 8-7. A metal appliance placed surgically in the posterior cervical spine for stabilization after an automobile accident is apparent. Patients with surgical procedures to the cervical spine may be at risk for postoperative dysphagia.

rior spine support at C2-C5 after a traumatic injury with accompanying anterior vertebral protrusions at C3-C4.

Abel et al.[26] provided demographic and outcome data for 73 patients with cervical spinal cord injury. Ten patients also sustained brain injury. Some patients required surgical intervention to stabilize the spine; others required intubation and tracheostomy. Oropharyngeal dysphagia was identified in 44% of patients. The authors concluded that surgical intervention was not related to dysphagia or the final outcomes but that the combination of tracheostomy and a rigid fixation device for postoperative stabilization (**halo**) predisposed patients to the most serious problems. Halo supports often put patients in a hyperextended position, which makes them more susceptible to tracheal aspiration.[27] Patients with dysphagia generally had longer hospitalizations and more medical complications.[26]

Surgical intervention into the cervical spine can cause injury to the pharyngeal plexus (CNs IX and X) with secondary pharyngeal weakness, edema in the prevertebral space resulting in loss of superior pharyngeal movement or, if the edema is extensive, the inability of the epiglottis to invert. In addition, retraction of the muscles and nerves in the neck to achieve exposure to the spine may result in peripheral nerve injury and vocal fold paralysis that contribute to dysphagia.[28] Patients with anterior cervical fusion (ACF) and swallowing disorders after surgery have received the most attention in the literature.

The incidence of dysphagic complications after ACF varies from 80%[29] to 6.5%.[30] The large variation is attributable to methods of detection (instrumental vs. patient report), definitions of dysphagia based on severity, and when the measurements were made. For instance, in a follow-up survey of patients at a mean duration of 3.3 years after surgery, 60% of the patients reported dysphagia, mostly with solids.[31] The evidence shows that dysphagia after ACF does improve with time. In a prospective study of 249 patients with ACF, Baraz et al.[32] documented the severity of dysphagic complaints by telephone at 1, 2, 6, and 12 months after surgery. The incidence steadily declined from 50.2% at 1 month to 12.5% at 6 months. Only patient gender (female) was related to an increased risk of dysphagia at 6 months. Other factors, such as age, type of procedure, level of surgery, and the type of stabilization hardware, were not related to the final outcome.

Buchholz et al.[33] used cineradiography to study patients who had ACF with cervical plates and dysphagic complaints (3 to 108 months later). The most common finding was a localized pharyngeal weakness at the site of the surgery with accompanying solid food dysphagia. They postulated that patients who initially had dysphagic complaints probably had some disruption in the pharyngeal constrictor muscles by way of the pharyngeal plexus and that a regeneration of those fibers was possible in those who totally recovered. Video 8-3 shows the same patient in Figure 8-7 on his fourth postoperative day. Note that the patient swallows thin liquids with some delay at the level of the piriform sinus, and what appears to be incoordination between pharyngeal contraction and pharyngeal esophageal segment (PES) relaxation is visible. As the bolus becomes increasingly thick, material collects at the vallecular level, causing the patient to report solid food sticking in the back of his throat. There is marked edema at the C3 level that restricts epiglottic inversion. The airway remains protected during all swallow attempts.

Bony changes (osteophytes) in the vertebrae of the cervical spine may push on the posterior pharyngeal wall or esophagus, creating mechanical (obstructive) disorders of swallow (Figure 8-8). Osteophytes are more common in older adults (20% to 30% of those who have them are in this age group) and most are asymptomatic.[34] In a series of 3318 patients referred for radiographic examination of suspected dysphagia, 1.7% had osteophytes that accounted for their symptoms.[35] Interestingly, 12 of the 55 patients with osteophytes had coexisting diseases, including histories of cancer surgery, thyroidectomy, and stroke. Osteophytes larger than 10 mm were associated with aspiration 75% of the time, whereas aspiration was found in 34% of those with osteophytes smaller than 10 mm. When they produce symptoms, osteophytes typically are at the C3 level, causing the epiglottis to not fully invert, or at the C6 level, resulting in disorders of flow through the PES and cervical esophagus. Osteophytes in both regions may result in aspiration. At the C3 level aspiration usually occurs during swallow, whereas at the C6 level it usually occurs after the swallow. In some cases osteophytes are associated with inflammation, edema, and fibrosis, all of which can affect pharyngeal swallow mechanics.[36] Treatment includes either neurosurgical intervention, postural changes such as chin-down, and/or avoidance of solid food boluses. The elimination of aspiration and subsequent pneumonia is paramount in the patient's care.

Esophagectomy

Cancer of the esophagus most often necessitates the need for total esophagectomy. Typically, the esophagus is removed and replaced with tissue either from the stomach or jejunum. This tissue is connected to a remnant in the cervical esophagus and is referred to as the *esophagopharyngeal **anastomosis***. For some

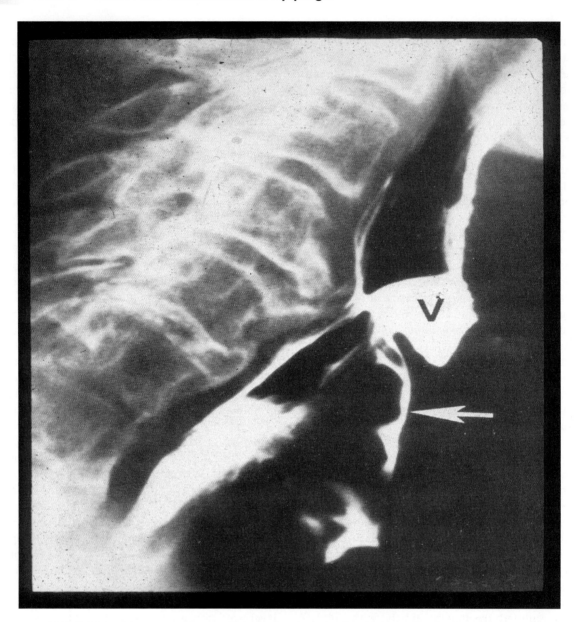

FIGURE 8-8. A large osteophyte at C3 is causing the bolus (in *white*) to collect in the vallecula *(V)* and eventually to spill into the airway *(arrow)*. (Reprinted from Jonas B, Donner MW: *Normal and abnormal swallowing: imaging in diagnosis and therapy,* New York, 1991, Springer-Verlag.)

patients, the anastomosis is made below this level in the thorax. In general, this procedure interferes with normal esophageal motility with presumed discoordination between the esophagus and pharynx and may secondarily impair vagal innervation (recurrent laryngeal nerve) to the pharynx, although all pharyngeal-based symptoms cannot be accounted for on this basis alone.[28] Therefore patients who undergo esophagectomy may be at risk for oropharyngeal- and esophageal-based dysphagia. When dysphagia is present postoperatively in patients who have undergone esophagectomy, it is predictive of pneumonia and

subsequent death.[37] Therefore early detection with fiberoptic endoscopy of swallow or videofluorographic swallowing studies and remediation before the initiation of oral feeding are important.[38,39] Atkins et al.[40] recommended serial evaluation of swallowing after esophagectomy to avoid the potential complications of aspiration. Using endoscopy, Leder et al.[38] found that immediately after surgery 21% of the 73 patients evaluated showed signs of vocal fold immobility and aspiration, implicating involvement of CN X. Patients with aspiration were not allowed to eat until examination results normalized. In a series of 26 consecutive patients who had undergone esophagectomy, Lewin et al.[39] found that 81% of the patients showed signs of liquid aspiration at a mean postoperative period of 13 days; most instances of aspiration were the result of poor anterior laryngeal movement that resulted in residue in the piriform sinuses, with spillage into the airway. These authors speculated that tongue weakness secondary to involvement of the ansi hypoglossal innervation (C1-C3) to the tongue may be a complication of the surgery. This would explain why the hyoid bone did not move anteriorly. In their study, the chin-down maneuver eliminated the aspiration in 17 of the 21 patients.[39] Kato et al.[41] also found a limitation of hyoid movement with resultant poor PES opening after esophagectomy regardless of the surgical reconstructive approach (retrosternal, posterior mediastinal, or intrathoracic). However, the poorest oropharyngeal biomechanics with subsequent aspiration were seen in patients who had the retrosternal reconstructive approach. Data on long-term outcomes in a significant number of those with esophagectomy and dysphagia are lacking. Martin et al.[42] found that in the 10 patients they studied, most had reduced or no swallowing difficulty in a range of 6 to 19 weeks after surgery. Heitmiller and Jones[43] studied 15 patients and found that their pharyngeal-based symptoms (aspiration/penetration, poor laryngeal elevation) had resolved at 1 month. Differences in these data can be attributed to the premorbid medical presentation, the surgical approach, and complications from aspiration or the surgery that would affect swallow recovery.

Patients in whom pulmonary complications develop after esophagectomy undergo swallowing studies to determine whether the source of their complication is related to aspiration. Typically, the first concern is that a leak has developed at the site of the anastomosis with resultant pulmonary complications. This situation is easily evaluated by radiographic studies. If a leak is not the source, then videofluoroscopic swallowing studies are conducted. A complication more common than an anastomotic leak after surgery is a stricture at the anastomotic site, often resulting in solid food dysphagia.[44] Such anastomotic strictures can be identified by standard radiographic studies. Video 8-4 shows a patient after a transhiatal esophagectomy. In the lateral view the patient shows aspiration during and after the swallow. The anteroposterior projection shows considerable bolus residue at the level of the anastomosis.

Skull Base/Posterior Fossa

Surgical procedures that involve the base of the skull and brainstem potentially can affect the peripheral cranial nerves important for swallowing (CNs V, VII, and IX through XII) and/or the central medullary controls for swallowing. Patients with dysphagia after posterior fossa surgery usually show bilateral pharyngeal impairment suggestive of brainstem, rather than peripheral nerve, injury.[28] Jennings et al.[45] detailed the swallowing disorders of 12 patients who had excision of skull base tumors with varying involvement of the key cranial nerves for swallow. They found oral and pharyngeal involvement in all patients, including oral-stage delay, unilateral pharyngeal weakness, reduced hyoid elevation, and pharyngeal retention after the swallow. In addition, 75% aspirated, three of them silently. Compensatory swallowing strategies allowed seven of the patients to eat orally. At discharge, all patients were eating orally except the patient with involvement of CNs IX through XII.

TRAUMATIC INJURIES

Trauma to the head/neck region has the potential to affect swallowing. Severe trauma (as to the spine) usually requires respiratory supports and issues of intubation and tracheotomy tubes that already have been discussed. Trauma involving the cortical controls over swallowing was discussed in Chapter 5. Local trauma to bones involved in swallowing, such as laryngeal and mandibular fractures, may interfere with swallowing. In laryngeal injury, the airway may be compromised, requiring tracheostomy, or the vocal folds may be injured, interfering with protection of the airway during swallow. Mandibular fractures of the jaw may need to be fixed (wired) in the closed position to promote healing. In some cases this may preclude oral ingestion or interfere with bolus preparation. Pineau and Ott[46] describe a case of isolated proximal esophageal injury from blunt trauma. The 52-year-old patient was in an automobile accident and had swelling in the left side of the neck, although a hematoma was ruled out. When the patient was unable to swallow solid foods the next day, an x-ray study revealed a stricture at the C6-C7 level. Pineau and Ott theorized that the trauma from the accident caused a disruption of the esophageal branches of the inferior thyroid artery that resulted in an ischemic stricture. The stricture was successfully dilatated.

Patients with burn injuries also may be vulnerable to swallowing disorders as a result of respiratory complications and direct injury to the tissue and structures in the mouth and pharynx. Burn injuries frequently are a result of a traumatic event such as an explosion or automobile accident.

I once saw a 22-year-old patient who had fractured his jaw in a fight. The oral surgeon wired the jaw closed to manage the fracture. However, he left one opening in the molar region on one side so that a small catheter could be inserted for feeding. The patient filled a syringe with pureed food and squirted the material onto his tongue, which he successfully swallowed. At first, he had numerous choking episodes because he emptied the syringe too fast, allowing the puree to enter the oropharynx faster than he could safely swallow. He quickly learned to avoid these episodes by controlling the rate at which he delivered the food.

Dental Trauma

Oral surgery may result in a temporary loss of normal swallow function caused by pain. The removal of teeth may affect oral preparation. Teeth that are in poor repair also may affect oral preparation. Patients with ill-fitting dentures may sustain trauma to the mandibular or maxillary arches, creating inflammation, and in some cases permanent injury, to the mucosa resulting in oral-stage preparation and delivery problems. Clinical examination of the dental arches reveals a reddened or whitish change in the mucosa at the point of denture contact where the patient feels the discomfort. Prolonged irritation can cause gingival hyperplasia, resulting in soft, sometimes flexible masses of tissue that appear markedly inflamed. Numerous studies have analyzed swallowing in older adults with and without their dentures in place.

Tamura et al.[47] found that dentures were important for older persons because they provided the posterior jaw stabilization necessary for a normal swallow. They also noted that older persons tend to have more xerostomia and that loss of saliva may affect patient perception of denture comfort. Furuya[48] and Yoshikawa et al.[49] found that the removal of dentures in the elderly affected only the oral stage (delay) of swallowing and that more penetration of the airway occurred when the dentures were out. Hattori[50] did not find any differences in timing of oropharyngeal mechanics with dentures in or out but did find increased hyoid bone movement with the dentures removed. In none of these investigations were the patients at risk for pneumonia from events of aspiration.

Thermal Burn Trauma

Traumatic events that lead to thermal burn injuries can affect the structures and supporting tissue for swallow by direct contact, through inhalation of toxic gasses with subsequent mucosal injury, and by the high incidence of respiratory complications requiring intubation and tracheostomy. Skin grafting procedures require intubation to achieve anesthesia with possible attendant injury to the upper airway. Grafts on the face may result in secondary fibrosis and restriction of facial and jaw musculature. Other respiratory complications that may compromise swallow include cough, hoarseness, stridor, **dyspnea**, increased mucus production, bronchospasm, necrosis, and ulceration. Video 8-5 on the Evolve site shows an endoscopic evaluation of the pharynx and larynx of a patient with an inhalation burn injury. There is generalized inflammation, particularly on the epiglottis, lateral pharyngeal walls, and in the interarytenoid space. Heavy mucus secretions are evident with ventricular fold edema. There is a visible ulceration on the right aryepiglottic fold. A feeding tube has been inserted through the PES.

Depletion of oxygen and carbon monoxide toxicity may result in diffuse brain injury that further complicates swallowing performance. Pain from burn injury is managed with sedatives and narcotics that compromise the levels of alertness needed for safe swallowing (see the section on medications). Severe burn injuries require immediate nutritional support by either **enteral** or **parenteral** routes. Hypermetabolic states are common, including increased oxygen consumption and cardiac demand, muscle wasting with a loss of lean body mass, and a compromised immune system. Because all these issues relate to swallowing and nutrition, stabilization of these medical problems often is a precursor to successful oral ingestion.

In a prospective review of 122 consecutively admitted patients to a burn unit, DuBose et al.[51] found that 18% had compromised swallowing. There were significant associations between the presence of oropharyngeal dysphagia and the number of days of mechanical ventilation, days to oral intake, age, length of hospitalization, and modified diet at discharge. The two highest predictors of dysphagia were age (odds ratio 2.18) and the presence of tracheotomy (odds ratio 26.9).

MEDICATIONS

Iatrogenic effects of medications may have negative effects on swallowing. In addition, they may negatively affect support systems needed for swallowing such as cardiac or respiratory function. Therefore it is important that the clinician review the medications a patient is taking because some may contribute directly to dysphagic conditions and others may exacerbate them. In general, side effects from medications that affect swallowing include those that interfere with cognition and/or motor performance, those that result in xerostomia, and those that affect gastrointestinal function. Side effects from medications that affect swallowing are not found in all patients and most likely will be found with higher doses. Combinations of drugs also may produce additive effects not found in single dosages. Even though the clinical examination may suggest that a medication is responsible for dysphagia, it is not always possible to either reduce the dosage or discontinue the medication for medical reasons.

Drugs that depress the central nervous system also may depress the activity of striated muscle with subsequent negative effects on swallowing. Delay in swallow or an inability to sustain motor performance because of drowsiness or inattention may affect swallowing safety. Major classes of drugs that may affect motor performance and states of arousal include antipsychotics such as haloperidol or chlorpromazine, anticonvulsants such as carbamazepine and phenytoin, opioids such as morphine, and antianxiety preparations such as diazepam and clonazepam. Long-term use of antipsychotic drugs may result in tardive dyskinesia, a condition characterized by uncontrollable, repetitive, regular movements of the tongue and lips. When severe, tardive dyskinesia may interfere with the oral preparatory and oral initiation stages of swallowing.

Drugs such as dantrolene (Dantrium), which are intended to relax muscles that are spastic, may secondarily weaken the muscles for swallowing. Side effects from drugs used to lower cholesterol levels and steroids used to treat inflammatory disease may cause generalized myopathies and difficulty swallowing.

Many classes of drugs inhibit the flow of saliva through their anticholinergic effects on the nervous system. The resultant xerostomia may affect oral preparation and initiation, taste, and the patient's ability to neutralize stomach acid. Commonly used antidepressants with known xerostomic effects include amitriptyline, doxepin, and desipramine.

Medications that affect gastrointestinal function and that secondarily lead to or exacerbate dysphagic complications include those that change or alter appetite and those that lower esophageal sphincter pressures with the possibility of contributing to gastroesophageal reflux disease (GERD). Most medications used to treat cancer and other chronic diseases of the internal organs reduce appetite. Although these medications may not directly cause dysphagia, patients with dysphagia may have mechanical difficulty with swallowing and may not swallow enough because of lack of appetite. Insufficient caloric intake leads to protein-calorie malnutrition, loss of muscle mass, and further compromised muscle (swallowing) strength.

CLINICAL CORNER 8-3

An 83-year-old man was admitted to the psychiatry unit with acute onset of paranoia. His schizophrenia had been controlled successfully for many years with chlorpromazine (Thorazine). Chlorpromazine use had caused tardive dyskinesia that interfered with speech intelligibility but not with swallow. After dinner the patient became combative and a 5-mg dosage of haloperidol (Haldol) was ordered to control his behavior before bedtime. At breakfast he was noted to be coughing and choking on his regular diet and a request for consultation was sent to speech pathology.

CRITICAL THINKING:

1. Based on the patient's history, what potential causes might be considered in the differential diagnosis of his new problem with swallowing?
2. Based on your answer, what would be your next steps in managing his problem?

Practice Note 8-4

An 81-year-old patient with a history of Parkinson's disease was admitted to the hospital with aspiration pneumonia that was believed to be attributable to increased oropharyngeal dysphagia. A progression of Parkinson's disease was suspected, and a nasogastric tube was inserted. A thorough medical history review revealed that the patient had recently seen his primary care physician because of increased pain in his right arm that had become progressively rigid. At that time he was given dantrolene sodium (Dantrium) to relax his arm and ideally relieve the pain. Because the patient had been eating fairly well before taking the Dantrium, I believed that the addition of the muscle relaxant was enough to remove any compensations he was making for his poor swallowing ability and probably led to his aspiration pneumonia. The Dantrium was discontinued while the man received treatment for his pneumonia, and he returned home to successful oral feeding. Although the intent to relieve his arm pain was well meant, the side effects of the treatment outweighed the advantages.

Medications used to treat respiratory disease, such as albuterol, beclomethasone, and theophylline, all reduce lower esophageal sphincter (LES) pressures, thereby increasing the risk of increased events of gastroesophageal reflux. The drug class of calcium channel blockers used to treat cardiac disease also may increase the patient's risk for GERD. For details on specific drug classes and drugs that affect patients with dysphagia, readers are referred to the work by Carl and Johnson.[52]

CHRONIC OBSTRUCTIVE PULMONARY DISEASE

As previously discussed, patients with respiratory-related disease may be at increased risk for dysphagia. One of the most prevalent disorders falls under the general category of chronic obstructive pulmonary disease (COPD). Subcategories of impairment include emphysema, chronic bronchitis, asthma, and cystic fibrosis. These diagnoses are characterized by airflow limitations, abnormalities in oxygen and carbon monoxide exchange, and lung hyperinflation characterized by failure to exhale sufficient amounts of carbon monoxide. Estimates of disease prevalence are difficult because of differences in measurement tools; however, the World Health Organization estimated that by 2020, COPD will be the third leading cause of death and the fifth leading cause of disability worldwide.[53] In 20% to 30% of patients with COPD their disease is complicated by congestive heart failure.[54]

Oropharyngeal swallowing performance has been studied in patients whose COPD is medically stable and in those with acute exacerbation. Mokhlesi et al.[55] used videofluoroscopy to compare the swallowing of 20 patients with stable COPD with 20 age-matched controls. No instances of aspiration were found in either group; however, those with COPD showed reduced hyoid bone elevation, earlier and longer airway closure durations, and earlier airway closure time relative to PES relaxation onset. The investigators noted that although no patient had evidence of airway protection problems, in instances of acute exacerbation these physiologic differences may become more pronounced, leading to swallow decompensation and the potential for airway protection disorders. Good-Fratturelli et al.[56] studied a group of 78 patients with COPD and other medical disorders such as stroke and myocardial infarction who were referred for suspected oropharyngeal dysphagia. Ninety-five percent were eating orally before evaluation and 42% aspirated, primarily on thin and thickened liquids, often with ineffective or absent cough responses. Half of the 42% aspirated silently. Colodny[57] studied the

swallowing and respiratory function of 15 patients with stable COPD. She found that only advancing age was the best predictor in those who aspirated. Interestingly, multisystem involvement did not predict aspiration in this cohort.

Coelho[58] studied 14 patients with COPD who were hospitalized for acute exacerbations. Thirteen had tracheotomies and five were dependent on ventilation support. On videofluorographic studies 3 of the 14 aspirated, although all patients showed swallow delay in both oral and pharyngeal stages suggestive of generalized muscle weakness.[58] Shaker et al.[59] studied the respiration and deglutition cycle relations in those with acute COPD whose condition eventually stabilized. During an acute exacerbation more swallows were initiated during inspiration than in normal subjects, and there were some differences in the relation between deglutition apnea and total swallow durations compared with normal subjects. When their condition was stabilized, the patients returned to swallow initiation on the exhalatory cycle, and respiration-to-deglutition timing measures returned to normal. Nishino et al.[60] noted similar changes in inspiratory/expiratory cycle relations in patients with COPD compared with normal subjects. These changes occurred most often during periods of **hypercapnia**.

Of concern in patients with COPD and dysphagia is the issue of whether acute exacerbations are the result of aspiration or if they are unrelated. Or does an acute exacerbation of COPD increase the risk for aspiration? In one third of patients with COPD, the reason for an acute exacerbation is unknown.[61] Kobayashi et al.[62] studied the timing of the swallow reflex in patients with stable COPD and in patients who averaged 2.4 exacerbations within 1 year. All patients were eating orally at the time of the study. There was a significant difference between the two groups. Those with exacerbations showed swallow reflex delay that could be associated with the potential for swallowing dysfunction. These data do not show a cause-and-effect relation between oropharyngeal dysphagia and acute COPD exacerbations but suggest the two could be related.

Other investigators have studied the changes of oxygen saturation levels during a meal. Presumably the work of eating may change saturation levels that secondarily may predispose the patient to aspiration. Brown et al.[63] found that not all patients with severe COPD experienced desaturation at mealtime. Only those whose baseline levels before the meal were below 90% desaturated. In 16 patients with severe COPD who had tracheotomies, Vitacca et al.[64] compared respiratory parameters during and after a

30-minute meal with and without ventilatory support. Respiratory rate, end-tidal carbon dioxide values, and an increase in dyspnea all were abnormally high when patients did not receive ventilatory assistance. This implies that in this specific group of patients that ventilatory support at mealtimes may be prudent to avoid the risk of aspiration.

Patients with COPD are at risk for aspiration from oropharyngeal sources as well as esophageal sources. It has been suggested that GERD may play a role in the exacerbation of COPD by three mechanisms: (1) direct infiltration of stomach contents into the lungs, (2) acid irritation to the esophageal vagal afferents with resultant bronchospasm and desaturation, and (3) primary disorders of the esophagus that secondarily affect PES physiology and subsequent airway protection.[65] Using videofluoroscopy, Stein et al.[66] studied 25 patients with severe COPD who were symptomatic for dysphagia. Disorders in flow through the PES were present in 21 of the patients. The authors suggested that the disorders in the PES for the older patients and those with more severe COPD may be related to compensatory activity of the PES resulting in its failure to adequately relax. This subgroup of patients was more likely to show signs of GERD. Using a questionnaire, Rascon-Aguilar et al.[67] found that 37% of 86 patients with COPD reported symptoms of reflux and that the rate of COPD exacerbations in those with such complaints was twice as high as in those with none.

This finding suggests that the presence of reflux-related symptoms may play a role in acute exacerbations in patients with COPD and that GERD control is important. Using 24-hour pH monitoring and measures of oxygen saturation, Casanova et al.[68] found pathologic reflux scores in 62% of patients with COPD. Of particular interest was that half of this group reported no GERD symptomatology. Kempainen et al.[69] found a similar prevalence of GERD in 41 (57%) patients with COPD, also noting that a high percentage reported no symptoms. In addition, 15% of the group with confirmed positive reflux studies had proximal esophageal reflux, suggesting there may be a threat to the airway. Readers are encouraged to reread the section on PES relations and GERD in Chapter 7 to fully appreciate the relations among GERD, the esophagus, and the potential for pharyngeal swallowing dysfunction.

The mechanism for the increased prevalence of GERD in patients with COPD is speculative. One theory is that the number of transient LES relaxations is increased because of failure of the crural diaphragm or LES fibers as a result of short or irregular respiratory cycles. The crural diaphragm provides a barrier during inhalation, whereas the LES provides a barrier during exhalation. Therefore interruptions in respiratory competence may allow increased movement of stomach contents across the LES barrier. Because of the known relaxation of LES pressures caused by medications used to treat COPD,[52] the patient with COPD is at great risk for GERD and its potential negative consequences on swallowing.

TAKE HOME NOTES

1. Disorders of breathing often affect swallowing because of the close relation between breathing and swallowing.
2. Patients who require placement of a tracheotomy tube may be at risk for aspiration, particularly if they have multiple medical complications.
3. Swallowing disorders resulting from medical or surgical interventions may be referred to as *iatrogenic*.
4. Surgical procedures such as carotid endarterectomy, cardiac bypass, thyroidectomy, cervical spine fusion, esophagectomy, and skull base surgery may involve key cranial nerves needed for swallowing.
5. Traumatic injuries that result in fractures of swallowing structures, dental trauma, and thermal burn injuries all may increase the patient's risk of swallow safety.
6. The side effects from medications used to treat medical conditions may be the primary causative factor of dysphagia or may complicate preexisting dysphagia.
7. Patients with chronic obstructive pulmonary disease are at risk for dysphagia, especially during periods of acute exacerbation, because of compromise to the respiratory system.

References

1. Butler SG, Stuart A, Pressman H et al: Preliminary investigation of swallowing apnea duration and swallow/respiratory phase relationships in individuals with cerebral vascular accident, *Dysphagia* 22:215, 2007.

2. Partik B, Pokieser P, Schima W et al: Videofluoroscopy of swallowing in symptomatic patients who have undergone long-term intubation, *AJR Am J Roentgenol* 174:1409, 2000.

3. deLarminat V, Montravers P, Dureuil B et al: Alteration in swallowing reflex after extubation in intensive care unit patients, *Crit Care Med* 23:486, 1995.

4. Ding R, Logemann JA: Swallow physiology in patients with trach cuff inflated or deflated: a retrospective study, *Head Neck* 27:809, 2005.

5. Bonano PC: Swallowing dysfunction after tracheostomy, *Ann Surg* 174:29, 1971.

6. Nash M: Swallowing problems in the tracheotomized patient, *Otolaryngol Clin North Am* 21:701, 1988.

7. Elpern EH, Jacobs ER, Bone RC: Incidence of aspiration in tracheally intubated adults, *Heart Lung* 16:527, 1987.

8. Eibling D, Diez Gross R: Subglottic air pressure: a key component of swallowing efficiency, *Ann Otol Rhinol Laryngol* 105:253,1996.

9. Sasaki CT, Susuki M, Horiuchi M et al: The effect of tracheostomy on the laryngeal closure reflex, *Laryngoscope* 87:1428, 1977.

10. Terk AR, Leder SB, Burrell MI: Hyoid bone and laryngeal movement dependent upon presence of a tracheotomy tube, *Dysphagia* 22:89, 2007.

11. Logemann JA, Pauloski BR, Coangelo L: Light digital occlusion of the tracheostomy tube: a pilot study of effects on aspiration and biomechanics of the swallow, *Head Neck* 20:52, 1998.

12. Leder SB, Ross DA, Burell MI: Tracheostomy tube occlusion status and aspiration in early postsurgical head and neck cancer patients, *Dysphagia* 13:167, 1998.

13. Dettelbach MA, Gross RD, Mahlmann J et al: Effect of the Passy-Muir valve on aspiration in patients with tracheostomy, *Head Neck* 17:297, 1995.

14. Leder SB: Effect of one-way tracheotomy speaking valve on the incidence of aspiration in previously aspirating patients with tracheotomy, *Dysphagia* 14:73, 1999.

15. Elpern EH, Borkgren Okonek M, Bacon M et al: Effect of the Passy-Muir tracheostomy speaking valve on pulmonary aspiration in adults, *Heart Lung* 29:287, 2000.

16. Suiter DM, McCulloch GH, Powell PW: Effects of cuff deflation and one-way tracheostomy speaking valve placement on swallow physiology, *Dysphagia* 18:284, 2003.

17. Leder SB, Joe JK, Hill SE et al: Effect of tracheotomy tube occlusion on upper esophageal sphincter and pharyngeal pressures in aspirating and nonaspirating patients, *Dysphagia* 16:79, 2001.

18. Donzelli J, Brady S, Wesling M et al: Effects of the removal of the tracheotomy tube on swallowing during the fiberoptic exam of the swallow (FEES), *Dysphagia* 20:283, 2005.

19. Buchholz DW: Oropharyngeal dysphagia due to iatrogenic neurologic dysfunction, *Dysphagia* 10:248, 1995.

20. Lombardi CP, Raffaelli M, D'Alatri L et al: Voice and swallowing changes after thyroidectomy in patients without inferior laryngeal nerve injuries, *Surgery* 140:1026, 2006.

21. Wasserman JM, Sundaram K, Alfonso AE et al: Determination of the function of the internal branch of the superior laryngeal nerve after thyroidectomy, *Head Neck* 30:21, 2008.

22. Pereira JA, Girvent M, Sancho JJ et al: Prevalence of long-term upper aerodigestive symptoms after uncomplicated bilateral thyroidectomy, *Surgery* 133:318, 2003.

23. Ekberg O, Bergqvist D, Takolander R et al: Pharyngeal function after carotid endarterectomy, *Dysphagia* 10:62, 1989.

24. Monini S, Taurino M, Barbara M et al: Laryngeal and cranial nerve involvement after carotid endarterectomy, *Acta Otolaryngol* 125:398, 2005.

25. Masiero S, Previato C, Addante S et al: Dysphagia in post-carotid endarterectomy: a prospective study, *Ann Vasc Surg* 21:218, 2007.

26. Abel R, Ruf S, Spahn B: Cervical spinal cord injury and deglutition disorders, *Dysphagia* 19:87, 2004.

27. Morishima N, Ohota K, Miura Y: The influences of Halo-vest fixation and cervical hyperextension on swallowing in healthy volunteers, *Spine* 30:E179, 2005.

28. Buchholz D: Dysphagia due to iatrogenic neurological dysfunction, *Dysphagia* 10:248, 1995.

29. Welsh LW, Welsh JJ, Chinnici JC: Dysphagia due to cervical spine surgery, *Ann Otol Rhinol Laryngol* 96:112, 1987.

30. Martin RP, Nery MA, Diamant NE: Dysphagia following anterior cervical spine surgery, *Dysphagia* 12:2, 1987.

31. Winslow CP, Winslow TJ, Wax MK: Dysphonia and dysphagia following the anterior approach to the cervical spine, *Arch Otolaryngol Head Neck Surg* 127:51, 2001.

32. Baraz R, Lee MJ, Yoo JU: Incidence of dysphagia after cervical spine surgery: a prospective study, *Spine* 27:2453, 2002.

33. Buchholz DW, Jones B, Ravich WJ: Dysphagia following anterior cervical fusion, *Dysphagia* 8:390, 1993.

34. Gamache FW, Voorhies RM: Hypertrophic cervical osteophytes causing dysphagia: a review, *J Neurosurg* 53:338, 1980.

35. Strasser G, Schima W, Schober E et al: Cervical osteophytes impinging on the pharynx: importance of size and concurrent disorders for development of aspiration, *AJR Am J Roentgenol* 174:449, 2000.

36. Granville LJ, Musson N, Altman R et al: Anterior cervical osteophytes as a cause of pharyngeal stage dysphagia, *J Am Geriatr Soc* 46:1003, 1998.

37. Atkins BZ, Shah AS, Hutcheson KA et al: Reducing hospital morbidity and mortality following esophagectomy, *Ann Thorac Surg* 78:1170, 2004.

38. Leder SB, Bayars S, Sasaki CT et al: Fiberoptic endoscopic evaluation of swallowing in assessing aspiration after transhiatal esophagectomy, *J Am Coll Surg* 205:581, 2007.

39. Lewin JS, Hebert TM, Putnam JB et al: Experience with the chin tuck maneuver in postesophagectomy aspirators, *Dysphagia* 16:216, 2001.

40. Atkins BZ, Fortes DL, Watkins KT: Analysis of respiratory complications after minimally invasive esophagectomy: preliminary observation of persistent aspiration risk, *Dysphagia* 22:49, 2007.

41. Kato H, Miyakaki T, Sakai M et al: Videofluoroscopic evaluation in oropharyngeal swallowing after radical esophagectomy with lymphadenectomy for esophageal cancer, *Anticancer Res* 27:4249, 2007.

42. Martin RE, Letsos P, Taves DH et al: Oropharyngeal dysphagia in esophageal cancer before and after transhiatal esophagectomy, *Dysphagia* 16:23, 2001.

43. Heitmiller RF, Jones B: Transient diminished airway protection following transhiatal esophagectomy, *Am J Surg* 162:422, 1991.

44. Rice TW: Anastomotic stricture complicating esophagectomy, *Thorac Surg Clin* 16:63, 2006.

45. Jennings SK, Siroky D, Jackson G: Swallowing problems after excision of tumors of the skull base: diagnosis and management in 12 patients, *Dysphagia* 7:40, 1992.

46. Pineau BC, Ott DJ: Isolated proximal injury from blunt trauma: endoscopic stricture dilatation, *Dysphagia* 18:263, 2003.

47. Tamura F, Mizukami M, Ayano R et al: Analysis of feeding function and jaw stability in bedridden elderly, *Dysphagia* 17:235, 2002.

48. Furuya J: Effects of wearing complete dentures on swallowing in the elderly, *J Stomatol Soc Japan* 66:361, 1999 [in Japanese].

49. Yoshikawa M, Yoshida M, Nagasaki T et al: Influence of aging and denture use on liquid swallowing in healthy dentulous and edentulous older people, *J Am Geriatr Soc* 54:449, 2006.

50. Hattori F: The relationship between wearing complete dentures and swallowing function in elderly individuals: a videofluoroscopic study, *J Stomatol Soc Japan* 71:102, 2004 [in Japanese].

51. DuBose CM, Groher ME, Mann GC et al: *The prevalence of swallowing disorders following thermal burn injury*, Unpublished manuscript, University of Florida Health Science Center, 2006.

52. Carl LL, Johnson PR: *Drugs and dysphagia: how medications can affect eating and swallowing*, Austin, TX, 2006, Pro-Ed.

53. Viegi G, Maio S, Pistelli F et al: Epidemiology of chronic obstructive pulmonary disease: health effects of air pollution, *Respirology* 11:523, 2006.

54. LeJemtel TH, Padeletti M, Jelic S: Diagnostic and therapeutic challenges in patients with coexistent chronic obstructive pulmonary disease and chronic heart failure, *J Am Coll Cardiol* 49:171, 2007.

55. Mokhlesi B, Logemann JA, Rademaker A et al: Oropharyngeal deglutition in stable COPD, *Chest* 121:361, 2002.

56. Good-Fratturelli MD, Curlee RF, Holle JL: Prevalence and nature of dysphagia in VA patients with COPD referred for videofluoroscopic swallow examination, *J Commun Disorders* 33:93, 2000.

57. Colodny N: Effects of age, gender, disease, and multisystem involvement on oxygen saturation levels in dysphagic persons, *Dysphagia* 16:48, 2001.

58. Coehlo CA: Preliminary findings on the nature of dysphagia in patients with chronic obstructive pulmonary disease, *Dysphagia* 2:28, 1987.

59. Shaker R, Li Q, Ren J et al: Coordination of deglutition and phases of respiration: effect of aging, tachypnea, bolus volume, and chronic obstructive pulmonary disease, *Am J Physiol* 263:G750, 1992.

60. Nishino T, Hasegawa R, Ide T et al: Hypercapnia enhances the development of coughing during continuous infusion of water into the pharynx, *Am J Respir Crit Care Med* 157:815, 1998.

61. Donaldson GC, Wedzicha JA: COPD exacerbations: epidemiology, *Thorax* 61:164, 2006.

62. Kobayashi S, Kubo H, Yanai M: Impairment of the swallowing reflex in exacerbations of COPD, *Thorax* 62:1017, 2007.

63. Brown SE, Casciari RJ, Light RW: Arterial oxygen saturation during meals in patients with severe chronic obstructive pulmonary disease, *South Med J* 76:194, 1983.

64. Vitacca M, Callogari G, Sarua M et al: Physiological effects of meals in difficult-to-wean tracheostomized patients with chronic obstructive pulmonary disease, *Intensive Care Med* 31:236, 2005.

65. Mokhlesi B: Clinical implications of gastroesophageal reflux disease and swallowing dysfunction in COPD, *Am J Respir Med* 2:117, 2003.

66. Stein M, Williams AJ, Grossman F et al: Cricopharyngeal dysfunction in chronic obstructive pulmonary disease, *Chest* 97:347, 1990.

67. Rascon Aguilar IE, Pamer M, Wludyka P et al: Role of gastroesophageal reflux symptoms in exacerbations of COPD, *Chest* 130:1096, 2006.

68. Casanova C, Baudet JS, Velasco MDV et al: Increased gastro-esophageal reflux disease in patients with severe COPD, *Eur Respir J* 23:841, 2004.

69. Kempainen RR, Savik K, Whelan TP et al: High prevalence of proximal and distal gastroesophageal reflux disease in advanced COPD, *Chest* 131:1666, 2007.

Chapter **9**

Clinical Evaluation of Adults

MICHAEL E. GROHER

OBJECTIVES

1. Describe the rationale for early detection of swallowing disorders.
2. Review the main components of the clinical evaluation of swallowing in adults.
3. Present the strengths and weaknesses of evaluation protocols.
4. Discuss noninvasive techniques for improving the diagnostic accuracy of the clinical examination.
5. Review standardized tests for dysphagia.
6. Present potential adjunctive measures of swallowing performance.

RATIONALE

A comprehensive evaluation of a patient with known or suspected dysphagia involves a number of medical and allied health disciplines. Data collected for patients in an outpatient setting who reported dysphagia revealed that the diagnostic process involved an average of 3.5 disciplines per patient.[1] Therefore for most patients, the comprehensive evaluation of the patient with dysphagia should be considered a team evaluation. Relevant disciplines were discussed in Chapter 1. For the speech-language pathologist (SLP) the evaluation is intended to assess factors that relate to swallowing function, not to diagnose the underlying disease, although it may either obviate or clarify the need for further studies. In some cases the clinical examination of swallowing confirms a particular diagnosis because the swallowing characteristics are consistent with other aspects of the disease, such as the repetitive tongue pumping in the oral stage of Parkinson's disease.

The clinical evaluation of swallowing often is referred to as the *bedside examination*. Although the bedside examination encompasses the same procedures, *clinical examination* is the preferred terminology because the examination is performed in any setting and is not restricted to the bedside. However, modifications in the standard clinical evaluation of swallowing may need to be made at the bedside—often because of poor patient cooperation. The clinical evaluation of swallowing is to be distinguished from the *instrumental evaluation* (see Chapter 10), which might include tests conducted outside the clinical environment, such as radiographic studies that require special space and equipment. Some patient settings, such as long-term care facilities, lack easy access to instrumental swallowing assessment environments. Patients must be transported to these settings. Therefore clinicians in these settings rely heavily on the clinical evaluation of swallowing to provide diagnostic and treatment information. Settings such as those in tertiary care hospitals can provide the instrumental support for advanced swallowing studies. In this environment the clinician may not always rely totally on the clinical evaluation. Rather, it is viewed as complementary to the instrumental evaluation. Interestingly, there are no **prospective data** that either support or refute the effect of each practice pattern on patient health outcomes.

The clinical evaluation of the patient with dysphagia has three main components: the medical history, the physical inspection of the swallowing musculature, and observations of swallowing competence with test swallows. Logemann[2] lists five reasons for performing a clinical (physical) evaluation for a swallowing disorder: (1) to define a potential cause (medical history), (2) to establish a working hypothesis that defines the disorder, (3) to establish a tentative treatment plan, (4) to develop a potential list of questions that may require further study, and (5) to establish the readiness of the patient to cooperate with any further testing. Not all elements of the physical evaluation may be completed because of patient cooperation or performance. In this circumstance, the clinician must rely heavily on the medical history or, if the patient is eating, observations of his or her swallowing ability. Another valuable use of the clinical examination is its use as an outcome measure, either in a research protocol or in clinical practice. Changes in physical status after treatment intervention can be easily measured with a clinical examination with numeric values associated with each finding. Skilled examiners use baseline clinical evaluation data to track dysphagia severity over time in patients with progressive neurologic disease.

Practitioners might choose to use an abbreviated portion of the clinical examination of swallowing as a method to screen for or detect dysphagia. Once a high suspicion for dysphagia is established, the entire clinical examination is administered. Early detection of dysphagia is important because complications from dysphagia increase patient morbidity, lengthen hospitalization (health care cost), and may ultimately increase patient risk for death.[3] Most "screening" tools for dysphagia do not meet the strict criteria of a screening device. A valid screening tool for dysphagia should be able to detect dysphagia in a large group of patients who are **not** symptomatic for dysphagia, but who may, in fact, have dysphagia.[4] The valid screening tool for dysphagia also should be able to show improved health outcomes as a result of its administration.[5] To establish that improvement in health status is a consequence of effective screening, the screening device should be tested in a group with dysphagia who did not receive the screening and a similar group who did.[5] Current practice with dysphagia screening tools presupposes that the screening tool is administered because the patient already has a high suspicion for symptoms. A good screening test for dysphagia will have high sensitivity (detecting dysphagia when it is present) and high specificity (determining accurately when it is not present), but it also should be predictive. For patients with dysphagia the screening tool should be predictive of positive health outcomes, such as fewer cases of aspiration pneumonia, better nutritional status, or positive quality of life scores as they relate to eating. Screening devices for dysphagia should be easily administered by any medical specialist in a short time. The clinical evaluation for swallowing as administered by the SLP is designed to provide a much broader perspective of the patient with dysphagia than a screening protocol would provide. The American Stroke Association has called for development of dysphagia screening devices. All patients, regardless of suspicion for dysphagia, will be screened for its presence. Currently, no clinical examination or portions of a clinical examination for swallowing have satisfied the statistical and application criteria needed to be called a screening instrument for dysphagia. One undoubtedly will be developed in the near future because of the importance of early detection.

Clinicians recognize that all clinical evaluations of patients with dysphagia are not the same, although clinician preference in selecting items for inclusion are items supported in the literature as discriminative.[6] Most clinicians combine data from the medical history, physical examination, and trial swallows.[6] The clinical examination for swallow suffers from lack of reliable methods of scoring and inconsistencies in agreement on observations, such as the definition of a wet-hoarse voice.[7] McCullough et al.[8] found that clinicians can reliably judge only 50% of items commonly administered in a clinical examination for swallow. The most reliable judgments were observation of the presence of tubes, oral motor data, and historical parameters. Inconsistency in recoding data carries the risk of diagnostic inaccuracy, which in turn will affect the treatment plan. Clearly there is a need to standardize the clinical evaluation of swallowing (see section on standardized tests later in this chapter).

SYMPTOMS OF DYSPHAGIA

Symptoms usually are defined as any perceptible change in bodily function that the patient notices. This change eventually leads the patient to seek medical help when it causes pain or discomfort or negatively affects his or her lifestyle. Some people have adverse medical symptoms and ignore them until the severity of the problem significantly affects their physiologic or mental health. Others seek immediate medical attention. Both groups may have a diagnosis of a disorder that is similar in type and severity.

Patient Description

The physical examination of a patient with dysphagia may begin by asking the patient to describe the symptoms. Some common symptoms are detailed in Table 9-1. Because dysphagia often is secondary to neurologic disease that also may compromise communica-

TABLE 9-1

Examples of Signs and Symptoms Associated with Dysphagia

Symptom	Sign
Difficulty chewing	Food spills from lips; excessive mastication time of soft food; poor dentition; tongue, jaw, or lip weakness
Difficulty initiating swallow	Mouth dryness (xerostomia); lip or tongue weakness
Drooling	Lip or tongue weakness; infrequent swallows
Nasal regurgitation	Bolus enters or exits the nasal cavity, as seen on radiographic swallowing study
Swallow delay	Radiographic study identifies transport beyond normal standard
Food sticking	Radiographic study identifies excessive residue in mouth, pharynx, or esophagus after completed swallow
Coughing and choking	Coughs on trial food attempts; material enters the airway on radiographic study
Coughing when not eating	Radiographic study shows aspiration of saliva or lung abnormality
Regurgitation	Undigested food in mouth; radiographic study shows food returning from esophagus to pharynx or mouth mucosal irritation on endoscopy; pH probe study positive for acid reflux
Weight loss	Unexplained weight loss; measurement of weight is below ideal standard

tion skills, not all patients can provide a report of their symptoms. Others may give unreliable or scant information because of cortical deficits. Anecdotal evidence suggests that many patients with dysphagia (particularly esophageal based) do not seek immediate medical attention. Rather, they make changes in their eating habits to accommodate their symptoms, such as chewing food more finely or eliminating troublesome items from their diet. Others know they have difficulty swallowing but cannot describe the specifics of their symptoms. Often it is difficult to remember how long the symptoms have been apparent; this may be from the inherent flexibility of the swallowing tract to accommodate changes in function. Only when these accommodations no longer provide relief or are too difficult to execute does the patient seek medical attention. Some patients may have symptoms of dysphagia but ignore them. For instance, one study of 56 older persons who did not report dysphagia found that a large majority had radiographic abnormalities during swallowing tests. Such abnormalities included poor esophageal motility and pharyngeal weakness.[9]

For those who are able to communicate symptoms of their dysphagia, a detailed description may be useful in helping establish a diagnosis. Detailed descriptions also may be used to help the examiner focus on the types of diagnostic tests that may be most useful in delineating the source of the complaint. The relation between the accuracy of a patient's complaint and the final diagnosis has not been investigated extensively. Whether the complaint is useful in guiding the diagnostic process also has not been experimentally verified. Nonetheless, asking the patient to describe the problem is a common point of departure in the dysphagia examination.

The literature suggests that asking patients to localize where they believe the problem exists is not always reliable and may not be useful in guiding the tests selected for patient examination, particularly when they report the problem is localized to the neck.[10] In one large study of patients who were found to have confirmed esophageal disease, most who pointed to the lower esophagus who had confirmed lower esophageal lesions were accurate. However, a significant number (30%) pointed to the upper neck and chest as the source of their discomfort.[11] Other investigators have found that a significant number of patients who described food sticking at the level of the pharynx did have abnormalities at this level; however, the primary source of that abnormality often was found to be in the esophagus.[12] This suggests that patients who report dysphagia localized to the neck and pharynx should not only have that specific region investigated, but also should have studies appropriate to the esophagus. Questioning patients about their disorder beyond localization often improves their accuracy. For instance, if the patient localizes the problem to the neck and reports coughing on fluids, the likelihood that the problem is pharyngeal based is high.[13] One study found that if patients who complained of food sticking in the region of the neck also reported respiratory symptoms (congestion, wheezing, cough), the sensitivity of dysphagia localized to the pharynx improved.[14] Another group of investigators found that subtypes of esophageal disorders (**motility** vs. **obstructive**) could be determined by patient report if the patient described a cluster of symptoms, such as heartburn with dysphagia, prior dilatation, pain, and weight loss, than if they reported heartburn alone.[15] In general, studies agree that the complaint (dysphagic symptoms) presented by the patient correlates better with the findings when the problem after diagnosis is judged to be severe. The fact that all studies do not agree on whether patient localization is accurate is largely attributable to inadequate numbers of subjects, the potential differences in final classification of the disease type, and the fact that some patients might have undergone other treatments and tests before being enrolled in the study.

Some clinicians find it useful to explore a patient's dysphagic symptoms by questionnaire. A sample questionnaire specific to patients with head/neck cancer that could be completed before their office visit is presented in Box 9-1. This method may help ensure that all relevant questions relating to the patient's symptoms are addressed by the examiner. It also gives the patient a chance to think carefully about the symptoms before responding. Other patient-specific questionnaires have been developed, including one specifically for stroke (the Burke Dysphagia Screening Test)[16] and one for patients with Parkinson's disease.[17] Wallace et al.[18] sought to develop a symptom severity assessment tool. Their tool is a 17-point questionnaire designed to evaluate initial dysphagic symptom severity that could be used to judge outcomes after therapy. Questions range from the patient's difficulty in swallowing various textures to issues of swallow initiation, episodes of choking, and how the disorder interferes with the patient's quality of life.

Regardless of which method is used—patient report to examiner questions or patient responses to a questionnaire—the patient's subjective complaint may not always fit the objective data gathered in the physical and instrumental evaluation. In another study, subjective complaints of patients with head/neck cancer and oropharyngeal dysphagia were compared with the objective findings from the instrumental examination.[19] In general, many of the objective findings did not always support the patient's complaint. However, in some cases other findings that the patient did not consider important were documented. Jensen et al.[19] concluded that subjective complaints may be useful in guiding the examination but should be confirmed with objective data. There have been no comparisons between the standardized dysphagia questionnaire and the structured clinical interview as it relates to diagnostic approach or accuracy.

Obstruction

One of the most common complaints from patients with dysphagia is that food or fluids "get stuck." Most frequently they report that the sticking sensation is

BOX 9-1	Sample Dysphagia Questionnaire

1. Do you have difficulty chewing your food?   Yes   No
2. If so, which foods give you the most trouble? Underline any that apply.
   A. Solids (e.g., meats)
   B. Liquids (e.g., water)
   C. Semisolids (e.g., cottage cheese, applesauce, cereal)
3. If you underlined a category in question 2, provide some examples:
   Specific solids:
   Specific liquids:
   Semisolids:
4. Do you have difficulty lining up your teeth?   Yes   No
5. Does food go all over your mouth, and is it difficult getting it together to swallow it?   Yes   No
6. Do you have trouble opening and closing your jaw?   Yes   No
7. Is the sensation in your mouth decreased?   Yes   No
8. Do you choke when eating?   Yes   No
9. If you answered "yes" above, do you choke before you swallow, when you are chewing, or after you   Yes   No
   swallow?
10. Is it hard for you to:
    A. Lift your tongue?   Yes   No
    B. Move it from side to side?   Yes   No
    C. Move it from front to back?   Yes   No
11. Do you eat or drink more slowly now than before surgery?   Yes   No
12. Do you eat or drink one category more slowly than others?
    Solids: Yes   No
    Liquids: Yes   No
    Semisolids: Yes   No
13. Does food catch in the:
    A. Left side of your throat?   Yes   No
    B. Right side of your throat?   Yes   No
    C. Left side of your mouth?   Yes   No
    D. Right side of your mouth?   Yes   No
    E. Behind your Adam's apple?   Yes   No
14. Do you need to pump your tongue many times to collect food to swallow?   Yes   No
15. Do you feel you have to swallow three or more times so all the food will go down?   Yes   No
16. Do you have trouble swallowing pills?   Yes   No
17. Do you cough up food?   Yes   No
18. If so, does the food come up:
    A. While chewing?   Yes   No
    B. After the food is swallowed?   Yes   No
19. Do small amounts of food or liquids ever fall out of your mouth:
    A. Before you swallow?   Yes   No
    B. After you swallow?   Yes   No
20. Do you have a gurgly voice after you eat?   Yes   No
21. Do you feel the need to clear your throat after swallowing or eating a meal?   Yes   No
22. Do you have trouble controlling drooling?   Yes   No
23. Does food or liquid leak out of your:
    A. Trachea?   Yes   No   NA
    B. Fistula?   Yes   No   NA
24. Do you ever have to clean your mouth out after eating because food has become stuck?   Yes   No
25. Do you ever have to "wash down" your food with liquids?   Yes   No
26. Do you eat as much now as you did before your surgery?   Yes   No
27. Have you changed your diet in any way that is not mentioned above?   Yes   No
You are encouraged to add additional helpful information.

From Baker BM, Fraser AM, Baker CD: Long-term postoperative dysphagia in oral/pharyngeal surgery patients: subjects' perceptions vs. videofluoroscopic observations. *Dysphagia* 6:11, 1991.
NA, Not applicable.

in the throat or esophagus. Some patients do not use the word *stuck* but may use the word *fullness*. Especially when they localize the feeling of obstruction to the throat, patients often describe their complaint as "a lump in the throat" when eating. The medical term for this feeling is *globus*. Some physicians have used the term *globus hystericus* to describe this sensation, because it was once believed that the description of a lump in the throat was usually associated not with **organicity** but with symptoms of **hysteria**. Technically, globus hystericus is reserved for patients who complain of a lump in the throat that is relieved by swallowing or talking, not as a cause for dysphagia. The globus sensation is usually relieved by swallowing. However, use of the term *globus sensation* often is associated with the dysphagic person who reports that food is sticking at the level of the cervical esophagus. Although early investigators reported that they rarely found a cause for the globus sensation (i.e., patients were hysterical), recent reports suggest that with the appropriate battery of diagnostic tests, most who report the globus sensation have identifiable disease.[20] Moser et al.[21] found that when patients reported the globus sensation with chest pain or heartburn, they were likely to have an esophageal motility disorder.

Liquids Versus Solids

Patients may report a change in their dietary habits that is associated with perceived dysphagia. For instance, patients who describe the globus sensation often have more difficulty swallowing solids than liquids. Classically, those with solid food dysphagia are more likely to have disorders of esophageal origin, whereas those with dysphagia for liquids are more likely to have oropharyngeal dysphagia. This dichotomy, however, may be artificial because it is well known that those with oropharyngeal dysphagia can have dysphagia for liquids and solids, and some forms of esophageal dysphagia evoke complaints regarding liquids and solids.[10] When patients report choking on liquids and/or solids, it suggests a more pharyngeal-focused cause, whereas those who report dysphagia for liquids and solids without choking episodes may have a more esophageal-focused cause. Gastroenterologists who suspect the esophagus as the source of dysphagia may use a decision tree such as the one presented in Chapter 7 (see Figure 7-9) to assist in diagnosis. Such a decision tree has not been validated against a large number of patients with confirmed diagnoses; however, the concept is useful because the symptoms related to the diseases represented are well known. Patients are asked questions related to diet (solids vs. liquids), intermittent versus progressive symptoms, and the presence of heartburn. In general, patients with solid food dysphagia are at risk only for more obstructive types of dysphagia in the esophagus. Those who report problems with both liquids and solids more frequently have disorders of esophageal motility. A decision tree for suspected oropharyngeal dysphagia has not been developed, primarily because of overlapping (and therefore nonspecific) symptoms and signs that may be related to many disease entities. Therefore using a decision tree approach based on patient complaints would have little precision in helping establish a diagnosis for those with oropharyngeal dysphagia.

Gastroesophageal Reflux

Some patients report episodes of gastroesophageal reflux (heartburn) associated with their report of dysphagia. Some patients describe pain or fullness in the chest associated with their reflux. Others may have reflux and dysphagia but may be unaware that they have reflux because the overt symptoms of chest pain, or acid taste, are not present. Not all patients describe episodes of reflux unless questioned by the examiner because they may not relate their reflux symptoms to their dysphagia. This is particularly true when patients describe the globus sensation in the neck because they might not think that reflux in the esophagus could be related to a problem in the throat (see Chapter 7 for a full discussion of gastroesophageal reflux disease [GERD] and dysphagia).

Eating Habits

Reporting on changes in one's eating habits may signal the presence of dysphagia, its level of severity, and its psychosocial impact. Complaints that center on elimination of specific food items, such as avoidance of liquids or solids, or items that are sticky or crumbly, may help the examiner focus the evaluation. Excessive chewing of solid food to avoid a sticking sensation may be more consistent with esophageal disease versus the pharyngeal-focused complaint that liquids always seem to come back through the nose. Tiring with foods that require mastication may be consistent with neurologic impairment. Patients who report excessive time to finish a meal often have dysphagia that requires careful evaluation. Patients who report they no longer feel comfortable eating in a restaurant because they have to regurgitate or choke should be examined with care. Patients who have experienced marked weight loss or no longer enjoy the pleasures of eating probably have dysphagia that has reached a high severity level.

SIGNS OF DYSPHAGIA

Signs are objective measurements or observations of behaviors that people elicit during a physical examination. In a patient with dysphagia who is cooperative, this entails an examination of the cranial nerves relevant to swallowing and, if appropriate, interpretation of any laboratory findings. Examples of patient symptoms and corresponding signs are presented in Table 9-1. Some signs are seen on observation when the patient is eating a meal. Signs and symptoms may overlap. For instance, a patient may report *(symptom)* liquid going into the nose and food sticking. Both may be seen by the examiner *(signs)* on the videofluorographic swallowing study. In this circumstance the patient's symptoms have been confirmed.

The physical evaluation of a patient may reveal signs consistent with dysphagia, such as drooling from the lip; tongue weakness; poor dentition; or loss of strength or range of motion in the tongue, jaw, or velum. Poor strength or coordination may result in choking on liquids during test swallows or in lack of bolus flow. The patient's cognitive status may affect swallowing; signs of cognitive deficit may include

CLINICAL CASE EXAMPLE 9-1

A 50-year-old woman comes to the clinic reporting a 6-year history of progressive weight loss. She tells the examiner it has become increasingly hard to swallow both solids and liquids. She denies heartburn. She reports that her dysphagia has interfered with her social life because it now takes an excessive time to finish her meal. The physical evaluation reveals a right facial weakness with atrophy of the left tongue. Her gag reflex is absent and her velum is weak on the left side. Her voice is weak and breathy. On test swallows of liquids and solids she coughs repeatedly.

By the patient's own report, her symptoms of weight loss and a change in social life because of increasing swallowing difficulty seem consistent with a diagnosis of dysphagia. On physical evaluation she has many signs consistent with dysphagia. This is manifest by the involvement of multiple cranial nerves that has resulted in misdirection of the food bolus into the airway, causing choking episodes that has made it embarrassing to eat in front of others. Her symptoms (complaints) are verified by the examination (signs).

failure to chew, talking while swallowing, or inattention to the feeding process. Patients who are hospitalized may have more overt medical signs such as the following: (1) feeding tubes already placed, (2) a tracheotomy tube, (3) respiratory congestion after eating, (4) need for excessive oral and pharyngeal suctioning, (5) eating refusals, (6) undernutrition and muscle wasting, (7) inability to maintain an upright feeding position, (8) an endotracheal tube, and (9) regurgitation of food.

MEDICAL HISTORY

The medical history can be assembled from prior or current medical records, from conversations with the medical staff if the patient is hospitalized, and verbally from the patient or family. Conversations with the patient often are needed to supply missing data or to elucidate or confirm data that are unclear. If the patient's mental status is not compromised, the physical examination often begins with the patient describing his or her dysphagic symptoms (see previous discussion).

Historical Variables

Figure 9-1 shows a sample medical history form. The form can be used to guide the examiner in gathering important historical elements that may affect the diagnosis and treatment of a person with dysphagia. This information can be obtained from the patient/caregiver or the medical record. Some patients, such as those who have had a stroke and dysphagia, make the connection between their neurologic impairment and their complaint. Others, however, such as those who may have dysphagia after surgery unrelated to the swallowing mechanism, may not make the connection between their surgery and dysphagia. For instance, their dysphagia may be related more to the **endotracheal tube** placed in the airway during surgery for their knee. A thorough medical history pertinent to dysphagia sometimes reveals important data that either had been ignored by other specialists or may lead to a path of evaluation that had not been considered.

The medical history as presented in Figure 9-1 is divided into nine parts: congenital disease, psychiatric disease, surgical procedures, cancer-related procedures, metabolic disorders, respiratory impairment, esophageal disorders, prior evaluations of swallowing, and **advance directive** status.

Congenital Disease

Disorders from childhood, particularly those of neurogenic origin such as cerebral palsy, should be noted.

Patient's name: _____

Date of birth: _____

Gender: _____

Medical record number: _____

Chief complaint: _____

_____

_____

Source of information:

——Patient

——Family

——Recent medical record

——Past history

——Other source

Congenital Family Illness:

Neurologic disease:

——Stroke

——Progressive disease

——Traumatic injury

——Other CNS disorders

——Medications taken for:

Psychiatric disease:

——Medications taken for:

——Movement disorder

Surgical procedures:

——Spinal fusion

——Myotomy

——Alimentary tract

Continued

FIGURE 9-1. Sample medical history form. *CNS,* Central nervous system.

___Fundoplication

___Head/neck cancer

___Thyroidectomy

___Cardiac

Cancer-related:

___Irradiation

___Chemotherapy

Systemic/metabolic:

___Nutrition/hydration status

___Current and ideal weight

___Laboratory values related to nutrition

___Infections

___Toxins

___Diabetes

Respiratory Impairment:

___Chronic obstructive pulmonary disease

___Prior history of aspiration pneumonia

___Cardiopulmonary disease

Esophageal Disease:

___Reflux/regurgitation

___Motility disorder

___Dilatation

Prior test results:

___Radiographic

___Manometric

___Scintigraphic

___Endoscopic

Current Advance Directive Status:_____

FIGURE 9-1, cont'd.

Practice Note 9-1

A 64-year-old man was referred to my outpatient swallowing disorders clinic and reported that he had been choking irregularly on liquids for 3 years. He told me that in each of the 3 years he had undergone a standard barium swallow examination and all results were normal. At this point I thought that perhaps his disorder had a pharyngeal focus and that the barium swallow only detailed his esophageal function. However, nothing in his history suggested he might have a reason for pharyngeal pathology until I asked if he had ever been hospitalized. There had been no record of a hospitalization in the medical file I had. He mentioned that 5 years earlier he fell down the basement stairs and was rendered unconscious. He was hospitalized and during his hospitalization had a tracheotomy for 2 months, even though he was discharged from the hospital after 3 weeks. I was unable to get any details about his tracheotomy tube tolerance, but I began to suspect that he might have sustained tracheal **malacia** with a subsequent tracheoesophageal fistula. I had a high suspicion for fistula because small ones frequently produce intermittent symptoms such as those the patient reported, and they may go undetected on standard barium swallow studies. A modified barium swallow study was ordered with particular attention to the anteroposterior projection. This projection provides the best opportunity to make the diagnosis. The radiologist confirmed a fistula, and the head and neck surgeons closed it.

These disorders may not have resulted in dysphagia in the past but may have more significance relative to the present complaint.

Neurologic Disease

Neurologic disorders are the most frequent cause of dysphagia. Stroke, head trauma, and progressive neurogenic diseases such as multiple sclerosis, amyotrophic lateral sclerosis, and Parkinson's disease often precipitate dysphagia. (For a full discussion of neurologic swallowing disorders in adults, see Chapter 5.) It is important to note any medical complications from the disease, particularly any side effects from medications to control the disease that may have adverse effects on swallowing. For instance, a patient who is taking a central nervous system depressant to control seizures may have a concomitant depression in motor function that affects swallowing.

Surgical Procedures

Any surgical procedure has the potential to create dysphagic symptoms, particularly if the patient underwent general anesthesia that required the placement of an endotracheal tube through the vocal folds. Damage to the vocal folds could interfere with airway protection, resulting in dysphagia. Any surgical procedure that involves the aerodigestive or respiratory tract should be noted. Patients who have undergone a surgical wrap (**fundoplication**) of the lower esophageal sphincter (LES) to control GERD may be dysphagic because the wrap is too tight. Patients who have undergone surgical relaxation (**myotomy**) of the upper or LES should have the circumstances of the outcome explored. Surgery to control cancer in the head, neck, or esophagus is of particular importance. Noting whether a patient's cancer was treated by chemotherapy or radiation therapy also may help explain common side effects from those therapies that may cause dysphagia (see Chapter 6). Other specific surgical procedures to note include cardiopulmonary surgery, thyroid surgery, surgery in the upper airway, and cervical spine surgery. The risk in these procedures of damaging cranial nerve (CN) X is higher than in other surgical procedures in these regions and therefore places the patient at greater risk for dysphagia (see Chapter 8 for a full discussion).

Systemic and Metabolic Disorders

Disturbance in the body's chemical balance that may result from toxins (as a result of medication intolerance) or infections may act on the central nervous system, resulting in symptoms of dysphagia. Disorders of metabolism may result in dehydration and undernutrition that compromise physical and mental performance. Physical weakness and mental confusion can be precursors to, or exacerbations of, the dysphagic condition. Asking the patient to comment on any recent weight loss or compare his or her current weight with previous weight may provide insight into the severity of the dysphagia. Diabetes is an example of a systemic, metabolic disorder that may affect swallowing, particularly esophageal peristalsis.

Respiratory Impairment

Because respiration and deglutition share common interactions, any compromise to the respiratory system may decompensate swallowing. Therefore it is important to ask patients if they have any respiratory disease such as chronic obstructive pulmonary disease (see Chapter 8) or asthma in their medical history. Patients who report being treated for suspected aspiration pneumonia already have shown signs of not being able to protect their airway adequately.

Esophageal Disease

Problems with esophageal motility or stenosis of the esophageal body can provide important clues in defining the dysphagic condition. Some patients may have a history of an enlarged heart that could be compressing the esophagus. Others may have a history of regurgitation or reflux that has required treatment such as dilatation. If patients have received specialized treatment or tests in the esophagus, the response to such treatment should be noted.

Previous Test Results

Results of any laboratory study, such as endoscopy of the upper airway, esophagus, or stomach, should be explored. The results of any radiographic results, such as a barium swallow, a modified barium swallow, or an ultrasound of the aerodigestive tract, also are of interest. Some patients with dysphagia and reflux may have undergone a scintigraphic evaluation in nuclear medicine to define the amount and extent of their reflux. Other patients may have undergone a 24-hour pH study to evaluate the presence and frequency of reflux.

Advance Directive

A patient may not have executed an advance directive stating his or her preference about tube feeding if dysphagia is severe. If an advance directive has been executed and is part of the medical record, it should be reviewed. If the patient has chosen not to have tube feeding under any circumstances, the need for further testing or treatments may be contraindicated (see Chapter 15).

PHYSICAL EXAMINATION

The physical examination specific to swallowing impairment typically includes observations of medical interventions that may affect swallowing, such as a tracheotomy tube, and an assessment of the patient's mental status and the cranial nerves involved in swallowing. If patients are eating, observations of their swallowing and feeding skills during test swallow attempts are made. A checklist of items of interest in the clinical evaluation of patients with dysphagia is presented in Box 9-2.

Investigators have sought to determine which elements in the clinical examination for swallow are more important in detecting and defining the disorder. Elements for which research evidence supports their importance, particularly in stroke patients, include dysphonia (harshness and breathiness), a wet-sounding voice, dysarthria, poor secretion management, cough on trial swallows, and decreased laryngeal elevation.[2,22,23] Some of these clinical markers were found to be more predictive of dysphagia and unsafe swallow if two or more of these features were found after clinical examination.[24] McCullough et al.[25] also found that a cluster of clinical findings was more predictive of aspiration than one sign alone. Their results suggested that dysphonia after trial swallows of 5 and 10 mL of thin and thickened liquids, unilateral jaw weakness, and failure on the 3-oz water test were most predictive of aspiration. One investigation found that in acute stroke patients, the clinical examination of swallowing compared with videofluoroscopic examination underestimated the detection of dysphagia but overestimated the frequency of aspiration.[26] During trial swallows, the most important elements in predicting airway safety included failure on thin liquids, a wet voice after swallow, failure on thick liquids, a cough after swallow, and inability to self-feed.

Clinical Observations

A portion of the physical examination can be completed with basic observations of the patient's medical status. These observations are particularly important for patients who are bedbound and undergoing medical or surgical treatment. Some assumptions can be made about swallowing performance based on observational data.

Feeding Tubes

Some patients may not be eating orally or may be taking part of their nutrition through a feeding tube. Nasogastric tubes, which are inserted through the nose and into the stomach, are easily visible (Figure 9-2). Feeding tubes come in various sizes. Larger tubes may be needed to pass medications without clogging. Smaller, more flexible ones (e.g., Dobhoff tubes, Sherwood Medical Supplies, Forest Hills, NY) are more comfortable for the patient. Evidence in healthy (normal) subjects indicates that the presence of a feeding tube through the nose may slow the sequence of the pharyngeal swallow regardless of tube size.[27] Feeding tubes placed in the stomach (gastrostomy) or **jejunum** (jejunostomy) may not be visible unless they are connected to a feeding pump or a bag hanging on a support stand (Figure 9-3). Other patients may be hydrated through intravenous feeding catheters placed in the arm and connected to a plastic bag containing specialized nutrients or medications.

BOX 9-2	Guidelines for the Clinical Evaluation of Swallowing

CLINICAL OBSERVATIONS

FEEDING METHOD
- Nasogastric
- Gastrostomy
- Jejunostomy
- Intravenous

RESPIRATORY STATUS
- SpO$_2$ level
- Tracheostomy
- Ventilator
- Rate

MENTAL STATUS
- Level of alertness
- Orientation
- Cooperation
- Sustained attention

COGNITIVE SCREENING
- Memory
- Language
- Perception

CRANIAL NERVE ASSESSMENT

CN V
- Jaw opening and closing
- Jaw lateralization
- Muscle strength, bite down

CN VII
- Facial muscles at rest
- Pucker, smile
- Raise eyebrow
- Lips closed against resistance

CN IX, X
- Gag reflex
- Velum
- Voice
- Cough
- Dry swallow

CN XII
- Tongue range of motion
- Tongue strength
- Fasciculations, atrophy

ORAL CAVITY INSPECTION
- Lesions, thrush
- Moisture
- Dentition

TEST SWALLOWS
- Thin liquid
- Thick liquid
- Pudding consistency
- Semisolid

CERVICAL AUSCULTATION RESULTS
- Normal sounds
- Abnormal sounds
- Swallow delay
- Respiratory changes

MEALTIME OBSERVATIONS
- Posture
- Ambiance
- Self-feeding skills
- Utensil use
- Assistance needed
- Diet level
- Respiratory pattern changes

CN, Cranial nerve.

Tracheotomy Tubes

The presence of a tracheotomy tube should be noted. Tracheotomy tubes are placed when the medical team requires access to the lungs to maintain pulmonary toilet. Often they are placed when the patient is in respiratory distress or when the upper airway is blocked after trauma or surgery. Readers are advised to review the discussion of tracheotomy tubes in Chapter 8.

Respiratory Pattern

Bedbound patients may be connected to a respirator to assist in the ventilation of the lungs and have a mask over the mouth or a cannula in the nose, both of which may supply oxygen. Most clinicians prefer for the medical team to achieve partial weaning of the patient from ventilator support before attempting oral feeding. Observations of the patient's ventilatory pattern can be made by watching the chest rise and fall. Rapid rates (more than 40 cycles/min) may make it difficult to close the airway for a sufficient time during the swallow. The respiration rate and oxygen saturation levels of some patients are measured by sensors attached to the skin. Oxygen saturation levels (ratio of oxygen to arterial blood) that drop below 90% may be an indicator for some patients that they are at risk for swallowing impairment. Respiratory rates and oxygen saturation levels can be monitored on a screen at the patient's bedside (Figure 9-4). For cooperative patients, a screening of vital and tidal

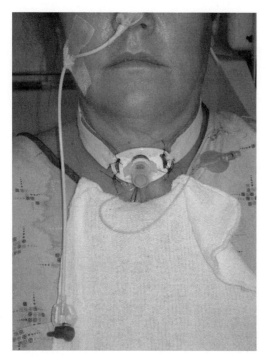

FIGURE 9-2. The patient has a small-bore feeding tube in place. The tube is taped away from her nostril to avoid nasal ulceration and taped to her cheek for comfort.

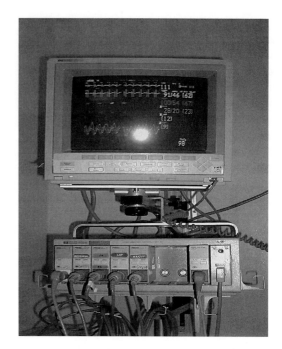

FIGURE 9-4. Bedside monitors track the oxygen saturation level (as a percentage), heart rate, and blood pressure on a single screen. The oxygen saturation level is monitored by a sensor that is attached to the hand or foot. On the lower right corner of this screen, the SpO_2 can be read as 98%.

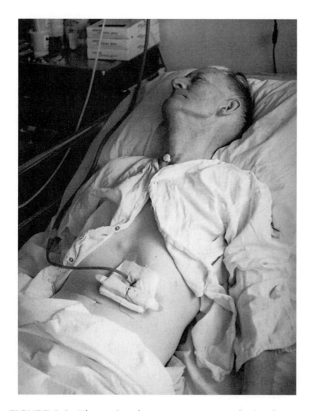

FIGURE 9-3. The patient has a gastrostomy tube in place. He is being fed specialized formula through the tube from a bag above his head.

respiratory capacities can be studied in the clinic or at the bedside with a portable respirometer. Declining respiratory capacities have been shown to be predictive of airway protection disorders in patients with amyotrophic lateral sclerosis.[28]

Mental Status

Observations of the bedbound patient may provide a preliminary indicator of mental status. For instance, patients who are alert often respond when the examiner enters the room, either visually by making eye contact or verbally with a greeting. These positive responses allow the examiner to assume that the patient may be able to cooperate with the remainder of the physical examination. Patients who are not readily alert to the examiner's presence or who are unable to sustain attention even after constant encouragement probably are not candidates for safe oral ingestion. The physical examination may be limited by the patient's inability to cooperate. Patients who are uncooperative, either from lack of attention or extreme agitation, or who are difficult to arouse should be reexamined periodically during the day. In some cases, the side effects of medications may interfere with normal mental status; in other cases, medications may improve mental status. If the patient is able to cooperate, orientation, linguistic skills, perceptual ability, and memory should be assessed. These learning modalities are important in giving the examiner an impression of the patient's ability to cooperate and learn during dysphagia treatment. For instance, patients who are confused and disoriented may need maximum assistance with eating, for feeding, and for reminders of how to perform therapeutic techniques needed for their care.

Practice Note 9-2

Patients with acute traumatic brain injury often are combative and are not able to cooperate with a formalized evaluation of their swallowing mechanism. A 24-year-old patient was in bed and restrained because he was combative with the nursing staff and at risk for pulling out his tracheotomy and feeding tubes. I needed to get him into a sitting position to attempt the physical examination. Positioning him required the restraints to be relaxed, but maintained. Once upright, it was clear he did not want to cooperate with the physical examination because of his poor cognitive status. However, he was attending to me and, although unintelligible, he was able to make a normal voice. He also showed signs of swallowing his own saliva. It seemed appropriate to try to see if I could get him to respond to a swallowing stimulus. I gave him a spoonful of crushed ice that he swallowed immediately without any cough or contents coming from the tracheotomy site. Sometimes, even with an uncooperative patient, information can be gathered about swallowing. Some patients do not have the cognitive skills to cooperate with a cranial nerve evaluation, but they do understand the learned behavior of taking a food item from a spoon.

Cranial Nerve Examination

Chapter 2 contains a review of the key cranial nerves involved in swallowing: V, VII, IX, X, XI, and XII. When smell and taste may be an issue, assessment of CN I is appropriate. The physical examination of the head and neck musculature for swallowing should focus on gathering information on the function of these cranial nerves. The examination begins by examining the muscles that can be seen easily and then proceeding into the oral cavity and oropharynx. The examination usually is focused on the motor aspects of relevant muscles, although gross, intraoral sensation may be of interest in patients who do not perceive a bolus once in the mouth. The examiner should look for any abnormality, including asymmetry, weakness, abnormal movements at rest, and abnormal movements during volitional efforts.

Facial Muscles

Observations of the facial muscles can be made with the patient at rest and during tasks such as lip pursing and smiling. Asking the patient to keep his or her lips closed against the examiner's attempt to pull them apart serves as a test for judging lip strength. The lower and upper facial muscles should be tested to differentiate between **upper and lower motor neuron** damage.

Muscles of Mastication

An assessment of the muscles of mastication begins by having the patient move the jaw up and down and laterally. Restrictions in mouth opening (**trismus**) should be noted. The strength of the masticator muscles can be appreciated by palpation as the patient bites down (Figure 9-5).

CLINICAL CORNER 9-1

A consultation was received for a 65-year-old patient who had a right brain stroke. He had left hemiplegia and left facial weakness. The patient was choking each time he drank liquids but did not seem particularly concerned. When attempting to eat solids he ate at a rapid rate and was asking when he could leave the hospital.

CRITICAL THINKING:
1. What could explain why this patient was not concerned about choking on liquids?
2. What other behavioral factors might need to be evaluated with this patient during his meal?

CLINICAL CORNER 9-2

A 58-year-old woman came as an outpatient with increased dysphagia and weight loss over the past 3 months. Five years ago she had completed a full course of radiation treatment for tonsillar cancer. The clinical evaluation revealed severe trismus, which made it very difficult to get a spoon in her mouth. She was treated with TheraBite (Atos Medical AB, West Allis, Wis.) for 3 weeks, resulting in improved jaw opening.

CRITICAL THINKING:
1. What is the probable source of her trismus?
2. What is TheraBite? How does it work?

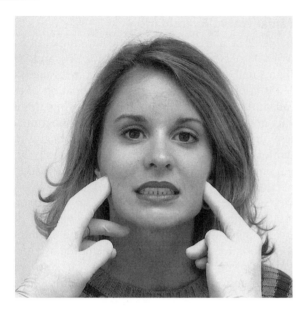

FIGURE 9-5. Asking the patient to bite down while palpating the response of the masseter muscles provides information about the integrity of the motor function of cranial nerve V.

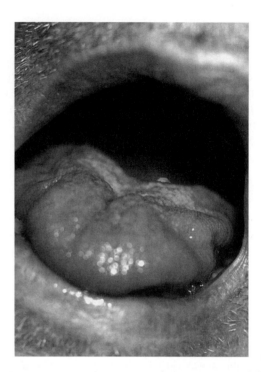

FIGURE 9-6. Lower motor neuron damage is assumed from the significant tongue atrophy (loss of tissue bulk) seen as deep grooves throughout the entire tongue surface.

Pathologic Reflexes

A number of brainstem-level primitive reflexes are associated with the chewing and swallowing mechanisms. Normally, these reflexes are inhibited in the adult by higher centers of the brain. Their presence in the adult patient suggests that these higher inhibitory centers are impaired. These pathologic reflexes are seen most commonly in patients with bilateral hemispheric or frontal lobe damage.

The suck reflex may be elicited either by tapping the upper lip with a reflex hammer or by stroking the lips rapidly with a tongue blade. Movement of the lips in the direction of the stimulus is an abnormal response.

The bite reflex is often elicited in patients with severe neurologic lesions by touching the lips, teeth, or gums with a tongue blade and observing a strong closure of the jaw. This reflex can be particularly troublesome for the examiner because it may prevent a good oral examination. Attempts to force a jaw open usually result in a stronger bite. The examiner should avoid strong resistance that could result in fracture or dislocation of the mandible. In some patients, spontaneous mouth opening will occur as a stimulus object, such as a spoon or food, is seen approaching the mouth. Although the bite reflex can interfere with feeding management, this mouth-opening reflex can be used to aid in the feeding plan.

Tongue Musculature

The examiner asks the patient to protrude the tongue and move it laterally. Rapid tongue movements may be assessed by asking the patient to repeat tongue-tip sounds such as "ta" rapidly. Ask the patient to move the tongue tip to the roof of the mouth, an activity important during bolus transfer. Protruding the tongue against a tongue blade gives the examiner a gross estimate of tongue strength. Inspect the tongue for atrophy, particularly along the lateral borders. Look for **fasciculations** if atrophy is seen (Figure 9-6). Both are consistent with lower motor neuron involvement. If the patient has had tongue resection because of cancer, note how much has been spared. Sensation can be tested with a tongue blade in the region of the reconstruction by asking the patient if there is a difference between touch in the reconstructed region and the region that has not been reconstructed. Knowing the most sensitive area may be important in food placement during treatment.

Oral Cavity

With the patient's mouth open, the examiner inspects the oral cavity for any lesions. The milky-white appearance of candidiasis (thrush) indicates a fungal infection (Figure 9-7). If left untreated, thrush may cause **odynophagia**, which is frequently seen in

CLINICAL CORNER 9-3

A 48-year-old told her dentist that she was choking on her saliva at night but not during the day. However, she did admit to choking on carbonated liquids. The dentist referred her to the speech pathologist for an evaluation of her swallowing. The physical evaluation was normal except for some atrophy on the left lateral border of her tongue.

CRITICAL THINKING:

1. What types of disorders might explain her tongue atrophy?
2. What referral should the speech pathologist make after this appointment?

Practice Note 9-3

Beginning clinicians find it particularly difficult to test the gag reflex. This usually stems from the fact that an active gag may cause temporary patient discomfort and in some patients actually stimulates emesis. The examination is accomplished best if it is done casually as part of the routine oral cavity inspection with a tongue blade. Use the tongue blade to test lateral tongue strength. Rather than announcing to the patient you are going to test the gag reflex, tell him or her you are going to test the sensation in the back of the throat. Quickly depress each side of the tongue dorsum below the level of the palatal curtain. This should take no longer than 2 seconds for the test and the judgment of the velar response. Using a good flashlight will help.

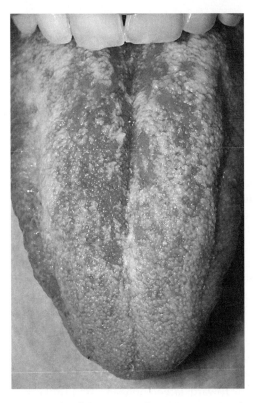

FIGURE 9-7. Whitish lesions on the tongue are consistent with thrush (oral candidiasis). (From Neville B, Damm DD, Allen CM et al: *Oral and maxillofacial pathology,* ed 2, Philadelphia, 2002, WB Saunders.)

those whose immune system has been decompensated by acute or chronic disease. Check to determine whether the amount of saliva is normal. Patients with xerostomia often have little moisture throughout the oral cavity and report poor taste. The tongue may appeared reddened and secretions thick. Inspect the

dentition. Teeth in poor repair or ill-fitting dentures may contribute to dysphagia.

Oropharynx

Observations of the velum at rest and during tasks of phonation should be made. The posterior dorsum of the tongue is stimulated on both sides with a tongue depressor to assess the gag reflex. If the patient has a gag response, it is important to note if the velum is elevated symmetrically and if the patient coughed. Some patients do not demonstrate a gag reflex until the tongue base is stimulated. Elicitation of the gag reflex accompanied by a cough provides information about the integrity of CNs IX (sensory) and X in the oropharynx (velum) and at the level of the larynx (vocal fold closure). The presence or absence of a gag reflex is not an indication that the patient has a normal swallowing response or is at risk for aspiration,[29] although for some examiners the absence of this reflex might suggest that the patient's swallow is compromised. The absence of a gag reflex as an isolated abnormal finding in the examination of the cranial nerves for swallowing may not be important.

Pharynx

There are no tests of pharyngeal function that can be easily appreciated during the physical evaluation of the swallowing response. In some patients, the activity of the superior pharyngeal constrictor muscle can be observed after an active gag reflex as the posterior pharyngeal wall contracts or during the production of a falsetto voice. The activity of the pharyngeal constrictor muscles is best visualized by endoscopy.

Larynx

Asking the patient to phonate or listening to his or her vocal quality in conversation provides useful information on the integrity of the airway protective mechanisms and on the coordination of articulatory structures during phonatory tasks. Speech is an extremely complex, overlearned behavior and as such serves as a barometer from which the examiner can assess the status of the neuromuscular system that also serves swallowing. Patients should be asked to sustain a vowel, with the examiner noting duration, quality (hoarseness, breathiness, and harshness), pitch, and intensity. Articulation should be assessed for precision and speed. The use of oral diadochokinetic tasks (forced rapid alternating movements) using consonant-vowel combinations is recommended. Both hypernasal and hyponasal resonance qualities should be noted. Hypernasality suggests impaired palatopharyngeal function. Hyponasality implies filling of the nasopharynx or occlusion of nasal passages. For patients with unimpaired voice and speech, the clinician may reasonably conclude that the swallowing problem either resides in the late pharyngeal stage (cricopharyngeal function) or is related to esophageal and LES function. The remaining physical examination should confirm the integrity of the peripheral sensory-motor swallowing mechanism.

Asking the patient to produce a "dry" swallow while palpating the larynx at the level of the thyroid notch (Figure 9-8) helps the examiner assess the presence and extent of laryngeal elevation. Normal elevation ranges from 2 to 4 cm.

Test Swallows

In a cooperative, alert patient, who up to this point in the examination has not demonstrated significant neurologic impairment and has been able to swallow secretions without significant airway compromise, the examiner may want to grossly assess the swallow response with real food items. This part of the examination is useful because it provides the examiner information about swallowing dynamics. Before this portion of the examination, each cranial nerve should be evaluated in isolation. Some investigators have suggested that the risk/benefit ratio of this part of the evaluation is poor[2,30]; however, it is commonly performed in most settings. Test trials provide the opportunity to see the coordinated integration of all the swallowing muscles. Most examiners use an array of items ranging from thin to thickened liquids, to pudding and softer items, to items that require mastication. Initially it is advisable to use a substance that

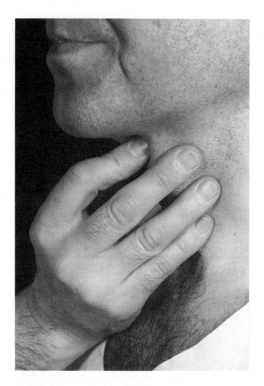

FIGURE 9-8. The examiner palpates at the level of the thyroid notch to feel for laryngeal elevation as a sign that a swallow response has been elicited.

is relatively safe if it is partially aspirated and to be absolutely certain that the patient is able to cough to protect the airway in situations of suspected aspiration.[31] A spoonful of crushed ice is relatively safe and provides a good medium for eliciting the chewing reflex because of its texture and cold stimulation to the gums.

Once it has been determined that the patient adequately elevates the larynx and that there is an adequate protective cough, the examination can proceed to other substances with different textures and consistencies. Volumes usually range from 5 to 10 mL, starting first with a smaller bolus and, if successful, moving toward larger boluses. Traditionally, changing volumes precedes changing textures. If successful with 10-mL boluses, the examiner may wish to test the swallow with a 20-mL bolus. Groher et al.[32] found that the most discriminative items to use in test trials if the examiner is interested only in using cough as a sign of aspiration were thin liquids in 5-mL amounts and thickened liquids in 5- and 10-mL amounts. Methods of delivery, such as cup versus straw, may yield important differences in performance since the latter requires longer and more coordinated airway closure mechanics. Clinicians should observe chewing and bolus preparation. One clinical method of making

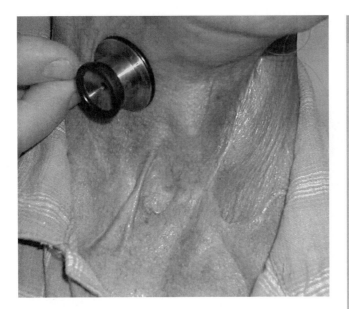

FIGURE 9-9. A stethoscope placed on the side of the neck can provide important acoustic information about the swallow response.

Practice Note 9-4

The three audible sounds associated with swallowing have both low- and high-frequency energy. The first two sounds are low-frequency energy, whereas the last sound (exhalatory burst) contains high-frequency energy. Microphones and accelerometers are capable of detecting the full frequency spectrum of these swallowing sounds; however, not all stethoscopes have this capability. Hamlet et al.[68] studied the frequency response characteristics of stethoscopes and identified two that had the capability of meeting these requirements: the Littman Cardiology II (3M, St. Paul, Minn.) and the Rappaport-Sprague pediatric size (Hewlett-Packard, Palo Alto, Calif.). There are two sides to a stethoscope—the flat, or diaphragm, side and the concave, or bell, side. Hamlet and colleagues found that the bell surface was best in detecting the sounds associated with swallowing.

a judgment of whether the swallow response is delayed is the use of cervical auscultation.[33,34] The examiner places a stethoscope on the neck at the level of the vocal folds and listens for the sounds associated with swallowing (Figure 9-9). Preswallow sounds can be heard before the swallow as the bolus size increases,[35] probably as a result of the tongue trying to contain a larger bolus. Larger boluses produce more intense sound.[35] Before the swallow, the examiner should be cognizant of the respiratory rate. Comparisons should be made between the predeglutitory and postdeglutitory patterns. Marked change in the respiratory rate or an increase in respiratory congestion may be a sign of airway compromise. During swallow, respirations should cease (period of apnea). Within the short apneic period, two bursts of sound are markers of the presence of a swallow; these can be heard by cervical auscultation. After listening to patients with normal swallows, the examiner can begin to appreciate what might constitute swallow delay in abnormal patterns, since the timing of the pattern from swallow onset to the first and second bursts of energy is consistent. Simultaneous videofluoroscopy and swallowing sound recordings have shown that the first burst of sound is associated with the bolus content that has entered the pharynx, whereas the second sound is associated with the bolus as it leaves the pharynx and enters the esophagus (Figure 9-10). After most swallows a short exhalation can be heard as a single, short burst of acoustic energy (release of subglottic air pressure). This exhalatory burst, or glottal release sign, is present in normal swallows and is affected by age and bolus volume.[36] Delay in detecting these sounds or failing to hear any of these sounds may serve as a potential marker of swallow abnormality.[36] In a series of patients with head/neck cancer, Uyama et al.[37] found that cervical auscultation could differentiate between normal and dysphagic swallows if the patient was asked to produce a voluntary exhalation after the swallow.[37] Changes in the frequency band from 0 to 500 Hz were more prominent in those with dysphagia compared with the changes in normal swallows. Although interrater agreement on swallow abnormality with auscultation alone is only fair, agreement on abnormality versus no abnormality improves with group discussion, suggesting that individuals are capable of making decisions about safe swallow using acoustic data.[34] Borr et al.[38] also found only fair interrater reliability when rating seven parameters of acoustic recordings of swallows in normal (healthy) subjects, older adults, and subjects with known dysphagia. However, experienced clinicians were able to detect reliably events of aspiration or penetration, with 70% sensitivity and 94% specificity. Interestingly, the significant distinguishing factor between normal aging swallows and dysphagic swallows was that the patients with dysphagia swallowed twice instead of once on small bolus sizes. Borr et al.[38] concluded that cervical auscultation may be a viable tool to screen for airway compromise as part of a complete clinical evaluation.

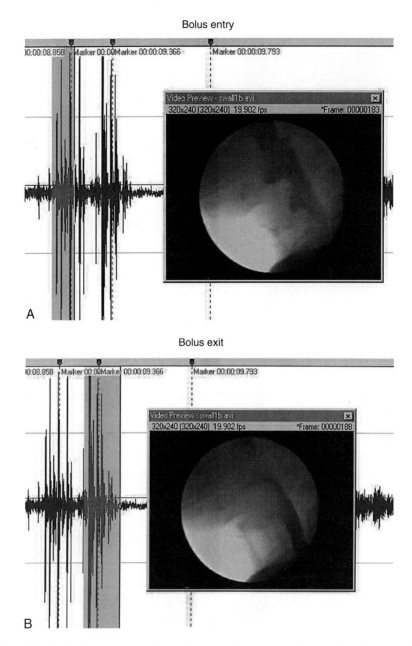

FIGURE 9-10. A, Simultaneous recording of the videofluoroscopic image of swallow and the corresponding acoustic pattern. The first swallow sound burst is associated with the bolus entry into the pharynx. **B,** The second sound burst should be associated with the bolus leaving the pharynx and entering the esophagus. (Courtesy T. Neil McKaig.)

An acoustic representation of an entire respiratory/swallowing sequence obtained with a microphone coupled to a computer with sound analysis capability is presented in Figure 9-11.

Feeding Evaluation

Patients who are unable to cooperate with a physical evaluation and who may be eating with suspected dysphagic complications can be partially evaluated through careful observation at the bedside. Bedside data should be gathered for three meals because the eating circumstance, including differing food items, may vary from breakfast to lunch to dinner. When possible, the entire meal should be observed because patients often fatigue. Swallowing competence therefore may change as the meal progresses.

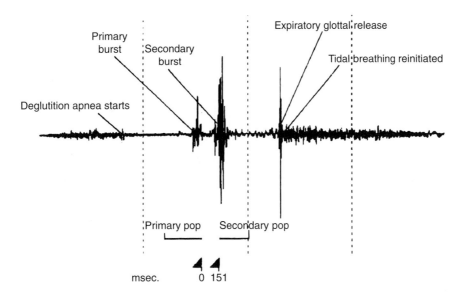

FIGURE 9-11. An acoustic representation of a normal swallow sequence. It is marked by the cessation of tidal airflow and two bursts of swallowing sounds within the apneic period (*first* and *last dotted lines*), followed by a burst of exhalation and the resumption of tidal breathing. (Courtesy T. Neil McKaig.)

Environment

Patients with cortical brain damage and dysphagia may be highly distractible. If the distraction causes the patient to talk while eating or to not focus on the process of feeding, swallowing safety may be sacrificed. Typical distractions include the feeding assistant asking the patient for a verbal response while eating, listening to the radio, and viewing television. Other distractions include those that are patient centered. For instance, the patient's glasses not being positioned properly, resulting in distraction, or attention being focused on an ill-fitting denture that is causing discomfort.

Feeding

If the patient is self-feeding, is he or she able to open all containers, find the food on the tray, and use the utensils properly? Can the patient use the utensils to transport food to the mouth? Is the feeding rate appropriate? Are bite sizes appropriate? Are there differences in swallowing performance between taking liquids using a straw and taking them by cup? If the patients is to use special feeding utensils, are they provided? If dentures are needed, are they in place and properly fitted?

Posture

Because an upright posture is best for swallowing, it is important to note whether the patient is in that position and if he or she can maintain that position throughout the meal. If the patient is to use a special posture such as chin-down as a method of airway protection (see Chapter 14), the examiner should observe whether this posture can be achieved. Even patients who are fed by gastrostomy tube should have the head of the bed slightly elevated to avoid the possibility of reflux from the stomach.

Eating

The diet level (soft, pureed, mechanical soft, or regular) should be noted. Some patients receive a diet level that is not appropriately matched to their disorder.[39] If fluids are to be altered by thickening, is the consistency appropriate? If thickened fluids are allowed to sit too long before serving, they may become too thick for safe ingestion. Does the patient have more difficulty with liquids than semisolids or vice versa? When the patient places a chewable item in the mouth, is adequate chewing motion evident, or does the food sit without any apparent attempt by the patient to start a swallow? Does the patient have choking episodes, either before a swallow attempt, during the swallow, or after the swallow has been completed? The use of cervical auscultation or observations of laryngeal elevation may assist the examiner in this determination. The examiner should observe whether the eating process is more efficient at the beginning or end of the meal because fatigue may decompensate safe swallowing in some patients. An estimate of the amount eaten and the total time to finish the meal are important markers of swallowing efficiency and may serve as useful functional outcome measures after swallowing treatment. Changes in respiratory status, taken from bedside monitors or from audible respiratory distress, such as wheezing or difficulty clearing secretions, should be part of the observational data pool.

Assistance

If prior recommendations have been made to improve the patient's feeding or eating performance, are these suggestions being followed by the patient? Or if the patient needs a feeding assistant who must provide reminders to accomplish safe feeding, are those reminders being provided?

CLINICAL CASE EXAMPLE 9-2

An elderly woman came to the hospital to have her hip replaced. Her medical history was remarkable for childhood polio from which she recovered, **hypertension**, and coronary heart disease. After the hip surgery a nurse noted she was choking on liquids and a request for a consultation was sent to Speech Pathology.

The physical evaluation revealed that the patient was alert, oriented, and cooperative. She was able to sustain a cogent conversation while sitting upright in bed. She told the examiner that because she was choking on liquids, they no longer put them on her meal tray, which consisted of a soft mechanical diet. She was noted to have an intravenous feeding line in her right arm. An evaluation of her oral peripheral speech mechanism revealed generalized weakness of the tongue and lips, more severe on the right than left side. Examination of the muscles of mastication was normal. Her oral cavity was xerostomic and she was **edentulous**. The gag reflex was present but not brisk. She was able to produce a voluntary cough and swallow response. Normal laryngeal elevation was noted during her dry swallow attempt. Her voice was markedly hoarse but not breathy. She did not show any signs of dysarthria. During test swallows of 5 mL of thin liquid, she coughed briskly, without delay, as the larynx was elevating. A commercial thickener was added to the thin liquid. During a test swallow with this consistency, the swallow was prompt without cough or delay. This was repeated with success on 10-mL and 20-mL boluses. The patient was then given a spoonful of pudding. This was swallowed without delay or cough. All swallow attempts were monitored with cervical auscultation so that a judgment of swallowing delay could be made.

In this case, the patient was able to express her difficulty swallowing thin liquids. Her difficulty was noted by the nurses, who reported that she coughed when swallowing thin liquids. Her problem was compensated by adding thickeners to the thin fluid. Failure to protect her airway on thin fluids could have been related to a temporary decompensation of her airway closure reflex related to the endotracheal tube from recent surgery. Airway closure problems frequently are most obvious with thinner fluids because of their speed of movement through the pharynx. This possibility was supported by the patient's severe hoarseness. An alternate explanation might be that she had generalized weakness in the bulbar musculature from her childhood polio that became more apparent at the laryngeal level after her surgery. That muscle weakness still was present was supported by diminished strength in the lip and tongue musculature. Her xerostomia was a side effect from medications to control her coronary artery disease. The patient started a diet of thickened liquids with a soft mechanical diet. The recommendation was made to discontinue her intravenous fluids because it was believed she could maintain her hydration with thickened liquids. The prognosis for returning to regular fluids was judged to be good because it was believed that the decompensation of her airway closure would be temporary. Continued monitoring of her respiratory status was recommended to ensure her safety on this dietary level. Because her complaint was explained and ultimately resolved by the clinical evaluation, no further testing was considered.

TESTS TO DETECT ASPIRATION

In studies comparing the utility of the clinical evaluation compared with videofluoroscopy to detect aspiration, most have shown that only 60% to 70% of the patients who aspirate are correctly identified after the clinical examination.[13,22,40] These findings have led to numerous investigations of tests to improve the accuracy of clinically based methods to detect tracheal aspiration. Another rationale to improve the accuracy of the ability of the clinical examination to detect aspiration is that many clinicians do not have easy access to instrumental examinations such as video-fluoroscopy and its capability to visualize aspiration. The presumed consequence of failing to detect aspiration is that aspiration pneumonia with its attendant morbidity and mortality will develop in these patients. Interestingly, no data have prospectively studied in homogeneous groups the health risk of not detecting aspiration with a clinical examination. For instance, screening examinations for the detection of aspiration may identify those with severe aspiration and not detect those with minor aspiration and that minor aspiration may not be a threat to health outcomes.[25]

Most studies of aspiration prediction have involved acute poststroke patients because they remain a population at risk for events of aspiration. Comparisons are made between the clinical examination's ability to detect aspiration with confirmation by an instrumental examination such as endoscopy or videofluoroscopy.

Mann and Hankey[41] used regression analysis and studied 23 clinical features related to swallowing in 71 poststroke patients to identify significant independent predictors of aspiration. Significant predictors of aspiration included an impaired pharyngeal response, male gender, disabling stroke (**Barthel score** <60), incomplete oral clearance, palatal weakness or asymmetry, and age greater than 70 years. They argued that together these six variables could be used to detect aspiration risk, potentially providing a more efficient approach to a clinical evaluation. In a group of patients referred for a swallowing evaluation as a result of burn injury, Edelman et al.[42] found that the standardized clinical examination was highly predictive of aspiration subsequently verified by videofluoroscopy.[42] However, this may be because their patients had severe oropharyngeal dysphagia from their pathology, biasing the results toward the high prediction accuracy of aspiration from the clinical examination. Leder and Espinoza[43] compared six clinical features from the clinical examination with endoscopic detection of aspiration. In 49 poststroke patients they concluded that the clinical examination underestimated those who aspirated and overestimated those who did not aspirate on endoscopy.

Water Tests

Water tests presumably are to be used in patients who are alert enough to accept a bolus of water as a method to clinically detect aspiration or risk for aspiration. The assumption is that water is chosen as the bolus of choice because, if aspirated, it is relatively innocuous in the lungs.

The first water test was the 3-oz (85-mL) water test in which the patient attempts to swallow 3 oz of water at any rate he or she chooses.[44] The examiner then makes a clinical judgment of aspiration based on the patient's response. DiPippo et al.[44] reported a sensitivity of 76% and specificity of 59%, with incorrect identification of aspiration in 34% of cases. The high number of false-negative results (41%) suggests a high number of silent aspirators in this cohort because cough is the feature judged to help make the prediction of aspiration. Garon et al.[45] expressed concern that the 3-oz water test would become the standard test for detecting aspiration.[45] They studied patients with mixed neurogenic causes, comparing the 3-oz water test with videofluoroscopy. In their study only 35% of the patients were correctly predicted as aspirating. However, it is important to note that this subject sample was different than the original sample reported by DiPippo et al.[44] (mixed neurogenic vs. stable stroke).

Sensitivity and specificity data similar to the 3-oz water test were found on the timed water test.[46] Patients are required to swallow 150 mL of water. Observations of cough, the number of swallows, the total time to finish the entire amount, and the amount of residue remaining if the patient could not finish are calculated. Accuracy of prediction is based on the speed of completing the swallow and amount of water swallowed.

Combinations of clinical evaluation procedures and water tests also have been studied. Mari et al.[47] combined a patient symptom checklist, a clinical examination, and the 3-oz water test as a method to detect aspiration compared with videofluoroscopy as the reference standard for aspiration documentation. The predictive value of the 3-oz water was 76% versus poor **predictive values** for the other two clinical measures. Sensitivity values were not as good as other studies because patients judged to have negative findings for aspiration showed silent aspiration on the videofluorographic study. Lim et al.[48] combined a 50-mL water test and oxygen saturation (SpO$_2$) data as a method of aspiration detection in acute poststroke patients with a 2% drop in saturation levels as the standard for abnormality and suspected aspiration during water swallows. The combination of the two tests showed 100% sensitivity and 70% specificity. Tohara et al.[49] designed a test battery that included a 3-oz water test, 4 g of pudding, and a standard plain x-ray film of the pharynx. They argued that some facilities may not have videofluoroscopy but probably did have the capability to obtain static images of the pharynx before and after swallow attempts. By summing the data from 63 patients on the three tests

CLINICAL CORNER 9-4

Investigators found that when patients with dysphagia were given 20 mL of a thickened liquid their eyes would tear ostensibly as a result of cough and congestion. They reported that their "eye-tearing test" had a sensitivity of 50% and a specificity of 40% at predicting aspiration.

CRITICAL THINKING:

1. How would you interpret the sensitivity data? Is this a good test to use to detect aspiration?
2. What is the consequence to the patient clinically given the 40% specificity of the test?

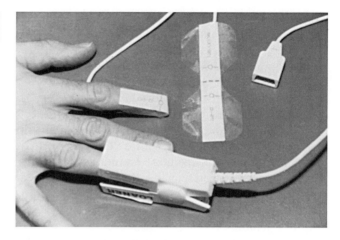

FIGURE 9-12. The pulse oximeter is usually attached to the finger in an adult and often is placed on the large toe in an infant. The device provides an estimate of the oxygenation in the blood as an indirect measure of respiratory status. Although oximetry is not as precise as an actual measurement of blood gases from a blood sample analyzed in the laboratory, it serves as a screening device for changes in respiratory status. (From Roberts J, Hedges J: *Clinical procedures in emergency medicine*, ed 4, Philadelphia, 2004, WB Saunders.)

they calculated 90% sensitivity in detecting aspiration and specificity of 56%.

Although water tests and combinations of tests using water may have some utility as screening devices for aspiration detection, all are hindered by design flaws that produce wide variability in results. Comparisons across studies are difficult because of differences in the diagnostic categories of subjects selected, differences in recruitment, time after onset of the patient's disease, variable(s) measured and how measured, the reference test for confirmation of aspiration, and the clinical examination chosen.[50] These discrepancies make it difficult for the clinician to know if any one test is better than another to detect aspiration by a clinical examination.

Oxygen Saturation Tests

Numerous studies have examined whether a drop in oxygen saturation (SpO_2) levels using a pulse oximeter (Figure 9-12) could reliably detect events of aspiration. The rationale for this assumption is based on the fact that changes in respiratory status may signal a change in airway protection during swallowing events. Early investigators concluded that a drop in SpO_2 was associated with events of aspiration.[51,52] More recently, Smith et al.[53] found that a 2% drop in SpO_2 levels had an 86% sensitivity in predicting aspiration but poor predictive value. They argued for a combination of a standard clinical evaluation and SpO_2 monitoring to improve the predictive value. Using simultaneous measures of oxygen saturation and fiberoptic endoscopy, Colodny[54] studied 104 patients with dysphagia and 77 patients with no dysphagia. In neither group did reduced SpO_2 relate to events of aspiration; however, the trend indicated that a drop in saturation levels was most likely to be found in patients symptomatic for dysphagia. Those at particular risk for **oxygen desaturation** aspirated on solid food.

Modified Evans Blue Dye Test

The modified Evans Blue dye (MEBD) test is another method used to detect aspiration at the bedside. The test is reserved for patients with tracheotomies who because of their illness may not be easily transportable to the radiographic suite for a videofluoroscopic swallowing study. The test protocol varies among institutions. The patient is given either a liquid or semisolid bolus that has been tinted with food coloring. The color is added so that any aspirated material is easily distinguished from other secretions. After the patient is given the test bolus, deep suctioning is performed through the tracheostomy site; suctioning is repeated in 15-minute intervals for an hour. The suction line is inspected for any coloration suggestive of aspiration.

Thompson-Henry and Braddock[55] reported on the MEBD procedure in five patients. On follow-up videofluoroscopic and endoscopic procedures, all patients showed signs of aspiration, whereas no patient showed aspiration after the MEBD procedure. These authors concluded that the MEBD should be used with caution because of the high false-negative rate in this small sample. Brady et al.[56] used simultaneous videofluoros-

Practice Note 9-5

Protocols for the MEBD vary greatly among medical centers. Variation includes the type and amount of coloring used, the size of the test bolus, and the period after the test swallows in which the suctioning is attempted. Suctioning usually is done immediately after the test but may be done at hourly intervals for 3 hours up to 24 hours. Suctioning is continued with the intent that initially the patient may not have aspirated, but residual content in the mouth or pharynx may become aspirated at a later time. The test also is confounded by agreement of whether colored, aspirated material is present in the suction line. If a patient aspirates only a small amount, visualization through a clouded suction tube to make a decision on aspiration is not always reliable and is subject to considerable debate.

copy and MEBD to study 20 patients. They divided their patients into two groups: those with only small amounts (trace) of aspiration and those with larger amounts of aspiration. Their results found 100% sensitivity in those with severe aspiration and 50% sensitivity in those with trace aspiration. It could be concluded from these data that MEBD is most useful in those with suspected severe aspiration. Although there is no experimental evidence to support it, even without the MEBD a standard clinical examination with inspection of trial swallows at the tracheostomy site might be as accurate in aspiration detection as the MEBD. O'Neill-Pirozzi et al.[57] also used simultaneous videofluoroscopy and MEBD with 50 patients. These investigators reported a sensitivity of 80% and a specificity of 62%. However, there was no association between aspiration on the MEBD and its severity as seen on videofluoroscopy, and the MEBD failed to detect some patients with severe aspiration. The differences across these studies are attributable to MEBD procedural differences, such as the bolus type and volume used, post-swallow suction intervals, and potential differences in the severity of acute illness of the patients studied.

STANDARDIZED TESTS

Most clinicians design their own clinical swallowing evaluations based on the elements they have determined are most useful in detecting and defining the dysphagic condition. The majority of these tests are scored with a plus/minus (+/−) scoring system, present no data on the reliability of scoring, and do not compare their usefulness with other related measures (validity). Standardization implies that the test developer presents reliability and validity data on a large sample of patients with varying severity levels of the target disease. Evidence of the process of test development (theoretical rationale), comparisons to reference tests, the type of statistics used to support the reliability and validity, and a clear statement of how the test should be administered should be stated in the test manual.

The *Mann Assessment of Swallowing Ability* (MASA) is the first clinical test of swallowing with psychometric integrity.[58] It has reported reliability and validity data, positive and negative predictor values, and positive **likelihood ratios** on a population of 128 first-time, poststroke patients. The MASA allows the examiner to make judgments of dysphagia and aspiration severity with clinical diagnostic criteria (an ordinal risk rating) or by adding individual subtest scores and comparing them with the study sample for dysphagia and aspiration severity. Scoring guidelines are provided in 24 areas of assessment: alertness, cooperation, auditory comprehension, respiration, respiration rate after swallow, aphasia, apraxia, dysarthria, saliva management, lip seal, tongue movement, tongue strength, tongue coordination, oral preparation, gag reflex, palatal movement, bolus clearance, oral transit, cough reflex, voluntary cough, voice, tracheostomy, the pharyngeal phase, and the pharyngeal response. The MASA has not been evaluated for its predictive ability in the postacute phase of recovery or with patients with nonneurologic disorders such as head/neck cancer.

The *McGill Ingestive Skills Assessment* (MISA) is a standardized test developed to clinically assess patients' functional eating skills in a natural environment.[59] It assumes that the patient is already eating but has dysphagic symptoms or, if the patient is not eating, the examiner prepares varied food items for consumption and records the patient's attempt to eat. The MISA is to be used in conjunction with any extant data from the patient's medical history. Conceptually, the test is designed for clinicians working with older adults in skilled nursing facilities. Scores are assigned to patients in five areas of eating performance: positioning, self-feeding, liquid ingestion, solid ingestion, and texture management (manages a variety of foods). Within each area of swallowing performance there are subtests for a total of 43 test items. Each subtest is scored on a 3-point scale with clear instructions on what behaviors fit the numeric assignments. Each numeric category contains a detailed description of the desired performance that easily leads the examiner to the functional activities one would select in treatment. The MISA also has predictive data relating to health outcomes.[60] Seventy-three patients from skilled nursing facilities had follow-up for 563 days after administration of the MISA. Statistical analyses revealed that selective subtests such as solid ingestion, self-feeding, and texture management were predictive of time to death.

SUPPLEMENTAL TESTS

Occasionally the examiner who is assessing a patient with dysphagia may be interested in gathering data specific to the patient's complaint. Usually these tests are easily administered and scored. Ideally the tests will have undergone the rigors of standardization. Data from these tests often serve as baseline measurement tools to assess outcome after intervention. Examples of supplementary testing include documentation of the patient's current dietary level, nutritional status, and documentation of the suspicion for GERD or laryngopharyngeal reflux (LPR).

A reliable and valid measure to document the patient's current dietary level is the *Functional Oral Intake Scale* (FOIS).[61] The FOIS is a 7-point ordinal scale that documents the patient's functional eating status ranging from total reliance on tube feeding to eating a diet with no restrictions or special preparation. Data are derived either from patient report or examiner observations. The FOIS is presented in Box 9-3.

A measure of nutritional status may be useful at the initial evaluation, particularly if the clinician does not have easy access to a dietitian. The *Mini Nutritional Assessment* (MNA) is a reliable and valid measure of nutritional status that can serve either as a screening device or, when used with additional test items, can provide a malnutrition indicator score.[62] The test items on the MNA are a mix of subjective examiner impressions, patient report, and objective measurements. The first five test items are used as a quick screening measure. Patients who score 11 points or below on this screening should be measured on 12 additional items. The only equipment the SLP needs to administer this test is the ability to measure mid-arm circumference, height, and weight.

Patients who present to the SLP with reports of food or liquid sticking at the level of the cervical esophagus should have a screening for GERD. Several reliable and valid methods for GERD screening have been developed, including the GERD score,[63] the

---

| BOX 9-3 | Functional Oral Intake Scale |

The Functional Oral Intake Scale is an ordinal scale that can be used to document the patient's functional eating status at the time of evaluation. It also is useful as a pretreatment and posttreatment outcome measurement tool.

Levels	Diet Level of Safe Oral Intake Meeting Nutritional and Hydration Needs
Tube dependent	1. Nothing by mouth (NPO)
	2. Tube dependent with minimal attempts at food or liquid
	3. Dependent with consistent intake of liquid or food
Total oral	4. Total oral diet of a single consistency
	5. Total oral diet with multiple consistencies but requiring special preparation or compensations
	6. Total oral diet with multiple consistencies without special preparation but with specific food limitations
	7. Total oral diet with no restriction

CLINICAL CORNER 9-5

A 58-year-old patient with myasthenia gravis reported increasing dysphagia with solid food. He underwent a modified barium swallow study with sEMG to measure the strength of his swallow. The patient had been taught to swallow hard to adequately clear his pharynx. By sEMG his swallow effort averaged 13 μV. During the study the examiner asked the patient to try to swallow with less force. The patient was still able to clear his pharynx with an average of 8 μV of effort.

CRITICAL THINKING:

1. How does the diagnosis of myasthenia gravis interfere with swallowing?
2. Why might it be important for this patient to swallow with less effort?

Reflux Disease Questionnaire (RDQ),[64] the *Gastrointestinal Symptoms Rating Scale* (GSRS), and Reflux Questionnaire (ReQuest).[65] ReQuest has a short (5-minute) version, and a longer (20-minute) version in which the patient answers questions to relevant questions using a 7-point Likert scale.

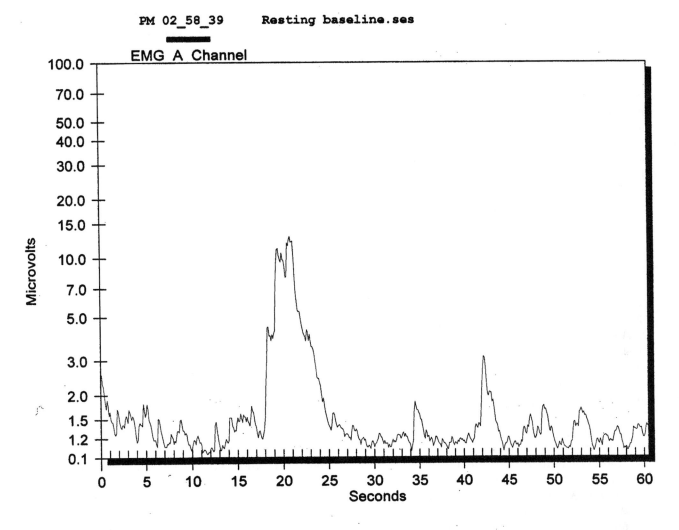

PM 02_58_39   Resting baseline.ses

FIGURE 9-13. Tracing of a swallowing event using surface electromyographic electrodes fixed to the lateral neck. The force of the swallow is measured in microvolts (µV) (vertical axis). The horizontal axis shows muscle activity below 2 µV for 18 seconds until a peak (15 µV) of activity representing the swallow is seen at 20 seconds. After the swallow, muscle activity returns to below 2 µV as the muscles relax.

Patients who present with the globus sensation, hoarseness, chronic cough, dysphagia or odynophagia, and chronic throat clearing should be screened for LPR. The easiest test to administer is the *Reflux Symptom Index* (RSI).[65] Patients are asked to answer questions about nine items that are sensitive to LPR detection. Each answer is scored on a 5-point scale.

An RSI score greater than 10 suggests the presence of LPR. Follow-up fiberoptic endoscopic examinations should be used for symptom confirmation.

Although the use of sEMG has not been studied empirically as a method for clinical evaluation of swallow, it may be useful in the detection of swallow events and in establishing baseline data for swallow strength. Submental muscle activity is associated with hyoid elevation and swallow initiation.[66] Both experienced and novice practitioners can use sEMG tracings to determine whether a swallowing event has occurred by looking at the visual representation.[67] Therefore measurement of swallow delay as detected by sEMG may be beneficial in determining the difference between normal and abnormal swallow responses because delay is associated with abnormality (Figure 9-13). Although there are no established normative data for the muscular strength needed to complete a swallow by bolus type or volume, sEMG technology can document the force needed to complete a successful swallow response.

TAKE HOME NOTES

1. Patients often wait for long periods before they report their dysphagia.
2. Patients may not always be able to describe each element of their dsyphagia.
3. Patients may not always realize that repeated bouts of pneumonia and weight loss may be a consequence of their dysphagia.
4. *Symptoms* are aspects of the swallowing process that the patient reports are problematic.
5. *Signs* are aspects of the swallowing process that are objectively measured and determined to connote a swallowing disorder.
6. Common dysphagic symptoms include the globus sensation, heartburn, loss of pleasure associated with eating, special preparation such as excessive chewing, regurgitation, and changes in diet level.
7. Common signs of dysphagia include drooling, choking, respiratory congestion after eating, increased need for suctioning, fatigue when eating, poor position when eating, loss of cognitive controls over the eating circumstance, undernutrition and muscle wasting, and the presence of feeding, tracheostomy, and endotracheal tubes.
8. The clinical examination of swallowing includes a review of the medical history, the physical evaluation and, if appropriate, test swallows.
9. The clinical examination fails to detect all patients who aspirate and patients who do not aspirate.
10. The physical evaluation includes observations of the patient in eating and noneating situations, evaluation of mental status, and an evaluation of the cranial nerves needed for swallowing.
11. Water tests, measures of oxygen saturation levels, cervical auscultation, and the Evans Blue dye test have been proposed as clinical methods to detect aspiration.
12. Standardized tests for oropharyngeal dysphagia are the Mann Assessment of Swallowing Ability and the McGill Ingestive Skills Assessment.

References

1. Ravich WJ, Donner MW, Kashima H et al: The swallowing center: concepts and procedures, *Gastrointest Radiol* 10:255, 1985.

2. Logemann JA, Veis S, Colangelo L: A screening procedure for oropharyngeal dysphagia, *Dysphagia* 14:44, 1999.

3. Smithard DG, O'Neill PA, Park C et al: Complications and outcome after stroke: does dysphagia matter? *Stroke* 27:1200, 1996.

4. World Health Organization: *Principles and practices of screening for disease*, Geneva, 1968, World Health Organization.

5. Martino R, Pron G, Diamant N: Screening for oropharyngeal dysphagia in stroke, *Dysphagia* 15:19, 2000.

6. McCullough GH, Wertz RT, Rosenbek JC et al: Clinicians' preference and practice in conducting clinical/bedside and videofluoroscopic examinations of swallowing in an adult neurogenic population, *Am J Speech Lang Pathol* 8:149, 1999.

7. Mathers-Schmidt BA, Kurlinski M: Dysphagia evaluation practices and inconsistencies in clinical assessment and instrumental examination decision making, *Dysphagia* 18:114, 2003.

8. McCullough GH, Wertz RT, Rosenbek JC et al: Inter- and intrajudge reliability of a clinical examination of swallowing in adults, *Dysphagia* 15:58, 2000.

9. Ekberg O, Feinberg MJ: Altered swallowing function in elderly patients with dysphagia: radiographic findings in 56 cases, *AJR Am J Roentgenol* 156:1181, 1991.

10. Cook IJ, Kahrilas PJ: AGA technical review on management of oropharyngeal dysphagia, *Gastroenterology* 116:455, 1999.

11. Edwards DA: Discriminative value of symptoms in the differential diagnosis of dysphagia, *Clin Gastroenterol* 6:5, 1976.

12. Jones B, Ravich WJ, Kramer SS et al: Pharyngoesophageal interrelationships: observations and working concepts, *Gastrointest Radiol* 10:225, 1985.

13. Logemann JA: *Evaluation and treatment of swallowing disorders*, ed 2, San Diego, 1998, Pro-Ed.

14. Lindgren S, Ekberg O: Swallowing complaints and cineradiographic abnormalities of the pharynx, *Dysphagia* 3:97, 1988.

15. Kim CH, Weaver AL, Hsu JJ et al: Discriminant value of esophageal symptoms: a study of the initial clinical findings in 499 patients with dysphagia of various causes, *Mayo Clin Proc* 68:948, 1993.

16. DiPippo KL, Holas MMA, Resing MJ: The Burke Dysphagia Screening Test: validation of its use in patients with stroke, *Arch Phys Med Rehabil* 75:1284, 1994.

17. Manor Y, Gilada N, Cohen A et al: Validation of a swallowing disturbance questionnaire for detecting dysphagia in patients with Parkinson's disease, *Mov Disord* 22:1917, 2007.

18. Wallace KL, Middleton S, Cook IJ: Development and validation of a self-report symptom inventory to assess the severity of oral-pharyngeal dysphagia, *Gastroenterology* 118:678, 2000.

19. Jensen K, Lambertsen K, Torkov P et al: Patient assessed symptoms are poor predictors of objective findings. Results from a cross sectional study in patients treated with radiotherapy for head and neck cancer, *Acta Oncol* 46:1159, 2007.

20. Ravich WJ, Wilson RF, Jones B et al: Psychogenic dysphagia and globus: reevaluation of 23 patients, *Dysphagia* 4:35, 1989.

21. Moser G, Vacariu-Ganser GV, Schneider C et al: High incidence of esophageal motor disorder in consecutive patients with globus sensation, *Gastroenterology* 101:1512, 1991.

22. Linden P, Kuhlemeir KV, Patterson C: Probability of correctly predicting subglottic penetration from clinical observations, *Dysphagia* 8:170, 1993.

23. McCulloch GH, Wertz RT, Rosenbek JC: Sensitivity and specificity of clinical/bedside signs for detecting aspiration in adults subsequent to stroke, *J Commun Disord* 34:55, 2001.

24. Daniels SK, McAdam CP, Brailey K et al: Clinical assessment of swallowing and prediction of dysphagia severity, *Am J Speech Lang Pathol* 6:17, 1997.

25. McCullough GH, Rosenbek JC, Wertz RT et al: Clinical swallowing examination measures for detecting aspiration post-stroke, *J Speech Lang Hear Res* 48:1280, 2005.

26. Daniels SK, Ballo LA, Mahoney MC et al: Clinical predictors and aspiration risk: outcome measures in acute stroke patients, *Arch Phys Med Rehabil* 81:1030, 2000.

27. Huggins PS, Tuomi SK, Young C: Effects of nasogastric tubes on the young, normal swallowing mechanism, *Dysphagia* 14:157, 1999.

28. Yorkston KA, Miller RM, Strand EA: *Management of speech and swallowing disorders in degenerative disease*, Tucson, AZ, 1995, Communication Skill Builders.

29. Leder SB: Videofluoroscopic evaluation of aspiration with visual examination of the gag reflex, *Dysphagia* 12:21, 1997.

30. Langmore SE, Logemann JA: After the clinical bedside examination: what next? *Am J Speech Lang Pathol* 9:13, 1991.

31. Miller RM: Clinical examination for dysphagia. In Groher ME, editor: *Dysphagia: diagnosis and management*, Boston, 1997, Butterworth-Heinemann.

32. Groher ME, Crary, MA, Mann GC et al: The impact of rheologically controlled materials on the identification of airway compromise on the clinical and videofluoroscopic swallowing examinations, *Dysphagia* 21:218, 2006.

33. Takahashi K, Groher ME, Michi K: Methodology for detecting swallowing sound, *Dysphagia* 9:54, 1994.

34. Leslie P, Drinnan MJ, Finn P at al: Reliability and validity of cervical auscultation: a controlled comparison using videofluoroscopy, *Dysphagia* 19:231, 2004.

35. Cichero JAY, Murdoch BE: Acoustic signature of the normal swallow characteristics by age, gender, and bolus volume, *Ann Otol Rhinol Laryngol* 111:623, 2002.

36. Cichero JAY, Murdoch BE: What happens *after* the swallow? Introducing the glottal release sound, *J Med Speech Pathol* 11:31, 2003.

37. Uyama R, Takahashi K, Michi Ken-ichi et al: Objective evaluation using acoustic characteristics of swallowing and expiratory sounds for detecting dysphagic swallow, *J Jpn Stomatol Soc* 46:147, 1997.

38. Borr C, Hielscher-Fastabend M, Lucking A: Reliability and validity of cervical auscultation, *Dysphagia* 22:225, 2007.

39. Groher ME, McKaig TM: Dysphagia and dietary levels in skilled nursing facilities, *J Am Geriatr Soc* 43:1, 1995.

40. Splaingard ML, Hutchins B, Sulton LD et al: Aspiration in rehabilitation patients: videofluoroscopy vs bedside clinical assessment, *Arch Phys Med Rehabil* 69:637, 1988.

41. Mann G, Hankey GJ: Initial clinical and demographic predictors of swallowing impairment following acute stroke, *Dysphagia* 16:208, 2001.

42. Edelman DA, Sheehy-Deardorff DA, White MT: Bedside assessment of swallowing is predictive of an abnormal barium swallow examination, *J Burn Care Res* 29:89, 2008.

43. Leder SB, Espinoza JF: Aspiration risk after acute stroke: comparison of clinical examination and fiberoptic endoscopic evaluation of swallowing, *Dysphagia* 17:214, 2002.

44. DiPippo KL, Holas MA, Reding MJ: Validation of the 3 oz water test for aspiration following stroke, *Arch Neurol* 49:1259, 1992.

45. Garon B, Engle M, Ormiston C: Reliability of the 3oz water test utilizing cough reflex as the sole indicator of aspiration, *J Neurol Rehabil* 9:139, 1995.

46. Nathadwarawala KM, McGroary A, Wiles CM: Swallowing in neurological outpatients: use of a timed test, *Dysphagia* 9:120, 1994.

47. Mari F, Matei M, Ceravolo MG et al: Predictive value of clinical studies in detecting aspiration in patients with neurological disorders, *J Neurol Neurosurg Psychiatry* 63:456, 1997.

48. Lim SH, Lieu PK, Phua SY et al: Accuracy of bedside clinical methods compared with fiberoptic examination of swallowing (FEES) in determining the risk of aspiration in acute stroke patients, *Dysphagia* 16:1, 2000.

49. Tohara H, Saitoh E, Mays K et al: Three tests for predicting aspiration without videofluoroscopy, *Dysphagia* 18:126, 2003.

50. Carnaby-Mann G, Lenius K: The bedside examination in dysphagia, *Phys Med Rehabil Clin North Am* 19:747, 2008.

51. Collins M, Bakheit A: Does pulse oximetry reliably detect aspiration in dysphagic stroke patients? *Stroke* 28:1773, 1997.

52. Sherman B, Nisenbaum JM, Jesberger ML et al: Assessment of dysphagia with the use of pulse oximetry, *Dysphagia* 14:152, 1999.

53. Smith HA, Lee SH, O'Neill PA et al: The combination of bedside swallowing assessment and oxygen saturation monitoring of swallowing in acute stroke: a safe and humane screening tool, *Age Aging* 29:495, 2000.

54. Colodny N: Comparison of dysphagics and non-dysphagics on pulse oximetry during oral feeding, *Dysphagia* 15:68, 2000.

55. Thompson-Henry S, Braddock B: The modified Evan's blue dye procedure fails to detect aspiration in the tracheostomized patient: five case reports, *Dysphagia* 10:172, 1995.

56. Brady SL, Hildner CD, Hutchins B: Simultaneous videofluoroscopic swallow study and modified Evans blue dye procedure: an evaluation of blue dye visualization in cases of known aspiration, *Dysphagia* 14:146, 1999.

57. O'Neill-Pirozzi TM, Lisiecki DJ, Momose KJ et al: Simultaneous modified barium swallow and blue dye tests: a determination of the accuracy of the blue dye test aspiration findings, *Dysphagia* 18:32, 2003.

58. Mann G: *MASA: The Mann assessment of swallowing ability*, Clifton, NY, 2002, Thomson Learning.

59. Lambert HC, Gisel EG, Wood-Dauphinee S, et al: *MISA: The McGill ingestive skills assessment and forms*, Ottawa, 2006, Canadian Association of Occupational Therapists ACE.

60. Lambert HC, Abrahamowicz M, Groher M et al: The McGill Ingestive Assessment predicts time to death in an elderly population with neurogenic dysphagia: preliminary evidence, *Dysphagia* 20:123, 2005.

61. Crary MA, Mann GDC, Groher ME: Initial psychometric assessment of a functional oral intake scale for dysphagic stroke patients, *Arch Phys Med Rehabil* 86:1516, 2005.

62. Guigoz Y, Vellas B, Garry PJ: Mini nutritional assessment: a practical assessment tool for grading the nutritional state of elderly patients, *Facts Res Gerontol Suppl* 2, 15, 1994.

63. Allen CJ, Parameswaram K, Belda J et al: Reproducibility, validity, and responsiveness of a disease-specific symptom questionnaire for gastroesophageal reflux disease, *Dis Esophagus* 13:265, 2000.

64. Shaw M, Dent J, Reebe T et al: The Reflux Disease Questionnaire: a measure for assessment of treatment response in clinical trials, *Health Qual Life Outcomes* 6:31, 2008.

65. Belafsky PC, Postma GN, Koufman JA: Validity and reliability of the reflux symptom index, *J Voice* 16:274, 2002.

66. Crary MA, Caraby Mann GD, Groher ME: Biomechanical correlates of surface electromyography signals obtained during swallowing by healthy adults, *J Speech Lang Hear Res* 49:186, 2006.

67. Crary MA, Carnaby Mann GD, Groher ME: Identification of swallowing events from sEMG signals obtained from healthy adults, *Dysphagia* 22:94, 2007.

68. Hamlet S, Penney DG, Formolo J: Stethoscope acoustics and cervical auscultation of swallowing, *Dysphagia* 9:63, 1994.

Chapter 10

Instrumental Swallowing Examinations: Videofluoroscopy and Endoscopy

MICHAEL A. CRARY

OBJECTIVES

1. Explain why it is important to "image" the swallowing mechanism and evaluate swallow function with an instrumental study. List some basic guidelines to help determine whether any instrumental swallowing examination is indicated.
2. Describe the basic components and potential modifications of a fluoroscopic swallowing examination and an endoscopic swallowing examination.
3. Describe some of the strengths and weaknesses of the fluoroscopic swallowing examination and the endoscopic swallowing examination.
4. Compare the endoscopic examination with the fluoroscopic examination, specifically regarding the identification of various dysphagia characteristics.

CONSIDERATIONS FOR AN INSTRUMENTAL SWALLOWING EXAMINATION

Many instrumental procedures may be used to evaluate different aspects of swallowing function. This chapter addresses the two most commonly used procedures: *videofluoroscopy* (also called *videofluorography*) and *flexible endoscopy* (also known as *fiberoptic endoscopy* or *transnasal endoscopy*). Procedures related to these primary methods are introduced and other instrumental techniques for swallowing evaluation are briefly mentioned. However, before these instrumental evaluation procedures are detailed, they should be placed in the context of the overall clinical evaluation of the adult patient with dysphagia. Frequent questions about these procedures include "What are they intended to achieve?" and "When is an instrumental procedure indicated?" The following information is derived largely from practice guidelines published by the American Speech-Language-Hearing Association.[1-3] The concept underlying the use of practice guidelines is that they result from the creative, clinical, and scientific input of many experienced professionals with thorough professional review. In that regard, although these views may change with the acquisition of new information at a given point in time, they represent a fair summary of existing knowledge and opinion.

Goals of Instrumental Swallowing Evaluations

Instrumental examinations of swallowing are only a part of the comprehensive examination of swallowing performance and function. In general, a thorough clinical examination (see Chapter 9) should precede any instrumental examination. The clinical examination can be important in tailoring specific questions to be addressed in an instrumental examination and provides a comprehensive clinical profile of patients in whom dysphagia is suspected. Thus instrumental examinations of swallowing may accomplish any number of objectives depending on the patient and the clinical situation. These examinations (1) provide valuable information on the anatomy and physiology of structures and muscles used in swallowing, (2) evaluate the ability of a patient to swallow various materials, (3) assess secretions and the patient's reaction to them, (4) document the adequacy of airway protection and the coordination between respiration and swallowing, and (5) help evaluate the impact of compensatory therapy maneuvers on swallowing function and airway protection. Although the fluoroscopic and endoscopic examinations of swallowing

function are not mirror images, they do share many common functions. In addition, each imaging study has specific attributes that the other may not possess. Furthermore, because each examination provides a permanent video record of the swallowing evaluation, both contribute to increased objectivity with enhanced documentation and the ability to review results of the respective studies.

Purposes of Instrumental Swallowing Examinations

Box 10-1 summarizes various purposes attributed to instrumental swallowing examinations. Perhaps the most overt purpose of any instrumental swallowing examination is the ability to image the structures of the swallowing mechanism and the movement of those structures during swallowing and other movements that may help assess their functional integrity. This assessment involves the lips, tongue, jaw, velo-

---

BOX 10-1	**Multiple Purposes Attributed to an Instrumental Swallowing Study**

- Image structures of the upper aerodigestive tract: oral cavity, velopharynx, pharynx, larynx, pharyngoesophageal segment, and esophagus.
- Assess movement patterns of swallowing-related structures in the upper aerodigestive tract to formulate inferences regarding physiologic integrity (e.g., speed of movement, symmetry, range, strength, sensation, coordination).
- Assess swallowing-related movement patterns of structures in the upper aerodigestive tract (e.g., effectiveness and safety of the swallow, accommodation to varying materials).
- Identify and describe any airway compromise (e.g., aspiration, penetration) and the circumstances under which these events occur.
- Evaluate the impact of compensatory maneuvers to improve swallowing safety and efficiency.
- Identify and describe any pooled secretions within the hypopharynx and larynx (or potentially other areas). Description should include the patient's ability to move or clear pooled secretions with swallows or coughing/clearing activities.
- Complete a cursory evaluation of esophageal anatomy and physiology to identify any overt esophageal contributors to dysphagia symptoms.
- Assist in forming clinical recommendations, including route of nutrition or hydration intake (i.e., oral, nonoral), safest or most efficient dietary level, need to make feeding modifications, or therapeutic interventions.

pharyngeal mechanism, pharynx, larynx, and esophagus. Evaluation of these structures should incorporate some indication of anatomic adequacy and movement capability. In some cases it is possible to assess or perhaps infer sensory integrity and motor functions. Beyond basic anatomy and movement of specific structures, coordinated movement among various components of the swallow mechanism should be assessed with reference to swallowing function. This assessment requires the patient to swallow materials of varying sizes and textures to allow inspection of adjustments (either positive or negative) within the swallowing mechanism. This component of the instrumental examination can help identify misdirection (specifically entrance into the airway) of a bolus and post-swallow residue as a result of inefficient swallowing. If aspiration is identified, the instrumental examination is helpful in differentiating situations when the patient is more likely to aspirate versus those when aspiration is less likely. By using a variety of swallowed materials and incorporating compensatory maneuvers, clinicians may make inferences regarding the safest and most efficient material to swallow and the need for any postural or other adjustments that improve swallowing safety and/or efficiency. Secretions pooled within the swallowing mechanism can be problematic for patients and contribute to respiratory complications. These fluids should be identified and described, including the patient's reaction to them and the patient's ability to remove them from the swallowing tract. In some situations the clinician may conclude that oral feeding is not safe or adequate and hence might use the results of instrumental examinations to recommend nonoral feeding sources (or to recommend discontinuation of nonoral feeding sources with reestablishment of oral feeding). In short, instrumental examinations of swallowing function provide objective imaging of the swallowing mechanism that assists dysphagia clinicians in determining the need for and the direction of swallowing rehabilitation. More details of the fluoroscopic and endoscopic swallowing examinations are provided in later sections.

Indications for Instrumental Swallowing Examinations

Box 10-2 addresses three important questions: (1) When *is* an instrumental swallowing examination indicated? (2) When *may* an instrumental swallowing be indicated? and (3) When is an instrumental swallowing examination *not* indicated?[1]

Perhaps the basic answer to when an instrumental examination *is* indicated is "when the clinical examination fails to answer the relevant questions." If the

---

BOX 10-2	Indications for an Instrumental Swallowing Examination

EXAMINATION DEFINITELY INDICATED

- The comprehensive clinical examination fails to thoroughly address the clinical questions posed by the patient and/or problem.
- Dysphagia characteristics are vague and require confirmation or better delineation.
- Nutritional or respiratory issues indicate suspicion of dysphagia.
- Safety or efficiency of swallowing is a concern.
- Direction for swallowing rehabilitation is needed.
- Help is needed to assist in identifying underlying medical problems that contribute to dysphagia symptoms.

EXAMINATION *MAY* BE INDICATED

- The patient has a medical condition that has a high risk for dysphagia.
- Swallow function demonstrates an overt change.
- The patient is unable to cooperate for a clinical examination.

EXAMINATION *NOT* INDICATED

- The patient no longer has dysphagia complaints.
- The patient's condition is too medically compromised or the patient is too uncooperative to complete the procedure.
- The clinician's judgment is that the examination would not alter the clinical course or management plan.

---

patient reports specific problems that are not clarified by the clinical examination, an instrumental examination is indicated. This examination may help clarify whether a significant dysphagia exists and delineate the parameters of that type of dysphagia—oral, pharyngeal, esophageal, or a combination of these components. Information from an instrumental examination may clarify airway protection issues that are potentially related to respiratory compromise or may elucidate swallow efficiency issues potentially related to nutritional decline. As previously mentioned, the impact of compensatory maneuvers may be verified during instrumental examination, and other information on swallowing movements may be garnered that facilitates direction in swallowing rehabilitation. Finally, in some instances information gained from an imaging study may contribute to a better understanding of the medical diagnosis contributing to dysphagia symptoms.

An instrumental swallowing examination *may* be indicated for various reasons, most of which are related to the condition of the patient. For example, some medical conditions pose a high risk for swallowing difficulty or may be complicated by swallowing difficulties that may not prompt a significant complaint from the patient. An instrumental examination provides an objective evaluation of swallowing ability that may facilitate early identification of problems and hence lead to improved care. In addition, clinical conditions may change over time because of changes in the underlying disease (i.e., progressive or recovering conditions) or changes in the patient (new treatments or new disease). Some patients present with clinical conditions that preclude adequate cooperation with a clinical examination (cognitive or communicative impairments). In this situation, an instrumental examination may help address the questions posed regarding swallowing ability.

Finally, in some clinical situations an instrumental examination is *not* indicated. Perhaps the most obvious is when the patient reports that he or she had difficulty in the past but no longer has any swallowing difficulty. Other situations might include the patient whose medical condition is too compromised to tolerate a procedure or who is too uncooperative to participate in a procedure. If the clinician judges that the patient's condition will result in an instrumental examination that provides no useful information, a valid decision may be to delay the examination until the patient's condition facilitates completion of a useful examination. The value of clinical judgment should not be underestimated. At times clinicians may simply feel that given all available information, the addition of an instrumental examination of swallowing function will not provide any further beneficial information.

Instrumental swallowing examinations—specifically fluoroscopic and endoscopic procedures that image swallow function—add an objective and valuable component to the comprehensive assessment of the patient with dysphagic symptoms. However, these examinations should not be isolated from the information obtained from a thorough clinical assessment. The combination of these tools is expected to provide the most complete clinical picture of the dysphagic patient, leading to the best possible treatment. Instrumental examinations of swallowing function address both the anatomy and physiology of structures within the swallowing tract and how movement of these structures may accommodate swallowing different materials. Clinicians also may assess the impact of immediate compensations with these examinations. Available guidelines offer suggestions for when an instrumental examination should, may, or should not be used; however, no guideline can account for all

clinical situations. The judgment of the clinician with direct knowledge of the comprehensive picture is valuable in deciding when and how to use an instrumental examination of swallowing function.

The following sections address the videofluoroscopic and fiberoptic endoscopic swallowing examinations separately and subsequently compare the two procedures directly to help clinicians decide whether one, both, or neither of these procedures is appropriate in various clinical situations.

VIDEOFLUOROSCOPIC SWALLOWING EXAMINATIONS

What's in a Name?

Various authors and health care institutions use different terms for what is essentially the same examination. Box 10-3 lists several name variants for this procedure. This list is not comprehensive but is probably representative of the variation that exists in nomenclature. The term *modified barium swallow,* initially coined by Logemann,[4] can be interpreted literally. The traditional barium swallow is focused on the esophagus and stomach and uses large amounts of liquid barium (**contrast agent**) and still-frame pictures to image the expanded esophagus and evaluate gastric emptying or other upper gastrointestinal functions. This examination is usually done with the patient in one or more combinations of lying positions. The adult patient with dysphagia is likely to be compromised both by the large amounts of liquid barium and by the lying position during swallowing attempts. Therefore this examination was modified to use smaller amounts of contrast material varying in size and consistency and to examine the patient in an upright position (whenever physically possible) to resemble the position most typically associated with eating. This procedure has become known as the *modified barium swallow* (MBS).

Some health care professionals and researchers held to different conventions in selecting a name for this relatively new procedure. Gastrointestinal (GI)

BOX 10-3	**Terminology Used to Describe the Videofluoroscopic Swallowing Study**

- Modified barium swallow (MBS)
- Upper gastrointestinal series with hypopharynx
- Videofluoroscopic swallow study (VFSS)
- Videofluoroscopic barium examination (VFBE)
- Videofluoroscopic swallow examination (VFSE)
- Rehabilitation swallow study

Practice Note 10-1

Different terms have been applied to the fluoroscopic evaluation of swallowing. Many clinicians who engaged in these examinations in the early 1980s may have been confused by the term *modified barium swallow*. In the author's experience, referring physicians would often order the more traditional "barium swallow" when they intended to order the "modified version." In an attempt to reduce confusion within the author's health care system, the term *rehab swallow* was adopted and later became the term *rehab barium swallow*. This term, negotiated between the speech-language pathologists and radiologists, was meant to reflect the importance of this study in "determining the need for and the direction of swallowing rehabilitation." Inclusion of the word *rehab* helped ensure that a speech-language pathologist was involved in each of these studies presented to radiology. Both the medical and the rehabilitative objectives of this examination were met by performing these studies in conjunction with a radiologist.

radiologists often referred to the procedure as an *upper GI series with hypopharynx*. This term reflects the traditional esophagram view but with the addition of a study of the hypopharynx. Other terms in the literature include *videofluorographic swallow study* (VFSS),[5,6] videofluorographic barium examination (VFBE),[7] and videofluorographic swallow examination (VFSE).[8] Presumably, each of these terms was intended to identify the unique radiographic procedure that evaluates oropharyngeal swallowing function. Clinicians in different areas may know or use other terms that refer to the same study. This chapter uses the more generic name variant, videofluoroscopic swallowing examination.

Objectives of the Videofluoroscopic Swallowing Examination

The videofluoroscopic swallowing examination can have multiple objectives. The *primary* objective is to obtain a video image of the upper aerodigestive tract during the act of swallowing. By manipulating what is swallowed, how it is swallowed, and patient positioning, clinicians can complete a comprehensive assessment of swallowing ability. Box 10-4 lists the more overt objectives of a videofluoroscopic swallowing examination. Additional objectives may be appropriate for individual patients and/or problems.[9]

Evaluation of the swallowing mechanism is initially approached by identification and description of

any deviations in the anatomy of structures within the swallowing tract. This presupposes the clinician's detailed knowledge of anatomy, including radiographic anatomy. Figure 10-1 depicts both lateral and anterior radiographic views of a normal swallowing mechanism. Review of anatomic detail and examples of normal swallow physiology may be found in narrated Video 2-3 on the Evolve site that accompanies this textbook. Basic physiology of the swallowing mechanism may be evaluated by asking the patient to phonate, breath hold, perform a Valsalva maneuver, produce falsetto phonation, or perform other activities that facilitate movement of the structures within the swallowing tract. This component of the evaluation is helpful in identification of potential movement deficits that may contribute to oropharyngeal dysphagia and in selecting appropriate compensatory maneuvers.

Swallow physiology is evaluated by asking patients to swallow various amounts and textures of contrast materials. Knowledge of both normal and impaired swallow physiology is implicit in evaluating this component of the fluoroscopic examination. Abnormal aspects of physiology typically are detailed in terms of reduced or altered movement patterns. In addition, the consequences of physiologic impairments such as aspiration or residue are documented. Finally, the impact of therapeutic compensations is evaluated. Compensatory postures or swallow maneuvers are useful both for introducing immediate improvement in the safety or efficiency of the swallow and for identifying potentially beneficial therapy strategies.

Symptom confirmation is an important objective of any instrumental examination, including the videofluoroscopic swallowing examination. If a patient reports food sticking in the lower neck area, the fluoroscopic study should thoroughly evaluate that area. If nothing of consequence is identified there, other potential contributors to that symptom should be

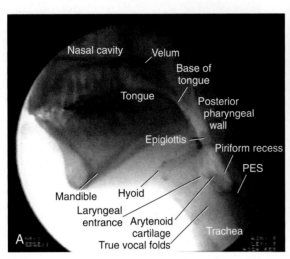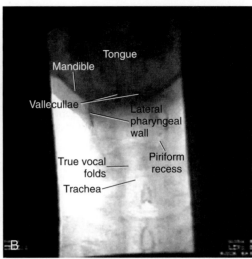

FIGURE 10-1. Lateral (**A**) and anterior (**B**) radiographic views of a normal swallowing mechanism. *PES,* Pharyngoesophageal segment.

evaluated (in this specific case, the esophagus and lower esophageal sphincter should be thoroughly evaluated). Addressing this objective relies heavily on the clinician's skill in focusing on the patient's complaints and descriptions of dysphagia symptoms and in directing the fluoroscopic study to adequately evaluate those components of the swallowing mechanism that may contribute to a specific set of symptoms.

Given that the fluoroscopic swallowing examination is a time-limited event and cannot possibly sample all foods that a given patient might eat, a certain amount of prediction is involved in interpreting this examination. For this reason, we include "prediction" as an objective of the fluoroscopic swallowing examination. After a thorough evaluation of the structure and function of the swallowing mechanism, swallow physiology and consequences of impaired movement, and the impact of compensatory maneuvers, the clinician must engage in a series of educated decisions regarding the functional swallowing performance of each patient. Examples of such decisions include the potential for future health complications, such as aspiration-related pneumonias and/or nutritional deficits, the level of functional eating ability and any recommended diet level changes, the need for swallowing therapy and, if indicated, the specific direction of that therapy, whether additional clinical or instrumental evaluations are indicated, and if consultations with other health care providers are needed to address the problems identified in the current examination. These are only a few of the potential areas of prediction in which clinicians may engage. Ultimately, questions of safe and adequate oral intake

of food and liquid must be directly addressed and based in part on the results of this examination.

Procedures for the Videofluoroscopic Swallowing Examination

A standard protocol is highly recommended for the fluoroscopic study.[5,6,9] Standardizing the protocol increases consistency and reproducibility of examinations both within and across patients. The use of a standard protocol does not preclude individual variations that may be required for specific patients or problems; however, it does provide a consistent framework from which reasonable variations may be accomplished. Several factors within the protocol must be considered, including patient positioning, materials to be swallowed, sequence of attempted swallows, and what to look for, including interpretation and documentation of the findings.

Patient Positioning

Positioning depends in large part on the physical abilities of the patient. In general, this study is accomplished with the patient in an upright, seated position with adequate support for the head and body. Patients with physical limitations from weakness, fatigue, disease, or other reasons may require special positioning systems during the examination. Various commercial positioning chairs are available to assist in optimal positioning of patients with physical limitations. Before purchasing or building a positioning chair, it is important to know the physical dimensions of the specific fluoroscopic system to be used. Often there is a fixed maximum distance between the table

Practice Note 10-2

During a recent visit to Japan, I observed a particularly innovative positioning chair used for videofluorographic swallowing evaluations. The patient (in this specific instance, the patient had significant physical limitations after a stroke) was seated in what looked like a modified, motorized wheelchair. The chair was then placed in the imaging field of a C-arm fluoroscope. By remote control, the examiner could raise or lower the patient, tilt the patient forward or backward, and tilt the patient from side to side. This chair was beneficial in this particular instrumental examination in that positioning variants could be evaluated for their impact on swallow function. Without this special chair, position variants likely would not have been evaluated or would have been evaluated only with extreme burden on both the patient and the examiner.

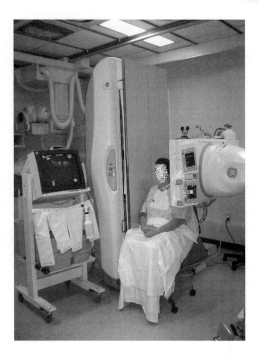

FIGURE 10-2. Patient positioned in fluoroscope for a lateral view image.

and tower of the fluoroscope. In addition, this study is typically completed in lateral and anterior views. The selected chair or positioning system should be adaptable to accommodate both views. Finally, specifically for lateral views, large patients may not fit easily into the fixed space between the table and tower of the fluoroscope. In such cases, it is possible to turn the patient slightly toward an oblique orientation while maintaining a lateral perspective as much as possible.

Typically, the videofluoroscopic swallowing examination begins with the patient in a lateral (or semioblique) position in reference to the fluoroscopic image (Figure 10-2). This perspective affords an excellent view of the swallowing mechanism from the lips to cervical esophagus and provides the best view of the trachea separate from the esophagus. This view is beneficial in determining whether material enters the upper airway. After examination of the swallow in the lateral perspective, the patient is turned for an anterior view. This perspective permits excellent evaluation of symmetry along the swallowing mechanism. When the esophagus is imaged with the patient in a sitting position the extent of the view is often limited. In these situations, imaging is done with the patient in a standing or lying position depending on physical limitations of the patient or specific aspects of the dysphagia presentation. In fact, for some patients who can tolerate standing during the fluorographic examination without compromise, the entire examination can be done with the patient in a stand-

ing position. This situation permits a great degree of control in moving and positioning the patient.

Material Used in the Fluoroscopic Study

The key material used in the fluoroscopic swallow study is barium sulfate suspension. This is a positive contrast agent that is **radiopaque**. As a result, barium sulfate appears as black on the fluoroscopic image compared with negative contrast substances, such as air, which appear as varying shades of gray. Tissue and bone appear as shades of gray depending on their density. Figure 10-3 depicts the shades of the bolus in the mouth, various bony structures (including the hyoid bone), and the air spaces in the pharynx and the trachea.

A popular point of discussion and even argument among clinicians is whether to use barium sulfate in isolation or in combination with real food items. No firm answer has emerged from these discussions and proponents of both perspectives have seemingly valid points. Individuals who focus on isolated barium products for this study claim that the range of food textures is so great that it would be impossible to image every possible food or liquid that a given patient might ingest. Another argument against using real food is the potential for complications resulting from aspiration of food products into the airway. Proponents of combining barium and real food items

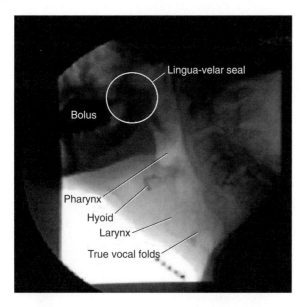

FIGURE 10-3. Lateral radiographic view with bolus held in mouth.

argue that barium products do not represent the consistencies noted in real food products.

Regardless of the outcome of this food-versus-barium discussion, the importance of using a range of textures and volumes during the study cannot be overstated. It is well known that a normal swallowing mechanism adjusts to changes in bolus volume and/or texture.[10-13] In the absence of this accommodation, a patient with dysphagia may demonstrate a variety of compensations or demonstrate the consequences of impaired physiology and the inability to compensate. Volumes used in fluoroscopic swallowing studies vary across published reports. One consideration is the average amount ingested in normal-swallowing adults. Published literature suggests that approximately 20 mL of liquid represents the average drink from a cup.[14] Moreover, an average teaspoon is approximately 5 mL. Therefore, based on a functional perspective, it seems reasonable that the majority of swallow attempts would include volumes somewhere within this range unless clinical indications exist to use less or more material. In fact, results of a recent study[15] suggested that swallows of a 5-mL bolus of thin barium liquid and a 5-mL bolus of nectar-thick barium liquid contributed the greatest amount of information to interpretation of 15 physiologic swallowing components. The author's standard protocol has been to use 5 and 10 mL of each material and then allow the patient to drink freely from a cup or by a straw whenever feasible or clinically indicated. This choice of volume and consistency is based in part on the functional considerations previously

mentioned and in consideration of a study suggesting that when using standard materials, 5-mL and 10-mL volumes of thin and thick liquid demonstrated the strongest associations between clinical signs of aspiration and observed aspiration during the videofluoroscopic swallowing study.[16]

In addition to varying volume, consistency—or **viscosity**—is varied across swallows. General categories of viscosity or textures include thin liquid, thickened liquid, paste or pudding, and masticated material.[7] One barium product line has attempted to standardize the viscosity of barium sulfate liquids into thin, nectar, and honey. A paste material also is available in this product line. One benefit of these standardized barium products is consistency and reproducibility of repeated examinations both within and across patients. In short, use of standardized materials reduces variability across examinations that might result from utilization of different materials.

Sequencing the Events in the Fluoroscopic Study

Different protocols have suggested different sequences of events during the fluoroscopic swallowing study. For example, Logemann[9] recommends beginning with thin liquids in progressive sequential amounts (1 mL, 3 mL, 5 mL, 10 mL). Once thin liquid swallows are completed, pudding and then masticated materials are evaluated. Palmer et al.[5] began their fluoroscopic swallowing protocol with 5 mL of thick liquids (this category includes pudding material in their protocol), followed by thin liquid and then masticated materials. Martin-Harris et al.[15] initiated their protocol with 5 mL of thin liquid followed by thicker liquids, pudding, and a masticated material. However, this group did caution that larger, thicker, and masticated materials were given to patients only if they demonstrated adequate airway protection and pharyngeal clearance on the thin liquid materials. The author agrees that a standard protocol is beneficial when completing the fluoroscopic swallowing, but recommends flexibility in the sequence of events to maximize the "diagnostic outcomes" for each patient. Described below is a general sequence of events used in the author's standard protocol for the videofluoroscopic swallowing study.

Initially the patient is seated and viewed from the lateral perspective. The first tasks often are simple speech or phonation activities to facilitate an impression of movement of structures in the swallowing mechanism (lips, tongue, velum, and pharyngeal wall). Subsequently the initial barium bolus is provided to the patient. Unless there is significant dryness (xerostomia), weakness, or anatomic deviation in the oral cavity structures, the initial bolus is typically

5 mL of thickened liquid. The next material would be 5 mL of thin liquid followed by 5 mL of pudding. This sequence is subsequently repeated with 10-mL volumes. The patient then is given a cup of thin liquid barium to drink freely and a masticated material coated with barium pudding (usually a cracker). Video 2-3 on the Evolve site shows examples of swallows of these and other materials by a healthy adult volunteer. Video 10-1 depicts examples of swallowing by patients with various dysphagia symptoms.

After this sequence of events is imaged from the lateral view, the patient is turned and viewed from the anterior perspective. From this view the patient is asked to sustain phonation or repeat the same vowel to visualize movement of the true vocal folds. Some patients are asked to phonate in a falsetto mode to evaluate medial movement of the lateral pharyngeal walls. Some are asked to perform a "trumpet" maneuver to evaluate potential weakness in the lateral pharyngeal walls. The trumpet maneuver is accomplished by asking the patient to lift the chin to provide a clear view of the entire pharynx. Then the patient is asked to puff the cheeks and blow as if playing a trumpet (Figure 10-4). Turning the head to each side during swallowing may assist in evaluating each hemipharynx and any effect on pharyngoesophageal segment (PES) opening. Materials used in the anterior view depend largely on the results of swallows examined with the lateral view. In general, not all materials are repeated with the change in orientation, but sufficient swallows are evaluated to assess symmetry, physiology, and the consequences of impaired movement.

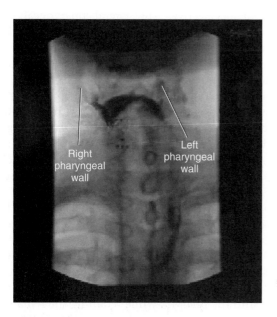

FIGURE 10-4. Anterior radiographic view of patient performing "trumpet" maneuver.

Either before or after the evaluation of the swallow from the anterior view, compensatory maneuvers might be introduced to evaluate their impact on any observed impairments in swallow physiology. Common compensatory maneuvers include the chin-down position, head turn, supraglottic swallow, and Mendelsohn maneuver (see Chapter 14). The impact of these maneuvers can be evaluated in terms of improved swallow safety (less aspiration or penetration) or efficiency (better timing or less residue).

Finally, the esophagus is evaluated whenever feasible. If the patient cannot be positioned appropriately or if the risk of aspiration is too great, esophageal inspection is not added to the standard oropharyngeal examination. Typically, a full esophageal study is not completed at the same time as the oropharyngeal study. However, a cursory examination of the esophagus may be completed to rule out overt blockages or poor passage of material through the esophagus into the stomach. If the clinical presentation indicates potential for a significant esophageal-based dysphagia and the oropharyngeal examination does not identify any overt difficulties, a more thorough esophagram should be completed.

Clinicians must decide how much of the standard protocol to complete for any given patient. Continuing to provide material to a patient who is aspirating a significant amount of each attempted bolus is unwise and contraindicated. Similarly, a study should not be continued if a patient becomes excessively fatigued or is otherwise unresponsive. Following a standard protocol blindly without consideration for the individual needs of the patient is poor practice. Box 10-5 lists the materials and sequence of presentation that may be included in a standardized fluoroscopic swallow study.

What to Look For

Despite recent attempts to "quantify" the interpretation of the videofluoroscopic swallowing study,[15,17] the prevailing interpretation for this instrumental examination is to describe various events associated with swallowing different materials. As noted with materials and sequencing of events during this examination, suggestions for interpretation vary across clinicians and authors. The following text presents a general approach to interpretation of the videofluoroscopic swallowing study.

The "short form" of what to look for is anatomy and physiology underlying swallowing activity. Initially, anatomic detail and any deviations from normal are to be noted. This includes not only the oral cavity structures, velopharynx, pharynx, larynx, pharyngoesophageal sphincter, and cervical esophagus, but

BOX 10-5	Materials and Sequence of Presentation That May Be Included in a Standardized Fluoroscopic Swallowing Examination

FROM LATERAL VIEW
- Short speech sample and vowel phonation
- 5 mL of thin liquid barium
- 5 mL of thick liquid barium
- 5 mL of barium paste (pudding)
- 10 mL of thin liquid barium
- 10 mL of thick liquid barium
- 10 mL of barium paste (pudding)
- Thin liquid taken freely from cup or through straw
- Masticated material (cracker coated with barium paste)
- Repeat thin liquid if residue from cracker

FROM ANTERIOR VIEW (ACTUAL MATERIAL DEPENDS ON RESULTS OF LATERAL VIEW)
- Repeated vowel phonation and falsetto
- Swallow with head forward and turned

COMPENSATORY MANEUVERS
- May be introduced at any time in the examination as clinically indicated

ESOPHAGEAL EVALUATION
- Cursory examination for overt obstruction or dysmotility

CLINICAL CORNER 10-1

Depending on the specific clinical presentation of the patient, it may be important to evaluate swallowing performance when the clinician provides the materials to be swallowed instead of when the patient self-feeds. This includes smaller, measured amounts and self-selected volumes by spoon, cup, or straw. The difference in performance may be staggering for some patients, particularly those with cognitive or movement impairments attributable to neurologic deficits. For example, if a patient does not initiate a swallow when the clinician places a bolus in the mouth, the clinician should give the same material in a spoon placed in the patients hand and assist him or her (if needed) in placing the spoon in the mouth. Although in some cases this simple modification is not informative, in others this adjustment may make a large difference in patient performance and hence clinical interpretation of the videofluoroscopic swallow study results.

CRITICAL THINKING
1. What clinical disorders or impairments might contribute to an absent swallow initiation?
2. What neurologic or cognitive mechanisms might have an impact on a change in patient performance when self-feeding versus being fed?
3. What clinical implications would result when swallow performance does change when the patient engages in self-feeding?

also the structure of the cervical spine. Depending on the clinical presentation of the patient, anatomy may be viewed from both lateral and anterior perspectives before any physiologic or swallowing assessment is initiated. The lateral view provides the best inspection of the movement within the swallowing mechanism. Box 10-6 summarizes the more salient observations obtained from both lateral and anterior views of the fluoroscopic study. Once the anatomy of the swallowing mechanism has been reviewed, basic movement patterns of structures within the swallowing mechanism should be evaluated without swallowing attempts. This practice aids in understanding any physiologic deficits within the mechanism that may contribute to swallowing problems. Typically this component of the examination is brief and involves short speech samples or vowel phonation. During these activities the clinician looks for appropriate movement of the lips, tongue, jaw, velum, larynx, and pharyngeal walls. Movement of the pharyngeal walls can best be evaluated by having the patient produce a falsetto phonation while viewed from the

anterior perspective. The lateral pharyngeal walls typically move toward the pharyngeal midline with this maneuver.

After assessment of the anatomy and basic movement capabilities of the swallowing mechanism, the clinician subsequently advances to a direct inspection of swallowing activity. Often the patient is asked to hold a bolus in the mouth before attempting to swallow. This affords the opportunity to evaluate lip seal anteriorly and lingual-velar seal posteriorly. Impairment in these functions results in anterior spillage of the bolus or posterior spillage potentially into an open airway. If a solid bolus is used, clinicians should observe the patient masticate the food material, form a cohesive bolus, and propel this material into the oropharynx. A larger masticated bolus may be swallowed in piecemeal fashion. In this pattern, the patient may deliver small amounts of masticated food into the pharynx while retaining the remaining food in the mouth for further preparation. Whether a liquid or solid bolus is used, the timing and effi-

BOX 10-6	**Observations That May Be Obtained from the Videofluoroscopic Swallowing Examination**

ANATOMY
- All structures

NONSWALLOW MOVEMENT (SPEECH OR VOWEL PHONATION)
- Lips
- Tongue
- Mandible
- Velum
- Larynx (vocal fold movement from anterior view)
- Pharyngeal walls (falsetto)

SWALLOW MOVEMENT (VARIES DEPENDING ON BOLUS SIZE AND CONSISTENCY)
- Oral containment of liquids anterior and posterior
- Mastication of semisolids and solids
- Oral transit of material into hypopharynx
- Oronasal separation
- Hyoid movement
- Laryngeal elevation and closure
- Pharyngeal constriction
- PES opening

CONSEQUENCES OF IMPAIRED SWALLOW PHYSIOLOGY
- Spillage (anterior or posterior)
- Residue
- Misdirection of bolus and airway compromise

IMPACT OF COMPENSATORY MANEUVERS (VARIES DEPENDING ON IMPAIRMENTS)
- Postural adjustment
- Head position changes
- Swallow timing changes (e.g., Mendelsohn maneuver)
- Breath-hold maneuvers
- Bolus changes

movement patterns—can result in entrance of food or liquid into the nasal cavity. This finding is commonly termed *nasopharyngeal reflux*. The hyoid bone and larynx typically move as a functional unit during swallowing attempts. Although extensive variation has been described in hyolaryngeal movement, most investigators and clinicians agree that the basic movement is upward and forward (elevation followed by anterior movement of both structures). Although this might seem to be a simple activity, appropriate movement of the hyolaryngeal complex involves adequate tongue base function and function of the muscles in the pharyngeal wall. Collectively these events lead to opening of the PES. In addition, movement of the hyolaryngeal complex is responsible for movement of the epiglottis during swallowing. This latter structure is positioned between the tongue base/hyoid bone and the larynx. As the larynx elevates and the tongue base moves posteriorly and inferiorly, the epiglottis retroflexes to assist in protecting the airway. Deficits in this movement often contribute to post-swallow residue in the valleculae anterior to the epiglottis. In addition to elevating within the pharynx, the larynx also closes during the swallowing attempt to protect the airway from the entrance of unwanted materials. On the lateral fluoroscopic view, this may be seen as a forward tilting of the arytenoid cartilages approximating the petiole of the epiglottis. As the larynx elevates, the pharynx constricts and along with tongue base retropulsion facilitates passage of the bolus through the hypopharynx into the PES. The PES opens behind the larynx and permits passage of the bolus into the cervical esophagus. Deficits in pharyngeal constriction and/or PES opening typically result in post-swallow residue along the pharyngeal walls and in the piriform sinuses.

If swallow physiology is impaired, clinicians should document the functional consequences of that impairment. Several consequences of impaired swallowing physiology were mentioned previously. Thorough descriptions of post-swallow residue and airway compromise in the form of material entering the laryngeal vestibule or aspirated below the true vocal folds should be incorporated. These descriptions should include the reason for residue or aspiration, the timing of each event, and the patient's reaction (or lack thereof) to residue or aspirated material. Finally, the impact of compensatory maneuvers should be investigated and documented. The effect(s) of these maneuvers should be considered in terms of changes in observed swallow physiology (i.e., faster swallow, more movement) and the functional consequences of these maneuvers (i.e., less residue, improved airway protection). Common compensa-

ciency of oral transit of the bolus should be documented. Poor temporal coordination of the oral component of swallowing might lead to entrance of material into an airway that has not yet closed. Alternatively, a prolonged oral component of swallowing may relate to prolonged mealtimes and thus reduced oral intake and nutritional risk for a patient. Reduced efficiency of oral transport might contribute to residue in and around the oral cavity after the swallowing attempt. This might result from poor motor coordination or from anatomic deficits.

Deficits in oral-nasal separation—whether from anatomic changes or physiologic deficits in velar tory maneuvers are described as therapy techniques in Chapter 14.

Clinicians often adopt or develop checklists to assist in the interpretation of the videofluoroscopic swallowing study. This practice may help organize the interpretation process, but clinicians should use such checklists only as assistive devices. Interpretation of the videofluoroscopic swallowing study involves more than a summary of items checked off on a list. Various attempts have been made to assist in the interpretation of the videofluoroscopic swallowing study. The Dysphagia Outcome and Severity Scale (DOSS)[18] is a 7-point **ordinal scale** that addresses multiple domains of dysphagia, including degree of functional deficit, diet recommendations, level of patient independence with feeding, and type of nutrition. This scale demonstrates adequate interrater and intrarater **reliability** but has no demonstrated **validity.** The Penetration-Aspiration Scale[19] is a unidimensional ordinal scale that describes the depth of entrance of material into the airway and the patient's ability to clear any entered material. Clinicians must be aware that this "pen-asp" scale is *not* a dysphagia severity scale. The scale addresses only a single aspect of dysphagia—material entering the airway. As such, this scale is biased toward patients who demonstrate laryngeal penetration or aspiration. Many patients may demonstrate significant dysphagia in the absence of either laryngeal penetration or aspiration of material below the vocal folds. Like the DOSS, the Penetration-Aspiration Scale has demonstrated reliability but has not been validated. More recently, both Martin-Harris et al.[15] (Modified Barium Swallow Impairment Tool [MBSImp]) and Han et al.[17] (Videofluoroscopic Dysphagia Scale [VDS]) have attempted to systematically develop and validate protocols and scoring procedures for the videofluoroscopic swallowing study. Although neither the MBSImp nor the VDS is presently used in general clinical practice, both protocols demonstrate excellent approaches to developing a standardized, validated protocol and scoring system for the videofluoroscopic swallow study.

Additional measures of swallow performance have focused on timing aspects of swallowing. Logemann[9] recommended evaluation of the duration of bolus movement during a swallow and suggested evaluation of oral transit time, pharyngeal transit time, pharyngeal delay time, and esophageal transit time. She further defines a summary measure of swallowing function, the oropharyngeal swallow efficiency (OPSE) score, as the ratio of the percentage of material swallowed into the esophagus divided by oral plus pharyngeal transit times. Given imaging technology used to capture video images, the assessment of timing measures is relatively easy to complete. An additional form of measurement—biokinematic assessment—focuses on measuring the movement of various structures during swallowing events or combined movement with timing analysis. A variety of swallow movements have been reported with this approach, including maximal excursion of the hyoid bone and the larynx, maximal opening of the upper esophageal sphincter, and amount of pharyngeal constriction.[20-22]

Timing and movement assessments of swallowing do add an objective dimension beyond basic descriptions of swallowing patterns. However, as emphasized by McCullough et al.,[23] a need exists to validate many suggested measures and to reduce in number and define the multitude of measures that have been proposed for interpretation of the videofluoroscopic swallowing study. In the author's experience, clinicians formulate impressions of speed of movement of a bolus through the swallowing tract, but objective evaluation of specific timing components is not commonplace in clinical practice. Perhaps future research will identify aspects of objective timing and movement evaluation that are most meaningful in the clinical interpretation of swallowing deficits.

Strengths and Weaknesses of the Fluoroscopic Swallowing Study

The videofluoroscopic swallowing examination is considered the gold standard in the clinical assessment of dysphagia. This examination has many strengths that merit this designation. It is a dynamic study that when captured on videotape or other medium provides a thorough evaluation of the biomechanics of oropharyngeal swallowing with unlimited review capability. In addition, it provides a comprehensive perspective on swallowing from the lips through the esophagus. Finally, within the hospital setting it is typically readily accessible for both patient and clinician.

Despite these strengths of the fluoroscopic swallowing study, weaknesses and questions remain. The use of radiation may be of concern in some instances, especially when multiple, repeated studies are conducted. However, the amount of radiation in a single examination is quite small. The fluoroscopic examination also is not the best examination to evaluate pooled secretions because these will not be visualized with this procedure. Other concerns or areas of question include the following: documentation of aspiration but not the effects of aspiration, difficulty in appreciation of airway closure mechanisms, possibly limited access outside the hospital setting, exami-

Radiologists have various methods to image the swallowing/digestive system. Two common techniques include the standard barium swallowing study and scintigraphy. The first of these studies, the barium swallow study, may be referenced as the *upper gastrointestinal examination* (upper GI, UGI, or an esophagram). The focus of this radiologic examination is on the esophagus. The hypopharynx and the stomach may also be imaged during this procedure. Although variations of this study have been described, the procedure is typically completed with the patient in a lying, usually prone, position. Liquid barium is ingested in large volumes through a straw. The radiologist views the dynamic study in real time but usually captures only still images that demonstrate specific pathologies in the esophagus.

The second study, scintigraphy, is actually a nuclear medicine procedure. Scintigraphic studies use a radionuclide, commonly technetium-99 sulfur colloid, mixed with another substance. In the author's facility this radionuclide is often mixed in an egg-white solution, and the study is known as a "tech-egg study." However, the radionuclide may be mixed with a variety of semisolid or thick liquid foods. In this study, radiation is emitted from the radionuclide and is measured by a scintillation camera and computer. In simple terms, the patient swallows a radioactive material (of very low dose) and stands, sits, or lies in front of a radiation detector. The benefit of this technique is that the timing, direction, and location of the swallowed materials or any objectively measured portion of the swallowed material can be assessed. Thus gastric emptying studies may be completed by this technique to determine how much of a swallowed material leaves the stomach in a specified time period. This technique also can quantify the amount and depth of aspirated material. Although scintigraphy has been used in studies of oropharyngeal dysphagia, it is not routinely used in the clinical evaluation of this problem.

CRITICAL THINKING

1. For what types of dysphagia symptoms would a UGI be preferred over a videofluoroscopic swallowing study?
2. Discuss some limitations of conducting both a videofluoroscopic swallowing study and an esophagram during the same evaluation.
3. Discuss potential strengths and limitations of using scintigraphy in the evaluation of oropharyngeal dysphagia.

nation of only a very short period in an abnormal environment and thus possibly not truly reflective of functional eating abilities, possible problematic transportation to the radiology department, and inconsistent interpretation among clinicians. This list is not intended to cast aspersions on the videofluoroscopic swallowing examination. Rather, it serves as a group of caveats that clinicians may consider when conducting and interpreting this instrumental study.

ENDOSCOPIC SWALLOWING EXAMINATIONS

Differences Between the Endoscopic Swallowing Examination and the Fluoroscopic Swallowing Examination

Like the fluoroscopic swallowing examination, the endoscopic procedure is referred to by a variety of names. Videoendoscopic evaluation of dysphagia (VEED),[24] videoendoscopic swallowing study (VESS),[25] and fiberoptic endoscopic evaluation of swallowing safety (FEESS)[26] have all been used to describe similar procedures. The American Speech-Language-Hearing Association[3,27] recommends use of the term *fiberoptic endoscopic evaluation of swallowing* (FEES) as the generic identifier of this procedure, with the exception of a specific procedure to assess upper airway sensitivity fiberoptic endoscopic evaluation of swallowing with sensory testing (FEESST).[28] However, in keeping with the discussion of the fluoroscopic examination, this chapter uses the generic descriptive term *endoscopic swallowing examination*.

The endoscopic swallowing examination is newer than the fluoroscopic examination in the clinical arena of dysphagia and, as a result, is used by fewer professionals. This instrumental examination is growing in popularity and application and shares both similarities and differences with the fluoroscopic study. Box 10-7 summarizes the more salient similarities and differences between these two instrumental procedures to assess swallowing function.

Similarities

Both fluoroscopic and endoscopic procedures have a similar purpose in the assessment of swallowing. Each is intended to provide an objective assessment of the anatomy and physiology of the upper aerodigestive mechanisms used in swallowing. Although each procedure has distinct advantages or disadvantages over the other, both are intended for a similar purpose. Materials used in both examinations vary in amount and texture. The fluoroscopic study uses barium sulfate as a visible contrast agent, whereas the endoscopic study uses liquids and foods of natural or added

<table>
<tr><td>**BOX 10-7**</td><td>**Similarities and Differences between the Fluoroscopic and Endoscopic Swallow Studies**</td></tr>
</table>

SIMILARITIES
• Purpose
• Materials
• Process of evaluation

DIFFERENCES
• Technique
• Image perspective
• Portability
• Repeatability
• Duration of examination
• Sensory assessment

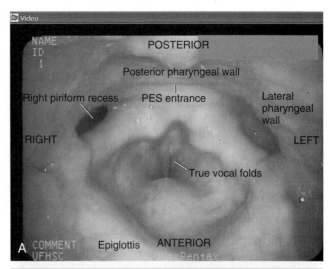

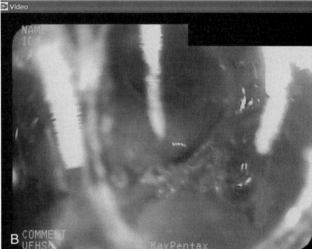

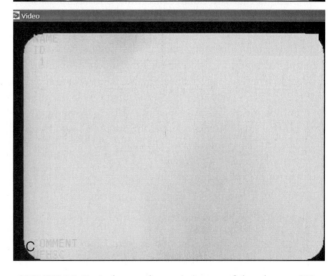

color to be visible. Thus both studies use a range of liquid and solid foods designed to be easily visualized by the respective examinations. Finally, both studies use a similar assessment process. Both procedures can evaluate the anatomy and physiology of the upper swallow mechanism, swallow function, and the impact of compensatory maneuvers.

Differences

Differences between the procedures include obvious technique differences. Aside from technique differences, the resulting images from the respective procedures differ. Fluoroscopy is considered to provide the more comprehensive perspective, including structures from the lips to the stomach. Endoscopy has imaging capability focused on the pharynx from the nasopharynx to the hypopharynx. Oral cavity and esophageal structure and function are not part of the typical endoscopic swallowing examination. In addition, although the endoscopic image is lost at the peak of the swallow or when material covers the end of the endoscope, the fluoroscopic image suffers no similar limitations. Figure 10-5 compares a clear endoscopic image, an image impaired by secretions on the endoscope, and a "whiteout" image that occurs at the swallowing peak. Despite the potential for image degradation during the endoscopic examination, this procedure is superior to fluoroscopy in the evaluation of anatomy and pooled secretion(s) within the swallowing mechanism. Another advantage of the endoscopic procedure is the potential for portability. Endoscopic systems are available that can be transported with relative ease to the patient in various locations, thus increasing access to this examination. Because endoscopy does not involve radiation,

FIGURE 10-5. A clear endoscopic image of the pharynx (**A**), an image obscured by secretions on the endoscope (**B**), and an example of "whiteout" (**C**). *PES*, Pharyngoesophageal segment.

repeated examinations are not viewed with as much concern as repeated fluoroscopic examinations. Also, because no radiation is used individual examinations can be somewhat longer than a fluoroscopic examination. Finally, with the endoscopic procedure sensory functions may be tested, albeit crudely, by touching the mucosa and asking the patient to acknowledge the tactile stimulus.

Procedures for the Endoscopic Swallowing Study

The endoscopic swallowing study is ideally suited to visualize the pharynx from nasopharynx to hypopharynx, the base of tongue region, and the larynx. Although slight variations have been described for this imaging study, certain elements are common across all variations.[24,28-30] In general the endoscopic swallowing study includes five components: (1) assessment of pharyngeal anatomy (including laryngeal structures), (2) evaluation of movement and sensation of pharyngeal structures, (3) assessment of secretions, (4) direct evaluation of swallowing function with liquid and solid material, and (5) evaluation of the impact of compensatory maneuvers.

Specialized equipment is required for this procedure. The minimal requirements for an adequate endoscopic system for evaluation of swallowing function include a fiberoptic endoscope, a light source, a camera, and a video recording system. These basic

elements are depicted in Figure 10-6. More advanced options include a recording device (videotape, DVD, or computer file), as seen in Figure 10-7. Video endoscopes are also available that provide excellent images as a result of placing the "camera" as a microchip at the distal end of the endoscope. Figure 10-8 shows comparison images from a regular endoscope and a videoscope.

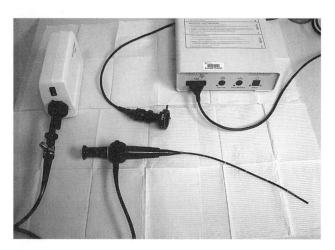

FIGURE 10-6. Basic equipment required for the endoscopic swallowing study: endoscope, light source, camera (video recording system not shown).

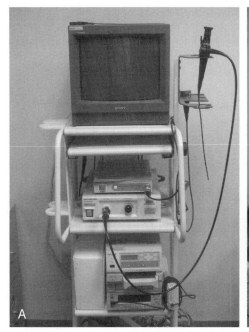 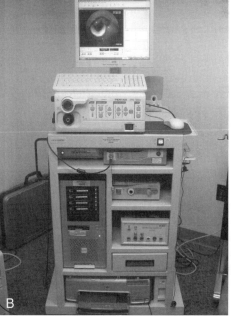

FIGURE 10-7. Complete endoscopy systems.

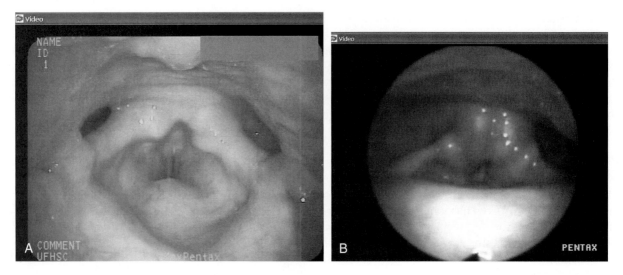

FIGURE 10-8. Examples of images from a videoscope (**A**) compared with a traditional scope (**B**).

The first step in the endoscopic procedure should be patient instruction. This is especially important for patients undergoing the examination for the first time. The **transnasal** endoscopic procedure is not painful, but it may be uncomfortable for some individuals. Whenever possible, the procedure should be thoroughly explained to the patient.

The next issue is whether to use nasal anesthesia. Historically, both a **vasoconstrictor** and anesthesia have been sprayed into the nose before the procedure. However, convincing evidence is available that neither medication is required for most examinations.[31,32] If used, these medications should be applied only under medical supervision and with appropriate administrative approvals because all medications have potential side effects.

Initially, the fiberoptic endoscope is passed through one nasal passage with care taken by the examiner to ensure that the scope stays in the **inferior nasal meatus** and away from the nasal septum. Once the scope is in the nasal **choana**, it may be positioned to view the velopharynx. (NOTE: Experienced endoscopists realize that the optimal view of the velopharynx is obtained with the scope placed in the middle nasal meatus. However, this can contribute to increased patient discomfort.) The function of the velopharyngeal mechanism can be examined by asking the patient to hum, produce vowels and consonants, and speak short sentences. Initially, a dry (saliva-only) swallow is completed to assess velar movement during swallowing. If nasopharyngeal reflux is suspected, this can initially be evaluated by looking for saliva passage through the velopharyngeal port during the dry swallow. It is preferable not to

Practice Note 10-3

Like many speech-language pathologists, I learned endoscopic techniques under the mentorship of an otolaryngologist. While working in the otolaryngology clinic it was customary to apply both a vasoconstrictor and topical anesthetic. Interestingly, many patients would tell me that this was the worst part of the examination and that the effects of the medications lasted well after the endoscopic examination was completed. Once I stopped using these medications, I would occasionally encounter a patient who had been first examined by a physician who used this technique. At times, they would say "Aren't you going to spray me first?" My response was to assure them that if a gentle approach was used, no medications were needed. Most, if not all of these patients, learned that the "numbing medications" were not necessary to perform this examination.

As a teacher and one who has conducted workshops on the endoscopic swallowing examination, I believe that clinicians should undergo this procedure themselves before they are allowed to use it to evaluate patients. This experience, though it should not be painful, usually gives the clinician a healthy respect for the gentle approach to transnasal endoscopy.

give the patient material to swallow at this point but to wait until the airway is clearly visualized.

After inspection of the velopharyngeal mechanism, the scope is advanced into the oropharynx with the tip positioned below the uvula and above the epiglottis. From this position the pharynx, including laryngeal structures, should be well visualized. Figure 10-9 presents the normal anatomic view from this position of the abducted and adducted larynx. Refer to narrated Video 2-4 on the Evolve site for more detailed information on normal swallowing viewed endoscopically. Assessment techniques for pharyngeal activities include falsetto phonation, performing the Valsalva maneuver, and swallowing various materials. Falsetto phonation facilitates medial movement of the lateral pharyngeal walls. This activity is a good method to identify hemipharyngeal weakness. The wall with little or no movement is likely to be paretic. The Valsalva maneuver is a method to expand the pharynx. This view may be helpful in identifying subtle anatomic deviations or as an indication of weakness on one side of the pharynx.

Assessment of laryngeal function includes activities for adduction and abduction, diadochokinesis, breath hold, and cough/clear actions. Simple phonation is adequate for laryngeal adduction. The vowel "ee" is most often used because it elongates the larynx and enhances the endoscopic view. Abduction may be evaluated by forced inhalation or sniffing. Laryngeal diadochokinesis may be assessed by alternating phonation and sniffing or by repeated productions of the syllable "see" or "he." Breath-hold maneuvers should include both a simple breath hold ("hold your breath") and a forced breath hold ("hold your breath and bear down"). It is well recognized that many adults do not completely close the larynx with a simple breath hold. Laryngeal closure is typically achieved with forced breath hold (barring significant anatomic or physiologic deficit). When a breath-hold maneuver may be incorporated into a therapy program, it is important to know whether a simple breath hold will achieve glottal closure or whether a forced breath hold is indicated. Finally, it is important to ascertain the patient's ability to execute a voluntary cough and whether that cough is sufficient to clear any pooled secretions or mucus from the vocal folds and/or laryngeal vestibule.

Attempted swallows should be completed with a range of materials that are clearly visible under endoscopic inspection. The selection and sequential presentation of materials to be swallowed follows concepts similar to the selection and sequential presentation of materials during the fluoroscopic examination. During each swallow, a period of whiteout occurs at the point of maximal pharyngeal constriction. After the swallow, the pharynx and larynx are again visible and assessment of airway compromise by penetration and/or aspiration and patterns of residue may be assessed. Again, although the view is different, the concepts of what to look for in the endoscopic examination are similar to those for the fluoroscopic examination. If impaired swallow physiology is identified, compensatory maneuvers may be implemented under endoscopic inspection to evaluate their impact on both the impaired physiology and the consequences of that impairment. Box 10-8 summarizes some salient techniques and observations to be included in the endoscopic swallowing examination. Clinicians are encouraged to seek formal training in this technique because it is relatively new in the dysphagia evaluation arena and not performed routinely by all practicing clinicians.

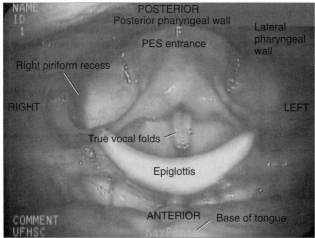

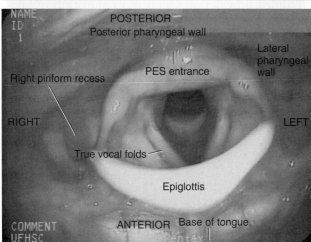

FIGURE 10-9. Normal endoscopic view of adducted (**A**) and abducted (**B**) larynx. *PES*, Pharyngoesophageal segment.

What to Look For

Much like the videofluoroscopic swallowing study, interpretation of the endoscopic swallowing study

BOX 10-8	Suggested Techniques and Observations for the Endoscopic Swallowing Evaluation

VELOPHARYNX
- Anatomic deviations
- Movement on phonation
- Movement on swallow
- Signs of material through sphincter during swallow

PHARYNX
- Anatomic deviations
- Secretions
- Movement on falsetto (medial movement of lateral pharyngeal walls)
- Valsalva maneuver—expand pharynx (pouches or other anatomic deviations)

LARYNX
- Anatomic deviations
- Secretions
- Movement on phonation—adduction
- Movement on breath hold/forced breath hold—adduction
- Movement on abduction—inhale or sniff
- Rapid alternating movement
- Cough

SWALLOW
- Vary volume and "consistency" of materials
- Oral containment: lingual-velar seal
- "Whiteout"—degree of pharyngeal constriction
- Residue
- Airway compromise—laryngeal penetration/aspiration
- Patient reaction to residue or airway compromise
- Impact of maneuvers and compensations

also is dominated by description.[29,30] A sample of descriptive observations from this examination is presented in Box 10-8. In general, examining clinicians should evaluate the anatomic integrity of each "level" (velopharynx, pharynx, larynx) of the swallowing mechanism. Basic movement characteristics of each level should be documented with specific reference to absent or reduced movement. Also, the presence of secretions should be noted. Secretions should be described in terms of location in the pharynx or larynx, amount and consistency (watery, thick, and so on), and movement during spontaneous swallows, throat clearing, or coughing. Once the basic anatomy and physiology of the swallow mechanism has been

evaluated, swallow attempts may be assessed. Much like the fluoroscopic swallow study, the patient should be observed attempting to swallow materials of different volumes and consistencies. Movements of swallowing structures should be described during swallow attempts. Airway compromise and residue should be described along with the patient's reaction to penetration, aspiration, or residue. Video 10-2 on the Evolve site presents a variety of abnormal swallow characteristics observed during the endoscopic swallow study.

In addition to basic descriptions, scales such as the Penetration-Aspiration Scale[19] that were initially developed for the videofluoroscopic swallowing study have been applied to interpretation of the endoscopic swallowing study.[33] Furthermore, similar to the fluoroscopic swallowing study, clinicians and investigators have considered a variety of timing measures to apply to the endoscopic swallowing study.[29] However, each measure presents the same strengths and limitations applied to the endoscopic swallowing study that were noted for the fluoroscopic swallowing study. Also similar to the videofluoroscopic swallowing study, recent attempts have emerged to quantify the interpretation of the endoscopic swallowing study and to identify those endoscopic observations that may be beneficial in clinical decision making about patients with dysphagia.[34-36] Still, as with recent similar attempts to quantify interpretation of fluoroscopic swallow studies, these protocols are not commonly used in general clinical practice.

Strengths and Weakness of the Endoscopic Swallowing Study

Like the fluoroscopic swallowing examination, the endoscopic procedure is a dynamic study that when recorded provides an objective examination of pharyngeal swallowing function with review capability. It provides a superior inspection of pharyngeal anatomy, sensation, laryngeal closure patterns, and secretions compared with fluoroscopy. Accessibility is deemed a strength of the endoscopic procedure because of the portability of equipment and no concern of x-ray exposure posed by repeated assessments. Some clinicians and researchers have used this technique in repeated applications as a biofeedback tool, often to teach patients airway protection strategies.[37,38] Finally, swallowing examinations with this procedure can be longer than with the fluoroscopic procedure because no radiation is involved.

Perhaps the biggest limitation of the endoscopic swallowing study is the relatively limited scope of view. Unlike the fluoroscopic study, this procedure does not provide imaging of the oral cavity, the PES, or the esophagus. The image and thus evaluation focus is clearly on pharyngeal aspects of swallowing. The issue of whiteout during the swallowing peak has been raised as a potential limitation of this procedure; however, in practice this brief period of image loss rarely affects the outcome of the evaluation and, in some instances, the absence of this normal finding implicates a weakened pharyngeal swallow.

Safety issues have been raised regarding this procedure; potential complications include nosebleed, **laryngospasm**, **vasovagal response**, and allergic reaction to medications when used. However, published reports of relatively large numbers of patients receiving this procedure have documented that it is a safe procedure with few complications.[29,39-42] As mentioned earlier in this section, additional research has demonstrated that neither anesthetics nor vasoconstrictors are necessary to complete this procedure.[31,32] Still, patient safety must be a primary concern in any clinical setting. Patients who may be combative or demonstrate movement disorders that might preclude completion of a safe examination or those patients with bleeding disorders might increase any risk factor associated with this procedure.

One final limitation of the endoscopic swallowing study merits consideration. Before engaging in either the application or the interpretation of endoscopic swallowing studies, clinicians must avail themselves of an appropriate degree of supervised training (of course, this same concern should be addressed for the fluoroscopic study). Published guidelines are available from the American Speech-Language-Hearing Association that detail the knowledge and skills required to undertake this procedure and suggest mechanisms to obtain appropriate training.[27,43]

DIRECT COMPARISONS BETWEEN FLUOROSCOPIC AND ENDOSCOPIC SWALLOWING EXAMINATIONS

Several investigations have undertaken direct comparisons between fluoroscopic and endoscopic swallowing examinations. Some comparisons have been practical suggestions for application based on clinical experience,[24,25] whereas others have been more rigorous comparisons of specific findings on the respective procedures in common groups of patients with dysphagia.[29,44] Recall that one advantage of the fluoroscopic procedure was a more comprehensive evaluation of swallowing from the lips to the stomach. Based on this advantage, the fluoroscopic procedure has been advocated as the preferred procedure for initial swallowing assessments and for instrumental assessment of dysphagia symptoms focused on the esophagus. Conversely, the endoscopic procedure provides a superior inspection of anatomy and secretions.[45] Based on this advantage, the endoscopic procedure has been advocated in cases involving paralysis secondary to cranial neuropathies, postsurgical or trau-

---

CLINICAL CORNER 10-3

This chapter has focused on the fiberoptic endoscopic swallowing study (FEES) procedure because this is the most common endoscopic procedure completed by dysphagia clinicians, including physicians and speech-language pathologists. However, other procedures, such as the commonly termed *esophagoscopy* (EGD or esophagogastroduodenoscopy) are frequently completely by gastroenterologists. A more recent procedure, *transnasal esophagoscopy* (TNE), is becoming increasing popular among otolaryngologists. Both procedures have the potential to evaluate the esophagus by using a longer and larger endoscope than the one used for the FEES procedure. The EGD procedure involves sedation of the patient, whereas TNE does not. During TNE the physician can also evaluate bolus transit though the esophagus because the awake patient can swallow various materials. TNE also affords the otolaryngologist the opportunity to evaluate the pharynx and larynx as the endoscope is passed transnasally in the awake patient.

Dysphagia clinicians may also encounter additional procedures such as capsule or pill endoscopy. As the name implies, this technique requires the patient to swallow a capsule (about the size of a vitamin pill) containing a wireless camera that transmits pictures to a small device worn by the patient. Video images are captured as the pill moves through the esophagus. In the author's experience to date, this procedure is not frequently encountered by clinicians working within the scope of oropharyngeal dysphagia.

CRITICAL THINKING

1. When would a patient benefit from a TNE procedure versus an FEES procedure?
2. Discuss specific symptoms that would suggest one examination over the other.
3. Discuss the reverse preference for FEES over TNE.
4. What other endoscopic imaging techniques can you identify that may be appropriate for patients with swallowing difficulties?

matic anatomic changes, or for any dysphagia in which the management and/or aspiration of secretions is problematic. Finally, because of the portability advantage of the endoscopic procedure and the absence of radiation exposure, this procedure has been advocated for patients who are not able to be transported (i.e., bedbound patients), for situations requiring repeated swallowing examinations, and for use as a biofeedback application in treatment. These advocated clinical preferences are summarized in Table 10-1.

Studies comparing specific findings between these two instrumental procedures have consistently identified a high degree of agreement. In general, agreement between these two imaging evaluations ranges between 60% and more than 90% across various items of interest. Table 10-2 summarizes the results of two studies comparing the same swallowing deficits.[46,47] Findings of residue or airway compromise reveal agreement averaging from 80% to 90% between these two procedures. However, Crary and Baron[48] offered a note of caution. These investigators compared endoscopic findings that were directly observed with those inferred from other findings with matched results from videofluoroscopic studies completed for the same patients. For example, if material was observed

entering the airway, this was a directly observed endoscopic finding. However, if residue was noted after a swallow on the endoscopic examination, the investigators may have inferred pharyngeal weakness, reduced laryngeal elevation, or reduced opening of the PES. Directly observed findings demonstrated much higher agreement with the fluoroscopic swallowing study than findings inferred from other endoscopic results. Crary and Baron concluded that when the endoscopic evaluation is dominated by inferred findings, a fluoroscopic examination should also be completed for the same patient. Thus depending on the requirements of the clinical situation, one procedure might be indicated over the other, or the two procedures might be used in a complementary fashion during the same dysphagia evaluation.

TAKE HOME NOTES

1. Instrumental studies of swallowing provide objective imaging of the anatomy and physiology of the swallowing mechanism and swallowing biomechanics across varying bolus and patient conditions.

2. Instrumental studies of swallowing should be strongly considered whenever a thorough clinical evaluation is insufficient to answer the pertinent clinical questions for a given patient. This may include delineation of dysphagia parameters, clarification of airway protection issues, the impact of compensatory maneuvers, and/or monitoring changes over time. These examinations may also provide information useful in understanding medical conditions that underlie dysphagia.

3. Commonalities exist between procedures for the fluoroscopic and endoscopic swallowing examinations. Both provide dynamic imaging of the swallowing mechanism and performance, use multiple bolus volumes and textures, and have the potential to evaluate the impact of compensatory maneuvers on swallowing safety and efficiency. In addition, each may be modified to address individual needs of specific patient groups or dysphagia characteristics.

4. Both instrumental swallowing examinations have strengths and weakness that might affect their optimal use. The fluoroscopic study offers the more comprehensive perspective of the swallowing mechanism, whereas the endoscopic study offers the superior view of anatomy and secretions. Certain weaknesses are common to both procedures. They may document the presence of aspiration but do not address the consequences of aspiration. They evaluate swallowing performance

TABLE 10-1

Relative Clinical Advantages and Uses of Fluoroscopic and Endoscopic Swallow Studies

Application	Advantage Fluoroscopy	Advantage Endoscopy
Initial evaluation	✓	
Esophageal dysphagia	✓	
Paresis/paralysis (cranial nerve)		✓
Anatomic deviations		✓
Evaluate secretions		✓
Patient cannot be transported		✓
Repeated use		✓
Biofeedback		✓

TABLE 10-2

Results of Two Studies Comparing Specific Findings of Fluoroscopic and Endoscopic Swallow Studies

Finding	Study 1	Study 2
Pharyngeal residue	80%	89%
Aspiration	90%	86%
Laryngeal penetration	85%	86%
Premature spillage (posterior)	66%	61%

Numbers reflect percent agreement between the two instrumental examinations.

in abnormal environments using procedures that do not resemble functional eating activities. Despite these potential criticisms, these examinations are important in the assessment of swallowing performance.

5. Published reports indicate strong agreement between the fluoroscopic and endoscopic swallowing studies—specifically, in the identification of individual dysphagia characteristics such as post-swallow residue and aspiration. Agreement in the identification of specific clinical findings along with consideration of the relative strengths and weaknesses of each procedure will help with the appropriate application of either and/or both procedures.

CLINICAL CASE EXAMPLE 10-1

An 85-year-old woman was seen in the outpatient dysphagia clinic. The patient currently resides in a long-term care facility. The facility staff were concerned because the patient is declining food and is beginning to lose weight. In addition, she has been reported to cough during mealtimes. Her adult son accompanied her to the evaluation and served as the primary informant. He visits his mother at least twice each week and has observed mealtimes and participated in feeding her. The patient is unable to self-feed because of severe arthritis in her hands. She has moderate dementia but is able to communicate her preferences and dislikes with simple responses. She is receiving a total oral diet of pureed foods and thickened liquids. She indicates that she does not like this diet and that the food has no taste. On occasion the family has brought regular food to her and observed her eat it without difficulty. Clinical examination revealed no gross abnormality in cranial nerve function or any anatomic deviations in the oral structures. Voice was deemed appropriate for her age and medical condition. Volitional cough was intact. The patient was provided a range of material to swallow based on the report of her daily oral intake. Initially thickened liquids were presented with a spoon. The patient was able to swallow these without difficulty or post-swallow voice change. Larger amounts of thickened liquid were provided from a cup. Again, no difficulties were detected. Subsequently thin liquid (fruit juice) was provided first by spoon, then by cup,

then by straw. A single cough was observed after cup drinking. No difficulties were observed during straw drinking. Pudding was presented in spoon-size amounts. Lingual mastication was evident and no difficulties were observed. Subsequently, a cracker was presented. Mastication was obvious, but oral residue was observed after swallow attempts. Thin liquid was presented by a straw to clear the oral residue. No overt signs of aspiration were noted and the voice was clear after drinking. Oral residue was cleared with straw drinking.

INTERPRETATION

This patient did not require any instrumental examination for swallowing function. Clinical examination with swallowing evaluation was sufficient in addressing the concerns regarding her refusal of food and occasional coughing during meals. Recommendations for this patient included upgrading her diet to soft mechanical or further depending on preference and tolerance and allowing her to drink thin liquids. An occupational therapy consultation was generated to fashion a cup-holding device to allow the patient to drink thin liquids (specifically water) through a straw at her discretion. Follow-up with this patient indicated that the recommendations were implemented; food and liquid intake increased and no dysphagia-related complications were encountered.

CLINICAL CASE EXAMPLE 10-2

A 64-year-old man presents to a dysphagia clinic after radiation therapy for a tonsillar fossa carcinoma. The patient reported dry mouth (xerostomia), which made it difficult for him to swallow dry, solid foods, and moderate pain in his throat that was worse with any swallow. He had no overt cranial nerve deficits, but his voice was mildly hoarse (he reported that this was a result of the radiation therapy). He reported that he consistently coughed to clear thickened secretions from his throat.

INTERPRETATION

This patient presented with several indications for completion of an endoscopic swallowing examination. He had received radiation therapy, which can contribute to xerostomia, mucositis, anatomic changes, and even physiologic changes in the pharyngeal structures used in swallowing. He demonstrated voice changes meriting inspection of the laryngeal valve, and he reported pooling of thickened secretions. Endoscopic swallowing study revealed thickened secretions bilaterally in the piriform sinuses and to a lesser degree within the laryngeal vestibule. The vocal folds were mobile but **edematous** and **erythematous**, suggesting irritation, and the left vocal fold was slightly bowed, creating a small glottal gap during phonation. Swallowing attempts of various consistencies revealed no difficulties with thin or thick liquids but mild post-swallow residue in the hypopharynx for pudding and masticated materials. This residue was completely cleared with subsequent swallows of thin liquid. Based on the results of this examination no fluoroscopic study was completed. Recommendations were to continue total oral feeding, to moisten the mouth before ingestion of pudding or solid materials, to use liquids to clear residue from more solid foods, and to consult his oncologist for treatment of mucositis.

CLINICAL CASE EXAMPLE 10-3

A 76-year-old man reports swallowing difficulty after a hemispheric stroke. His primary complaint is that food sticks; he localizes the problem to the base of the neck just above the sternum. He complains of having excess saliva that causes him to cough. His cough is weak, and his voice is dysphonic and breathy.

INTERPRETATION

This patient has dysphagia complaints that require both endoscopic and fluoroscopic swallowing examinations. Difficulty managing secretions, weak cough, and voice changes are indications for an endoscopic examination of pharyngeal and laryngeal functions. Reports of food sticking at the level of the neck base indicate the need to complete a fluoroscopic examination. Endoscopic examination revealed a left vocal fold paresis with incomplete glottal closure, and pooled "foamy" secretions throughout the hypopharynx and in the laryngeal vestibule. Falsetto maneuver revealed a paretic left hemipharynx. Swallow attempts revealed post-swallow residue in the left piriform sinus that

increased as the viscosity of the swallowed material increased. Fluoroscopic swallowing study confirmed a left hemipharyngeal paresis and incomplete opening of the pharyngeal esophageal segment with less opening on the left side. Recommendations initially focused on referral to an otolaryngologist for consideration of vocal fold medialization and procedures to improved pharyngoesophageal segment opening.

References

1. American Speech-Language-Hearing Association: *Clinical indicators for instrumental assessment of dysphagia [guidelines]*. Available at www.asha.org/policy.

2. American Speech-Language-Hearing Association: *Guidelines for speech-language pathologists performing videofluoroscopic swallowing studies [guidelines]*. Available at www.asha.org/policy.

3. American Speech-Language-Hearing Association: *Role of the speech-language pathologist in the performance and interpretation of endoscopic evaluation of swallowing: guidelines [guidelines]*. Available at www.asha.org/policy.

4. Logemann J: *Evaluation and treatment of swallowing disorders*, San Diego, 1983, College-Hill Press.

5. Palmer JB, Kuhlemeier KV, Tippett DC et al: A protocol for the videofluorographic swallowing study, *Dysphagia* 8:209, 1993.

6. Martin-Harris B, Jones B: The videofluorographic swallowing study, *Phys Med Rehabil Clin North Am* 19:769, 2008.

7. Roberts MW, Tylenda CA, Sonies BC et al: Dysphagia in bulimia nervosa, *Dysphagia* 4:106, 1989.

8. Peruzzi WT, Logemann JA, Currie D et al: Assessment of aspiration in patients with tracheostomies: comparison of the bedside colored dye assessment with videofluoroscopic examination, *Respir Care* 46:243, 2001.

9. Logemann JA: *Manual for the videofluorographic study of swallowing*, ed 2, Austin, TX, 1993, Pro-ED.

10. Buchholz DW, Bosma JF, Donner MW. Adaptation, compensation, and decompensation of the pharyngeal swallow, *Gastrointest Radiol* 10:235, 1985.

11. Kahrilas PJ, Lin S, Logemann JA et al: Deglutitive tongue action: volume accommodation and bolus propulsion, *Gastroenterology* 104:152, 1993.

12. Kahrilas PJ, Lin S, Chen J et al: Oropharyngeal accommodation to swallow volume, *Gastroenterology* 111:297, 1996.

13. Kendall KA, Leonard RJ, McKenzie SW: Accommodation to changes in bolus viscosity in normal deglu-

tition: a videofluoroscopic study, *Ann Otol Rhinolaryngol* 110:1059, 2001.

14. Adnerhill I, Eckberg O, Groher ME: Determining normal bolus size for thin liquids, *Dysphagia* 4:1, 1989.

15. Martin-Harris B, Brodsky MB, Michel Y et al: MBS measurement tool for swallow impairment—MBSImp: establishing a standard, *Dysphagia* 23:392, 2008.

16. Groher ME, Crary MA, Carnaby-Mann GD et al: The impact of rheologically controlled materials on the identification airway compromise on the clinical and videofluoroscopic swallowing examinations, *Dysphagia* 21:218, 2006.

17. Han TR, Paik NJ, Park JW et al: The prediction of persistent dysphagia beyond six months after stroke, *Dysphagia* 23:59, 2008.

18. O'Neil KH, Purdy M, Falk J et al: The dysphagia outcome and severity scale. *Dysphagia* 14:139, 1999.

19. Rosenbek JC, Robbins JA, Roecker EB et al: A penetration-aspiration scale, *Dysphagia* 11:93, 1996.

20. Crary MA, Butler MK, Baldwin BO: Objective distance measurements from videofluorographic swallow studies using computer interactive analysis: technical note, *Dysphagia* 9:116, 1994.

21. Kendal KA, McKenzie S, Leonard RJ et al: Timing of events in normal swallowing: a videofluoroscopic study, *Dysphagia* 15:74, 2000.

22. Kendall KA, Leonard RJ: Pharyngeal constriction in elderly dysphagic patients compared with young and elderly nondysphagic controls, *Dysphagia* 16:272, 2001.

23. McCullough GH, Wertz RT, Rosenbek J et al: Clinicians' preferences and practices in conducting clinical/bedside and videofluorographic swallowing examinations in an adult, neurogenic population, *Am J Speech Lang Pathol* 8:149, 1999.

24. Bastian RW: Videoendoscopic evaluation of patients with dysphagia: an adjunct to the modified barium swallow, *Otolaryngol Head Neck Surg* 104:339, 1991.

25. Bastian RW: The videoendoscopic swallowing study: an alternative and partner to the videofluoroscopic swallowing study, *Dysphagia* 8:359, 1993.

26. Langmore SE, Shatz K, Olsen N: Fiberoptic endoscopic examination of swallowing safety: a new procedure, *Dysphagia* 2:216, 1998.

27. American Speech-Language-Hearing Association: *The role of the speech-language pathologist in the performance and interpretation of endoscopic evaluation of swallowing; [technical report].* Available at www.asha.org/policy.

28. Aviv J, Kim T, Sacco R et al: FEESST: a new beside endoscopic test of the motor and sensory components of swallowing, *Ann Otol Rhinolaryngol* 107:378, 1998.

29. Langmore SE: *Endoscopic evaluation and treatment of swallowing disorders*, New York, 2001, Thieme.

30. Murray J: *Manual of dysphagia assessment in adults*, San Diego, 1999, Singular Publishing.

31. Leder SB, Ross D, Briskin KB et al: A prospective, double blind, randomized study on the use of a topical anesthetic, vasoconstrictor, and placebo during transnasal flexible fiberoptic endoscopy, *J Speech Lang Res* 40:1352, 1997.

32. Singh V, Brockbank M, Todd G: Flexible transnasal endoscopy: is local anesthetic necessary? *Laryngol Otol* 111:616, 1997.

33. Colodny N: Interjudge and intrajudge reliabilities in fiberoptic endoscopic evaluation of swallowing (fees) using the penetration-aspiration scale: a replication study, *Dysphagia* 17:308, 2002.

34. Farneti D: Pooling score: an endoscopic model for evaluating severity of dysphagia, *Acta Otorhinolaryngol Ital* 28:135, 2008.

35. Farneti D: Endoscopic scale for evaluation of severity of dysphagia: preliminary observations, *Rev Laryngol Otol Rhinol* 129:137, 2008.

36. Dziewas R, Warnecke T, Olenberg S et al: Towards a basic endoscopic assessment of swallowing in acute stroke—development and evaluation of a simple dysphagia score, *Cerebrovasc Disord* 26:41, 2008.

37. Denk DM, Kaider A: Videoendoscopic biofeedback: a simple method to improve the efficacy of swallowing rehabilitation of patients after head and neck surgery, *ORL J Otorhinolaryngol Relat Spec* 59:100, 1997.

38. Leder SB, Novella S, Patwa H: Use of fiberoptic endoscopic evaluation of swallowing (FEES) in patients with amyotrophic lateral sclerosis, *Dysphagia* 19:177, 2004.

39. Warnecke T, Teismann I, Oelenberg S et al: The safety of fiberoptic endoscopic evaluation in acute stroke patients, *Stroke* 40:482, 2009.

40. McGowan SL, Gleeson M, Smith M et al: A pilot study of fiberoptic endoscopic evaluation of swallowing in patients with cuffed tracheostomies in neurological intensive care, *Neurocrit Care* 6:90, 2007.

41. Aviv JE, Mury T, Zschommier A et al: Flexible endoscopic evaluation of swallowing with sensory testing: patient characteristics and analysis of safety in 1,340 consecutive examinations, *Ann Otol Rhinol Laryngol* 114:173, 2005.

42. Cohen MA, Setzen M, Perlman PW et al: The safety of flexible endoscopic evaluation of swallowing with sensory testing in an outpatient otolaryngology setting, *Laryngoscope* 113:21, 2003.

43. American Speech-Language-Hearing Association: Knowledge and skills needed by speech-language pathologists providing services to individuals with swallowing and/or feeding disorders, *ASHA Supplement* 22:81, 2002.

44. Périé S, Laccourreye L, Flahault A et al: Role of videoendoscopy in assessment of pharyngeal function in

oropharyngeal dysphagia: comparison with videofluoroscopy and manometry, *Laryngoscope* 108:1712, 1998.

45. Schröter-Morasch H, Bartolome G, Troppmann N et al: Values and limitations of pharyngolaryngoscopy (transnasal, transoral) in patients with dysphagia, *Folia Phoniatr Logop* 51:172, 1999.

46. Langmore SE, Shatz K, Olson N: Endoscopic and videofluoroscopic evaluations of swallowing and aspiration, *Ann Otol Rhinolaryngol* 100:678, 1991.

47. Wu CH, Hsiao TY, Chen JC et al: Evaluation of swallowing safety with fiberoptic endoscope: comparison with videofluoroscopic technique, *Laryngoscope* 107:396, 1997.

48. Crary MA, Baron J: Endoscopic and fluoroscopic evaluations of swallowing: comparison of observed and inferred findings, *Dysphagia* 12:108, 1997.

Chapter 11

Special Considerations in Evaluating Infants and Children

JO PUNTIL-SHELTMAN AND HELENE TAYLOR

OBJECTIVES

1. Identify and understand the five subsystems of the premature infant.
2. Identify and understand four types of premature infant stress cues.
3. Identify and understand the three stages of premature infant development.
4. Identify three oral reflexes typically seen in infants.
5. Understand the purpose of the outpatient clinical feeding evaluation.
6. Understand the individual roles of the caregiver and feeding specialist in the clinical feeding evaluation.
7. Describe the sequence of activities in the clinical feeding evaluation.

INFANTS

Evaluation of the term infant and the preterm infant is quite different. Infants born prematurely with congenital or acquired medical conditions are at higher risk of developing feeding and nutritional problems than term, healthy newborns.[1] The preterm infant presents an interesting model for the understanding of sensory stress on the developing brain. Neurobehavioral and neuroelectrophysiologic studies show that the preterm infant is prone to deficits. These may include attention deficits; sensory and motor disorganization; difficulties in self-regulation; and modulation of autonomic, motor, sensory, and affective interactive state systems that can continue well into preschool years.[2] The subsystems of a preterm infant play a vital role in feeding. These systems include (1) physiologic stability, (2) motor performance, (3) state systems, (4) attention, and (5) self-regulatory systems. The infant's subsystems require continuous regulatory and facilitative structuring in their environment (usually the neonatal intensive care unit [NICU]) to support effective learning and maturation.[3] Feeding specialists need to assist the preterm infant in regulating these systems to achieve successful oral ingestion. The time from the initiation of oral feedings to **ad lib** oral feedings in the preterm infant may be days to several weeks or months.

INFANT SUBSYSTEMS

Human development is shaped by dynamic, continuous interactions between biology and experience. In the evaluation of any infant, all subsystems should be continuously observed to assess the infant's response to external stimuli. Preterm infants may have difficulty synchronizing and integrating all these subsystems. Similar patterns with integration may be seen in healthy term infants.

Physiologic Support Systems

Assessing these systems includes monitoring the infant's respiratory patterns, heart rate, and skin color. The clinician should observe the intensity or severity of the signs present, not their absolute numeric values. Automatically mediated movements include tremors, startles, reflexive eye movements, and sounds such as whimpers and cries. The behavioral indications of decreased visceral control include hiccups, spitting up, gagging, and bowel movements. It is important to observe the baseline color of the infant's skin during quiet sleep. Any changes from normal to dusky, pale gray or blue are abnormal.

Motor System

Assessing the motor system includes observations of the infant's posture at rest and how it is modulated during movement in his or her environment or when stimulated. When observing the infant's posture, the clinician should check for flaccidity, abnormal flexion and extension patterns, and tone that varies abnormally between hypertonicity and hypotonicity. Well-organized motor systems in infants demonstrate **modulated tone** and an ability to maintain flexion. Their movements are controlled without variability. Infants remain in a tucked position, maintaining flexor posture when grasping. Normal motor organization in infants includes the ability to brace, suck, and stabilize their posture in an appropriate position without swaddling. Motor disorganization in an infant is characterized by splaying of the arms or legs and arching movements with increased muscle tension during stimulation. Arms and legs may be hyperextended and hypertonic with rigid extensions or overly flexed with arms tight in to the chest. The clinician should note whether motor movements are diffuse, overly abrupt, or lack movement after effort. Further assessments of motor organization should be made while the infant is in transition from a sleep to an alert state, during routine medical procedures, when feeding, and while being held.

State System

Observations of eye movements, eye opening, facial expressions, gross body movements, and respiratory patterns should be made when the infant is in a sleep state, in transition from sleep to awakened, and when fully awake. The ability to transition from one state to another without disruption of physiologic homeostasis is a precursor to normal cognitive and motor development. When the state systems are well organized, infants usually have periods of restful sleep with easy transition from one state to another. Organized infants also normally show periods of quiet alert and demonstrate a relaxed, calm, awake state. The cortically disorganized infant may sleep with frequent squirms, irregular activity, irregular respirations, and abrupt changes from awake to sleep or sleep to awake. Such infants may be fussy, irritable with sudden arousal, and abnormally reactive to environmental stimuli and appear fragile. At times the brightness of the room may interfere with the infant's ability to regulate external stimuli. Because of these distractions some infants may look away or avert their gaze when stimulated with face-to-face contact. The alert state is assessed by observing their interaction with caretakers during an alert state.

Disorganization in state systems can range from mild to severe. Mild sleep disorganization is characterized by generalized jerky movements, facial twitching or grimacing, or an irregular respiratory pattern. The transition from a sleep to awake state with mild drowsiness and diffuse movements with whimpers may be common. When awake, infants are alert and quiet with minimal motor activity or they are briefly fussy. Moderate disorganization is characterized by frantic movements while infants are awake with an unsteady respiratory and heart rate. Often they are irritable and fussy. Severe disorganization is characterized by hyperalert states with a look of panic or fear, which may be followed by motor flaccidity and inactivity. Once infants are overwhelmed by external stimuli they may not respond to any further stimuli.

Attention System

Close observation of the duration and quality of the alert state and the degree to which the infant is available to interact with his or her environment are important. Disorganized patterns of attention are often consistent with eye gaze aversion or closing, poor attention to task, or hyperactivity followed by inactivity during periods of stimulation. Other issues that should be addressed include whether the infant attends to social stimuli and inanimate objects or if the infant is able to transition to an alert state independently or needs assistance. In addition, does the infant actively inspect the environment, and is the attention to that environment controlled?

Self-Regulatory System

Self-regulation is demonstrated by how well the infant can maintain a deep or quiet sleep state or maintain a calm state when alert. It is important to observe the strategies the infant uses to accomplish the task of maintaining a calm state. Baseline measures of how long the infant is able to maintain this state should be made. Observations of the amount of effort needed to achieve this state and the amount of external support needed should be documented.

DEVELOPMENTAL STAGES

Premature infants normally develop the ability to interact as their nervous system matures. Gorski et al.[4] termed this process "neurosocial, behavioral development." The initial stage in this development is known as *in-turning*. Infants in this stage are generally younger than 32 weeks' postconceptional age (PCA) and respond to the environment in a purely physiologic manner. Infants are mainly in a sleep state, with no ability to regulate arousal. They demonstrate involun-

tary and jerky movements and are unable to engage socially. They can be easily stressed, may need ventilatory support, and generally devote all energy to autonomic stability and homeostasis. The second stage is termed *coming out*. This stage is characterized by improved physiologic stability. Infants are between 32 and 35 weeks' PCA and demonstrate more frequent periods of alertness. They may maintain color, oxygen saturation, and respiratory stability and a consistent heart rate during some interactions. These infants continue to be easily stressed, although they may participate in brief interactions demonstrating visual, auditory, and social responses. Infants at this stage slowly begin the feeding process. The third stage is known as *active reciprocity*. Infants in this stage are generally 36 weeks' PCA and older. Infants have the capacity for self-arousal and self-soothing. They actively seek stimuli and may tolerate some stressful interactions without a loss of physiologic stability. This stage is indicative of neurobehavioral maturation and tolerance for mutually satisfying experiences with caregivers.

BEDSIDE DEVELOPMENTAL AND/OR FEEDING EVALUATION

Neurodevelopmental assessments are designed to consider factors that influence early development, such as whether the infant is born at term or preterm or whether the infant is at risk for developmental delay. Many tests have been developed and researched to assess feeding the term and preterm infant. Most institutions use a combination of tests that measure physiologic, motor, state-regulatory, attentional-interactive, self-regulatory, and feeding processes. Several published clinical assessment scales have been developed.[5-10] It is wise to review all these and ascertain the best assessment tool for the infant being evaluated. Regardless of the test choice, the developmental specialist should be careful to observe the threshold at which an infant shifts from an organized to a disorganized response. Testing conditions should be standardized to prevent excessive variability over multiple testing sessions.

History

A comprehensive history should be completed, including gestational age, adjusted age, birth weight, and any abnormalities associated with the birth. **Apgar scores**, perinatal complications, hospitalization history, cardiopulmonary history, any radiologic or ultrasound procedures, and laboratory values should be reviewed for any abnormality.

State Systems

The sleep, transition to awake, and awake states should be assessed as previously described.

Posture and Tone

These factors include the infant's posture and tone in various positions. Infants who are born at 28 to 32 weeks are more hypotonic in the upper and lower limbs. As infants mature they demonstrate increased tone—increased flexion in the lower extremities followed by the upper extremities. The developmental specialist assesses reflexes and positions expected at certain maturity levels, which hopefully correlate with the estimated gestational age of the infant. Clinicians look at active tone in prone suspension, **slip through**, trunk support, neck flexors and extensors, and lower extremity abilities. Posture and passive tone positions include the infant's posture when supine, in a heel-to-ear maneuver, **popliteal angle**, **scarf sign**, and return to flexion of the forearm to determine the age of the infant. It is also important to observe midline orientation, head and neck control, overall postural control, and movement patterns to ascertain the effects of the tone on feeding.

Reflexes

Certain reflexes are seen early in the infant's life, and others emerge later in maturity. By 28 to 32 weeks' gestational age, the infant demonstrates the rooting, sucking (weak at 28 weeks), plantar grasp, flexor withdrawal, extensor thrust, and poor responses to the crossed extension and **Moro reflexes**. By 32 to 36 weeks' gestational age, the infant demonstrates a more refined root (including head turning), suck (inconsistent irregular), palmar grasp, the Moro reflex in the lower extremities, Galant reflex, neonatal neck righting (at 34 weeks), proprioceptive placing of legs (35 weeks), neonatal positive support (35 weeks), and the emergence of the tonic neck (asymmetric tonic reflex [ATR]). All these reflexes are more refined and present by 36 to 40 weeks' gestational age.

Adaptive Responses

An infant's response to touch during bedside care and procedures and during feeding become more organized and mature the older the gestational age. From 32 to 34 weeks' gestational age, infants may respond poorly to handling and be easily stressed. They may be difficult to console and are unable to self-regulate without external support. They may be inattentive or demonstrate brief responses to stimuli. Infants at this age may not focus or can only briefly follow a stimulus. Some stress signs may include hiccups, sneezes, passing gas or having bowel movements, nasal flaring, cries, splaying of arms and/or legs, arching, gaze aversion, and no apparent response to external stimuli. As infants mature, their responses become more controlled.

Physiologic Stability

In general, the earlier the gestational age the more unstable the infant's ability to regulate physiologic stability. The clinician should observe the infant's baseline cardiac and respiratory function (rate and depth of breathing), and color. When testing motor activity during feeding, it is important for the clinician to observe the infant's physiologic response to the potential stress of this activity. This includes assessing possible changes in respiratory patterns resulting from the work of breathing. Increased signs of stress such as nasal flaring, use of respiratory accessory muscles, respiratory fatigue, an ability to modulate nonnutritive suck patterns, cry, and postural retractions should be documented. It may be important to monitor the patterns of oxygen saturation during feeding versus sleep. Evaluating the sounds of respiration is important. Normal breathing is smooth and effortless. Extraneous noises may indicate a problem of dynamic airway compliance. Observations of changes in skin color or cardiac rate and rhythm should be made because they may change as respiratory patterns change due to the demands of any external task involving motor activity.

Oral Reflexes

Assessment of the sensory and motor components of the facial and intraoral structures is essential before the infant attempts oral feedings. The clinician should observe the infant's oral structures at rest and in response to light touch on the face, lips, and intraorally. Normally infants enjoy playful/light touching in their mouths. Their response to the placement of a finger or pacifier in the mouth should be observed. Was the response one of pleasure or did it markedly alter the infant's baseline homeostatic state? Reflexes that are present in utero, at birth, and throughout one's lifetime are the gag, cough, **transverse tongue**, and swallow. Oral reflexes that should be present after birth are the rooting (32 weeks up to 6 months), sucking (17 weeks up to 4 months), palmomental (see below, birth to 3 or 4 months), Santmyer (see below, 34 weeks to 1 to 2 years), and phasic bite (28 weeks to 9 to 12 months). These reflexes assist in the acquisition of food but disappear or are integrated by muscle function at the aforementioned intervals.[11]

The *rooting reflex* is elicited by stroking the perioral area, which normally results in the infant turning toward the stimulus and opening the mouth. Notation of the presence, inconsistency, or absence of the rooting reflex should be made. The *suck* is assessed with a gloved finger placed in the infant's mouth to feel the strength and rhythm of the suck as well as the function of the tongue. The *gag reflex* is elicited by placing a little finger in the posterior oral cavity. Observe if the reflex is present, diminished, or absent. The *palmomental reflex* is elicited by providing bilateral, quick pressure on the palms. The normal response in newborns is depression of the mandible and an accompanying sucking motion. The *Santmyer reflex* is tested by delivering a quick puff of air to the perioral area of an infant who is awake. Normally, this elicits a swallow. The phasic bite reflex is elicited by stimulating the molar region on the mandibular ridge. Normally this results in a rhythmic up-and-down movement of the mandible. The characteristics of the tongue are evaluated by noting the shape of the tongue, the frenulum, symmetric movements, and if the tongue moves up, down, and laterally. The shape of the hard and soft palates, the buccal musculature, and pharynx should be inspected before any feedings.

Nonnutritive Suck

The nonnutritive suck is the key to neurologic readiness for feeding and neurologic integrity. The nonnutritive suck is elicited by using either a little finger or a pacifier inside the infant's mouth. The normal rate should be 2 sucks per second, and if possible, sucking should be evaluated for at least 1 minute to evaluate any signs of fatigue. It is important to look and feel the strength, rhythm, endurance, impact on breathing, speed, and general motor organization. Does the infant demonstrate a strong, sustained, and rhythmic suck, or is it weak, irregular, and interferes with normal respiration?

Nutritive Suck

Before assessing a nutritive suck the infant needs to be in a quiet, alert state and hungry. Ideally this evaluation should be done in a quiet setting without potential distractions. The clinician should see if the infant is rooting and shows an interest in feeding. Some institutions orally feed an infant with a nasogastric tube in place, and some remove the tube and reinsert it after feeding if necessary. The preterm infant should be swaddled in a blanket for proper containment and positioning during the feeding. The clinician assesses which feeding position is most beneficial. Positions vary from the cradle hold, upright facing away from the caretaker, facing the caretaker, or side-lying. The infant's lower lip or corner of the mouth is touched with a nipple from a breast or bottle to elicit a rooting reflex. Once the infant provides the open-mouth gesture, the nipple is placed on top of the tongue. Normally, the infant leads the progression and length of feeding, including pauses from and resumption of sucking. It is important to document the strength, rhythm, endurance, speed, and motor organization of the suck. The clinician notes again if the feeding process affects the infant's breathing patterns, the coordination of the dynamics of the suck and swallow bursts, and the overall pattern of sucking. Normal nutritive sucking occurs at a rate of 1 suck per second. The sucking "bursts" can be as many as 10 to 30 followed by a pause for breathing. The healthy term infant demonstrates continuous sucking and swallowing bursts and integrates breathing effortlessly within the bursts. A full feeding should last from 15 to 20 minutes. This time frame allows the feeding specialist time to evaluate the infant's response to the feeding and stability of all the subsystems that support normal feeding.

INSTRUMENTAL EVALUATION

The details of the instrumental evaluation of swallowing in adults were described in Chapter 10. Similar examinations are used with infants, although positioning during the examination and the stimuli used may differ. Because of the potential risks of x-radiation in infants, the videofluorographic swallowing study is used more judiciously than in adults. Therefore radiographic studies may be shorter in duration. Issues of cooperation during the study may also differ. In general, the oral, pharyngeal, and esophageal phases of swallow are studied in all persons with dysphagia. In infants, children, and adults, the lower gastrointestinal tract also may require evaluation.

Videofluoroscopic Swallowing Study

The videofluoroscopic swallowing study (VSS) for preterm and term infants is usually completed in the upright lateral position using special supportive devices for proper positioning. A Tumble Form seat (Patterson Medical/Sammons Preston, Bolingbrook, Ill.) can be placed on a chair and adjusted to upright and semi-upright positions. For preterm and term infants, only liquid barium is used to ascertain the safety of oral feedings. At 5 to 7 months it is common to use a variety of pureed foods and fluids. Once the infant is 12 months old, more textures and viscosities are used in the assessment. The infant is tested with thin liquid barium with a bottle and nipple. A variety of nipples and bottles with variable flow rates may be used to determine whether the infant can tolerate liquids safely. The clinician may need to pace the infant throughout the procedure for safe swallowing, and at times the liquid barium may need to be thickened for the infant to tolerate oral feedings safely. Assessment of the oral phase includes observations of the organization of the suck-swallow-breathe sequence, the amount of bursts the infant is capable of performing, the position of the lips and tongue on the nipple, and head position. Infants may channel barium into the valleculae before initiation of the swallow; this is considered part of the normal swallow.[12,13] If the pharyngeal phase is slow or demonstrates reduced motility, the child may be at risk for aspiration. Infants may not show overt signs of coughing during aspiration. Usually aspiration is seen in the anterior trachea. When the infant is positioned properly, the esophageal phase can be evaluated. Ideally there will be a strong primary peristaltic wave that clears all material through the lower esophageal sphincter into the stomach. A normal secondary wave may be seen (independent of a swallow) to clear any residual material through the lower esophageal sphincter. The esophageal phase should be completed in 6 to 10 seconds. The radiologist should document any dysmotility, obstruction, stricture, or tracheoesophageal fistula.

Videofluoroscopic Swallowing Study and Upper Gastrointestinal Series

A combination of the VSS and an upper gastrointestinal series may be completed during the same procedure (Video 11-1). This can provide the medical team with a more comprehensive evaluation of the entire deglutitive process. The procedure starts with the infant in the upright position using a bottle filled with barium using the appropriate nipple flow rate that the infant can tolerate for safe oral feedings. The flow rate is determined by the clinical evaluation. Once the clinician ascertains that the infant is not aspirating or is unable to feed without aspiration, the infant is placed in the supine position and fed with the same bottle and nipple. This position allows the clinician and the radiologist to assess the integrity of the esophageal phase without gravity and to determine whether the infant shows signs of gastroesophageal reflux. If the infant is unable to take orally the total amount needed for the assessment, the barium may be syringed into the nasogastric tube to fill the stomach with the appropriate amount of barium to evaluate the lower gastrointestinal tract to demonstrate possible gastroesophageal reflux. Premature infants commonly demonstrate reflux. The following points are important for the clinician to consider:

1. Counting the suspected number of reflux events seen within the first 5 to 10 minutes of the feeding

2. Observing whether the infant is able to protect the airway if the reflux flows to the level of the upper esophageal sphincter

3. Documenting any change or lack of change in behavior as a result of these events

The radiologist will then view the fluid passing through the stomach, pyloric valve, and the ligament of Treitz. Physiologic instability tied to reflux events such as changes in heart rate, respiratory rate, or oxygen saturation levels also should be documented.

Fiberoptic Endoscopic Evaluation

Flexible nasopharyngoscopes are designed especially for infants to visualize the upper aerodigestive tract directly. Fiberoptic endoscopic evaluation (FEES) is a practical way to evaluate swallowing in infants.[12] The assessment usually is completed by the pediatric otolaryngologist, speech-language pathologist, or neonatologist.

The infant is positioned on the feeding clinician's or mother's lap in the infant's normal feeding position. The assessment starts with the infant sucking on a pacifier to assist in calming while the endoscope is passed transnasally. Some physicians may administer a local anesthesia to the infant's nasal mucosa to decrease the discomfort of the scope. As soon as the scope is in place, the anatomy and physiology of the hypopharynx and larynx are assessed. Special attention is directed to the infant's ability to manage his or her own secretions. Pharyngeal and laryngeal sensation can be evaluated if the scope is equipped with a channel to deliver air puffs.[13] The feeding clinician presents the infant with colored breast milk or formula in a bottle with the appropriate nipple so that these materials can be easily visualized. Because FEES does not require any radiation exposure, it allows the clinician time to assess the infant with a variety of flow nipples and a various swallowing stimuli. Interpretation of the test results after the swallow is similar to that described in Chapter 10.

OLDER CHILDREN

The evaluation and treatment of an older child with a feeding disorder must be made with as much background information as possible. An older child who presents as *typically developing* with no apparent underlying medical difficulties may, in fact, have a history of multiple medical or psychosocial disorders that affect feeding. Many such disorders were discussed in Chapter 4. Most diagnoses and classification systems for feeding disorders define the feeding disorder as existing only in reference to that child. The context in which the child exists (e.g., emotional, developmental, social, medical, and nutritional) is "at most implied but left undefined or, if defined, contextual factors tend to be ruled out as exclusionary criteria."[14] Successful diagnosis and treatment of a child's feeding disorder must include addressing parental functioning, the parent-child relationship, other family relationships, and other social relationships within and outside the family.[15] Therefore the holistic approach in addressing a child's feeding challenges includes coordination of many disciplines[16-18] as discussed in Chapter 1.

CLINICAL FEEDING EVALUATION

The clinical feeding evaluation examines the child's oral structure and function, behavioral and sensory responses to the feeding process, self-feeding skills, oral capabilities relating to liquids and solid foods, and the caregiver's feeding skills. Other aspects of the evaluation include examination of the impact of feeding on postural control, general movement patterns, cognition, speech and language, and sensory system development.[19,20] With this information the evaluation should also explore therapeutic strategies that may improve function. As in most types of therapeutic interventions, the evaluation should be a dynamic process that assists in the reevaluation and modification of treatment goals. The information in this chapter provides a broad base of information for the evaluation and treatment of a wide range of children and their feeding challenges. Expected outcomes of the clinical feeding evaluation for infants and older children include (1) a determination of the child's current level of feeding, (2) identification of areas in which a child shows potential for progress, (3) the implementation of a treatment plan that addresses therapist and family goals, and (4) the development of a home program for continued feeding practice.

The assessment and treatment of children with feeding disorders must involve the child and family. In addition to the physical evaluation, multiple factors such as culture and level of parental understanding of the child's disorder must be assessed.[14,15] A vital component in the evaluation is an assessment of the goals of the family. Family goals often may guide the evaluation and treatment plan. Typical family goals are summarized in Box 11-1. Caregiver perceptions of the child's skills in these areas and satisfaction with these skills must also be evaluated.[21] Of note, the parents of a child with a feeding disorder often will come to the evaluation with a sense of anxiety related to their child's performance and the recommendations of the feeding specialist.

As previously discussed, children who have clinical feeding evaluations usually present with a wide range of medical disorders[22] that may have been successfully

BOX 11-1	Family Feeding Goals

- The need to eat safely
- The need to maintain weight and growth patterns
- The need to increase the acceptance of food and liquid in varying amounts and types
- The need to eat in natural social situations
- The need to self-feed
- The need to reduce or eliminate tube feedings
- The need to be trained in the best way to assist their child with feeding

addressed or are still present. Children with feeding disorders also may be referred as typically developing without an identified medical diagnosis. These children require a detailed review of their medical and psychosocial history, family history of feeding-related concerns, and evaluation of the child's feeding difficulties.

Children who may not yet be ready for these evaluations include those with moderate to severe illness that may interfere with feeding therapy, those with a decreased level of consciousness or awareness, and those who receive treatment such as chemotherapy. The evaluating therapist should have access to the prescribing physician for a determination of the appropriateness of the evaluation.

Preparing for the Evaluation

Before the feeding evaluation begins, a review of the case history, medical record, and other referral information is necessary. It is helpful to provide the family with information to help them be prepared for their child's appointment. Questions that may be asked at the time of scheduling the appointment are summarized in Box 11-2.

Often there is additional information that should be requested from the family at the time of scheduling. The family should bring an array of the child's preferred foods and foods that they would like the evaluating therapist to examine with the child during the evaluation. If the child is taking breast milk or formula, the family needs to bring it with them. It is important that the family bring the child hungry. Typically this means not feeding the child for at least 3 to 4 hours before the evaluation. For children with tube feedings, the parents may turn off (with physician approval) the continuous tube feedings for 2 to 3 hours. For bolus feedings, alimentation should be withheld until the child's appointment time. The family also should be informed to bring the child's preferred utensils, including bottles, special nipples, and cups.

BOX 11-2 **Important Questions to Ask Caregivers**

- What is your main concern about your child's feeding needs?
- Does your child have a specific medical diagnosis? (It is important to obtain all past diagnoses because some may affect the child's feeding skills.)
- Is your child breastfeeding (for children younger than 5 years)?
- Does your child have difficulty swallowing liquids or any particular texture?
- Does your child take all nutrition orally?
- Does your child have chronic respiratory concerns?
- Does your child have any food allergies? Are there allergies to any medications? (If there are food allergies in the child's history, the clinician should confirm that the parents know how to manage an adverse reaction. If they do not have this knowledge, then no new foods should be given during the evaluation.)
- Is the child taking any medication(s)? If so, which one(s)?

Practice Note 11-1

All clinical feeding evaluations with children should be conducted with a high degree of sensitivity. For the parents of an infant, their primary roles are to feed and nurture the child. Feeding their baby often is the largest piece of this role. The parents have hoped for the moment when they can feed their baby without potential complications. Feeding a newborn is at the core of a parent's dreams, especially for the mother. Their dreams of easy feeding change quickly as they encounter a baby who is irritable, unable to take enough breast milk or formula, or at risk for other medical problems if fed. If the child fails the feeding evaluation, the feeding specialist faces presenting a treatment plan that is necessarily slow and must proceed in graded steps. Although the family may initially be disappointed in this approach, it may relieve some of the pressure they feel to have to feed their baby *now*. Understandably, parents may feel a sense of hopelessness. After the evaluation, it is important for the feeding specialist to offer parents something they can immediately implement to help their child.

CASE HISTORY

The case history may be gathered through the use of standardized case history forms, review of the medical chart, and family interview. A complete case history assists in the development of the evaluation session and the subsequent treatment plan for the child and parent. It also may provide direction for referrals to related services.[23] Pertinent information from the case history useful in completing the evaluation of a child with a feeding disorder is summarized in Box 11-3.

BOX 11-3 **Pertinent Case History Information**

1. The family's primary concerns, including coughing and choking episodes, a history of aspiration pneumonia, the need for transition to other food types, or the need for transition from bottle to cup or to the use of utensils.
2. Family priorities for feeding such as enjoyment, nutrition, or safety.
3. Results from previous swallowing studies.
4. Length of pregnancy, including child's birth weight and length.
5. If the child was born at less than 37 weeks' gestation, was NICU admission required? If so, for how long? How long has the family been home since the NICU stay?
6. A review of medical diagnoses and types of physicians or clinics attended.
7. Has the child had any surgery or specific medical procedures such as **bronchoscopy**?
8. Is there a history of respiratory complications? If so, what type?
9. Is there a history of gastroesophageal reflux? If there is a positive history of reflux, how is this managed and by whom?
10. Do the parents perceive the feeding problem as ongoing or do they believe there was a single event that triggered the feeding difficulties?
11. Does the child have any nasopharyngeal reflux?
12. Is there a family history of feeding problems, gastroesophageal reflux, or food allergies?
13. Has the child received any previous feeding therapy? If so, for how long and by whom? And what were the goals?
14. Does the child use any special equipment to eat?

15. Is there a history of tube feeding?
16. If the child is currently tube fed, ask about the type of tube, the formula type, the formula calorie concentration, the feeding schedule and rate, and the parents' perception of the child's tolerance of the tube feedings.
17. Has the child been breastfed in the past? If so, what are the parents' perceptions of success with breastfeeding? If breastfeeding was not successful, information regarding the mother's breast health, child's sucking patterns, mother's milk supply, and feeding schedule may be helpful.
18. If the child is currently being breastfed, has a lactation consultant been involved?
19. What is the child currently being fed? This includes food type, favorite foods, number of foods in the child's diet, texture and flavor preferences, and food consistencies accepted. It may be helpful to inquire which foods are eaten by category—proteins, fruits and vegetables, and starches. For children 2 years and older with less than 10 accepted items per category, further assessment may be needed in the areas of sensory system development and nutritional status.
20. What is the child's current feeding schedule? Include all bottles, tube feedings, small snacks, and nibbles in this schedule.
21. Ask the family to describe the environment in which the child is fed. Specifically, in which room does the child eat, in which type of seat, and if anything else is happening during the child's mealtime?
22. Who feeds the child? Who else is present? Does the child eat better for any one person?
23. Does the child have a need for distractors, rewards, and/or contingencies so that he or she will eat? If so, what are they?
24. Are there any other behavioral concerns or stressors specific to the child or in the family?
25. What is the family's daily and weekly schedule as it might relate to the feeding circumstance?

Ask the family to complete the *Sensory Profile* to examine sensory-based challenges that may be contributing to the feeding difficulties.[24] For speech-language pathologists, scoring and interpretation of the *Sensory Profile* should be completed in consultation with an occupational therapist. Consideration of sensory system dysfunction is an important component in the evaluation and treatment of children with oral feeding disorders.[25]

Finally, screening for nutritional concerns is important. A referral should be made to a dietitian if the child's history or evaluation results suggest the following: (1) failure to gain weight, (2) dietary restrictions that eliminate large parts of or an entire food group; (3) need for a calorie count, a change in formula, or the need for nutritional supplementation; or (4) a home-prepared tube-feeding regimen that may not be nutritionally adequate.

The case history may be gathered while the child is in the evaluation room with the family and clinician. Ideally this setting should be an eating-type setting such as a kitchen. The room should be arranged so that the child identifies the area as an "eating place" rather than as a location for a medical examination. If the child is older than 12 months, he or she may be prepared for the session with play or other developmentally appropriate activity to familiarize the child with the setting and the person performing the evaluation. The procedure to be used for the evaluation should be discussed with the child (if appropriate) and the parents.

PREFEEDING ACTIVITIES

Prefeeding activities include play activity that is useful in the evaluation. This play time is important because it allows the child to become more comfortable with the clinician. This time also allows the clinician to observe the language, muscle tone and movement patterns, and other developmental patterns of the child. Respiratory status (type of breathing, rate of breathing, need for assistance) also can be observed. If a child is receiving supplemental oxygen, it is important to know the flow rate and how often the child receives oxygen. The frequency of oxygen use may include all day, sleep time only, or during periods of greater exertion (such as feeding).[26] If a child has a tracheostomy, the need for suctioning should be identified. Parents often are very accustomed to suctioning their child's apparatus and may not be able to identify suctioning frequency. During the evaluation it is important to observe whether suctioned secretions or secretions at the tracheostomy site contain food or liquid residue.[27]

Seating options should be determined at this time. Appropriate seating should minimize the child's work of sitting. Infants and children with neurologic disorders may be unable to hold their head up or sit easily without support. A child first places energy in sitting, creating a need to focus on positional stability rather than eating. Various seating options are summarized in Box 11-4. In addition to these suggestions, additional support of the head, trunk, or legs may be

BOX 11-4	Seating Options for the Clinical Feeding Evaluation

FOR INFANTS
Bouncy seat
Infant car seat
Reclined high chair
Tumble Form seats

FOR TODDLERS (SEATING TYPE IS DETERMINED BY THE CHILD'S DEVELOPMENTAL LEVEL)
Reclined high chair
Upright high chair
Reclined car seat
Booster seat
Tumble Form seats

BOX 11-5	Prefeeding Materials That Can Be Used During Play Activities

Chewy Tubes*
Mini-massagers
Unflavored toothettes
Tooth brushing with a wet toothbrush (only if this is reported as an accepted activity)
Warm, moist washcloths
Use of food-shaped toys
Whistles and other musical instruments that involve the mouth, such as a kazoo
Oral play toys and games such as bubbles and blowing cotton balls

*Speech Pathology Associates, LLC, South Portland, Maine.

needed. If additional supports are needed, they should be used in consultation with the physical or occupational therapist. If the child is able, he or she may assist the clinician in setting up the food and utensils for the evaluation. This places the evaluation into a play context for the child, avoiding the appearance of a medical evaluation. For children who may demonstrate reduced sensory system integrity when eating, assistance with this setup as a play activity is a first step in their acceptance of the evaluation. Prefeeding activities also may be used for toddlers, preschoolers, and older children, although they should be approached at the appropriate age and maturity level. Suggested prefeeding play materials are presented in Box 11-5. The clinician should be an equal participant in this activity so that the child perceives that the activity is done *with* and not *to* them. The evaluation setup time also provides the opportunity to decide who will do the feeding. Optimally, the parents should feed the child. Much information can obtained by watching the manner in which the parents feed their child. This is also a time when improved feeding strategies may be taught in a more natural manner. Rather than appearing as a formal evaluation, it should become an opportunity for learning for both the therapist and caregiver(s).

Safety considerations should be discussed with the parents and monitored throughout the entire feeding evaluation. The assessment for safe swallowing, such as overt coughing or choking or gagging, or an obvious change in respiratory status, always should be noted. The clinician should continuously monitor the child for allergic responses. New foods should be introduced carefully, especially in a child with possible or known food allergies. The child should be assessed continuously for stress level and tolerance for interventions. It is helpful to identify these areas in coordination with the parents because multiple causes of stress responses may exist. These may be related to possible or known psychosocial diagnoses, such as anxiety, previous events such as a history of a choking incident, a long history of gastroesophageal reflux, or sensory system dysfunction. It is important to identify the need for suctioning equipment before the evaluation so that suctioning equipment is available. Standard universal health precautions are necessary. In some circumstances, gowns or other protective equipment may be needed according to the patient's medical diagnosis.

TECHNICAL ASPECTS

Regardless of whether the child is fed by the parents, the clinician, or self-feeds, the clinician should be prepared to record observations of multiple factors occurring simultaneously, such as motor control patterns, sensory reactions to food ingested, acceptance of utensils, and behavioral reactions to any part of the feeding process. The clinician will organize information from each of these areas and evaluate any interaction of these factors to determine the type of treatment plan necessary to address the feeding issues. It is important that the judgment of "normalcy" of these behaviors be based on a complete understanding of the typical developmental milestones at each age with respect to oral motor and feeding skills, typical dietary recommendations for age, self-feeding skills, fine and gross motor skills, respiration, and communication. With this information the feeding specialist is able to interpret evaluation observations and create a treatment plan based on the child's overall functioning level rather than on age alone.

Examining Oral Structure and Function

The oral structural and motor function evaluation is completed by the clinician. The child often considers this an invasive procedure. At times, a portion of this information may be completed during the play portion of the evaluation or during the feeding process itself. Each structure and related movement pattern should be examined for symmetry of movement, noting smoothness of movement patterns, rhythm, rate of movement, range of movement, and strength of movement. In addition, the clinician should be careful to evaluate each structural or functional difference with respect to the functional impact of this difference. Children may have a strong ability to accommodate to differences with very functional performance. Box 11-6 presents a suggested format for performing the examination of oral structure and function.

BOX 11-6 **Suggested Format for Performing the Evaluation of the Oral Mechanism in a Child**

OBSERVATION OF FACIAL STRUCTURE
- Facial symmetry (e.g., **hemifacial microsomia** or the later effects of **torticollis**)
- Head size and shape appropriate for age: Look for macrocephaly, microcephaly, or evidence of **plagiocephaly**
- Abnormalities of the eye area
- Abnormalities of the nose
- Observations of oral-facial muscle tone

JAW, MANDIBLE, CHEEK MUSCULATURE
STRUCTURE
- Position (protruded, **micrognathia**, neutral position, deviation)
FUNCTION
- Stability of jaw movements in feeding and speech (deviations to the left or right)
- Activation of the cheek musculature during sound production and eating (well-defined, flaccid, bunched)
- Mouth posture at rest (open versus closed)
- Judged strength of muscle movement during sucking and chewing
- Endurance for repeated patterns of sucking and chewing

TEETH
- Misalignment of individual teeth may affect biting
- Misalignment of upper to lower may affect biting and chewing
- Condition, including eroding enamel, decay, caries, capped teeth

LIPS
STRUCTURE
- Shape and contour (normal, retracted upper lip, bow-shaped upper lip, full upper or lower lip, protruded lower lip, appearance of **columella**)
- Symmetry (left to right, proportional to face, relation of upper to lower lip)
- Structural integrity (evidence of repaired cleft, other type of notch, trauma to lip)
FUNCTION (IN ISOLATED AND COMBINED MOVEMENTS)
- Lip rounding (purse, protrude, round)
- Retract, as in smiling
- Press together and maintain closure

TONGUE
STRUCTURE
- Inspect the frenulum for ankylosis
- Symmetry and position in the mouth (Does the tongue remain relaxed in the lower portion of the oral cavity? Is it bunched [contracted in the center]? Is it retracted or deviated to the left or right? Does the tongue rest outside the lower lip?)
- Size in relation to the oral cavity, such as microglossia or macroglossia
- Definition of the tongue tip: pointed (normal) or rounded, square, heart shaped (all abnormal)
- Appearance of fasciculations
FUNCTION
- Transverse tongue reflex (necessary for management of liquids and formed solids)
- Full excursions to the left and right (necessary for management of liquids and formed solids)
- Licking around lip circumference
- Tongue tip elevation
- Cupping and grooving during feeding (necessary for bolus formation, control, and propulsion)

PALATE AND RELATED STRUCTURES
STRUCTURE
- Arch of palate (adequate, high, central notch)
- Visible pharynx-oropharyngeal space (adequate, large)
- Repaired cleft and/or presence of a palatal prosthesis
- Appearance of uvula (typical, short, long, bifid, absent)
- Presence and appearance of tonsils (Do they create an obstruction for breathing or swallowing?)
FUNCTION
- Soft palate and uvular movement on phonation (symmetric, restricted, absent)

It is important to assess other effects on feeding by observation before, during, and after feeding. Subjective assessment of dysphagia must be made during this time. Common symptoms of dysphagia include generalized feeding difficulty, such as poor feeding efficiency, food refusal, and failure to thrive. Specific symptoms include choking, coughing, food or liquid refusal, significant anterior loss of oral material, decreased control of oral secretions, unexplained temperature spike within 24 hours, frequent bacterial upper respiratory tract infections, eyes tearing during feeding, changes in breathing and cardiac patterns, changes in vocal quality such as "wet" vocalizations, and facial color changes. The possibility of dysphagia can be identified by a thorough feeding history and careful observation. Aspiration in the infant, toddler, and child can be present without outward signs.[28] If swallowing dysfunction is suspected, the feeding specialist should recommend further assessment of swallowing. The most objective assessment of swallowing can be completed by a videofluoroscopic swallow study or by FEES.

OBSERVATION OF THE FEEDING PROCESS

Liquids

Evaluation of liquids is made according to the age and functional level of the child and caregiver needs. For infants who are breastfeeding or bottle feeding, the clinician observes for initiation of feeding toward the breast or bottle nipple, lip closure on the nipple, ability to draw in liquid, and the ability to sequence the suck-swallow-breathe pattern. For evaluation of liquids during cup drinking, the clinician observes lip closure on the cup, the presence of the tongue under or in the cup, the child's ability to draw in liquid, the general position of the cup, and the need for different types of cups. In all children, the clinician evaluates the ability to maintain liquid in the mouth without excessive loss, swallow control, speed of drinking, tolerance of variation in liquid type (including thickness), the need to adjust liquid thickness, and the effect of change in position during these activities of swallowing performance.

Foods

Evaluation of foods also is based on the age and functional level of the child. Although children take liquid nutrition from infancy, the ability to manage solids is based on age and the level of gross motor development. A typically developing child is introduced to solid foods (infant cereal and stage 1 infant foods) at approximately 6 months. The introduction of these foods at this age is based on the maturity of oral- and pharyngeal-stage function and the maturity of the gastrointestinal system. Correction for prematurity, as previously described, must be made when choosing which solid foods to introduce.

SPECIAL CONSIDERATIONS FOR THE INFANT

Evaluation of the infant should include identification of whether the infant is breastfed, bottle fed, or both. Observation of each type of feeding method is preferable, although it is often difficult to evaluate bottle feeding if the child has been breastfeeding only. If the child is to be evaluated while breastfeeding, it is important that the clinician has been trained as a certified lactation specialist. Identification of concerns relating to breastfeeding must be separated from infant-specific issues. Many times, such as in the case of tongue tie, the issues may be interrelated.

Feeding difficulties in an infant may signal other underlying medical problems. The feeding specialist should be aware of the child's overall respiratory rate; more than 60 breaths/min is considered abnormal and poses difficulty with the suck-swallow-breathe sequence. A baby should be able to breathe after every three to five sucks. The infant may need some pacing from the feeder to assist with a safe suck-swallow-breathe sequence.[6] The therapist examines the child for color changes during feeding; such changes may indicate possible respiratory or cardiac concerns associated with the feeding process. Babies who actively resist feeding, cry, or are fussy during or immediately after feeding should be examined for gastroesophageal reflux. Babies who use a pacifier should be observed for the strength and endurance during this nonnutritive suck pattern. Babies who are able to efficiently show nonnutritive sucking patterns generally do not demonstrate underlying oral motor difficulties.

SPECIAL CONSIDERATIONS FOR THE TODDLER

Solid Foods

General guidelines exist for the introduction of solid foods in the evaluation of the toddler, preschooler, and early elementary school child. It is important to examine the child for the food textures tolerated with respect to sensory acceptance and ability to show safe and functional management of the food. Food types also are evaluated in regard to the following:

- Method of presentation (type of spoon, fork infant training devices)
- Responses to variations in taste and temperature
- Lip closure on the utensil
- Lip closure during chewing and swallowing
- Type of chewing pattern (mashing, munching, diagonal, rotary)
- Level of chewing competency (ability to maintain the food in the mouth until the food is properly masticated)
- Strength of bite and chew
- Any anterior oral cavity loss
- Tongue-thrusting patterns
- Lateral tongue movements in food management (key to the development of efficient management of formed solids)
- General oral range of motion
- Effect of overfilling of the mouth
- Pacing of feeding
- Effect of changing the feeding position on feeding efficiency

The clinician also observes the manner in which the caregiver(s) present food, their ability to adjust their feeding patterns in response to the child's skills, and their own behavioral responses to the child's feeding abilities.

Food Types

The goal of most aspects of feeding therapy is to achieve appropriate nutrition to support growth. Choices of foods and the manner in which they are offered should be made with that goal in mind.[29] Examination of eating responses should include proteins, starches, and fruits and vegetables. Consideration of food choices also should be made regarding flavor, color, texture, and temperature. Food texture should be within the child's mechanical skill range. When possible, the feeding evaluation should examine dry meltable solids, purees, other mechanical soft solids, hard munchables, and mixed textures.

During early and middle childhood, family environments are the basis for the development of food preferences, patterns of food intake, eating styles, and the development of activity preferences and patterns that shape children's developing weight status. These environments affect children in whom failure to thrive has been diagnosed and those with obesity. Practical instruction for parents during the feeding evaluation and subsequent treatment should include how to foster a child's preferences for healthy foods and how to promote acceptance of new foods. Parents need to understand the cost of coercive feeding prac-

tices, including force-feeding practices, and be given alternatives to pressuring children to eat. These practices often are a function of the family's desperate efforts to help the child achieve appropriate levels of nutrition.[30]

SPECIAL CONSIDERATIONS FOR THE OLDER CHILD

Evaluation of the older child includes consideration of many factors. The older child may present as a typically developing child with a history of significant food refusal. The older child may be a child with cerebral palsy who appears to be showing changes in food preferences or food management, or a child with a history of typical feeding who has sustained brain injury.[30] The older child also may be high functioning on the autism spectrum and is now showing signs of food refusal. A thorough medical history is required, especially for the child who has never received any therapeutic feeding intervention but continues to show signs of feeding disability. The evaluation proceeds in a manner similar to that of younger children but hopefully with more input from the child. Although the family will have specific goals, it is important to determine the older child's desire to eat. If necessary, the older child and family may benefit from psychological intervention because the older child most likely can be an active participant. It is possible that the feeding concerns are longstanding and have resulted in specific stressors for the child and family.

SHARING THE RESULTS

At the conclusion of the clinical feeding evaluation, the feeding specialist discusses the results of the evaluation with the caregivers and makes specific recommendations for home program activities, additional evaluations, the need for treatment, and the frequency of treatment. In some cases the clinician may uncover a new cause for the child's feeding disorder that requires medical confirmation. Whenever possible, printed information (specific suggestions and handouts) should be provided. Frequency and type of treatment may be considered according to the cause of the feeding disorder (acute or chronic), the child's assessed ability to make rapid versus slower change(s), the extent and severity of the feeding disorder, the caregiver's need for therapeutic support, and the response and treatment of any underlying medical conditions that may affect treatment approaches.

Practice Note II-2

The feeding specialist often is the first professional to note features of a syndrome or the effects of a syndrome on feeding. This is another opportunity for the feeding specialist to provide information to the family without overwhelming them. If the therapist believes that a child demonstrates features of a syndrome that has not yet been identified, it is vital to discuss these findings with the child's primary care physician. There is a delicate balance between providing helpful information and too much information. Parents who are given the name of a syndrome typically want more information. They may go home and search for this information on the Internet. For example, the therapist may state that the child has features of velocardiofacial syndrome. With an Internet search, information on this syndrome is readily available. Parents will note that researchers have identified at least 168 different problems associated with this syndrome. Some problems may be alarming, such as schizophrenia, cardiac anomalies, learning disabilities, or cleft palate. A misdiagnosis causes unnecessary worry for the family. In most cases, the feeding specialist should discuss the findings with the primary care physician, who will be able to order the appropriate tests for a definitive diagnosis and coordinate the child's care based on test results.

CLINICAL CORNER 11-1

Emily is a 14-month-old girl with a history of effortful swallowing and limited weight gain and is described as a picky eater. She enjoys limited quantities of purees and very soft foods. She was born after a term pregnancy and is developmentally within normal limits. Her oral structure and function are also within normal limits. Her mother reports that Emily is a restless sleeper, and she hears Emily snoring at night.

CRITICAL THINKING

1. What would you look for during Emily's physical examination and during the clinical feeding evaluation?
2. What other evaluations will you discuss with Emily's pediatrician?
3. What types of foods might you recommend to Emily's mother until further assessments are completed?

CLINICAL CORNER 11-2

A toddler of 20 months accepts only small amounts of food and drink. His diet (allowed foods) is very limited because he has short-gut syndrome. He receives PediaSure (Abbott Nutrition, Columbus, Ohio) feedings by gastrostomy tube. He enjoys meltable solids and selected strongly flavored purees. He has started to enjoy a small selection of mechanical soft solids that includes soft-boiled eggs, strained baby food meats, and potato chips.

CRITICAL THINKING

1. What types of foods may be examined during the clinical feeding evaluation?
2. What is the rationale for trying these foods?
3. What types of eating skills (including self-feeding) might you see with this child?
4. What may be some of your initial home program recommendations? Why?
5. What therapy frequency might be appropriate for this child?

CLINICAL CORNER 11-3

A mother has been trying to feed her 1-year-old child with a squeezable sippy cup and has offered stage 2 baby foods. He takes up to 40 minutes to eat a 4-oz container of this food. He takes varying amounts of liquids but shows fatigue during drinking. The mother states that she has been given a thickening agent for the formula to be thickened to a nectar consistency but has not been able to try this yet. The child's nasogastric feedings are bolus feedings every 3 hours with the volume based on his oral intake. The recommendation is for this child to take 32 oz of formula per day. He weighs 25 pounds.

CRITICAL THINKING

1. What seating system may be best used to evaluate this child's feeding?
2. What is the benefit of this position?
3. What food types, textures, and flavors should be tried during the evaluation? Why?
4. What utensils should be used for eating? For drinking?
5. Are there any additional evaluations that may be needed to complete the feeding picture? What will be the benefit of these evaluations?
6. What types of parental support may this family need?

CLINICAL CORNER 11-4

John is a typically developing 4-year-old boy. He was referred for a clinical feeding evaluation because of decreased appetite and self-induced vomiting. His parents noted this approximately 6 months before the evaluation. John has had significant weight loss. He has a diagnosis of gastroesophageal reflux. He is taking lansoprazole (Prevacid) and metoclopramide (Reglan) for this disorder. He has a history of anxiety. He is an alert and curious child at the onset of the evaluation. He appeared to be very reluctant to communicate with the feeding specialist initially, although when allowed to play he began to interact. John is able to sit independently in a regular chair and shows knowledge of the use of typical eating utensils. He has been exposed to a variety of "fast" and convenience foods. His speech and other developmental skills are within normal limits. His feeding schedule at home is quite varied, with frequent snacks. His parents are very concerned about his intake so they give him snacks whenever he requests them.

CRITICAL THINKING

1. What approaches may benefit this child before the "eating" part of the evaluation?
2. What types of additional evaluation questions may be appropriate to ask the parents? The child?
3. How would you approach the introduction of food for this child?
4. Would you expect to see oral motor feeding delays in this child? Why or why not?

TAKE HOME NOTES

1. The developmental specialist and NICU team work together to understand and monitor the five critical subsystems and how they play a vital role in infant feedings.
2. The premature infant's feedings are evaluated by the entire team, which makes the decision regarding the appropriate time to start or discontinue oral feedings.
3. Assessment of the infant's tone, reflexes, physiologic stability, and state is imperative before the initiation of oral feedings. Close observation of the infant's development often provides the feeding specialist with important prefeeding cues.
4. Instrumental evaluations of an infant are scheduled after team consultation, usually when the clinical evaluation or presentation does not fully

explain the infant's feeding difficulty. If a radiology procedure is necessary, it is important to evaluate the entire aerodigestive tract.

5. Successful diagnosis and treatment of a child's feeding disorder must address parental functioning, the parent-child relationship, other family relationships, and other social relationships within and outside the family.
6. The evaluation of a child's feeding disorder may include coordination of information from many disciplines, including the speech-language pathologist, occupational therapist, physical therapist, dietitian, gastroenterologist, otolaryngologist, pulmonologist, surgeon, psychologist, and social worker.
7. The outcomes of the clinical feeding evaluation relate to the child's ability to safely gain nutrition orally, the parents' ability feed their child, and the child's ability to self-feed.
8. The information gained from the clinical feeding evaluation often results in the need for referrals to other specialties. The feeding specialist needs to be aware of other pediatric specialists from the medical and therapeutic communities. This information should also be coordinated with the child's primary care physician.
9. Clinicians should be prepared for the child whose skills surprise them. The diagnosis and case history serve as a preparatory guide for the evaluation, but a child's motivation to eat may allow him or her to surpass the expected skills. In other words, "never say never."

References

1. Ross E, Browne J: Developmental progression of feeding skills: an approach to supporting feeding in preterm infants, *Semin Neonatol* 7:469, 2002.
2. Als H, Butler S, Kosta S et al: The assessment of preterm infants' behavior (APIB): furthering the understanding and measurement of neurodevelopmental competence in preterm and full term infants, *Mental Retard Devel Dis Res Rev* 11:94, 2005.
3. Shaker C: The early feeding skills assessment for preterm infants, *Neonatal Netw* 24:7, 2005.
4. Gorski PA, Davison MF, Brazelton TB: Stages of behavioral organization in the high risk neonate: theoretical and clinical considerations, *Semin Perinatol* 3:61, 1979.
5. Sheppard J: Assessment of oral motor behaviors in cerebral palsy, *Semin Speech Lang* 8:57, 1987.
6. Wolf L, Glass R: *Feeding and swallowing in infants and children: pathophysiology, diagnosis and treatment*, San Diego, 1995, Therapy Skill Builders.

7. Palmer M, Crawley K, Blanco L: Neonatal oral-motor assessment scale: a reliability study, *J Perinatol* 13:28, 1993.

8. Arvedson J: Oral-motor and feeding assessment. In Arvedson J, Brodsky L, editors: *Pediatric swallowing and feeding: assessment and management*, San Diego, 1993, Singular.

9. Shaker C, Woida A: An evidence-based approach to nipple feeding in a level III NICU: nurse autonomy, developmental care, and teamwork, *Neonatal Netw* 26:77, 2007.

10. Ross CS, Browne JV: *The baby regulated organization of systems and sucking*. Abstract presented at the Physical and Developmental Environment of the High-Risk Infant Conference, 2003, Clearwater Beach, FL.

11. Rommel N: Assessment for babies, infants, and children. In Cichero J, Murdoch B, editors: *Dysphagia, foundation, theory and practice*, Chichester, UK, 2006, John Wiley.

12. Leder SB, Karas DE: Fiberoptic endoscopic evaluation of swallowing in the pediatric population, *Laryngoscope* 110:1132, 2000.

13. Link DT, Willging J, Miller CK et al: Pediatric laryngopharyngeal sensory testing during flexible endoscopic evaluation of swallowing: feasible and correlative, *Ann Otol Rhinol Laryngol* 109:899, 2000.

14. Davies WH, Berlin KS, Sato AF et al: Reconceptualizing feeding disorders in interpersonal context: the case for a relational disorder, *J Fam Psychol* 3:400, 2006.

15. Garro A, Thurman SK, Kerwin ME et al: Parent and caregiver stress during pediatric hospitalization for chronic feeding problems, *J Pediatr Nurs* 20:268, 2005.

16. Martin C: The importance of a multifaceted approach in the assessment and treatment of childhood feeding disorders, *Clinical Case Studies* 7:79, 2008.

17. Williams S, Witherspoon K, Kavsak P et al: Pediatric feeding and swallowing problems: an interdisciplinary approach, *Can J Diet Pract Res* 67:185, 2006.

18. Manikam R, Perman JA: Pediatric feeding disorders, *J Clin Gastroenterol* 30:34, 2000.

19. Ayres AJ: *Sensory integration and the child*, Los Angeles, 2005, Western Psychological Services.

20. Morris SE, Klein MD: *Pre-feeding skills: a comprehensive resource for feeding development*, San Antonio, TX, 2000, Psychological Corporation.

21. Greer AJ, Gulotta CS, Masler EA et al: Caregiver stress and outcomes of children with pediatric feeding disorders treated in an intensive interdisciplinary program, *J Pediatr Psychol* 33:612, 2008.

22. Miller CK, Willging JP: Advances in the evaluation and management of pediatric dysphagia, *Curr Opin Otolaryngol Head Neck Surg* 11:442, 2003.

23. Schwarz SM, Corredor J, Fisher-Medina J et al: Diagnosis and treatment of feeding disorders in children with developmental disabilities, *Pediatrics* 108:671, 2001.

24. Dunn W: *The sensory profile*, San Antonio, TX, 1999, Pearson.

25. Kranowitz CS: *The out-of-sync child: recognizing and coping with sensory integration dysfunction*, New York, 2005, Perigree.

26. Klein MD, Delaney TA: *Feeding and nutrition for the child with special needs: handouts for parents*, San Antonio, TX, 1994, Therapy Skill Builders.

27. Bell HR, Alper BS: Assessment and intervention for dysphagia in infants and children: beyond the neonatal intensive care unit, *Semin Speech Lang* 28:213, 2007.

28. National Dysphagia Diet Task Force: *The national dysphagia diet: standardization for optimal care*, Chicago, 2002, American Dietetic Association.

29. Birch LL, Davidson KK: Family environmental factors influencing the developing behavioral controls of food intake and childhood overweight, *Pediatr Clin North Am* 48:893, 2001.

30. Tomlin P, Clarke M, Robinson G et al: Rehabilitation in severe head injury in children: outcome and provision of care, *Devel Med Child Neurol* 44:828, 2002.

Chapter 12

Treatment Considerations, Options, and Decisions

MICHAEL E. GROHER

CHAPTER OUTLINE

OBJECTIVES

1. Introduce the concept of how evidence-based practice guides treatment decisions.
2. Discuss general factors that influence therapy decisions.
3. Provide examples from the three major classes of therapeutic interventions for dysphagia.
4. Discuss how the evaluation results will affect treatment planning.
5. Present a decision tree for selecting and implementing dysphagia therapy.

EVIDENCE-BASED PRACTICE

The selection of any treatment for the patient with dysphagia should be based on the best available evidence from the published literature, the patient's wishes, and the clinician's experience with similar problems. The combination of these three variables in preparing a treatment plan is referred to as *evidence-based practice* (EBP). Given any individual patient, clinicians will assign different weights to each variable. For example, if the clinician has had excellent success with an unconventional form of therapy for which there is no research support, he or she may, with the patient's consent, choose to apply that treatment strategy. Or if a patient did not feel able to cooperate with a recommended plan of treatment, another course of action may need to be implemented. EBP differs from traditional clinical management because it does not rely solely on clinical intuition and experience but also values patient desires and a critical appraisal of published research.

In all fields of health care, clinicians have been challenged to evaluate and use available research evidence to solve clinical problems and provide the best patient care possible in the most cost-efficient manner. Examples of how EBP affects patient care are numerous. For example, assume that a clinician had been using the tactile-thermal stimulation technique (see Chapter 14) with patients who show swallowing onset delay because of experimental evidence suggesting its application with that particular group of patients. However, when reviewing additional evidence in multiple studies with similar patients, the investigators reported that the effect was minimal. In this circumstance the clinician might be hesitant to apply the treatment. However, before changing practice, the clinician must evaluate the strength (believability) of the new evidence before he or she alters the treatment approach. Even in the face of strong evidence, some clinicians find it hard to abandon their own experience and intuition. Complete reliance on experimental evidence runs the risk of setting patient care guidelines and paths of care that experience suggests may not be in the patient's best interest. The intersections of experimental evidence, clinical experience, and patient desires ultimately lead to the best treatment approach. When using an EBP model it is incumbent on the clinician to consult the research literature to evaluate treatment **effectiveness** or **efficacy** in patients similar to the one requiring evaluation or treatment.

Astute clinicians recognize that failure to implement EBP runs the risk of overusing familiar and comfortable treatments that might be less effective in achieving desired outcomes. Similarly, clinicians could be using what they perceive to be the most effective treatment strategy, but they are applying it incorrectly—for example, recommending that an exercise be done 10 times a day when the experimental evidence suggests that the best outcomes are achieved when it is done 100 times a day.

Practice Note 12-1

In 1998 the Dutch Neurological Society published guidelines for the treatment of neurogenic dysphagia developed from an evidence-based review. The following pathway of care was to be used when encountering a patient with dysphagia from a neurogenic source.

1. Dysphagia should be detected with 50 mL of water because this is the most useful screening test.
2. If dysphagia is present, a nasogastric tube should be placed.
3. If after 2 weeks dysphagia is still present, a **percutaneous gastrostomy tube** should be placed.
4. There is no scientific support for evaluation with videofluoroscopy.
5. There is no scientific support for swallowing therapy.

Although these guidelines may seem stringent and not in the patient's best interest, at the time they were developed the published research supported this pathway of clinical care.

EVALUATING EVIDENCE

After the clinical and/or instrumental evaluation the clinician should be able to formulate questions (hypotheses) about which treatment approach might fit the patient's profile. For example, if the patient was having difficulty protecting the airway during the swallow sequence, could he or she benefit from learning a swallowing maneuver, and would a change in posture be beneficial? A more focused question might be "Does the combination of a postural change and a swallowing maneuver help protect the airway, or is one intervention better alone?" Another relevant question might be "How long does the patient need to maintain these interventions before complete swallowing safety is achieved?"

The search for answers to questions could come from multiple sources, including personal experience ("It worked before so I will try it again"); textbooks (although these are rarely opened once the course is completed); expert advice through continuing education opportunities ("the expert said it, so it must be true"); commercial sales ("this is exactly what you will need"); and journal articles (although research has shown that the frequency of professional reading declines with years away from the university). All these sources, with the exception of the published journal articles, represent *information* that can be gathered. Information is different from evidence, because *evidence* results from a controlled approach to a clinical question.

Assuming the clinician wants to review the evidence pertaining to a clinical question, the next step would be to consult relevant databases using key search terms that might help answer those questions. Terms such as "posture," "swallowing," "outcomes," and "treatment" might be used in the initial search. Finding the relevant evidence can be accomplished by using databases such as MEDLINE or PubMed, or Web sites that summarize data such as the Cochrane Library or the American College of Physicians. Typing terms in a Web search such as "evidence based" and "clinical trials" can lead to other relevant databases. Government-based Web sites such as www.guideline. gov (National Guideline Clearinghouse) can be a useful starting point in an evidence-based search. If the search is directed toward a specific disease such as Parkinson's, accessing a specific organization's official Web site also is a valuable point of departure.

After the evidence is accessed, the clinician must evaluate the relevance to the patient in question and its strength (believability) and clarity in guiding treatment. Judging the strength of the evidence is done through an analysis of the study's design characteristics. Some Web sites (e.g., the Cochrane Library) are designed to provide critical reviews of the extant evidence on a multitude of diagnostic and treatment questions. Because these systematic analyses are designed to gather and grade the strength of many studies on a single topic, they are very useful for the busy clinician who may not have the time to do an extensive search. In the small subspecialty of oropharyngeal swallowing disorders, not every clinical question will have been reviewed systematically.

Because the study's design often determines the relative strength of the evidence, it is important to know what constitutes weak evidence for any given outcome and what constitutes stronger evidence for the same outcome. Table 12-1 presents a classification system for grading levels of evidence according to the study's design characteristics. For instance, the highest level of evidence (grade A or 1) is associated with study designs that are randomized, controlled trials

TABLE 12-1

Classification System for Grading Levels of Evidence

Evidence Grade	Level of Evidence	Type of Evidence
A	1a	Systematic review of RCTs
	1b	Individual RCT
	1c	All or none
B	2a	Systematic review of cohort studies
	2b	Individual cohort study
	2c	Outcomes research
	3a	Systematic review of case-control studies
	3b	Individual case-control study
C	4	Case series (and poor-quality case-control and cohort studies)
D	5	Expert opinion without critical appraisal or based on physiology or "first" principles

Grading levels of evidence. The *far right column* shows the study design designations. Depending on the design of the study, it is assigned a strength level *(middle column)*. The strongest designs are at level 1, and the weakest designs are level 5. Within each level the strength of evidence can be graded, such as levels 2a to 3b, with a study graded at 2a being stronger than 3b. Because it is not always possible to make fine distinctions between studies based on their design, investigators grade studies with more general categories such as A through D *(far left column)*. *SR*, Systematic review; *RCT*, randomized controlled trial. Adapted from Oxford Centre for Evidence-Based Medicine, 2001. *RCT*, Randomized controlled trial.

(RCTs). A lower grade (grade D or 5) is associated with studies that report on a series of patients. Investigators who use the RCT design to study a question are bound by much stricter criteria to answer their question. In general, these criteria try to eliminate any bias in the study that might shed doubt on the believability of the results. Some of these criteria include a large sample size in an experimental and control group with subjects assigned randomly, measurements made by investigators who are **blinded** to the study, and accounting for the outcomes of all study subjects at the end of the experiment. Study designs at levels B, C, and D may meet some of these criteria, but not all of them. The fewer criteria met, the weaker the evidence. In general, a clinician would have more confidence in studies graded at grade A than at grade D. Therefore the applicability of the findings from RCTs would be applied clinically with more confidence than findings from studies that reported on similar outcomes with a case series design. Such criteria can help the clinician decide which diagnostic or treatment approach might fit the patient and how much confidence to place in the outcome. An extensive discussion of each level of evidence and its corresponding characteristics is beyond the scope of this chapter. Readers are referred to *The Handbook of Evidence-Based Practice in Communication Disorders* for a thorough discussion.[1]

Judgment of the strength of the experimental evidence must be complemented by other analytic methods. For example, were the relevant studies done with patients similar to the patient in question, or were the characteristics in the reference sample different—such as age or gender? Was the treatment protocol in the study described precisely enough so that it could be replicated? Do you have the skills needed to replicate the treatment? For example, if the treatment described the use of certain equipment, do you have the equipment and are you trained to use it? And, finally, are the outcomes in the study similar to the ones you and your patient envision? Even the best-designed, grade 1 study may not be applicable to your clinical question. One also must judge whether the study under scrutiny has clinical significance. That is, if the conclusion from a study was that technique "X" improved hyoid elevation by 2 mm in a group of acute poststroke patients, is that change clinically significant or was it only a statistically significant difference? In this example, unless the study reported that a 2-mm change in hyoid elevation actually made a difference in airway protection or in an improvement of dietary intake, one may choose to ignore the data even though statistically technique "X" made a difference. Chapter 14 provides a more detailed discussion of study designs as they relate to answering clinical questions.

GENERAL TREATMENT CONSIDERATIONS

Two common considerations inherent to all aspects of dysphagia are airway protection and nutrition and hydration. Clinicians often face the important question, "Can the patient safely resume or increase adequate oral intake?" Dissecting this question reveals critical considerations in dysphagia treatment. The primary concerns for patients with dysphagia may be found in the words *safe* and *adequate*. Safety is often expressed in terms of airway protection. Patients who aspirate most of any given bolus of food or liquid are not considered safe in reference to the risk of aspiration and subsequent respiratory infection or, possibly, the risk of airway obstruction from more solid foods. The reference to *adequate* refers to the individual's ability to ingest sufficient food or liquid by mouth to maintain (or increase, if required in the situation) nutrition and hydration. A patient who engages in total oral feeding only to ingest inadequate volumes of food or liquid is a patient who is at risk for future

---

CLINICAL CASE EXAMPLE 12-1

A 69-year-old woman had a respiratory arrest after cardiac bypass surgery. After extubation she gained strength and a swallowing study was ordered. The videofluoroscopy revealed a delayed oral stage with good airway protection on all materials and volumes. It was recommended that she be given a soft mechanical diet with regular fluids and that the speech-language pathologist (SLP) monitor her at the bedside the next day. During breakfast it was noted that the patient ate half of her meal, complaining of fatigue and lack of appetite. The doctor ordered a 3-day calorie count because he was concerned about her nutritional and hydration status. The dietitian calculated that the patient's caloric need per day was 2000 calories. On the second day of oral feeding her respiratory status changed, as did her mental status. The calorie counts revealed that she was taking in only about 1100 of the 2000 calories needed. At that time the team believed that she could not sustain nutrition orally and that the secondary changes in respiratory and mental status were attributable to poor nutritional and hydration status. A nasogastric tube was placed so that nutrition and hydration could be maintained until her overall strength improved to the point where she could ingest enough calories to meet her metabolic needs.

---

health problems. When patients are fed by nonoral routes, treatment should be focused on the potential to resume oral intake of food and liquid. If the patient is taking a total oral diet, the focus may be on expanding the amount of intake to enhance nutrition or on expanding the variety of the diet to improve social aspects of eating and presumably quality of life. In planning treatment, it is important to have a clear grasp of the patient's present situation and a clear vision of where both clinician and patient want to be in the future and the factors that may help or hinder that direction.

In selecting any therapy, consideration must be given to the objective of that therapy. For example, in medicine one goal of therapy might be to cure a disease. How do clinicians "cure" dysphagia? Does curing dysphagia suggest that clinicians must return patients who are fed nonorally to oral feeding? This outcome is not always possible. Do clinicians want to prevent recurrence of a dysphagia-related **comorbid-**

BOX 12-1	Treatment Considerations Focusing on the Nature of the Swallowing Deficit

- Feeding or swallowing deficits (or both)
- Voluntary or involuntary processes
- Stage of deficit
- Deficit or compensatory activity

---

ity? One potential objective might be to diminish or eliminate recurrent chest infections. This goal certainly provides direction in treatment planning. In some situations clinicians may focus on limiting functional deterioration or facilitating recovery. To adopt this focus, clinicians must have a clear understanding of the underlying conditions contributing to dysphagia in individual patients. Certainly, clinicians hope that interventions do not contribute to later complications and that they, in fact, contribute to prevention of complications such as chest infections and malnutrition.

Beyond specific goals of treatment, clinicians must consider the nature of the swallowing deficit and the treatment options available to them and the patient (NOTE: these are not always the same). Box 12-1 summarizes some issues that might be addressed regarding the swallowing deficit. A basic question might revolve around feeding versus swallowing processes: Are there physical or cognitive factors that preclude successful feeding but that do not interfere with swallowing function? Are both of these factors present and, if so, do they interact in a positive or negative manner? Certain dysphagia-causing diseases might demonstrate differences between voluntary or involuntary motor processes. If differences are present, are there swallowing activities that may be used to tap into voluntary versus involuntary motor processes? Stage of deficit is an artificial delineation often used for convenience. Are the swallowing deficits primarily located within the oral, oropharyngeal, pharyngeal, or esophageal component? Clinicians must also remember that not only are these "stages" artificial, but that the swallowing mechanism is interactive—events occurring in one anatomic area have the potential to affect performance in another area (see Chapter 2). A difficult clinical task can be attempting to separate the specific swallowing deficit from any compensatory activities used by individual patients. For example, consider the patient who attempts to swallow but immediately begins to expectorate, or a patient who demonstrates a pattern of multiple, incomplete swallows interspersed with throat clearing, resulting in only a minute amount of material

Practice Note 12-2

A 34-year-old patient had sustained severe burns to his head, neck, and upper torso. Because of the severe pain that typically accompanies such injuries, he was on narcotics that made it difficult for him to remain awake. He had improved to the point where his physician believed he could start to eat orally. During the clinical evaluation the SLP noted he could only remain totally alert for 5 minutes and questioned whether he could stay awake long enough to eat an entire meal. The clinical examination also showed that although he coughed on liquids, he did not cough if he held his breath through the entire swallow sequence. Because this method required concentration for each attempt, it was questionable if the patient's alertness level would allow this compensation. After reading the report, the physician decided to begin weaning the patient from his medications, keeping the patient on his nasogastric tube. After 1 week the patient was reevaluated by the SLP. His marked change in level of alertness made her confident that he now could tolerate oral feeding and cooperate with any needed compensations during the meal. This case illustrates how a change in medical management might affect the success of a behavioral intervention.

actually swallowed. Does this pattern reflect a specific pattern of impaired physiology? Does it reflect the presence of compensations intended to protect the airway, or are there other possibilities? In some cases, this distinction may not be important. However, in others, it may be important to understand what might be changed as a result of therapy versus what might not be changed. This consideration may affect the decision to engage in therapy and, if so, the direction of therapy.

Another noteworthy point is that dysphagia treatment is rarely unifocal. Dysphagia is the result of underlying disease or disorder processes. Consequently, patients with dysphagia often receive therapies from medical, surgical, and/or behavioral realms. Clinicians who are treating patients with dysphagia should be aware of concomitant treatments, as well as dysphagia treatments in other realms that may either work together or in place of behavioral treatment strategies the SLP may provide. Figure 12-1 is a schematic reminder of how these therapy categories may interact. In certain clinical situations one category may comprise the primary or sole treatment approach. In other situations two or all three catego-

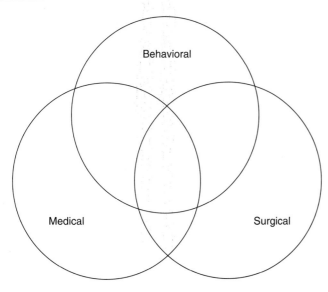

FIGURE 12-1. A schematic representation of potential interactions of behavioral, medical, and surgical treatment options in dysphagia.

BOX 12-2	Treatment Considerations Focusing on Patient Characteristics

- Etiology (underlying cause/disease or disorder)
- Severity
- Eating history
- Psychosocial factors
- Anticipated medical course
- Caregiver factors

ries may interact to form the most beneficial intervention.

PATIENT-SPECIFIC TREATMENT

Patients bring to any clinical situation a variety of unique circumstances. Box 12-2 provides a list of potential patient-related considerations that may have an impact on dysphagia treatment options and decisions. Because dysphagia is the result of underlying disease processes, the cause of dysphagia should be understood as best as clinically possible because the underlying disease presents a clinical course that has direct impact on swallowing function and benefits from various intervention strategies over time.

The severity of dysphagia is a more complex concept than might first be imagined. How is the severity of dysphagia graded? Some clinicians and investigators have used impairment of swallowing physiology based on instrumental examination,[2]

Practice Note 12-3

A 37-year-old woman came to the outpatient clinic with a diagnosis of suspected dysphagia secondary to multiple sclerosis (MS). She had just been discharged from the hospital, where she received the diagnosis of MS. Her modified barium swallow study showed minor penetration of the airway with a strong cough on thin liquids only. The SLP recommended that she continue the present diet; however, the focus of the appointment was on the possible progression of the MS and how that might affect swallowing. Because some types of MS show periods of exacerbation and remission, it was important to tell the patient that if swallowing became suddenly worse, it might be a signal of a new exacerbation; however, with medical and behavioral treatment, it should improve. Another area of discussion was whether the patient would ever want a feeding tube, and in which circumstances she would want it. The discussion of executing an advance directive to guide her future medical care was important because most likely she would have additional problems with swallowing in the future. The concept of an advance directive is discussed in Chapter 15.

whereas others have used more functional measures such as amount of food or liquid taken by mouth.[3,4] Some clinicians may believe that patients who take no food by mouth also have the poorest swallowing physiology. Unfortunately, this is not always the case. Patient status may change over time, and some patients who receive only nonoral feeding may actually have adequate swallowing physiology to ingest some food or liquid by mouth. Thus severity of dysphagia should not be considered a unitary concept because many factors are involved.

Eating history may provide clinicians with some idea of a patient's motivation and willingness to push toward increased oral intake. This interacts directly with certain psychosocial considerations. For example, the patient who reports that he "lives to eat, not eats to live" and who engages in the practice of chewing food that cannot be swallowed just for the taste may be more compliant with a rigorous therapy plan than the patient who uses only nonoral sources and never attempts any oral intake of food or liquid. In addition, eating history may provide the clinician with cultural biases in food selection (i.e., the patient never ate that food or always ate that food) or limitations in specific food availability associated with the patient's environment. Social aspects of eating should also be considered in terms of the patient's current situation ("I attempt to eat alone in my room") and future goals ("I would like to eat in a restaurant"). Finally, for patients who engage in both oral and tube feeding, eating history may explain the timing of one form of feeding relative to the other. This factor may be important in reaching functional goals in therapy.

The patient's anticipated medical course is an essential factor for the clinician to understand. It may affect the consideration of whether to initiate therapy as well as which types of therapy to undertake. In some clinical scenarios it may be better to wait and monitor the patient's condition (e.g., stability, endurance). In other situations aggressive therapy is indicated. Clinicians must keep in mind that therapeutic strategies should change as the patient's underlying condition (and potentially dysphagia) changes.

Caregiver considerations are an extension of patient considerations, especially for patients (at any age) who are unable to perform self-care (including feeding). Whether the caregiver is a nurse, other qualified health care provider, spouse or other family member, or friend, caregiver performance can have a direct impact (positive or negative) on the performance of the patient with dysphagia. Mealtimes can become complicated by a caregiver who is uninitiated in proper feeding strategies for the dependent patient. Positioning of the patient, rate and manner of food presentation, and other variables need to be clearly understood by caregivers.

Practice Note 12-4

A 78-year-old woman who lived alone had just had a second stroke that left her immobile and dysphagic. Her swallowing improved in the hospital to the point where she could safely eat a blended diet. She also needed oral supplements six times a day to receive a sufficient amount of calories. Her neighbor and best friend volunteered to take her home. Before leaving the hospital the neighbor received training from the dietitian on how to prepare the patient's food. After 6 months, the neighbor said that the time to prepare the food was becoming a burden and that her friend really could not afford the supplemental feedings. She did not want to put her friend in a nursing home. The physician, friend, and patient agreed that a gastrostomy would allow the patient to receive the majority of calories through her tube. It also was determined that a few of her favorite food items that did not require special preparation could be taken orally for pleasure.

The patient's residential environment also can affect the nature of dysphagia interventions (see Chapter 1). The needs of the patient in the intensive care unit are different from those of the individual receiving outpatient therapy. In addition, the resources available in different environments differ dramatically. Clinicians working in academic medical centers often have more resources available than do clinicians working in rural long-term care facilities.

APPROACH-SPECIFIC TREATMENT

Treatment techniques (including medical, surgical, and behavioral), like individual patients, require specific consideration in planning intervention. As previously mentioned, treatment options change as the patient's condition changes over time. From this perspective the decision of when to intervene, as well as how to intervene (choice of technique), changes according to the patient's condition. In general, treatment strategies may be considered in reference to the degree of interaction with the patient and/or the intent of treatment. A common approach to patients who are severely debilitated or in the acute phase of an illness is a prophylactic or preventative approach. Such approaches often tend to be passive, not requiring substantial activity from the patient. Oral hygiene, passive movements, and perhaps diet changes might be considered passive interventions. Active interventions are those in which the patient is required to engage in direct maneuvers or compensations to change some aspect of swallowing performance. Another dichotomy that may overlap with active versus passive interventions is that of patient-centered versus environment-centered interventions. Patient-centered interventions may be active or passive, but all focus on the patient. Environment-centered interventions are primarily passive, with the focus on changing some aspect of the patient's environment. Dining rooms or special mealtimes for patients with dysphagia are examples of environment-centered interventions.

Treatment Choices

Box 12-3 presents a list of considerations that apply in choosing any specific treatment technique. Clinicians must consider which treatment options are realistically available. In determining this, the following should be considered: the physical presence of technology/equipment required to use a specific technique (e.g., surface electromyography [sEMG] biofeedback), the clinician's knowledge of and skill in performing a specific technique, and the patient's acceptance of the technique. (Does the patient under-

BOX 12-3	Considerations in Choosing a Specific Treatment Technique
Options	→	What?
Clinical indicators	→	Why?
Anticipated risks and benefits	→	Immediate
Functional outcome	→	Long term
Patient empowerment	→	Compliance

BOX 12-4	Common Medical Options for Dysphagia Treatment

DIETARY MODIFICATIONS
- Special diets
- Regulation of nutrition and hydration
- Possible interaction with feeding route (oral vs. nonoral)

PHARMACOLOGIC MANAGEMENT
- Antireflux medications
- Prokinetic agents
- Salivary management

stand the instructions? Is he or she able to perform the technique? Can the patient afford the technique? What are the demands on the patient to adequately perform the technique?)

Clinical indicators address the question, "Why choose this particular technique?" For example, how does the technique under consideration relate to the specifics of the patient's dysphagic complaints or symptoms? Is the technique clinically and biologically plausible? Should the technique be performed in isolation or in combination with other techniques? These considerations are important in selecting any specific technique. Seeking the answers to these questions forms the basis of an evidence-based literature search.

Anticipated risks and benefits to the patient should be considered in reference to the immediate outcome of the proposed technique. Some techniques that appear to be relatively benign may complicate certain comorbid conditions in some patients. For example, techniques that emphasize a prolonged **apneic pause** during swallowing attempts might be problematic for some patients with significant respiratory diseases (see Chapter 8 for a discussion of respiratory-related issues). Techniques that require significant muscular effort during repeated swallow attempts might be counterproductive in certain patients with muscle wasting or weakness. In addition to identifying the risks, clinicians also must identify the potential immediate benefits to the patient from any given technique. Some techniques have been shown to be immediately effective in reducing or eliminating certain swallowing deficits (e.g., head turn to compensate for hemipharyngeal weakness leading to residue and aspiration (see Chapter 14). Clinicians should always consider the potential risks of any technique in reference to the potential benefits to the patient.

Functional outcome refers to the long-term benefit of the proposed technique. This is often considered in reference to the goal(s) of therapy. A technique that results in an immediate change in swallowing performance may or may not have a long-term positive impact or it may not be functional for the daily environment. Similarly, some techniques may not have an immediate impact but may produce long-term functional benefit after intensive practice. Therefore choice of technique should be considered in reference to long-term functional outcome in addition to the potential for immediate impact.

Patient *empowerment* may be interpreted in different ways. One focus of this term is patient involvement in the design of the treatment plan. Involving patients implies their understanding of the proposed plan of treatment and their willingness to participate in that particular plan. This process makes the patient a partner in treatment rather than only a recipient. Patients who are empowered in this process are known to be more compliant with treatment activities, hence increasing the probability for successful outcomes.

OVERVIEW OF TREATMENT OPTIONS

Clinicians should be aware of multiple options for dysphagia intervention, including medical, surgical, and behavioral treatment. Such knowledge increases pertinent communication with other health care providers and facilitates selection of the best treatment options for individual patients. This section provides a brief overview of some of the more recognized medical, surgical, and behavioral treatment options for dysphagia. Chapters 13 and 14 provide a more detailed review of behavioral treatment techniques.

Medical Options

Box 12-4 offers an introduction to common medical options for dysphagia intervention. Medical options in this context refer to dietary modifications or pharmacologic management.

Dietary adjustments might seem a strange inclusion under medical treatment options; however, clinicians should be aware that the patient's diet (oral or nonoral route) may need to be modified to accommodate an underlying disease or condition. Common examples of this occur in diabetes or **hypertension**, which are both related to stroke. Other examples are found among patients who do not tolerate certain tube feedings well, resulting in diarrhea or constipation. A different example is the patient who requires a minimal (or maximal) amount of caloric intake or hydration for health reasons that may or may not be related to dysphagia. Even if the dietary requirements are tangentially related to the condition contributing to dysphagia, the fact that a specific regimen is required will interact with planning dysphagia intervention.

Pharmacologic management of dysphagia refers to the use of medications to improve some aspect of swallowing function. The most commonly encountered medications are those used to combat reflux, improve gastric motility, and alter secretions. A hierarchy of medications is available to combat reflux symptoms. On the lower end of the hierarchy are approaches such as over-the-counter antacids and certain chewing gum products. The next level of medication is the class of **histamine-receptor antagonists**. These medications are reported to eliminate approximately two thirds of stomach acid. The strongest level of medication is the **proton-pump inhibitor**. These medications are reported to eliminate nearly all stomach acid and represent the strongest pharmacologic approach to acid suppression (see Chapter 7). Multiple drugs are available within each class of medications, and often the choice of medication is based on patient tolerance (fewer side effects) and symptom reduction.

Few medications to improve gastric motility are available.[5] These so-called prokinetic agents are intended to improve esophageal motility, increase lower esophageal sphincter pressure, and promote gastric emptying.

Salivary secretions are important to swallowing functions. They provide important lubrication to the swallowing mechanism and contain important chemicals that protect the teeth and assist with digestive functions. In general, two components of saliva may be considered. One is the watery saliva that emerges from the sublingual and other salivary glands during chewing or other oral movements. The other is the thicker coating of the internal mucosa. Many medical conditions and medical treatments can alter saliva. Some medical treatments such as radiotherapy (see Chapter 6) and certain medications reduce the amount of watery saliva, leaving the patient with a dry mouth and reports of thick, adhering mucus in the mouth and throat. Depending on the cause of the condition, certain medications (mucolytics) might be used to thin the thicker secretions, making them easier to swallow (or expectorate if necessary). In addition, certain medications are available that attempt to increase the volume of watery secretions. Alternatively, substances are available (most do not require prescription) that can provide lubrication to the mouth from external application. Medical conditions rarely increase salivary flow. Careful examination of the patient who reports excessive saliva often reveals a reduction in the frequency of swallowing as the cause for salivary retention in the mouth or pharynx.

Surgical Options

Box 12-5 summarizes common surgical interventions for dysphagia. Surgical interventions can be divided into three categories: those that improve glottal closure, those designed to protect the airway, and those designed to improve opening of the pharyngoesophageal segment (PES).

Improving Glottal Closure

Two basic approaches have become popular to improve glottal closure: medialization thyroplasty and injection of biomaterials. Before these techniques are described, it should be noted that which patients will benefit from these procedures is not always clear. Clinical experience has revealed that some patients who aspirate receive direct and immediate benefit from improving glottal closure, whereas others have negligible benefit even in combination with other therapies. In this regard, these techniques should be included within the conceptual background of the

---

BOX 12-5	Common Surgical Options for Dysphagia Treatment

- Improved glottal closure
  - Medialization thyroplasty
  - Injection of biomaterials
- Protection of the airway
  - Stents
  - Laryngotracheal separation
  - Laryngectomy
  - Tracheostomy tubes
  - Feeding tubes
- Improved pharyngoesophageal segment opening
  - Dilatation
  - Myotomy
  - Botulinum toxin injection

dysphagia clinician, but with the caveat that the techniques need to be considered realistically in the context of individual patients.

Medialization thyroplasty is a surgical technique that requires the patient to be sedated but not under general anesthesia. A small incision is made in the lower neck over the thyroid cartilage. A small window is made through the cartilage just behind the vocal fold. The vocal fold is moved toward the midline, and a small piece of medical-grade plastic is placed behind the vocal fold between it and the thyroid cartilage. Because the patient is awake during the procedure, transnasal endoscopy is used to monitor the degree of medialization of the vocal fold, and the patient may be asked to phonate so that the surgeon can assess glottal function for voice production. Using patient swallowing symptom report, Kraus et al.[6] found that all their patients reported improvement in swallowing function after thyroplasty. In a modified version of thyroplasty in 15 patients with vocal fold paralysis after thoracic surgery (see Chapter 8), all patients reported improvement in or a reduction of dysphagia symptoms.[7]

Biomaterials may be injected directly into a weakened vocal fold in an attempt to "bulk up" the tissue, thus improving glottal closure. Historically, Teflon was a common material injected into the vocal fold; however, in recent years Teflon has fallen out of favor and has been replaced by **autologous fat** (taken from the patient's anterior belly) or collagen (commercially available). Most commonly (although variations exist), materials are injected into the vocal fold while the patient is under general anesthesia. Typically, injection of biomaterials is used to reduce a smaller glottal gap, whereas medialization thyroplasty is used for larger gaps. However, different surgeons may prefer one technique over the other.

Protecting the Airway

Although glottal closure techniques are intended to enhance airway protection during swallowing, certain medical conditions may require more dramatic airway protection approaches. Some of these surgical approaches are intended for short-term use until a crisis passes, whereas others may be permanent. A *laryngeal stent* has been described as a "plug" within the larynx to prevent material from entering the airway. Because the glottis is blocked, this procedure requires a tracheostomy. *Laryngotracheal separation* is a self-describing surgical procedure. The trachea is surgically separated just below the larynx and brought forward to a tracheostoma, and the remaining trachea inferior to the larynx is sutured closed. Thus the larynx is in place but is separated from the airway.

Both stents and laryngotracheal separation have been described as temporary surgical interventions until patients recover from acute aspiration risk.[8] However, data on the success of reversibility are mixed. In a series of patients with amyotrophic lateral sclerosis, Mita[9] reported a reduction in the rates of aspiration and rehospitalization; however, only 21% of the patients were able to eat orally. Pletcher et al.[10] performed laryngotracheal separation for a patient with severe aspiration after a brainstem stroke. The patient recovered to a point where oral ingestion and voice could be restored, and the procedure was reversed. In a 5-year follow-up the patient continued to eat safely and had good voice. Zocratto et al.[11] provided follow-up data on 60 patients who underwent laryngotracheal separation, 12 of whom had surgical reversals. The complication rate in the group without reversals was 43%, although aspiration was successfully managed. In the group with reversals, the complication rate was 58%. The authors concluded that although the benefits of aspiration reduction were positive, the postsurgical complication rate was unacceptably high. A *total laryngectomy* represents a potential permanent surgical solution to dysphagia and aspiration. Although a dramatic approach, in some circumstances patients will have better overall function without the larynx (see Clinical Case Example 15-1). Permanent separation of the airway and food tracts may allow the individual to ingest food and liquid safely, and techniques for voice restoration in laryngectomy may facilitate spoken communication.

The use of tracheostomy tubes or feeding tubes in attempts to protect the airway from prandial aspiration has been questioned. Available research suggests that this may not be valid reasoning, and that in some patients tracheostomy tubes can further impair swallowing function and increase the risk of airway compromise (see Chapter 8). Placement of a feeding tube (nasogastric or gastrostomy) does not necessarily reduce aspiration and may increase the rate and/or severity of aspiration, often from reflux mechanisms (see Chapter 15). Therefore although both surgical options are valid and helpful in individual patients, caution and clear reasoning should be exercised in their consideration.

Improving Pharyngoesophageal Segment Opening

Three general surgical approaches are available to improve opening of the PES: stretching, cutting, or paralysis. Stretching is accomplished by the process of dilatation. Dilatation may be accomplished by more than one technique, but the goal is to stretch the lumen of the PES. If PES opening is restricted by scarring, dilatation tears tissue to create a larger opening.

However, the risk is twofold: (1) The tear may extend beyond the esophageal tissue, and (2) the effect is often temporary, requiring repeated procedures and, at times, reaching a plateau of benefit. PES limitations resulting from physiologic processes may also respond to dilatation.[12] Although dilatation is used less often than other techniques, reports have demonstrated benefit from this procedure in cases of physiologic stenosis of the PES.

Surgical myotomy is a technique in which the fibers of the cricopharyngeal muscle within the PES are separated.[13] As with many surgical techniques, variations exist and little evidence suggests that one technique variation is superior to any other. Myotomy may be used in combination with other surgical techniques such as supraglottic laryngectomy or total laryngectomy. Applied judiciously to the appropriate patient, surgical myotomy may provide significant benefit to the individual with dysphagia.

Injection of *botulinum toxin* (Botox) has been described as an effective technique to "relax" the PES. Botulinum toxin works by the process of **chemodenervation**, in which the chemical communication between the motor nerve and the muscle is interrupted. The result is a paresis in the muscle. Injection of botulinum toxin has been shown to improve PES opening and hence swallowing function in selected patients.[14-16] A general rule for selecting patients for this technique (as well as for other techniques focusing on the PES) is that swallowing mechanics above the PES should be optimized. Significant esophageal reflux might be considered a contraindication to these techniques because weakening the PES may result in supraesophageal complications to voice and the airway.

Behavioral Options

More options exist for behavioral interventions for dysphagia than both medical and surgical options combined. Box 12-6 summarizes five general categories of behavioral intervention that may be used in dysphagia intervention. These categories are not meant to be either exhaustive or specific (see Chapters 13 and 14 for specifics on techniques); rather they are intended to serve as an overview to behavioral therapy approaches.

Food Modifications

Food modifications are among the most widely used behavioral interventions in dysphagia therapy. Food and liquid may be modified in many ways to compensate for a swallowing deficit or in an attempt to alter the swallow pattern toward the goal of improved function. Several aspects of food and liquid modifications may be considered.

Rheology. Modifying the **rheologic** properties of foods and liquids is a common strategy. Thickening liquids with commercial products or purchasing thickened liquids such as nectars is often done in an attempt to slow liquid-bolus transit and form a slightly more cohesive bolus. It is believed that these rheologic changes give patients a better opportunity to swallow without (or with less) airway compromise. This practice has attained a quasi-scientific level at which multiple degrees of thickening have been advocated. The issue also is complicated by the fact that the rheologic properties of test swallow materials used at the bedside are not the same as those used for the modified barium swallow studies.[17,18] Therefore swallowing success on materials used in the modified barium swallow study may not be a rheologic match with what the patient actually receives on the meal tray. Current evidence on the benefits of thickened liquids is limited, and there is some suggestion that patients may not enjoy, and thus may not comply with, a regimen of thickened liquids.[19] Solid foods may also be rheologically modified. A common example of this is pureed food. Experienced clinicians recognize that the concept of puree is highly variable. As one clinician commented, "One man's puree is another man's soup." Nonetheless, clinicians, caregivers, and patients chop, mix, blend, and puree foods to reduce the need for chewing, reduce the particulate nature of certain foods, and enhance the ease of swallowing. Another example in this category is the soft mechanical diet. This diet level requires mastication, but foods are soft and often form a cohesive bolus when swallowed. A related question is *"How* soft?" Some patients are able to masticate certain foods with their teeth or tongue without significant reduction in functional eating ability. Little evidence exists to help formulate guidelines to identify which patients should receive which diet level. Thus clinicians must consider this decision in reference to each individual patient. Dysphagia experts from the American Speech, Language, and Hearing Association and the American Dietetic Association have developed the National Dys-

BOX 12-6	Five General Categories of Behavioral Interventions for Dysphagia

- Food modification
- Modifying feeding activity
- Patient modifications
- Swallow modification
- Mechanism modifications

phagia Diet.[20] Liquid materials have been described with specific rheologic ranges (in **centipoise**) to define thin, nectar thick, and honey thick. Other recommendations on what types of semisolids and solids would be considered safe and unsafe for the patient are described.

Volume. This bolus modification is self-explanatory. Some patients require smaller bolus volumes to be able to control and safely transit the bolus through the swallowing mechanism with minimal post-swallow residue. Others may require a larger bolus for various reasons, such as increased sensory input. The average bolus size (±1 standard deviation) of a liquid bolus taken from a cup ranges from 15 to 26 mL and differs between men and women.[21,22] Bolus volume is one factor that may alter swallow physiology. Thus when small bolus volumes are used, either in assessment or in treatment, swallow physiology may be altered. The important clinical issue is to take all available steps to ascertain that physiology is altered in a positive direction to enhance swallow function through changes in bolus volume.

Temperature. Temperature manipulation is an interesting, multifocal consideration in dysphagia intervention. Cold materials are believed to enhance awareness of a bolus and may have an impact on oropharyngeal swallowing physiology. How cold a bolus should be is an unanswered question. Hot materials (and very cold materials) typically are ingested in smaller amounts and thus may interact with bolus volume. Both hot and cold materials may affect esophageal function. Anyone who has ingested either very hot or very cold materials recognizes the discomfort as that material passes through the esophagus. In those with myotonia, cold may interfere with the rapid musculature contraction need for sequential swallows. In **diffuse esophageal spasm**, extreme pain may be triggered by hot or cold materials within the esophagus. The presence of this condition (or other conditions) may be a contraindication for using hot or cold materials in dysphagia intervention. There are reports of swallow **syncope** (vasovagal reflex) triggering **bradycardia** associated with the temperature (hot) of the bolus.[23]

A different perspective on temperature is that of the patient who does eat by mouth but eats inefficiently. These individuals may face the inconvenience and frustration associated with a warm meal getting too cool before the meal is finished. Such patients often report that they use microwaves, ovens, hot plates, or other means to maintain a desired temperature of food over the course of a meal.

Taste and Smell. The senses of taste and smell are not part of the traditional evaluation of swallowing function, and patients are often left to the culinary skills of caregivers or kitchen staff in reference to the palatability of food. However, taste and smell are both essential features of eating. These senses are interrelated because the four basic tastes are supplemented by flavors (mediated by odor) to provide sensory input during meals. Taste and smell alterations may affect appetite, motivation, and swallowing physiology. Furthermore, taste enhancement (which is typically accomplished by increasing flavor) has been shown to have a positive effect on oral intake in older adults and in certain clinical populations.[24] Hence, taste and smell manipulation may contribute to changes in swallow physiology, appetite, motivation, and enjoyment of meals. The positive aspects of these sensory manipulations may be improved ingestion of food and liquid, contributing to improved health status. Figure 12-2 shows the same pureed meal presented in different aesthetic contexts. Inasmuch as a picture is worth a thousand words, these images should speak loudly.

What a patient sees on a plate might be as important as how it smells or tastes. Certain pureed foods can be visually unappealing and may depress or, at best, not facilitate appetite or motivation to eat. Although aesthetics of food presentation is still an aspect requiring clinical investigation, available clinical research has focused on enhancing the visual appeal of meals as a factor in improving intake.

Modify Feeding Activity

Mealtime activity may require modification to accommodate the needs of individual patients. Examples of mealtime modification include changing the meal schedule, oropharyngeal cleansing or hydration, and/or the use of feeding aids.

For some patients, the meal schedule may be extremely important—for example, the importance of timing meals to the maximal benefit cycle of medications in certain diseases such as Parkinson's disease. Other examples include the patient who is satiated with small amounts of food and requires multiple meals per day to maintain adequate nutrition. Finally, a common recommendation for timing of oral feedings in patients who are being weaned from feeding tubes is for the patient to ingest the oral meal before tube feeding to take advantage of biologic motivation (hunger) during the oral meals (see feeding tube weaning in Chapter 15).

Other mealtime adjustments may be warranted in various situations. For example, patients who reside in care facilitates may require special dining arrangements to minimize distractions during meals. These "dysphagia dining rooms" often afford the patient a

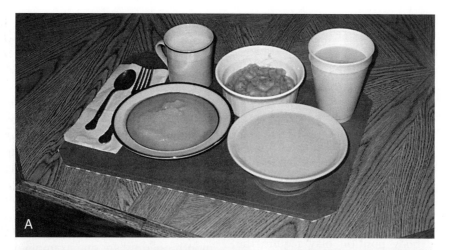

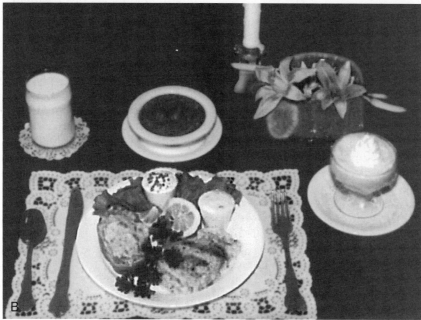

FIGURE 12-2. **A** and **B** are photographs of pureed meals with different aesthetic presentation.

better caregiver/patient ratio and thus the potential for increased cueing or other strategies that may facilitate a positive meal experience.[25] This arrangement may interact with other mealtime modifications, including rate of feeding, specific placement of a bolus, and various clearing strategies to minimize residue and enhance airway protection. During mealtimes, these tactics may be more successful with enhanced clinician or caregiver supervision in an area with reduced distraction.[26]

Patients who have poor oropharyngeal clearance when swallowing certain foods may benefit from alternating food swallows with liquid swallows. The intent here is to use the subsequent liquid as a "wash"

or cleansing mechanism to remove residue from the prior swallow. If a patient has xerostomia (dry mouth), preswallow hydration of the oral cavity may be beneficial. This may be accomplished by swallowing liquid, by sucking on gauze soaked in liquid, by spraying water into the mouth, or by using synthetic saliva.

Feeding aids may benefit patients with any number of physiologic or anatomic limitations. Occupational therapists (see Chapter 1) may be invaluable in fashioning devices to accommodate limitations in hand and limb function. Such devices may make the difference between the patient achieving independence as a self-feeder or remaining a dependent feeder. Other modifications may be required in cases of trauma or surgical restructuring of the oral mechanism. Possible alternatives may include the use of nipples, flow-controlled feeders, straws, specialized utensils (e.g., glossectomy spoons), or catheters.

Patient Modifications

The most common strategies used in this category are positioning strategies. These might involve head-position strategies such as head-turn or chin-tuck maneuvers or whole-body–positioning strategies. Chapters 13 and 14 address head position strategies in more detail. This section addresses whole-body positioning.

An initial caveat is the reminder that for certain patients, changing body position may require the consultation of other dysphagia team members, specifically the physical therapist (see Chapter 1). In general, the patient should be positioned such that physical capabilities are maximized and accommodations to improve swallowing can be incorporated. With that in mind, common position adjustments might include the patient tilting to the side or back, side-lying, or maintaining an upright posture.

Patients with hemipharyngeal weakness may benefit from tilting the upper body such that the stronger side is lower and able to benefit from gravity to assist bolus transit. This positioning technique may be combined with a head turn toward the weaker side of the pharynx. An exaggerated example of this approach is the side-lying position. This technique may be used in circumstances in which patients want to maximize residual pharyngeal muscle function, while at the same time reducing bolus speed by removing the influence of gravity. If pharyngeal asymmetry exists, the stronger side is typically lower.

Tilting the patient backward may be beneficial when oral movements reduce transit of the bolus through the mouth or when significant residue remains in the piriform sinuses after a swallow. One consideration for this technique should be airway protection ability.

Upright posture may be an important consideration in patients with oropharyngeal or esophageal deficits. Residue in the proximal esophagus may reflux into the hypopharynx during or after meals. Keeping the patient upright adds the potential protective mechanism of gravity in an attempt to minimize the upward movement of esophageal residue. In cases of severe reflux, upright posture during and after meals may be important even if the patient receives nutrition from a gastrostomy tube. Finally, it is well known that elevating the head of the bed is beneficial in combating nocturnal reflux.[27]

Mechanism Modifications

Attempts to modify the swallowing mechanism include motor exercises, sensory stimulation, and prosthetic adjustments to compensate for physiologic or anatomic deficits. Motor exercises typically address one of five features of motor function: strength, range, tone, steadiness, or accuracy. Depending on the underlying disease and the overt movement dysfunction, various techniques may be applied. Common approaches to improve strength may include resistance activities in which the patient attempts to move against resistance. Range of movement may be increased by stretching activities. Stretching activities used by patients with trismus in an attempt to increase mouth opening are one example of increasing range of movement. Accuracy and steadiness affect coordination. Depending on the specific attributes of the movement dysfunction, various techniques may be used, ranging from altering the rheologic properties of swallowed materials to using a contained bolus manipulated around the mouth but not swallowed.

Sensory stimulation activities may involve changes in taste, temperature, or the application of pressure. Limited experimentation has occurred with the use of electrical stimulation as a sensory approach to improving movement associated with swallowing (see Chapter 14). Finally, improved oral hygiene, when indicated, may facilitate improved sensory functions and reduce disease risks.

Prosthetic management may be accomplished in conjunction with a maxillofacial prosthodontist as a member of the dysphagia team. Prosthodontists can fabricate palatal lifts, obturators, and other devices to fill anatomic deviations that might exist in certain patients with dysphagia.

Swallow Modifications

Swallow modifications focus primarily on altering the physiology of the attempted swallow. These activities often require active participation from the patient and intensive practice to induce movement change. Chapters 13 and 14 provide a detailed review of the more common behavioral techniques to modify swallow physiology in children and adults.

MAKING TREATMENT DECISIONS

Many approaches may be followed in developing intervention plans. This section offers a framework detailing steps in clinical decision making that may be helpful to dysphagia clinicians. Three aspects are considered: (1) sources of information used in treat-

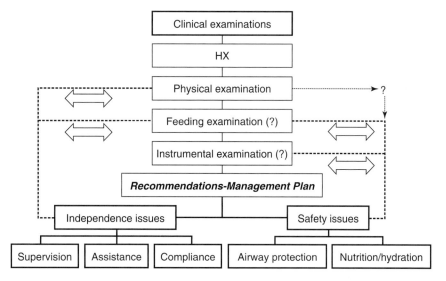

FIGURE 12-3. Flowchart depicting potential sources of treatment-planning information based on various components of the dysphagia evaluation. *HX,* Medical history.

ment planning, (2) formation of meaningful clinical questions, and (3) development of individual treatment plans.

Sources of Information

Figure 12-3 presents a flowchart detailing potential sources of clinical information that may address treatment issues. In this depiction, treatment issues are divided into "independence issues" and "safety issues." Independence issues include supervision, assistance, and compliance. *Supervision* refers to the patient's need for direct supervision during mealtime, perhaps to monitor food intake and use of compensations or for other reasons. *Assistance* refers to the use of direct physical assistance during mealtime. *Compliance* refers to the patient's adherence to an intervention plan. Safety issues include airway protection and nutrition and hydration. *Airway protection* refers to the overt presence of aspiration or the risk of aspiration from excessive residue or other factors. This term should also consider airway obstruction from solid foods. *Nutrition and hydration* refer to the patient's ability to ingest sufficient calories and fluids. Independence and safety issues often interact. For example, the patient who requires but does not receive adequate assistance may have reduced airway protection or may ingest insufficient amounts of food or liquid.

The diagram in Figure 12-3 attempts to estimate the source(s) of assessment information relative to independence and safety issues. Independence issues may be addressed more from the physical examination and the feeding examination. Instrumental examinations may not be needed to address inde-

pendence issues. Conversely, instrumental examinations seem essential in making safety determinations, especially airway protection issues. Nutrition and hydration issues are better addressed through a combination of the instrumental examination and the feeding examination.

Forming Meaningful Questions

Once relevant clinical information has been gathered and organized into some conceptual framework (such as that depicted in Figure 12-3), a next logical step is to pose the question "Which treatment technique(s) are best suited to this individual patient or problem?" This becomes part of an evidence-based approach to treatment of dysphagia. The framework depicted in Figure 12-4 offers one potential method from which to formulate meaningful clinical questions pertaining to treatment options.

Starting with the focus on the patient or problem, clinicians should first frame the question. The example in Figure 12-4 presents a patient with neurogenic pharyngeal dysphagia resulting from nonprogressive disease. This patient demonstrates residue and aspiration on examination. Based on the examination, a treatment option is considered—in this case, the use of sEMG biofeedback. Next, treatment alternatives are considered—in this case, teaching the Mendelsohn maneuver in isolation. Finally, expected outcomes are framed as a question. Can the use of biofeedback in addition to the clinical maneuver improve functional outcome (e.g., better swallow) while reducing the number of treatment sessions (i.e., increasing efficiency of therapy)? After forming this question, clini-

	Patient or Problem	Therapy Technique	Other Options	Outcomes
Focus Your Question	Starting with your patient, ask: "How would I describe a group of similar patients?"	Ask: "Which technique am I considering?"	Ask: "What is the main alternative or option?"	Ask: "What can I hope to gain?"
		Be specific	Be specific	Be specific
Example	In patients with neurogenic pharyngeal dysphagia in nonprogressive disease with residue and aspiration....	"Would use sEMG biofeedback"	"Compared with only a Mendelsohn maneuver"	"Improve the functional outcome of therapy and decrease the number of therapy sessions"

FIGURE 12-4. One framework from which to pose meaningful clinical questions regarding best treatment options. *sEMG,* Surface electromyography.

cians need to survey the evidence on these techniques to find the answer. For this specific example, evidence supporting the use of biofeedback would be research indicating that use of this technique enhanced functional outcomes of therapy with less time investment than therapy without this technique.[28-30] If such evidence was identified, the clinician should consider using this technique.

Planning Individual Therapy

Once the treatment question is formulated and treatment options have been systematically considered (based on available evidence), the individual treatment plan may be developed. One format for the treatment plan is depicted in Box 12-7. *Goals* are statements of anticipated outcome based on the patient's pretreatment functional level with consideration of the clinical examination results (presumably identifying some or all of the reasons for the pretreatment functional level). Beginning clinicians are encouraged to keep in mind that goals can change as the patient's status changes. In addition, it may be prudent clinical practice to focus on a single functional goal, especially in the initial aspects of therapy. Goals should be simple statements that are understood by the patient and caregivers. For example, a goal statement for a patient who is taking no food or liquid by mouth may be "to establish the safe and consistent oral intake of any substance in any amount." Conceptually, if the patient cannot reach this functional level, further advances in oral intake are unlikely. Setting goals that

---

BOX 12-7   One Format for Developing Individual Treatment Plans for Dysphagia

GOALS
- Statement(s) of anticipated functional outcome

OBJECTIVES
- Target aspects of the swallow and/or patient that require change to reach the functional goal

ACTION PLANS
- Activities in which the patient and clinician engage; procedures and progress monitors to be used in therapy are specified

---

are too ambitious may reduce patient (and clinician) motivation and compliance with a treatment program. Surpassing goals most likely will not contribute to that scenario.

Objectives target items regarding the swallow and/or the patient that require change for the functional goal to be reached. These may be specific aspects of swallow physiology such as increased hyolaryngeal elevation or patient-related aspects such as rate of eating. If objectives are met, goals will be reached.

Action plans reflect activities in which the patient and/or clinician will engage. These are direct statements of procedures. Action plans should include instructions to the patient reflecting technique, frequency of practice, amount to be swallowed, or other

Practice Note 12-5

Two months after his brainstem stroke and being fed by gastrostomy, the patient came for an evaluation to determine whether he was a candidate for dysphagia treatment. The SLP thought the patient could begin therapy and in the discussion asked the patient what he hoped to achieve in therapy. The SLP used the 7-point Functional Oral Intake Scale (see Chapter 9) and asked the patient to point to a number on the scale that he believe would be a reasonable goal. Because he was completely tube fed at the time of the evaluation, the patient's current level was at 1. He immediately pointed to 7 (total oral diet with no restrictions). Having treated similar patients in the past and based on the current evaluation, the SLP believed that a total oral diet without restrictions was unreasonable. Instead she asked the patient if he would be satisfied as an initial goal to reach level 4 (total oral diet of one consistency). She pointed out that reaching that goal would mean he would be free of the tube feeding. The patient agreed that this goal would provide him great relief and add immensely to his quality of life. Use of the Functional Oral Intake Scale can be valuable in reaching agreeing on therapist and patient expectations.

CLINICAL CORNER 12-1

A new clinician was told by her supervisor that patients who demonstrate swallow delay may benefit from the therapeutic intervention of a sour bolus. The clinician was told that the hospital kept a large supply of lemon ice on each floor for this purpose. The clinician was working with a patient who showed swallow delay as a result of a partial tongue resection secondary to cancer. After 6 days of therapy with the lemon ice, the clinician did not believe that the swallow delay had improved.

CRITICAL THINKING:
1. What are some potential reasons why the sour bolus did not help trigger a faster swallow in her patient?
2. Do a literature search on sour bolus and swallow delay and decide when, how, and with whom you would use this technique.

CLINICAL CORNER 12-2

After radiation treatment to the tongue base, the patient was working on hard swallow techniques to improve laryngeal elevation. Attempts in therapy using 5 and 10 mL of water showed considerable swallow delay, double swallows on most boluses to clear them from the oral cavity and pharynx, and considerable post-swallow coughing with approximately 30 seconds between swallow attempts before the coughing subsided.

CRITICAL THINKING:
1. Physiologically, speculate on why the patient was coughing after the swallow.
2. In addition to measuring the number of expectorations, what other simple behavioral measurements could be made to show progress in therapy?

directly overt aspects of the therapy program. In addition, action plans should include techniques to monitor the immediate impact of the treatment technique(s). These monitors do not need to be elaborate, nor do they require repeated instrumental examinations to evaluate progress. However, often based on instrumental examinations, monitors may be behaviors that indicate change in the swallow performance. For example, consider the patient who expectorates after each swallowing attempt. One potential monitor of performance change in swallowing might be a reduction in the frequency of post-swallow expectoration. Actions plans affect objectives, which in turn affect functional goals and therefore overt swallowing performance.

FRAMEWORK FOR TREATMENT PLANNING

Figures 12-5 and 12-6 depict one organizational framework for planning dysphagia treatment. Using pharyngeal dysphagia as an example, these flowcharts present the general organization of the treatment planning concepts in this chapter, followed by a spe-

cific clinical example. At the top of the hierarchy (see Figure 12-5), pretreatment functional level is determined. As previously indicated, severity of dysphagia or functional level is a complex issue. One perspective might be to consider the amount and type of food and liquid a patient is safely ingesting by mouth at the time of evaluation. Although simplistic, this approach may be the most meaningful to the patient. Extending from this functional level are swallowing

Making Clinical Decisions
Steps in Developing a Treatment Plan

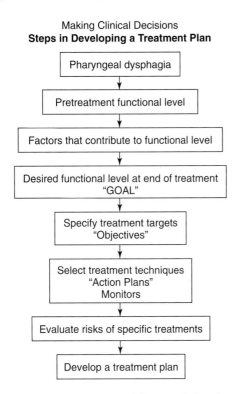

Pharyngeal dysphagia

↓

Pretreatment functional level

↓

Factors that contribute to functional level

↓

Desired functional level at end of treatment
"GOAL"

↓

Specify treatment targets
"Objectives"

↓

Select treatment techniques
"Action Plans"
Monitors

↓

Evaluate risks of specific treatments

↓

Develop a treatment plan

FIGURE 12-5. An organizational framework for planning dysphagia treatment.

factors believed to be contributing to the reduced function. Next, a goal for therapy is established. This is an outcome statement and, whenever possible, it should be developed in conjunction with the patient and/or caregivers. Objectives and specific actions are selected as stepping stones by which the patient may reach the functional goal. Finally, risks of the respective treatment techniques are considered in reference to the anticipated benefit(s).

Figure 12-6, *A,* uses the example of pharyngeal dysphagia, and specific decisions that might be made during the planning process are detailed. Early in the planning process, the clinician must decide whether the patient is a good candidate for therapy. This decision involves a prognosis. Several considerations for treatment candidacy were discussed earlier in this chapter; however, prognosis for therapy response is not an exact science for dysphagia. The best course of action may be to overtly recognize the basis for any prognostic decision based on available evidence.

If the patient is considered a good therapy candidate, goals and objectives are developed. Figure 12-6, *A,* presents four objectives that may be considered in pharyngeal dysphagia: laryngeal elevation, pharyngeal contraction, airway protection, and PES opening. The next step is to select action plans for each of these objectives. Figure 12-6, *B,* takes one of the objectives—

laryngeal elevation—and considers three potential action plans. The Mendelsohn maneuver facilitates sustained laryngeal elevation and thus is an appropriate action plan. On the negative side, this maneuver may prolong the apneic pause during swallowing and thus may be contraindicated for some patients with compromised respiratory function. In addition, it is difficult to teach this maneuver to certain patients. Clinicians should consider the available evidence supporting use of this maneuver for the specific problem and patient under consideration (see Chapters 13 and 14). Finally, the decision to use (or not to use) a technique is made along with any special considerations. An example of a special consideration for this maneuver is using biofeedback to help teach what may be a difficult maneuver. Similar considerations apply to the "hard swallow" technique and the surgical technique of laryngeal suspension. The clinician must consider the following questions: What is the intended impact of the technique? Are there any potential contraindications or risks? Is there any available evidence to support use of the technique?

A 78-year-old woman had a left cerebrovascular accident 6 months ago and has no known family; she is now residing in a long-term care facility. She has a possible history of a prior stroke but no details are available. The patient is ambulatory with a walker and physical assistance; however, she spends most waking hours in a wheelchair or in bed. She is currently receiving a total oral diet, which is modified to pureed and thickened liquids. She is able to self-feed. She was referred for dysphagia evaluation and treatment because of continuing weight loss and reports of coughing during meals. A review of her chart indicates a recent history of repeated urinary tract infections. Clinical examination reveals a small woman who is interactive but with subtle signs of impaired mental status and possible mild aphasia. She demonstrates no overt corticobulbar deficits. The right arm and leg are paretic, with the leg more involved than the arm. When asked about swallowing, she replied that she swallows "just fine." When asked about the food at the facility, she indicated that it is "okay." Fluoroscopic swallowing evaluation indicated mild physiologic deviations, including slow oral transit, reduced hyolaryngeal elevation, reduced

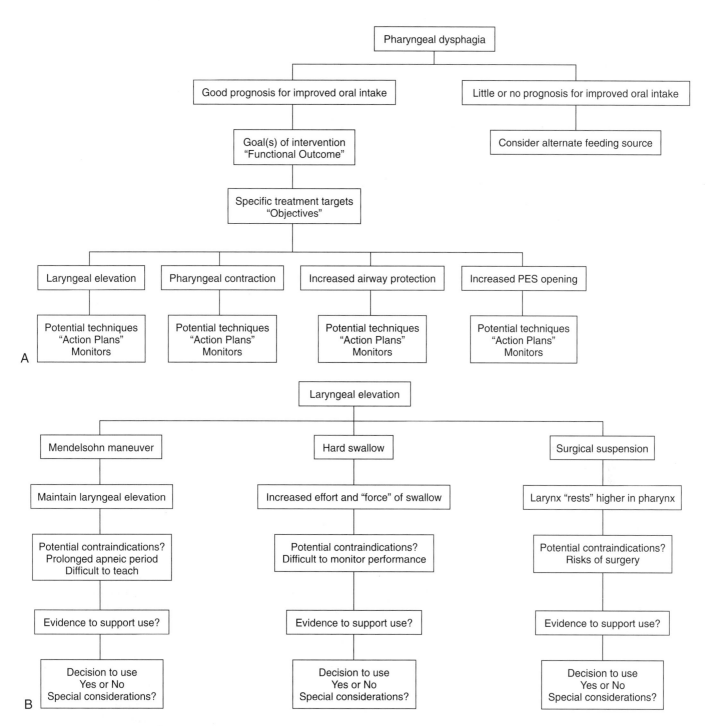

FIGURE 12-6. A and **B** show a specific example of an organizational framework for planning dysphagia treatment based on a hypothetical case of pharyngeal dysphagia. *PES,* Pharyngoesophageal segment.

pharyngeal contraction, and reduced PES opening. Post-swallow residue was noted in the valleculae and the piriform recesses, primarily on thicker materials. When liquid was used to remove residue, a minute amount of aspiration was noted after swallow. The patient demonstrated a consistent reactive cough with aspiration. Maneuvers such as the chin tuck or head turn had no effect on this pattern of swallowing. The patient was able to chew a cracker but had difficulty forming a cohesive oral bolus and removing the material from her mouth.

The first consideration for treatment planning is the current functional eating level of the patient. In this particular case, the patient is self-feeding and taking all food and liquid by mouth but with a restricted diet of pureed and thickened liquids. A primary concern is continuing weight loss. A related concern might be the recurring urinary tract infections.

The next consideration is that of factors that may contribute to the existing functional level. Both the weight loss and the recurring infections may relate to an insufficient intake of nutrition and hydration. This point should be addressed through communication with the long-term care facility. Predisposing factors may not always be overt and clear, so many issues should be considered. A few factors to consider in this case include swallow physiology, physical status, appetite, and the patient's environment. The clinician must consider the functional eating level in reference to the observed swallow physiology as seen fluoroscopically. This patient demonstrated slow transit and mild reduction in pharyngeal components of the swallow. She had more difficulty with dry, particulate materials (cracker). She did aspirate mildly in certain circumstances and had a strong reactive cough. This last observation may relate to the observed coughing during meals. The relation of the physiologic deviations to the functional eating pattern is more difficult to understand. Overall slowness may be related to prolonged mealtimes and thus to reduced food intake. Is it possible that this patient is demonstrating mild cognitive changes that may reflect early-stage dementia and the swallowing changes that may accompany the cognitive change (see Chapter 5)? This might be one area for further clinical examination.

Are there other possibilities that may help support or refute a possible relation between the observed swallow physiology and the functional eating pattern? Physical status may help explain some of the reduced intake of food and liquid. Recall that this patient is self-feeding. In addition, recall that she has some weakness in the right upper limb and may have had a previous stroke. It would be beneficial to observe her eating a meal to help determine the extent to which physical limitation may restrict intake of food and liquid. Appetite loss may be another factor in reduced intake. Although the patient described the food as "okay," she did not indicate high motivation for eating. This may be related to cognitive or environmental (social) issues. Depression should also be considered. The current dining situation may be distracting, noisy, or unpleasant to the patient. She may require cues to continue eating or other adjustments that are not provided in her current situation. Under these circumstances, she may have reduced intake. All these factors must be considered to derive the best possible intervention for this patient.

The primary goal for this patient might be to stop weight loss and subsequently to increase weight to appropriate levels. A related goal may be to reduce urinary tract infections (if these result from reduced hydration). To address these goals, the factors contributing to the current functional level must be addressed, and treatment objectives must be selected for factors that may be altered to improve functional status. One obvious objective is to increase the amount of nutrition and hydration taken by mouth. The methods by which this is accomplished should relate directly to those factors perceived to contribute to reduced oral intake.

Selecting specific action plans in this particular case may require a period of further observation under differing conditions. For example, it might be prudent to observe this patient eating a more rheologically complex meal, observe her eating meals of varying amounts, enhance taste properties, increase mealtime cues, and/or change the dining environment. The best intervention approach may be a combination of these strategies. One monitor for improvement might be the amount of calories and hydration consumed daily. The functional outcome would be weight gain to appropriate levels and reduced urinary tract infections.

TAKE HOME NOTES

1. Evidence-based practice is the use of combinations of published research, clinician expertise, and patient wishes in establishing the most effective treatment plan.
2. Primary considerations for dysphagia treatment include airway protection and nutrition and hydration. These may be influenced by multiple factors related to the patient, the underlying disease or disorder, the clinician, and/or the health care environment.
3. Dysphagia treatment is often multifocal and multidisciplinary. Clinicians should be familiar with multiple treatment options across medical, surgical, and behavioral domains.
4. Choice of a specific therapy technique may depend on the specifics of the patient's health care status, the skills of the treating clinician, the health care environment, or other factors.
5. Clinicians must make sure to evaluate health care risks and potential obstacles when considering treatment options.
6. A comprehensive therapy plan should include a statement of functional goals, objectives to meet those goals, and specific actions to initiate for each objective.

References

1. Dollaghan CA: *The handbook of evidence-based practice in communication disorders*, Baltimore, 2007, Paul H Brookes.

2. Leonard RJ, Kendall KK, McKenzie S et al: Structural displacements in normal swallowing: a videofluoroscopic study, *Dysphagia* 15:146, 2000.

3. O'Neil KH, Purdy M, Ralk J et al: The Dysphagia Outcome and Severity Scale, *Dysphagia* 14:139, 1999.

4. Crary MA, Carnaby GC, Groher ME et al: Initial psychometric assessment of a functional oral intake scale for dysphagia in stroke patients, *Arch Phys Med Rehabil* 86:1516, 2005.

5. Storr M, Allescher HD: Esophageal pharmacology and treatment of primary motility disorders, *Dis Esophagus* 12:241, 1999.

6. Kraus PH, Orlikoff RF, Rizk SS et al: Arytenoid adduction as an adjunct to type I thyroplasty for unilateral vocal fold paralysis, *Head Neck* 21:52, 1999.

7. Grant JR, Hartemink DA, Patel N et al: Acute and subacute awake injection laryngoplasty for thoracic surgery patients, *J Voice* 22:245, 2008.

8. Isshiki N: Progress in laryngeal framework surgery, *Acta Otolaryngol* 120:120, 2000.

9. Mita S: Laryngotracheal separation and tracheoesophageal diversion for intractable aspiration in amyotrophic lateral sclerosis—usefulness and indications, *Brain Nerve* 59:1149, 2007.

10. Pletcher SD, Mandpe AH, Block MI et al: Reversal of laryngotracheal separation: a detailed case report with long-term follow-up, *Dysphagia* 20:19, 2005.

11. Zocratto OB, Savassi-Rocha PR, Paixao RM et al: Laryngotracheal separation surgery: outcome in 60 patients, *Otolaryngol Head Neck Surg* 135:571, 2006.

12. Scolapio JS, Gostout CJ, Schroder KW et al: Dysphagia without endoscopically evident disease: to dilate or not? *Am J Gastroenterol* 96:327, 2001.

13. Kelly JH: Management of upper esophageal sphincter disorders: indications and complications of myotomy, *Am J Med* 108(suppl):43S, 2000.

14. Crary MA, Glowasky AL: Using botulinum toxin A to improve speech and swallowing function following total laryngectomy, *Arch Otolaryngol Head Neck Surg* 122:760, 1996.

15. Murray T, Wasserman T, Carrau RL et al: Injection of botulinum toxin A for the treatment of dysfunction of the upper esophageal sphincter, *Am J Otolaryngol* 26:157, 2005.

16. Shaw GY, Searl JP: Botulinum toxin treatment for cricopharyngeal dysfunction, *Dysphagia* 16:161, 2001.

17. Cichero JA, Jackson O, Halley PJ et al: How thick is thick? Multicenter study of the rheological and material property characteristics of mealtime fluids and videofluoroscopy fluids, *Dysphagia* 15:188, 2000.

18. Groher ME, Crary MA, Carnaby Mann G et al: The impact of rheologically controlled materials on the identification of airway compromise on the clinical and videofluoroscopic swallowing examination, *Dysphagia* 211:218, 2006.

19. Low J, Wyles C, Wilkinson T et al: The effects of compliance on clinical outcomes for patients with dysphagia on videofluoroscopy, *Dysphagia* 16:123, 2001.

20. National Dysphagia Diet Task Force: *National dysphagia diet: standardization for optimal care*, Chicago, 2002, American Dietetic Association.

21. Adnerhill I, Ekberg O, Groher ME: Determining normal bolus size for thin liquids, *Dysphagia* 4:1, 1989.

22. Steele CM, Van Lieshout P: Influence of bolus consistency on lingual behaviors in sequential swallowing, *Dysphagia* 19:192, 2004.

23. Omi W, Murata Y, Yaegashi T et al: Swallow syncope, a case report and review of the literature, *Cardiology* 105:75, 2006.

24. Schiffman SS: Intensification of sensory properties of foods for the elderly, *J Nutr* 130(suppl):927S, 2000.

25. Shanley C, O'Loughlin G: Dysphagia among nursing home residents: an assessment and management protocol, *J Gerontol Nurs* 26:35, 2000.

26. Musson ND, Kincaid J, Ryan P et al: Nature, nurture, nutrition: interdisciplinary programs to address the prevention of malnutrition and dehydration, *Dysphagia* 5:96, 1990.

27. de Carle DJ: Gastro-oesophageal reflux disease, *Med J Aust* 169:549, 1998.

28. Crary MA: A direct intervention for chronic neurogenic dysphagia secondary to brainstem stroke, *Dysphagia* 10:6, 1995.

29. Huckabee ML, Cannito MP: Outcomes of swallowing rehabilitation in chronic brainstem dysphagia: a retrospective evaluation, *Dysphagia* 14:93, 2002.

30. Crary MA, Carnaby Mann GD, Groher ME: Functional benefits of dysphagia therapy using adjunctive sEMG biofeedback, *Dysphagia* 19:160, 2004.

Chapter 13

Treatment for Infants and Children

JO PUNTIL-SHELTMAN AND HELENE TAYLOR

CHAPTER OUTLINE

OBJECTIVES

1. Identify and understand why a premature infant needs positional boundaries.
2. Understand the potential benefits of skin-to-skin care.
3. Identify the cues indicating when an infant might be ready to eat.
4. Understand the benefits of using a pacifier for the premature infant.
5. Discuss the formulation of child- and family-oriented goals for feeding therapy.
6. Describe prefeeding therapy strategies for the child with oral motor dysfunction.
7. Describe prefeeding therapy strategies for the child with a sensory-based feeding disorder.
8. Describe a potential sequence of activities for feeding therapy sessions.
9. Discuss three theories of outpatient feeding therapy.

The key to developmental approaches to treatment of swallowing disorders in infants is to foster the neurodevelopmental skills that will lead the infant from a state of mature sucking to a state of mature feeding. Coordinated oral feeding is difficult work for most premature, sensory and motorically disorganized, structurally impaired, and medically fragile infants. Swallowing management of infants usually requires individualized treatment planning and approaches. This approach depends on the infant's physiologic stability, alertness levels, neural organization, and available levels of energy (see Chapter 4). Infants need to be able to maintain physiologic, motor, sensory, and state stability to have pleasurable and successful feeding. The combined goals of the feeding specialist and parents for management and treatment usually include improving the infant's overall stability with integrated developmental care, proper positioning in an incubator or crib, proper positioning during feeding, use of appropriate latching skills and positioning for breastfeeding, and use of appropriate bottles and nipples. The entire process should be positive for the infant and caregiver with minimal stress and maximal social enjoyment.

FOSTERING STABILITY AND ORGANIZATION

Several common techniques can be used to foster the development of physiologic stability and neurodevelopmental organization in infants. All these interventions serve as precursors to successful feeding.

Developmental Supportive Care

Infant development is a process that involves an individual's ability to integrate new demands and new information, achieving stability at each new developmental level (see Table 4-2). The goal of facilitating the development of feeding skills in the neonatal intensive care unit should be directed toward assisting the infant in achieving stability at each level and should be viewed as important steps leading to a more complex process such as oral ingestion.[1] Developmentally supportive care promotes the importance of compassionate touch, cluster care (see Chapter 1), proper positioning during feeding and nonfeeding activities, and controlling environmental stimuli such as excessive noise and light.[2] Developmental supportive care also should assist the infant in maintaining organization that will help the infant in attaining safe and positive feedings throughout the day. The key to successful feedings is to recognize the infant's cues that may disrupt his or her stability and to minimize negative experiences during feeding.

Positioning

Proper positioning while the infant is in the incubator or crib is important in encouraging physiologic stability and mature neural development and organization. Because the premature infant is outside the uterus early, it is necessary to be "nested" or swaddled while in the incubator or crib. There are several ways to provide boundaries (containment) for the infant. Commercial products such as "Bendy Bumpers" (Philips Children's Medical Ventures, Philips Healthcare, Andover, Mass.) can stabilize infants in positions that are tucked and flexed. This allows them to "feel" and sense these boundaries around their arms and legs. The bumpers reduce the total space for movement and, when combined with swaddling, maintain the infant in a flexed position. It is important to place a "halo" or bean bag under the infant's head to promote the development of a uniform, round shape to the head. Allowing the infant to sleep nested for 3 hours between care activities in an appropriate position (supine, prone, side-lying) helps promote physiologic, motor, and state stability. Noise and all interruptions should be minimized to allow the infant to complete a full sleep cycle while contained in the close environment.

Skin-to-Skin Care

Skin-to-skin (also known as "kangaroo care") is contact between an infant and parent that usually is chest to chest with the infant in an upright and prone position. The infant's arms and legs are flexed close to the baby's body with the hands near the mouth. Usually a blanket is wrapped around both the parent and infant (Figure 13-1). Skin-to-skin posturing ideally should last 60 to 90 minutes or as long as the infant remains stable. Skin-to-skin usually is started at the completion of a feeding or during **gavage** feeding. The environment should be quiet with the lights dimmed throughout the session. Skin-to-skin care can be done with the most medically fragile infant, even one who is supported by mechanical ventilation. Skin-to-skin care is a beneficial developmental intervention for the infant and the parent. Skin-to-skin touch benefits the infant by stabilizing physiologic parameters such as heart and respiratory rate, oxygen saturation, and oxygen consumption. It also encourages sleep, a higher mean daily weight gain, and breastfeeding success as well as fosters neurobehavioral development.[3-5] It provides a direct benefit to the caregiver because bonding often produces relaxation, which in turn decreases the stress associated with hospitalization. Skin-to-skin contact allows parents and their infant to learn each other's smells, scents,

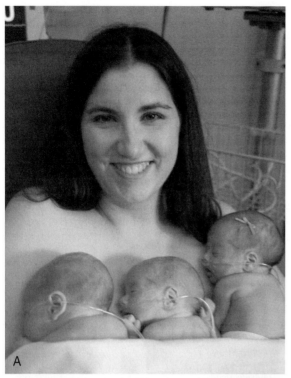

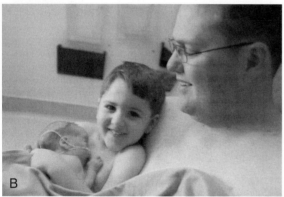

FIGURE 13-1. A and **B,** Skin-to-skin contact can involve a single parent or an additional family member.

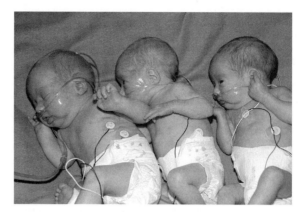

FIGURE 13-2. Triplets are co-bedded with cardiopulmonary monitors and respiratory support.

and voices. For some mothers it increases breast milk production and prolongs the duration of breastfeeding.[6]

Co-bedding

Research has demonstrated that children at a very young age often bond when positioned together, as in the case of multiple births. It has been demonstrated that co-bedding of multiples of infants may encourage self-regulation, thermoregulation, respiratory regulation, and improved growth.[7-9] When this circumstance is possible, it is helpful to have an incubator with dual temperature probe capability, adequate-sized open cribs, and a receiving blanket large enough to swaddle more that one child to assist in co-regulation (Figure 13-2). Considerations with co-bedding include whether the physical environment can support dual monitoring, the size of the support staff, the size of the blankets and incubators, and the need for infant support lines such as those to support nutrition and respiration. If co-bedding involves twins, there should be maintenance of identification to track changes in each infant's developmental skills.

READINESS TO EAT

When the feeding specialist wants to ascertain if an infant is ready to feed, it is important to attend to the infant's cues as they might relate to changes in neurodevelopmental milestones. As infants adjust to their environment, the speed and intensity of swallowing interventions change. The feeding specialist must pay particular attention to the infant's reaction to environmental stimuli, recognizing which stimuli either disrupt the physiologic state and which stimuli are best tolerated. Overwhelming the infant leads to physiologic instability and potential difficulty in feeding. Medically fragile infants require pacing according to their ability; often these infants are overwhelmed with too many ill-timed interactions that interfere with the feeding process. They need to be provided with enough support to maintain their behavioral organization skills, but not so much as to interfere with the development of their ability to self-regulate. The feeding specialist must pay attention to patterns of feeding performance when deciding whether an infant can sustain nutrition orally. For instance, infants generally are not messy eaters; if they are thrusting fluid from their mouths there usually is a reason. Perhaps the nipple flow is too fast or the pace of delivery is too fast.

During feeding attempts it is important to monitor the infant's physiologic state, including color and respiratory patterns. Before feeding attempts the feeding specialist must be sensitive to the infant's physiologic stability, motor responses to the environment, and his or her ability to self-regulate. During feeding it is important to note whether the infant can sustain his or her attention to the task without disruptions from either a change in physiologic state or external stimuli that interfere with feeding success. Positive cues help establish when the infant may be ready to sustain oral feeding; negative cues mean to stop the feeding. It is important to remember that a successful feeding session should be measured by the overall positive experience or the ability to maintain a stable physiologic state—and not by the quantity of fluid swallowed.

PACIFIERS, BOTTLES, AND NIPPLES

Pacifiers are commonly used with preterm infants to assist in the nonnutritive sucking process. Pacifiers also may assist in strengthening the suck and in providing a more rhythmic suck pattern. Pacifiers come in various shapes, lengths, and sizes. The size should match the size of the infant's oral cavity, sensitivity, gag response, and sucking needs (Figure 13-3). Pacifiers may help calm the infant during stressful situations and provide positive oral stimulation during gavage feedings.[10]

Bottles are made of hard or soft plastic. Softer plastics are flexible and can be squeezed to assist in the rate of flow (Figure 13-4). Softer bottles are commonly used in children with cleft palate (see Chapter 4). Ideally, bottles should be clear so that the fluid inside is visible.

Nipples (or teats) are characterized by the material composition that determines the nipple's shape, size,

and flow rate. A variety of nipples are available for term and preterm infants (Figure 13-5). Some nipples are made of silicone that is clear, firm, and less likely to collapse. A plastic nipple may be tan colored and will collapse easily under pressure. The shape of the nipple is either straight or orthodontic. The *straight nipple* requires more tongue cupping by the infant and more pressure before it will collapse. It also provides a consistent flow rate, although it may make it more difficult for the infant to draw the tongue posteriorly to the pharynx. An *orthodontic nipple* is useful when the infant has a flatter and larger tongue, requires less pressure to collapse, has a less predictable flow rate, and can draw the infant's tongue back to the pharynx. Similar to pacifiers, the size of the nipple should match the size of the infant's oral cavity. Standard and small sizes are available for premature infants.

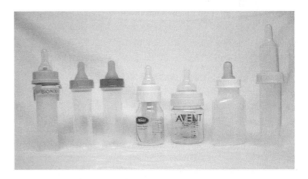

FIGURE 13-4. Various types of bottles can be used. *Left to right:* Bionix (very slow to regular flow; Bionix Controlled Flow Baby Feeder, Bionix Medical Technologies, Toledo, Ohio); hard plastic neonatal intensive care unit bottle with slow-flow nipple (Enfamil, Mead Johnson Nutrition; Glenview, Ill.); hard plastic, fast-flow nipple (Enfamil); Dr. Brown's (vented bottle; Handi-Craft Co., St. Louis, Mo.); variable-flow nipple (AVENT; Philips AVENT, Suffolk, UK); squeeze bottle with a pigeon nipple for cleft palate babies (Mead Johnson); Haberman cleft palate feeder (Medela, McHenry, Ill.).

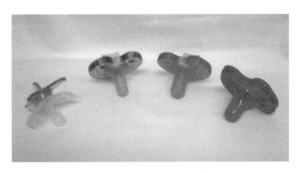

FIGURE 13-3. Examples of pacifiers. *Left to right:* Micro-preemie pacifier, preemie pacifier (infants <32 weeks' gestation), preemie pacifier (>32 weeks' gestation if the oral cavity can tolerate it), pacifier for a term infant.

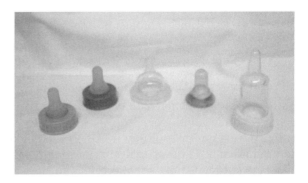

FIGURE 13-5. Various type of nipples. *Left to right:* Green slow-flow (Enfamil); blue fast-flow (Enfamil); clear variable-flow (Avent); dark yellow pigeon cleft palate nipple; Haberman variable fast-flow cleft palate nipple.

One rule of thumb for nipple choice is that if the infant is able to suck on your finger, he or she usually will tolerate the standard-size nipple. There are many varieties of flow rates for nipples. Flow rates need to be adjusted as the infant matures. The flow rate usually depends on the infant's sucking strength and the viscosity of the fluid. For instance, breast milk has a higher flow rate than formula. Nipples for premature infants generally tend to flow more quickly. Variable-flow–rate nipples should be used with caution because the slowest rates with this type of nipple are generally faster than most fast-flow straight nipples. Selecting the correct nipple for a premature infant is similar to the process of selection for a term infant. Flow rate adjustments are made by assessing the maturity of the suck, the coordination of the swallow, breath, burst control, and the overall respiratory status of the infant before and during feeding.

FEEDING POSITIONING

The breastfeeding process is more successful if the infant is positioned by supporting the head and body. The infant may be placed in a variety of positions for feeding at the breast or with a bottle. Some of the more common positions that maintain stability are the cross-cradle hold, cradle hold, and the football hold. An infant needs to latch on correctly for successful breastfeeding. *Latching on* refers to the way the infant takes the breast into the mouth. The infant is correctly latched on when the mother's nipple and a good portion of the surrounding breast tissue is at the back of the infant's mouth. There are also a number of positions that stabilize the infant for bottle feeding. The mother or caregiver may feed the infant in a cradle hold, upright facing the feeder, in a right or left side-lying position, or facing away from the feeder. The side-lying position is beneficial because it reduces the infant's ability to see the feeder while eating, thereby reducing distractions and maintaining the infant's overall neurodevelopmental organization.

ORAL SENSORY AND FACIAL STIMULATION

Oral and facial stimulation may be needed for infants with neuromuscular disorders, oral aversions, prolonged endotracheal tube placement, long-term placement of tubes in the head or neck, and gastroesophageal reflux. For the infant to be able to tolerate a nipple or teat in the mouth, the feeding specialist may have to provide oral and sensory stimulation. Such stimulation helps the infant become accustomed to opening the mouth wide enough to latch on to a nipple with the tongue forward and in the down position and to begin to develop the compression and suction pressures necessary to extract milk from a breast or bottle. Stimulation by stroking the outside of the mouth with gradual steps toward the inside in varying lengths of time and with differing pressure should help facilitate the infant's acceptance of the nipple.

CUE-BASED FEEDING SCHEDULE

Determining the readiness for advancement in oral feeding is an individualized approach. If the infant is older than 34 weeks' gestational age, the feeding specialist will initiate cue-based feedings, allowing the cues from the infant to drive the schedule (see the section on readiness to eat above). Infants may be able to feed before 34 weeks if cueing, ready, and able to maintain some physiologic stability. Typically infants start with one feeding per 12-hour shift and advance as the infant tolerates the schedule. Two evidence-based approaches using a cue-based program for oral feeding by bottle or breast are presented in Figures 13-6 and 13-7.

THEORIES OF FEEDING TREATMENT

Feeding therapy has become an area of specialization for occupational therapists, developmental specialists, and speech-language pathologists (SLPs). Feeding therapy approaches have been developed with a focus on behavioral therapy, sensory integration, and oral motor treatment.

Sequential Oral Sensory Approach

The Sequential Oral Sensory (SOS) approach to feeding is a transdisciplinary therapy program for evaluating and treating children with feeding and weight and growth concerns. The approach stems from studies of multidisciplinary intervention programs for infants and young children demonstrating poor growth as a result of disordered feeding. The SOS approach was developed over a 15-year period through the clinical work of psychologist Kay Toomey in conjunction with SLPs, occupational therapists, dietitians, and physicians. The program emphasizes the "whole child" approach to feeding, integrating sensory, motor, oral motor, behavioral/learning, medical, and nutritional factors. It is based on achieving feeding competency according to developmental skills found in typically developing children. This program is based on the premise that each child has specific levels of eating and food acceptance based on past experience, rather than the assumption that eating is an instinct based solely on biologic needs.

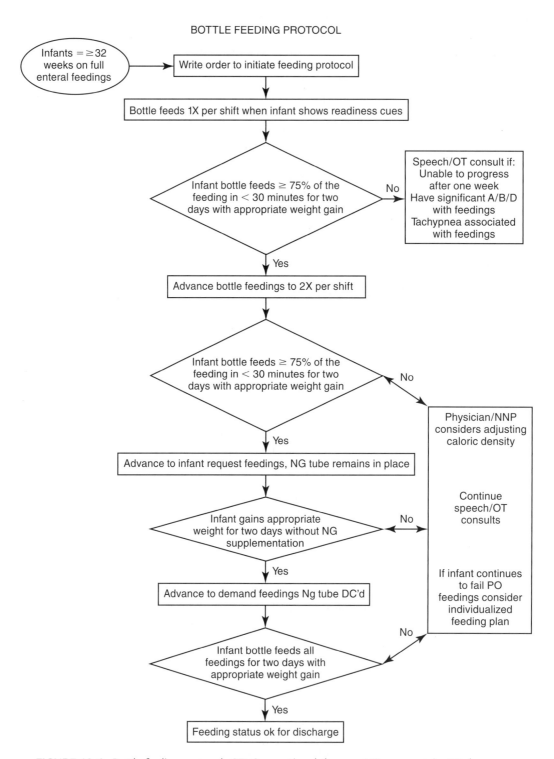

FIGURE 13-6. Bottle feeding protocol. *OT,* Occupational therapy; *NG,* nasogastric; *PO,* by mouth; *DC,* discontinued. (From Kirk A, Adler SC, King JD: Cue based oral feeding clinical pathway results in earlier attainment of full oral feeding in premature infants, *J Perinatol* 27:572, 2007.)

BREAST FEEDING PROTOCOL

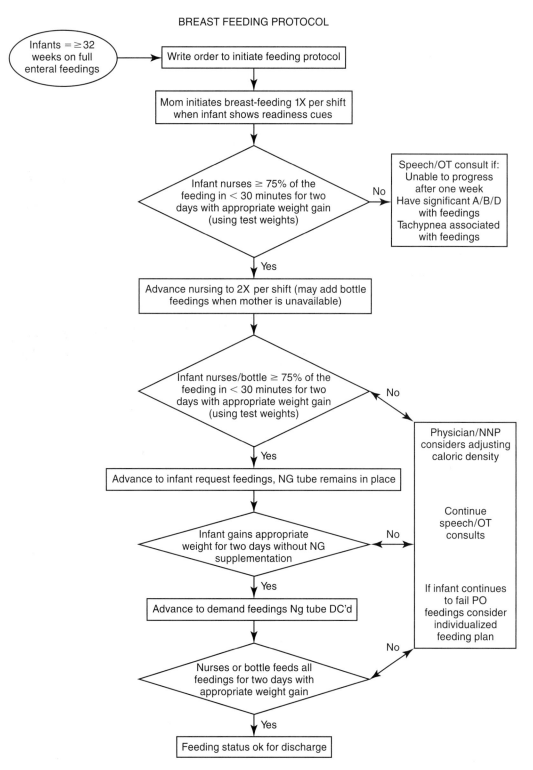

FIGURE 13-7. Breastfeeding protocol. *OT,* Occupational therapy; *NG,* nasogastric; *PO,* by mouth; *DC,* discontinued. (From Kirk A, Adler SC, King JD: Cue based oral feeding clinical pathway results in earlier attainment of full oral feeding in premature infants, *J Perinatol* 27:572, 2007.)

The SOS approach uses systematic desensitization to help a child build new skills. This includes the implementation of the "Steps to Eating," which includes substeps of tolerating the presence of food, interacting with food, the ability to smell food, touching food, tasting food and, finally, eating. This approach has been used with individuals and in group treatment settings. Studies of group programs have shown gains in both weight and height and a 41% increase in expanding food variety.[11,12]

Structured Behavioral Feeding Approach

Children develop many feeding behaviors as a result of negative experiences surrounding food and feeding related to medical complications. However, once the medical problem is under control or is resolved, the child is left with learned experience and behaviors, often as a protective response that may interfere with normal feeding. The child may establish a strong avoidance pattern that continues between the child and the caregiver whenever food is presented. Treatment should include behavioral principles that reward positive behaviors and decrease negative behaviors.[13]

Behavioral feeding programs have been developed by several centers and specific practitioners. Behavioral feeding programs have been successful for up to 67% of children with feeding disorders stemming from a variety of causes.[14] The goal of a structured behavioral feeding program is to increase acceptance of oral intake through behavioral reinforcement strategies. Aversive behaviors that should be addressed include food stuffing or holding, spitting food out, food selectivity or refusal, tantrums or crying, refusal of the high chair, blocking, grimacing, and intentional vomiting or gagging. The Structured Behavioral Feeding Program, established by Krisi Brackett, was developed to address these areas.[13] The program fully integrates all the child's medical and therapeutic background and needs with a behavioral intervention plan. The program begins with appropriate supportive positioning. Progressive applications of spoon placement are used with a prescriptive approach to what may be on the spoon (often using a dry spoon) and a specified number of trials. Rewards are used consistently throughout the program. Rewards may include a short turn with a toy (lasting less than a minute), praise, a few seconds of music, or the reading of a portion of a page in a favorite book. At first, rewards may be given each time the child accepts the spoon, gradually reducing the number as acceptance increases. Acceptance of the spoon could be paired with the child being allowed to play with a toy. The toy is then put away and the child is again offered the spoon. This sequence is repeated until the child accepts the spoon 10 times. The Structured Behavioral Feeding Program progresses through a series of structured steps with practice sessions two to four times per day. As the child progresses, the feeding specialist moves toward increasing food variety and volume.[15]

Beckman Oral Motor Approach

Many individuals with impaired oral motor skills are not able to follow a command for oral movement. To better serve these individuals, Debra Beckman developed specific interventions that provide assisted movement to activate muscle contraction and to provide movement against resistance to build strength. The focus of these interventions is to increase functional response to pressure and movement, range, strength, and variety and control of movement for the lips, cheeks, jaw and tongue. The interventions needed are determined by using the Beckman Oral Motor Protocol.[15] The protocol uses assisted movement and stretch reflexes to quantify response to pressure and movement, range, strength, variety and control of movement for the lips cheeks, jaw, tongue, and soft palate. The assessment is based on clinically defined functional parameters of minimal competence and does not require cognitive participation. Because these components of movement are functional and not age specific, the protocol is useful with a wide range of ages (birth to geriatric) and diagnostic categories. Oral motor skills affect basic survival such as sucking and swallowing by infants. These skills begin by the third month of gestation. Development of these skills enhances the progression from breast milk or formula, then to pureed foods and to table foods, as well as the skills needed to progress from sucking a nipple, to using a wide variety of utensils, including straws, cups, spoons, and forks. These areas of performance are scored with three trials in each area of motor performance based on movement consistency. Although there are no published norms for performance, the test is used to document individual progress in specific areas, including improved oral motor function. Beckman recommends that a primary therapist be designated (typically a licensed SLP) to assess the oral motor skills, plan the oral motor interventions needed, and work closely with other team members.

MODELS OF THERAPY

The choice of the model of feeding therapy should be made with consideration of the child and family needs. At times, the ideal clinical recommendation may need to be modified so that the family is able to attend therapy sessions that will help them achieve consistency in their own intervention skills or allow them to use recommended treatment strategies.

Individual Therapy

Individual feeding therapy is considered the traditional manner of most treatment. Feeding therapy sessions typically last 1 hour, with part of this session used for caregiver education. Therapy is scheduled within a designated time frame, such as for 3 to 4 months, with a structured plan for family and child skill development that is modified according to measured progress. Therapy frequency is determined by individual child and family needs (e.g., weekly, biweekly, monthly). It is important that the family take ownership of this plan to ensure treatment compliance.

Group Therapy

Group therapy is typically used with groups of four to six children of similar ages and needs. Most group therapy programs consist of weekly group sessions for 10 to 12 weeks. Group therapy is a model that often includes more than one feeding specialist (usually an SLP and an occupational therapist) and often includes the psychologist. In most cases, group therapy is considered an optimal program to provide parent support, child-to-child modeling, and broad-based teaching on a variety of feeding related areas.

Intensive Day Treatment

Intensive day treatment and intensive inpatient programs are designed for children with needs that require a higher degree of medical and therapeutic monitoring. These programs are held in a hospital setting. Typically they are advanced programs designed for quick transition from tube feedings to oral feedings during the course of several weeks. Children who participate in these programs have been evaluated previously and are referred for intensive treatment programs only after a team of specialists have completed the evaluation and agreed on the plan of care.

FAMILY-FRIENDLY GOALS

Families come to the feeding therapy setting with many different experiences derived from culture, education, personal experiences with food and eating, family pressure, and the experiences and expectations that they have already had with their child. The family of a child with a feeding disorder experiences emotional and other psychological stressors on a daily basis. Parents blame themselves for their child's poor eating, even in the presence of a known physical problem over which they have no control. For the parent of an infant, their sense of "success" is directly tied to the child's feeding skills and weight gain.[16,17] Parents of children of all ages often blame themselves for their child's poor feeding. Some consequences of these "failures" include depression, anxiety, anger, and frustration. It is important that the feeding specialist refer the family to a qualified psychologist if any of these problems are observed or reported. It is not uncommon that families arrive at the clinical feeding evaluation and subsequent treatment sessions with a certain degree of stress. An important component of evaluation and treatment involves working with that stress through appropriate levels of information provided to the families and identification of areas in which the child and family are showing progress. High stress levels contribute to negative parent-child interactions, especially within the feeding environment. It is crucial for health care providers to help parents identify specific stressors and develop coping strategies to deal with these stressors as effectively as possible. Decreases in stress are noted when the families realize their goals are being met, their perceptions of their child's eating problems are validated, and specific feeding or medical problems are clarified.[17] Integration of the caregiver in feeding therapy plays a critical role in intervention. Effective management of feeding disorders should always be seen as a partnership between the caregiver and the interdisciplinary feeding team. The additional gain is an increased feeling of competency by the caregiver who is appropriately trained in feeding the child with special needs. Providing caregivers with appropriate feeding training, setting of realistic goals, regular instruction for home practice, and the expectation for periodic setbacks can help the child and the caregiver achieve the greatest benefit from feeding therapy.[18] Assisting the family with the importance of objective documentation of feeding activity using a food diary (see Appendix 13-A) can facilitate the communication between the feeding specialist and the family in discussions of how therapy is progressing. The completion of a food diary provides information on the type and quantity of food consumed, the timing of tube and oral feedings, and the adequacy of hydration. The feeding specialist should instruct the family to keep a detailed record for three consecutive days. This information allows the feeding specialist to determine whether a dietary consultation is necessary.

Treatment goals should be written with parental needs in mind and with a focus on reasonable achievement for the child and family. Issues important in developing a realistic plan for feeding include (1) the amount of time the family can realistically spend on feeding intervention on a daily and weekly basis; (2) the number of other siblings in the home, who also require family attention; (3) additional therapies the child may be receiving at home; (4) the distance from the therapy center (for example, a family who lives 90 minutes away may want to come to therapy weekly, but may only be able to attend two sessions a month); (5) the cognitive level of the caregivers; (6) the extent and complexity of the child's feeding disorder; and (7) any related medical conditions, including allergies.

It is helpful to define the period in which the goals will be addressed. Families who are given defined periods (deadlines) to focus on a goal are more likely to address the goal with a greater degree of intensity. It is helpful to ask the family what they believe may be a reasonable goal(s) for a 1-, 3-, or 6-month period. Goals should be functional and must be measurable by the parent and therapist. Typical basic goals with varying time frames that are child dependent may include (1) decreasing the tube feeding by 25%; (2) eliminating the tube feeding; (3) increasing oral food variety to 20 consistently accepted food items; (4) increasing the child's weight and growth; and (5) being able to eat safely and comfortably with no evidence of coughing, choking, or gagging.

SHORT-TERM GOALS

Short-term treatment goals are based on preestablished longer term goals. These goals are developed by the feeding specialist in consultation with the family. Short-term goals should be achievable in no more than 3-month periods and should be reviewed regularly with the family to support their efforts and successes with their home programs. The feeding specialist also monitors other goals established by the medical team that may be related to the feeding process, such as working on trunk and position stability. Most short-term goals are limited to four and are set with the assumption that the child can meet these goals within a specific time period. Feeding therapy goals often address the following areas: (1) oral motor movement, (2) sensory acceptance of food, (3) the ability to allow food to remain on the high chair or plate, (4) the child's ability to remain in the high chair for a designated time, (5) self-feeding skills, (6) cup drinking skills, (7) tasting new foods, (8) eating a specific number of bites per meal, (9) increasing the number of foods within designated food categories, and (10) increasing the amount of food eaten between meals.

Cultural Considerations

Cultural considerations should be addressed during the evaluation and feeding therapy process. A variety of cultures live in the United States, and each has a unique lifestyle and customs. Different cultures have their own beliefs and traditions regarding the appropriateness of specific foods, the role of food in celebrations, foods that may be served in a particular order, foods that are given only to older children and adults, foods that may not be served with other foods, the location of food on a plate, the time of day when certain foods are served, foods that are typically served (or not served) on specific days of the week, and foods that may or may not be seasoned.[19] For example, typically the food on an infant's plate is unseasoned in the United States. However, many other cultures offer pureed versions of "adult food" that is liberally seasoned to their infants with excellent tolerance. Culture-specific foods may be examined as well. Whenever possible, the feeding specialist should ask the family to bring food from home for the evaluation and treatment sessions.

Cultural considerations in therapeutic feeding also include the role of the primary caregiver. In many ethnic groups the father is considered the individual in charge of most family decisions, although the mother is primarily in charge of the children. These considerations also affect where children may sit to eat and whether they eat their meals with adults or separately. These individual differences need to be addressed in treatment. If the feeding specialist is unfamiliar with a particular culture, he or she should enlist the help of the family in selecting foods and in any nuances of the eating process. Interpreters for families who do not speak English are important for conveying information.

DEVELOPING A CARE PLAN

The development of a therapeutic feeding plan begins by reviewing the details of the feeding evaluation. If goals were established at that time, they should be reviewed or modified as necessary. The development of a feeding care plan should address any or all of the following: (1) therapist and family goals based on the initial evaluation and any past attempts at treatment; (2) a review and discussion of all medical precautions and recommendations to include all food sensitivities, positioning guidelines, dietary recommendations, and food or liquid restrictions; (3) a demonstration or review of any special equipment, such as utensils that are to be used in the feeding process; (4) feeding goals that are functionally based, measurable, and within the family's capability; and (5) a detailed review and rationale of the day's therapeutic activities.

Preparing the Child for Eating

Feeding interventions always are targeted toward developmentally appropriate activities based on the initial evaluation recommendations and current observations. For example, gross motor play, or interactive play without food for a child reluctant to participate, or "pretend feeding" activities using play food could be implemented. General sensory system activities are often helpful in preparing the child for the therapy session and often are provided in conjunction with the occupational therapist. When possible, sensory feeding activities should include food; however, it need not be an *eating* activity. Nonoral proprioceptive and tactile activities, such as playing with scented modeling compound and painting with pudding, may be included. Food preparation activities may be helpful in this aspect of therapy. Before the treatment session begins it is important to determine who will feed the child; this may be done by the parent, therapist, child, or all three. Whenever possible, the caregiver and child should be included as soon as possible in the therapy sequence. If needed, the therapist should plan for oral motor or oral sensory preparation activities. This type of therapy may include use of items such as Chewy Tubes (Speech Pathology Associates, LLC, South Portland, Me.) (Figure 13-8), NUK Massage Brushes (Super Duper Publications, Greenville, SC) (Figure 13-9), minimassagers, and oral-safe tubing. Careful evaluation of the child's acceptance of these tools is necessary to create a positive therapeutic experience.

Introducing New Foods

For the majority of foods, a child's preferences are shaped by repeated experience. The predispositions that shape food acceptance patterns may include neophobia (avoidance or refusal of "new" foods) and the ability to learn to prefer and accept new foods when offered repeatedly. Foods presented in positive social and environmental contexts often are more accepted than those offered in negative contexts.[20]

It is important that the person feeding the child begins with a previously accepted food, with continued modifications of taste, texture, or quantity, always working on just one change at a time. The changes should be small and may be related to previous food presentations. A change can be as simple as moving from food that is pureed to a fork-mashed version of the same food, to a chopped version, and then to small pieces. Food property links should be present when moving from one food type to the next food type. These links may include food color, taste, temperature, texture, form, size, and shape. The developmental hierarchy—rather than the age of the child—should guide decisions when advancing to the next level.[21]

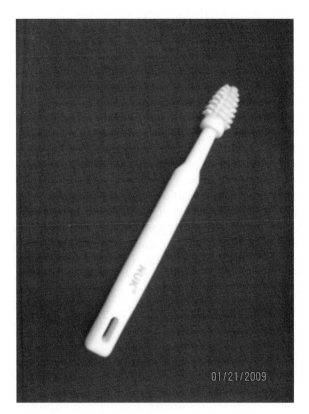

FIGURE 13-9. The NUK brush is used to stimulate sensation and movement before and during feeding.

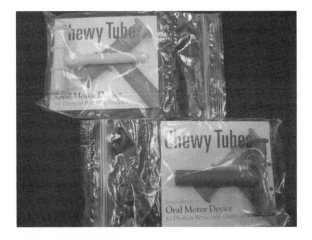

FIGURE 13-8. Chewy Tubes (Speech Pathology Associates, LLC) may be a minimally invasive and productive tool to use in feeding preparation if the child is able to maneuver the tube independently. They are available in two different sizes and two densities.

Making the Transition to New Foods

Moving to a new food may be simple for some patients and more complex for others. The key is to provide the "smallest noticeable difference." An example of moving a child through very small steps toward the goal of eating cooked carrots is provided. It is important to note that the child may be at each level for a day, or sometimes for a week, and that each step should not be rushed. In this example, the child has been accepting only jarred infant stage 2 carrots. The following steps should be followed in order.

1. Jarred/purchased infant food pureed carrots.
2. Pureed (smooth) steamed carrots made in a food processor with no added flavoring. The appearance and texture should be identical to processed stage 2 food.
3. Pureed steamed fresh carrots (ground with a small amount of texture) made in a food processor with no added flavor. Once this step has been achieved, it may be helpful for the child to observe the parent taking the carrots from whole, cooked form to purees.
4. Fork-mashed steamed carrots.
5. Sliced carrots cut into age-appropriate bite sizes.
6. Steamed and cooled baby carrots that the child can pick up using fingers or a fork if able.
7. Introduce flavoring such as butter, brown sugar, cinnamon, or other family-preferred flavorings. If flavorings are used, the next step in food texture should be delayed pending acceptance of the new flavor.

Once a new food is readily accepted, it can be added at mealtimes and can continue to be introduced during feeding therapy. For example, if a child is unable to advance beyond jarred purees, moving to home-prepared purees may be a next step so that the child begins to adapt to the change in consistency. Once accepted, the texture of the purees can be increased and fork-mashed foods may be introduced.

For children who do not tolerate any food by mouth, treatment may require developing sensory tolerance and acceptance for feeding. These food experiences may include sitting in a high chair, acceptance of utensils, and acceptance of the smells of various foods. During the feeding skill acquisition period, the complexity of the task and environmental stresses should be minimized. Procedures to teach a child a new skill include modeling, hand-over-hand prompting, shaping of responses to food and food interactions, and feedback. Young children may learn best through the modalities of sight and touch. Therefore showing them appropriate behaviors (modeling), such as how to select foods, may be useful. Hand-over-hand prompting is provided by therapists by placing their hand on the child's hand, guiding the child through desired motor behaviors using utensils. Providing additional practice and reinforcement during these tasks increases the speed and accuracy. It is important to develop consistent baseline behaviors before advancing the feeding therapy program. The feeding therapist should change only one aspect of the desired targeted skill at a time. For example, if moving from an outpatient therapeutic setting to a home setting, the parent should have the opportunity to feed in the therapeutic setting, under observation, before trying the skill at home. Similar to the therapeutic clinic session, the family should be educated to move slowly when introducing new foods.[22]

Matching Skills with Texture and Taste

The introduction of foods for each child should match the child's level of development rather than their chronologic age. This continuum of food introduction should be coordinated with information discussed in Chapters 4 and 11 with respect to foods that are able to be safely ingested. Foods can then be managed in the most efficient and enjoyable manner.[16,21] For example, children who have not yet acquired complete head control will be most efficient and safe with the introduction of smooth purees, such as stage 1 and stage 2 infant foods.[23] The move to the next developmental stage generally requires competency in a previous step. Certain foods may be continued while new foods are introduced in the transitional period. Other foods, such as hard munchables (see Box 13-3), may be used to improve oral exploration and increase specific oral motor skills such as tongue lateralization, tongue cupping and grooving, and tongue-tip elevation. The choice of a hard munchable depends on the child's flavor preferences as well as foods that have been targeted for nutritional purposes.

As previously discussed, it is necessary to examine each child's history and help make food choices. The feeding specialist can provide important guidance in this area. Families often feel pressured to move to the next level of food choice before their child's readiness for that food. General guidelines showing the sequence of food readiness based on a child's developmental

BOX 13-1	Suggested Guidelines for Food Readiness Based on a Child's Developmental Level

Food Type	Readiness Age Level
Breast/bottle	Birth
Thin infant cereals/infant cereals mixed with formula or breast milk to a soupy consistency	5 to 6 months
Slightly thicker infant cereals and the first thin baby food purees/stage 1 foods	6 months
Thicker infant cereals and thicker baby food purees/stage 2 foods	7 to 8 months
Soft, mashed table foods and table food smooth purees	8 to 9 months
Hard munchables (for typically developing children)	9 to 10 months (see Box 13-3)
Meltable solids	9 to 10 months (see Box 13-3)
Very soft single-texture solids/ moist solids that mash readily in the mouth	(10 months)
Other single-texture **mechanical soft solids**	(11 months)
Mixed-texture foods	(12 months)
Soft table foods	(12 to 14 months)
Advanced mechanical soft solids	(16 to 18 months)

level are presented in Box 13-1.[16,21,24] It is important to note that some children will advance to foods earlier or later than others.

Changing Taste and Texture

Humans have eight senses, all of which become involved in the process of managing food. The senses of touch, taste, smell, and vision are easily understood in the eating experience. The hearing, proprioceptive, vestibular, and kinesthetic senses also provide strong input toward food acceptance and management. Children, regardless of developmental age, develop feeding skills through the use and integration of all these senses. They hear a food "crunch," can tell if a food is mushy or chewy, and have varying responses to seeing food move (such as gelatin). They want to be involved in food preparation and serving. Children older than 10 months begin to develop preferences for taste and texture. Children with specific diagnoses, such as those with low muscle tone, almost always prefer stronger flavors (usually savory or salty foods) over milder flavors. Contrary to traditional dietary

considerations, many children with a history of gastrointestinal disorders also prefer foods with a higher degree of flavor. The feeding specialist must be ready to provide guidance in this area. For example, seasonings may be added to smooth purees for added flavor. A NUK brush (see Figure 13-9) may be used to provide a safe introduction to texture until the child develops oral motor skills for independent management of higher levels of food texture.[25] Matching a child's sensory needs for food is as important as making accurate decisions for food types. Suggestions for food selection for toddlers are presented in Box 13-2.

Meltable Solids

For therapeutic purposes, specifically related to dysphagia and overall feeding safety, the definition of a *meltable solid* is a dry, formed food that when placed in the mouth will dissolve (in the presence of enough saliva) with only a minimal mashing pattern needed, versus actual chewing. These types of foods reduce the risk of choking on a solid but still offer the opportunity for the child to progress beyond purees and liquids and use some chewing movements. A list of meltable solids is presented in Box 13-3.

Hard Munchables

Hard munchables are defined as food items that are meant for oral exploration only, are designed to develop prechewing skills, tongue lateralization, and to assist in moving the sensitivity of the gag response further to the back of the mouth. These items must be thick enough that the child cannot bite through the food. A list of hard munchables is presented in Box 13-4.

Therapy Guidelines

Throughout the treatment process the following questions may help guide the treating therapist:
1. What is the best coordination of available treatment approaches (relevant to age and cause of the feeding problem)?
2. What does the child need to function better and allow the achievement of acceptable levels of nutrition? Changes may be made in the position of the feeder, the child, or the food. Changes may be made in food type, food consistency, feeding schedules, and food flavor. Changes may need to be made in the tube feeding schedule.
3. What can be changed first to affect nutrition and mealtimes? The changes that are made should be easy for the child to accept and for the caregiver to implement. Most children have firmly developed eating patterns. A different spoon may be a

BOX 13-2	Food Suggestions for Toddlers*	
PROTEINS	**STARCHES**	**FRUITS**
Lunch meat, chicken	Fruit bars	Cubed kiwi
Lunch meat, turkey	Banana muffins, blueberry muffins	Mandarin oranges
Canned meats:	Banana bread	Small cubed watermelon
Gerber meat sticks	Donuts	Spreadable fruits (in jars)
Spam	Pancakes (softened with butter and syrup)	Gerber Graduate fruits
Deviled ham or chicken		Small cubed canned peaches
Tuna fish	Graham crackers	
Canned chicken	Town House crackers	Small cubed canned pears
Cheese (grated or American)	Puffy Cheetos	Cubed bananas
Yogurt (custard style, whipped)	Wheat toast strips	Blended fruits in smoothies
	Waffles	
Refried beans	French toast (softened with butter or syrup)	Soft cubed cantaloupe and honeydew
Smashed lentils		
Hummus		
Ricotta cheese	Well-cooked pasta (rigatoni, cavatelli, ziti, spiral, ravioli, tortellini)	Quartered grapes
Cottage cheese		Soft cubed mango
Cream cheese as a dip		Adult applesauce
Soft scrambled eggs	Cubed cooked potato	**VEGETABLES**
Poached white fish (flounder, sole, orange roughy)	Dry cereal	Cubed avocado
	Polenta	Overcooked carrots
	Nabisco character Cheese Nips (softer than typical cheese nips)	Canned green beans
Smooth peanut butter		Gerber Graduate veggies
Tofu		
Veggie dogs (quartered and sliced)	Zucchini bread	Ingredients from vegetable soups
		Beets
		Cubed cooked squashes
		Well-cooked broccoli
		Cooked peas
		Tomatoes (cooked, canned)
		Sweet potatoes
		Cooked zucchini
		Cooked cauliflower or broccoflower

*These toddler food ideas are for toddlers 13 months and older. A child requires a tablespoon of food from each group above for each year of age. For example, a 3-year-old needs 3 tablespoons of protein, 3 tablespoons of starch, and 3 tablespoons of fruit or vegetable with a 4- to 6-oz cup of whole milk at each meal and snack. This food list is compiled from information received from Dr. Kay Toomey and revised by Prat et al.[12] in 2004.

BOX 13-3	Examples of Meltable Solids

- Town House or Ritz crackers (*not* saltines or club crackers)
- Puffy Cheetos or cheese puffs (*not* the crunchy variety)
- Lorna Doone cookies (shortbread)
- Gerber Graduates dissolvable wagon wheel- and star-shaped snacks
- Small pieces of soft muffin (no nuts, seeds, or fruit pieces; no crust pieces)
- Trix cereal (dry)
- Kix cereal (dry)
- Cotton candy

These items may be found in the "health food" section of a grocery store:
- Pirate's Booty
- Fruity Booty
- Veggie Booty
- Veggie Stix

BOX 13-4	Suggested Hard Munchables

Slim Jim
Beef jerky
Turkey jerky
Thick, well-cooked strips of roast beef
Celery sticks
Thick, raw carrot sticks (not baby carrots)
Dried papaya spears
Frozen bagel strips, cut thickly
Jicama cut into thick strips
Licorice and red vines (ideally a few days old so they are harder in texture)
Broccoli stalks (no flowers)
Frozen melon strips

significant change for the child. Changing the position of feeding may be difficult for the parent. Each change should be made with a focus on the progression and sequence of changes that will need to be made and the maximum potential for each change.

4. How can routine help the family's eating? Incorporating family mealtime routines and consistency in scheduling such as what happens before the family sits down to eat can have an impact. Eating routines are a key factor in the child's feeding skill development. The child may gain positive sensory

experiences and anticipatory behaviors through inclusion in meal preparation. A regular meal and snack routine, with meals and snacks separated by 2 to 3 hours, also will allow the child to develop adequate hunger and satiety for appropriate nutritional intake. The feeding specialist may help the family work with their existing schedules to achieve these beneficial interactions.

5. How can modeling of appropriate eating have an apparent effect on the family? The goal is to have the child eat with the family. Eating is a social time, and the modeling of appropriate eating gives the child cues as to the positive aspects of eating. The child can learn appropriate social cues and specific eating patterns by participating actively in mealtimes with other family members.

6. How can one help modify the caregiver interactions before, during, and after the meal? The manner in which therapists and caregivers interact with a child during meals is critical to the development of feeding skills. Words and actions that instruct and not threaten help the child learn appropriate feeding behaviors.[25] Caregivers and therapists should use positive phrases such as "you can," "we're going to have a … ." and "we can (describe the action to be completed)." The child may be given choice questions assuming there is a clear, and correct choice—for example, "do you want a cracker or a pretzel?" Caution also is necessary to questions requiring a yes or no response. It is important to not ask a question if "no," is not the desired response. "Do" language allows the child to know what is expected. For example, the child who is told "don't throw the food on the floor" will learn to throw the food on the floor. The child may alternatively be told what the caregiver or therapist "does" want them to do. For example, the child may be told, "Keep the food on your tray" or (while pointing) "You can put it there." Neutral or positive language focused on teaching the child the sensory properties of food (smell, color, shape, size, texture, temperature, taste, appearance) and the mechanics of how the food moves or breaks apart will allow the child to become familiar with foods. If the child is not able to talk or interact with his or her food, the therapist or caregiver may do so. For example, if the child is struggling with the food (in regard to sensory or oral motor skills), the caregiver or therapist may show and tell the child, in specific detail, how to manage the food.

7. What position should the child be in for the best positional and postural stability so that he or she can focus on the "work" of eating? A child who is working to sit fully upright will be unable to adequately focus his or her energy on eating. Simple positioning devices, such as small towel or blanket rolled and placed in the high chair or slightly reclining the high chair may increase eating efficiency for the developing child.

8. What is the child's tolerance for stimulation? The child's sensory tolerance and needs for environmental input should be addressed. The feeding environment may be too noisy (TV, radio, other people, pets), too bright, or have too much activity, such as the parent cooking while the child is eating. Minimizing these sensory distractions may help increase the child's organizational skills and attention to eating.

Choosing Utensils

The choice of utensils for eating and drinking is made according to the child's age, functional needs, oral structure, and self-feeding skills. Caregivers are frequently overwhelmed by the number of choices offered in infant and toddler specialty stores. Each company claims product superiority. Although there is not always a specific criterion for the choice of each bottle, bottle nipple, cup, and spoon, some guidelines exist. A match then may be made between the child's skills and needs and the benefit of the utensil. Guidelines that should be addressed include the following issues.

Mouth Opening (Size and Range)

A larger base of a bottle nipple may not always be a good match for a child with a very small mouth or restricted mouth opening. The bowl of a spoon should be approximately one third to two thirds the length of the child's lower lip; it should not reach from corner to corner of the mouth. Open cup diameter should be viewed similarly to allow for activation of the lips in controlling the flow of liquid from the cup. Different options for spoon sizes are shown in Figure 13-10.

Sucking Strength

Bottle nipples have variable flow rates. Some nonspill cups require more suction than others. Children with cleft palate and children with velopharyngeal dysfunction may require specialized nipples such as the Pigeon Nipple (Children's Medical Ventures, Monroeville, Pa.) or the Haberman bottle system (Medela, Baar, Switzerland). For the development of straw drinking, a honey bear feeder (Figure 13-11) with clear aquarium tubing may be constructed with a clean "honey bear" or a squeeze bottle used to dispense mustard or ketchup.

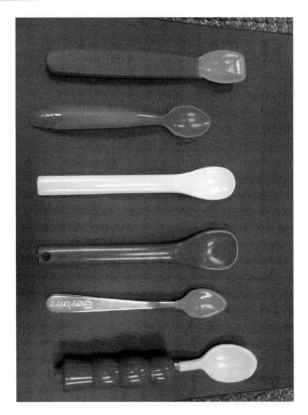

FIGURE 13-10. Spoons come in many shapes and sizes to match the age and needs of the child.

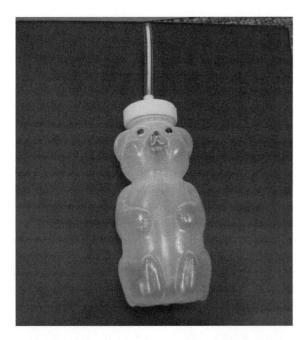

FIGURE 13-11. The components of the honey bear feeder are easily obtained and replaced. Either the caregiver or child may squeeze the bear to disperse liquid or any other material through the straw attachment.

Swallowing Skills

Bottle nipples and certain cups with variable flow rates usually are labeled as such. A child with difficulty coordinating swallowing may require a slower flow rate. Children who are drinking thicker liquids may require a faster flow rate. Specially shaped cups such as the Flexi-Cut Cup (AliMed, Dedham, Mass.) may be used to maintain a neutral head position rather than having the child tilt the head back as the cup empties (Figure 13-12).

Age

For many families, 12 months is the traditional age for transition from the bottle to the cup. Many children with feeding difficulties require a carefully sequenced transition from bottle to cup to maintain oral feeding skills and nutrition. Some children may not be able to make the transition to a nonspill sippy cup or an open cup. For these children, alternative drinking methods may be explored rather than continued use of the infant bottle into adolescence and beyond. These alternatives include cups with lids, sports bottles, and the use of a honey bear feeder. Suggestions for food selection for toddlers with feeding disorders are presented in Box 13-2.

Reinforcement

Ideally, the feeding therapy session should end on a positive note when the child has successfully completed a task. Positive responses in feeding therapy are sometimes difficult to identify, although *any* positive response should be reinforced. Positive responses may include a short time in the high chair, a child swallowing one taste of food, or the child's ability to touch

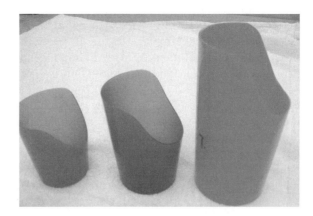

FIGURE 13-12. The Flexi-Cut cup (AliMed) is sometimes called a "nosey" or "cutout" cup. It is available in three different sizes and levels of plastic density to allow for modification and advances in drinking skills.

the food. It is important to identify, in advance, the amount of time to be spent in direct interaction with food. If the amount of time spent with food inside or outside the mouth is prearranged, the level of stress surrounding attempts at feeding can be limited for the therapist and caregiver.

TUBE FEEDING

For all families the goal is to help their child achieve and maintain the ability to eat by mouth. The discussion regarding tube feeding may be viewed by the parent as failure in their attempt to feed their child orally. The discussion of evaluation for tube feeding must be made sensitively and with objective informa-

tion in mind. The child for whom a feeding tube is recommended usually is not able to take adequate nutrition by mouth to support growth. Use of a feeding tube does not mean that the child always will be unable to eat. Many children are able to take some nutrition by mouth as long as they demonstrate safety in swallowing. Children who may be candidates for feeding tubes include children who are born prematurely, those with anatomic abnormalities that challenge efficient feeding, those with accompanying neurologic disorders, those with evidence of pulmonary aspiration, or those with failure to thrive because of medical complications. The evaluation for considering placement of a feeding tube is made by a number of medical professionals. For example, the dietitian

---

CLINICAL CORNER 13-1

A toddler and his parents/caregiver come for a feeding evaluation. The child appears to have some interest in food presented to him, although he shows some apprehension to foods that are wet or sticky. He prefers foods that are considerably stronger in flavor than is typical for a child of this age. This preference is more specific for salty foods. He shows the ability to bite and chew foods, which are of a meltable soft solid to mechanical soft solid texture. He demonstrates reduced intraoral awareness because he frequently overfills his mouth with food. He does manage to continue to chew, swallow small boluses, and empty his mouth. He is able to drink from a bottle and has shown increasing interest in drinking from a cup. He is able to sit independently and stand with support. He plays with toys using both hands. He is not saying any words. The family's goal is for the child to eat a larger variety and quantity of food so that they may decrease his tube feedings.

CRITICAL THINKING:
1. What may be the initial treatment goals for intake of liquids and solids?
2. What type of seating system may be used during eating time?
3. What sequence of foods should be offered in therapy?
4. How will you work toward increasing food and liquid quantity without compromising gastrointestinal function?
5. What reinforcement strategies may be appropriate?
6. What will be your criteria for discharge?

CLINICAL CORNER 13-2

Evaluation of a 1-year-old shows poor head control with no trunk control. The boy requires maximal support in all positions. The child is visually interactive and is able to vocalize clearly. Active sucking movements are not noted with either a bottle or sippy cup. The mother must squeeze liquid into his mouth. Evaluation of jaw movements varies from too small to too large a mouth opening. "Choppy" movements are noted in spoon feeding. He has limited activity of the cheek musculature. The tongue appearance is "bunched" (constriction of muscles along the central longitudinal aspect of the tongue), creating a narrow appearance with limited function for bolus formation and control. The child responds positively to moderate pressure on the blade of the tongue with the spoon, with greater flaring and flattening of the tongue. Initiation of all oral responses is slow but increases with tactile and pressure input. He enjoys food, including infant purees and pureed, table foods such as yogurt.

CRITICAL THINKING:
1. What may be the initial treatment goals for intake of liquids and solids?
2. What sequence of foods may be given in the first and subsequent sessions?
3. What types of home program strategies may be taught to increase oral function and food management?
4. What types of family mealtime strategies may be helpful?
5. How will you decide how to guide this family toward increasing quantities and types of liquids, solid foods, and general nutrition?
6. What will be your criteria for discharge?

determines the nutritional need for the feeding tube on the basis of growth factors. The dietitian also determines the type of feeding formula used in the feeding tube. This may include breast milk, infant formula, or a specialized formula based on the child's current medical status, age, and nutritional needs. Tube feedings may be provided by pump or syringe. The rate of the tube feeding depends on the age of the child, the stomach's ability to tolerate specific amounts of formula, and the rate at which the stomach empties. Families should be educated about the care of the tube, how to provide feedings, and how to assist the child with tolerance of the tube.

A nasogastric (NG) tube passes through the nose, pharynx, and the lower esophageal sphincter and into the stomach. NG tubes are placed most often as a temporary measure when supplementary feedings may be needed or for longer term needs when a gastrostomy tube (GT) cannot be placed. Children with NG tubes are in an acute phase of feeding difficulty. Feedings by NG tube are typically delivered by gravity over a short time or more gradually by a timed feeding pump. Some children with difficulty tolerating volumes of formula in their stomach may also receive continuous feedings administered by a feeding pump. Many children with NG tubes show intermittent swallowing discomfort and may have breathing problems related to the tube's placement in the nose. They also may show facial-tactile sensitivity because of the tape placed on the face to secure the tube. Some children may attempt to dislodge the tube, requiring replacement by parents or professionals. Frequent dislodgment may create further discomfort in the nose and pharynx.

Nasojejunal (NJ) tubes are tubes that pass through the nose, pharynx, the lower esophageal sphincter, through the stomach, and into the jejunum. Feedings delivered by NJ tubes are used when supplemental feedings are needed for children with severe reflux, cardiac conditions, and certain gastric disorders. NJ feedings are always delivered continuously by feeding pump. GT feedings are given directly into the stomach. The rationale for choosing GT placement and feeding is that it may avoid the complications of NG tube placement, but more often it is used for children who will require longer periods to achieve complete oral feeding competency.

TAKE HOME NOTES

1. Because oral feeding may be difficult for the infant, the *quality* of the process is more important than the *quantity* of intake. Stress signals from the infant often are an indication of the need to stop feeding,

---

CLINICAL CORNER 13-3

Robert is a typically developing 4-year-old boy. He was referred for a clinical feeding evaluation because of decreased appetite and self-induced vomiting. His parents noted this approximately 6 months before the evaluation. He has had significant weight loss and a diagnosis of gastroesophageal reflux. He is taking lansoprazole (Prevacid) and metoclopramide (Reglan) for this disorder. He has a history of anxiety. He appears to enjoy eating selected foods. He was able to eat two mini-corn dogs (familiar food), two chicken nuggets (familiar food), a fruit cup (new food), tasted pizza rolls with great reluctance (new food), and ate ⅓ cup of boxed macaroni and cheese (new food). He was initially very apprehensive of the macaroni and cheese but when asked to help prepare it, he ate the quantity given readily. He was also able to finish a drink box quantity of orange juice. He did not appear to have any challenges with wet or sticky foods. He gagged once during the evaluation but did not vomit. The initial recommendation included working on only one new food item each week, scheduling meals and snacks (no "grazing"), increasing the family's awareness of target portions, and avoidance of yes and no questions such as "do you want to eat?" The parents' goals are for him to be able to eat without vomiting and to reduce his anxiety surrounding the eating circumstance.

CRITICAL THINKING:

1. What therapy goals may be reasonable for this child with respect to food quantity and variety?
2. What sequence of foods may be given in the first and subsequent sessions?
3. What types of home program strategies may be taught to increase oral function and food management?
4. What types of family mealtime strategies may be helpful?
5. How will you explain each week's strategies to the child?
6. What types of reinforcement strategies may be appropriate?
7. What will be your criteria for discharge?

---

even if there is only small amount remaining to complete the task.

2. Providing comprehensive, developmentally supportive care throughout the infant's process of feeding is paramount to successful eating.

3. Skin-to-skin contact is an important part of treatment for regulating the premature infant. It plays a vital role for the parents and the infant.

4. A cue-based feeding clinical pathway provides the team an evidence-based approach to allow the infant to drive the feeding schedule to achieve the most efficient outcomes.

5. Most families are highly invested in the potential of their child as a successful eater. Approach the formulation of goals and strategies with small steps that create positive advances toward safe oral feeding.

6. Families must be integrated into all aspects of treatment; this is key to their child's progress. Each therapy session should involve the feeding specialist demonstrating therapy strategies, followed by the therapist watching the caregiver use these same strategies. This approach instills a greater degree of confidence in the caregiver and ensures more effective carryover.

7. Feeding therapy does not use a "one size fits all" set of strategies. Multiple strategies and programs are available and should be applied according to the needs of the child. Strategies may be used alone or in combination with others.

8. Integration of therapy services between occupational therapy and speech therapy provides the most effective balance of intervention strategies that address sensory, motor, cognitive, oral structural, and other developmental areas relating to feeding.

9. The introduction of a feeding tube may feel like a safety net or a failure to families. Therapists should approach discussion of this intervention carefully, with a positive outlook toward improved nutrition for the child.

References

1. Ross E, Browne J: Developmental progression of feeding skills: an approach to supporting feeding in preterm infants, *Semin Neonatol* 7:469, 2002.

2. Als H, Lawhon G, Duffy FH et al: Individualized developmental care for the very low birth weight preterm infant: medical and neuro-functional effects, *JAMA* 272:853, 1994.

3. Ludington-Hoe SM, Anderson GC, Swinth JY: Randomized controlled trial of kangaroo care: cardio-respiratory and thermal effects on healthy preterm infants, *Neonatal Netw* 23:39, 2004.

4. Ludington-Hoe SM, Swinth JY: Developmental aspects of kangaroo care, *J Obstet Gynecol Neonatal Nurs* 25:691,1996.

5. Eichel P: Kangaroo care: expanding our practice to critically ill neonates, *Newborn Infant Nurs Rev* 1:224, 2001.

6. DiMenna L: Considerations for implementation of a neonatal kangaroo care protocol, *Neonatal Netw* 25:405, 2006.

7. Byers JF, Yovaish W, Lowman LB et al: Co-bedding versus single-bedding premature multiple-gestation infants in incubators, *J Obstet Gynecol Neonatal Nurs* 32:340, 2003.

8. Polizzi J, Byers JF, Kiehl E: Co-bedding versus traditional bedding of multiple gestation infants in the NICU, *J Healthc Qual* 25:5, 2003.

9. Touch SM, Epstein ML, Pohl CA et al: The impacts of cobedding on sleep patterns in preterm twins, *Clin Pediatr* 41:425, 2002.

10. Hill A: The effects of nonnutritive sucking and oral support on the feeding efficiency of preterm infants, *Newborn Infant Nurs Rev* 5:133, 2005.

11. Boyd K: The effectiveness of the sequential oral sensory approach group feeding program. In Toomey K, editor: *When children won't eat: advanced topics in the use of the SOS approach to feeding*, Denver, 2007, Toomey and Associates.

12. Toomey K: *When children won't eat: advanced topics in the use of the SOS approach to feeding*, Denver, 2006, Toomey and Associates.

13. Clawson B, Purcell D: The role of psychology on a pediatric feeding team. In Brackett K, editor: *Pediatric feeding and swallowing disorders: a medical, motor, and behavioral approach*, Fort Mill, SC, 2004, Motivations.

14. Shadler G, Suss-Burghart H, Toschke AM et al: Feeding disorders in ex-prematures: causes-response to therapy-long term outcomes, *Eur J Pediatr* 166:803, 2007.

15. Beckman D: Oral motor assessment and intervention. Available at www.beckmanoralmotor.com. Accessed February 9, 2009.

16. Toomey K: *When children won't eat: the SOS approach to feeding.* Presented at symposium at Primary Children's Medical Center, Salt Lake City, UT, 2002.

17. Garo A, Thurman SK, Kerwin ME et al: Parent and caregiver stress during pediatric hospitalization for chronic feeding problems, *J Pediatr Nurs* 20:268, 2005.

18. Ayoob KT, Barresi I: Feeding disorders in children: taking an interdisciplinary approach, *Pediatr Ann* 36:478, 2007.

19. Davis-McFarland E: Family and cultural issues in a school swallowing and feeding program, *Lang Speech Hear Serv Sch* 39:119, 2008.

20. Birch LL: Psychological influences on the childhood diet, *J Nutr* 128:407S, 1998.

21. Murray N, Pratt C, McDonald K: *General guidelines for normal feeding development: birth to two years of age*, unpublished document, Salt Lake City, UT, 2004, Primary Children's Medical Center.

22. Pressman H, Berkowitz M: Treating children with feeding disorders, *ASHA Leader* 8:10, 2003.

23. Wolf LS, Glass RP: *Feeding and swallowing disorders in infancy*, Tucson, AZ, 1992, Therapy Skill Builders.

24. American Dietetic Association: *The National Dysphagia Diet: standardization for optimal care*, Chicago, 2002, American Dietetic Association.

25. Girolami PA, Boscoe JH, Roscoe N: Decreasing expulsions by a child with a feeding disorder: using a brush to present and re-present food, *J Appl Behav Anal* 40:749, 2007.

APPENDIX 13-A

FOOD DIARY FOR _____

Meal	Time	Food Offered	Amount Eaten
		Formula:_____	Oral:
			Pumped:
Meal	**Time**	**Food Offered**	**Amount Eaten**
		Formula:_____	Oral:
			Pumped:
Meal	**Time**	**Food Offered**	**Amount Eaten**
		Formula:_____	Oral:
			Pumped:
Meal	**Time**	**Food Offered**	**Amount Eaten**
		Formula:_____	Oral:
			Pumped:
Meal	**Time**	**Food Offered**	**Amount Eaten**
		Formula:_____	Oral:
			Pumped:

APPENDIX 13-B

Useful Resources Of Materials And Contact Information For Treatment Of Children With Feeding Disorders

The Reflux Book
Beth Pulsifer-Anderson
Intensive Care Parenting, LLC
5257 Buckeystown Pike #308
Frederick, MD 21704
www.refluxbook.com

The Pediatric Feeding and Dysphagia Newsletter
Krisi Brackett, MS, CCC-SLP
Hiro Publishing
3106 S. Lincoln Street
Salt Lake City, UT 84106
feedingnews@earthlink.net

The Food Allergy & Anaphylaxis Network
11781 Lee Jackson Hwy., Suite 160
Fairfax, VA 22033-3309
www.foodallergy.org

Dr. Kay Toomey and Toomey & Associates, Inc.
1780 S. Bellaire Street, Suite 515
Denver, CO 80222
(303) 344-1460

Cleft Palate Foundation
1504 East Franklin Street, Suite 102
Chapel Hill, NC 27514
http://www.cleftline.org

The Sensory Processing Disorder Network
(Formerly The Kid Foundation)
5655 S. Yosemite Street, Suite 305.
Greenwood Village, CO 80111
www.SPDNetwork.org
Sensory Integration International-The Ayres Clinic
200 Second Avenue South, Suite 447
St. Petersbug , FL 33701-4313
1-888271-2-SII
www.sensoryint.com

A Parent's Guide to Understanding Sensory Integration (1991)
Published by Sensory Integration International, Inc. (see contact information above)

Chewy Tubes
Speech Pathology Associates, LLC
P.O.Box 2289
South Portland, ME 04116
www.chewytubes.com

Treatment for Adults

MICHAEL A. CRARY

OBJECTIVES

1. Describe some of the basic differences between compensatory techniques and rehabilitative techniques. Tell how this distinction applies to specific therapy techniques.
2. Describe the impact of various therapy techniques on the swallowing mechanism.
3. Identify the expected functional benefits associated with various behavioral treatment strategies.
4. Describe risks from specific therapy techniques that may be posed to patients.
5. Explain strategies that may be helpful in evaluating the appropriateness of existing or novel interventions for a specific patient.

WHICH TECHNIQUES AND WHAT TO CONSIDER

As indicated in Chapter 12, practicing clincians should avail themselves of evidence supporting (or refuting) the application of any therapy technique. Beyond evidence, however, clinicians will benefit from a conceptual framework from which any clinical technique might be considered. Following this line of reasoning, some common questions to consider might include (1) "What is the purpose of the technique?" (2) "What are the details of the technique?" and (3) "What is the impact on the swallowing mechanism?"

Clinicians may have different intentions for applying various intervention techniques. For example, the term *management* might be an appropriate descriptor when techniques are chosen to maintain the status quo and reduce the risk of **morbidity** in patients with dysphagia. In this scenario, the clinician is not actively attempting to change the swallowing mechanism, but rather is using strategies to prevent the development of dysphagia-related complications while maintaining adequate nutrition and hydration. Techniques that might be used in a management scenario include compensations. Compensations are considered to be short-term adjustments that facilitate improved swallowing function but do not have a lasting impact on swallow physiology. If a compensatory technique is not used, the patient will not be expected to swallow successfully. Conversely, the term *treatment* might be an appropriate descriptor when techniques are chosen in an attempt to effect a lasting improvement on the swallowing mechanism that will continue beyond the intervention period. The term *rehabilitation* would be appropriate here because the intent of intervention is to improve an impaired swallow mechanism by the systematic application of techniques focused at the specific impairments identified in the swallowing evaluation. Rehabilitation techniques are anticipated to enact lasting changes in swallowing performance that will remain even after a technique is discontinued. Given this distinction, clinicians may ask whether a technique is intended to have short-term or long-term impact, accommodate various bolus characteristics, change the swallow physiology, or have other influences on the patient or the swallow mechanism. Clinicians would use different techniques depending on the purpose or intent of the clinical intervention (manage versus treat).

Details of any technique are essential for appropriate clinical application. Even simple techniques may become confused by the clinician and/or the patient. For example, a recent survey[1] reported poor agreement in the details of the chin-down posture. This seemingly simple compensation may be more variable than conceived and variants have been described using different terminology. Variability may be clinically important as different postures are likely to have different physiologic and hence functional impact on the swallow mechanism. Thus, a basic question is whether published articles, presentations, or other sources of information provide clear descriptions on how to perform or teach the technique under consideration. This information might incorporate a clear description of the technique and specific instructions for how to apply the technique clinically. This information should include how often and under what conditions the technique should be used. Furthermore, it is important to determine whether the published evidence was gathered from a group of patients similar to the patient being considered for a given technique. For example, evidence supporting the use of a given technique for stroke patients may not be applicable to patients with head/neck cancer.

An additional consideration for any therapy technique would be to understand the intended impact on the swallow mechanism. The impact of any technique relates to the outcome of the intervention using that technique. Ultimately, intervention should result in functional benefit for any patient, but what are the specifics of the intended functional benefit? Following terminology from Chapter 12, the technique would be the *action plan* used by the clinician. Techniques would have expected physiologic impact(s) on the swallow mechanism that are related to the *objectives* of treatment. If successful, the *goal* or functional outcome of therapy would be realized. Thus it is important for the clinician to understand how the specific technique relates to the intended physiologic impact on the swallow mechanism and how this change will relate to the functional benefit sought by intervention.

Box 14-1 lists common swallow therapy techniques described in dysphagia treatment literature. Each technique has some degree of supporting evidence in subgroups of patients with dysphagia. The following information is presented (if available) for each technique: (1) purpose of the technique, (2) details of the technique, and (3) impact on the swallow mechanism.

MANAGING DYSPHAGIA SYMPTOMS: ADJUSTMENTS, COMPENSATIONS, AND MODIFICATIONS

General Postural Adjustments

Postural adjustments may involve the entire body or only the head. In general, changes in head and/or

BOX 14-1	List of Therapy Techniques

- Postural adjustments
  - Body posture
  - Head posture
- Modifying liquids and solids
- Oral motor exercises
- Supraglottic swallow
- Super-supraglottic swallow
- Mendelsohn maneuver
- Effortful swallow
- Multiple swallows
- Tongue-hold maneuver
- Head-lift exercise
- Thermal-tactile application
- Applying exercise principles
- Adjunctive modalities

body posture are considered effective in reducing aspiration in various patient groups.[2,3] Reported results suggest that change in posture has the potential to redirect the bolus and may change the speed of bolus flow, thus giving the patient more time to adjust the swallow. Generally, changes in body posture are considered compensatory and thus fall under the category of dysphagia management. In some clinical situations, notably in patients who have abnormal postures because of physical reasons, adjustments in body posture to facilitate safe swallowing may be long term. However, even in these situations, adjustments in body posture are considered compensations rather than attempts to change the dynamics of the abnormal swallow. Furthermore, Logemann[4] appropriately notes that no single posture improves swallowing function in *all* patients. Thus, depending on the specific swallowing deficits presented by an individual patient, the treating clinician may use one or more compensatory postures to facilitate safer swallowing function. Beyond posture, clinicians may find it necessary to use additional compensations to facilitate safe swallowing function in some patients.[5]

Typically, body posture changes involve lying down and/or side-lying. Both changes are expected to reduce the impact of gravity either during the swallow or on post-swallow residue. The side-lying technique may be applied when a difference in pharyngeal function is noted between the right and left sides. In this situation, conventional wisdom suggests that the stronger side be the down side. This position uses gravity to direct the bolus (or residue) toward the stronger hemipharynx. The direct clinical impact of altering body posture on the swallow, specifically on airway protection, may be assessed during the instrumental swallowing examination. One physiologic result of lying down during swallowing may be increased hypopharyngeal pressure on the bolus, contributing to increased maximum opening of the **pharyngoesophageal sphincter** (PES) and reduced duration of sphincter opening during the swallow.[6] These physiologic changes may be helpful in strengthening the swallow in some patients.

Postural adjustments may not be the ideal intervention for patients who are at risk for noncompliance due to physical or cognitive limitations. Also, change in body posture, specifically any variant of lying down, may affect esophageal motor functions.[7,8] An additional functional consideration may be the impact of supine position on reflux episodes.[9] Patients with severe reflux (even those being fed via tube) may benefit from maintaining an upright posture during and after feeding. The upright posture helps reduce or prevent reflux that may contribute to aspiration. In addition, nocturnal head of bed elevation has long been advocated for patients with nocturnal reflux.

Practice Note 14-1

The impact of altering body posture on the swallow may be assessed during the instrumental swallow examination. Because this compensation is often used to reduce or eliminate aspiration, the fluoroscopic swallowing study is well suited to evaluating the impact of postural adjustments. When considering side-lying or other lying-down positions, the patient may be appropriately positioned on the fluoroscope table to examine the impact of various "down" positions. Furthermore, fluoroscopy tables can be tilted to different degrees to determine whether a flat or inclined position provides the greatest benefit. One issue with inclined positions is how to make the transition from the radiology suite to the patient's daily environment. Clinical creativity is the best advice here.

When fluoroscopic evaluation is simply not possible, clinicians may attempt to evaluate the impact of altering body posture using endoscopy or by change(s) in clinical signs associated with aspiration. Endoscopy offers an advantage over use of clinical signs because the airway is observed before and after each swallow attempt. If clinical signs alone are used, we strongly suggest inclusion of cervical auscultation to monitor airway sounds before and after swallowing attempts. This clinical approach has several limitations, but in some instances it may be the only avenue available to assess the impact of postural alterations on swallow safety.

This simple postural adjustment is highly effective in promoting acid clearance from the esophagus.[10] Thus clinicians should evaluate the impact of body posture variations on esophageal functions during the instrumental swallow examination. This guideline especially applies to patients with clinical symptoms or signs of esophageal deficit.

Head Postural Adjustments

Changes in head posture may include extension, flexion, or rotation. Each of these postural adjustments is considered compensatory and hopefully is used for a limited time. Although in the same category of intervention, each adjustment has a different impact on the swallow mechanism and thus each is used for a range of specific clinical indications. Videos 14-1 through 14-4 show endoscopic and fluoroscopic examples of each head posture adjustment.

Head Extension

Head extension may be accomplished by raising the chin. This has the anatomic effect of widening the oropharynx (Figure 14-1) and may be helpful in moving a bolus from the mouth into the pharynx when oral/lingual deficits are present. Thus patients who have received a glossectomy, other oral resection, reconstruction, or patients who have significant lingual paralysis may benefit from use of a head extension technique. The basic concept is to elevate the chin and use gravity to assist in oral bolus transit toward the pharynx. The patient should be determined to have adequate pharyngeal function and adequate laryngeal closure for airway protection. Clinical benefit (reduced aspiration) from the head extension posture used during the fluoroscopic swallow examination has been demonstrated in a small number of patients treated for oral cancer.[2] Conversely, with head extension, defective laryngeal closure was observed in appoximately one third (10/35) of patients demonstrating normal laryngeal closure during swallowing in a head neutral position.[11]

Head extension may also affect the PES and the coordination between pharyngeal and PES activity. Specifically, head extension increases **intraluminal** pressure (less relaxation), decreases duration of relaxation in the PES, and changes the temporal coordination between pharyngeal and PES swallow pressures as measured manometrically.[12] These changes may complicate an existing swallowing problem. Thus head extension may be a useful clinical technique in patients with difficulty transporting a bolus from the mouth to the pharynx, but it may contribute to swallowing difficulties in patients who have airway protection or PES deficits. Like most compensatory maneuvers, the impact of head extension on swallow function may be evaluated during the instrumental swallow examination.

Head Flexion–Chin Tuck

Head flexion has been suggested as a technique to facilitate improved airway protection in patients who demonstrate deficits in airway protection during swallowing.[11] Flexing the head (chin tuck) has the anatomic effect of improving laryngeal vestibule closure,[11] narrowing the oropharynx[13] (Figure 14-2), and reducing the distance between the hyoid bone and the larynx.[14]

The physiologic effects of head flexion (chin tuck) in patients with dysphagia are reported as minimal.

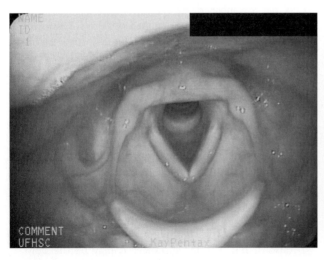

FIGURE 14-1. Oropharyngeal widening resulting from head extension (chin raise).

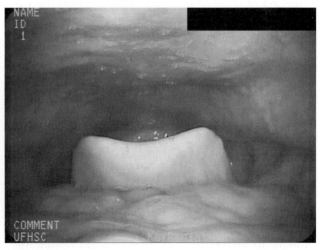

FIGURE 14-2. Oropharyngeal narrowing resulting from head flexion (chin tuck).

In patients with pharyngeal dysphagia, no manometric differences were found between control swallows and swallows using the chin-tuck maneuver.[14,15] Furthermore, in a small sample of healthy volunteers, weaker pharyngeal contractions were observed during swallows using the chin-tuck position.[16] Moreover, the combination of a reclining posture (60 degrees) with a chin tuck (60 degrees) may significantly increase the duration of **swallowing apnea.**[17] This change in respiratory pattern may contribute to increased respiratory stress in some patients. At the very least, clinicians should monitor pharyngeal residue and any respiratory changes induced by introduction of the chin tuck or any swallowing maneuver.

Clinical benefit from the chin-tuck maneuver has been desribed primarily in reference to improved airway protection. Shanahan et al.[18] reported elimination of aspiration with the chin tuck in 15 patients with dysphagia resulting from neurologic damage. These investigators also reported that this postural maneuver was not useful for patients who demonstrated delay in swallow initiation and post-swallow residue in the piriform recesses. From a larger, heterogeneous sample, Rasley et al.[3] reported that the chin-tuck position eliminated aspiration on all tested volumes in 21 of 84 (25%) patients. Logemann, Rademaker, and Pauloski[2] reported that 5 of 6 (83%) patients with head and neck cancer–related dysphagia were able to eliminate aspiration on at least one bolus volume of liquid barium during the fluoroscopic swallowing study. Lewin et al.[19] reported elimination of aspiration for liquids using the chin-tuck position during the fluoroscopic swallow examination in 17 of 21 patients after esophagectomy. Finally, Logemann et al.[20] conducted a large randomized study to evaluate the effectiveness of the chin-down posture (chin tuck) compared with thickened liquids in the reduction of aspiration in patients with dysphagia related to dementia or Parkinson's disease. Results indicated that the chin-down posture was less effective than thickening liquids in reducing aspiration events during the fluoroscopic swallow examination.

Note that each of these studies evaluated the impact of the chin-tuck position within the confines of the fluoroscopic swallow examination. Thus each study describes the effect of this posture as a short-term compensation. Zuydam et al.[21] reported that compensatory maneuvers (chin tuck and supraglottic swallow) used as therapy techniques were effective in 50% of patients who aspirated. In a companion paper to the effect study of chin tuck versus thickened liquids,[19] Robbins et al.[22] monitored a subgroup of the original patients for 3 months after the initial swallow

examination. Patients were randomly assigned to one of the three interventions (chin tuck for thin liquids, nectar-thick liquids, or honey-thick liquids) as a management strategy and the rate of new pneumonia (**incidence**) was evaluated as the primary outcome. Results indicated no significant differences in the rates of pneumonia across the three interventions.

The chin-tuck position may be helpful in reducing or eliminating aspiration in some patients with dysphagia. However, it does not produce benefit in all patients and may be inferior to thickened liquids in some patients. Although anatomic adjustments have been demonstrated in response to this posture, physiologic changes reportedly are minimal. Furthermore, at least one study raises the possibility that this posture, especially combined with a reclining body position, may alter the coordination of swallow and respiration. Finally, it is possible that this technique may need to be combined with other strategies, including other postures or bolus changes, to produce maximum benefit.[2] Because this is such a simple task to perform, its impact on appropriate patients should be evaluated during instrumental swallow studies.

In this chapter we have used the term *chin-tuck* to refer to a specific compensatory posture. We have also used terms from published descriptions including *head flexion* and *chin-down posture*. This variability in terminology is given a practical focus by the survey results of Okada et al.,[1] who remind us that different postures may result in different physiologic or functional results. Thus what may seem simple to clinicians may be confusing to patients. In evaluating research on any technique, clinicians need to look beyond the terminology and be certain of the technique. Furthermore, when evaluating the impact of any technique or instructing patients, clarity and consistency are very important.

Head Rotation–Head Turn

Head rotation or the head-turn maneuver is another postural adjustment that can function as an effective short-term compensation to improve swallowing function. The head-turn posture has been advocated primarily in cases of unilateral pharyngeal deficit.[23,24] Conventional wisdom suggests that patients turn the head toward the weaker side in cases of hemilateral impairment. The anatomic result of this postural maneuver is a narrowing or closing off of the swallowing tract on the side toward which the head is turned. This effect is demonstrated in Figure 14-3 in which the head is turned to each side with the corresponding change in oropharyngeal configuration. However, this closure effect may not extend throughout the hypopharynx but may be restricted to the

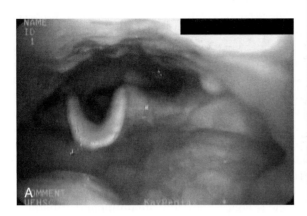 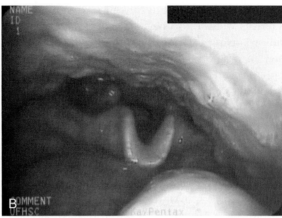

FIGURE 14-3. Changes in oropharyngeal configuration resulting from head rotation. **A**, Right; **B**, left.

level of the hyoid bone at the superior hypopharynx, which leaves the inferior aspects of the pharynx open in some patients.[25]

Physiologic effects of head rotation include a drop in PES pressure and corresponding increase in PES opening.[24] Additional physiologic effects of the head-turn position include increased pharyngeal manometric swallow pressures on the side of the pharynx toward which the head is turned, a drop in PES resting pressure opposite the direction of head turn, and a delay in PES closure (e.g., longer relaxation of the PES).[26] These physiologic findings suggest that the head rotation technique should be considered for patients with reduced PES opening. The combined anatomic and physiologic changes resulting from turning the head are anticipated to facilitate an increase in the amount swallowed with less residue and reduced risk of airway compromise.

Clinical benefit from the head-turn position has been reported in a variety of patient groups. Logemann et al.[24] reported improved swallow function (larger amount of bolus swallow/less residue) in all 5 patients (100%) patients with dysphagia after lateral medullary stroke. Within a sample of patients with various causes of dysphagia, Rasley et al.[3] reported that liquid aspiration was eliminated for all tested volumes in 20 of 77 (26%) of patients. In a group of postsurgical head and neck cancer patients, Logemann, Rademaker, and Pauloski[2] reported 75% effectiveness (9/12 patients) in the elimination of liquid aspiration in at least one volume.

Like many postural maneuvers, head rotation should be considered a compensatory technique, not a lifelong adjustment in swallowing. Also, like other techniques in this category, effectiveness may be

Practice Note 14-2

Evaluating the impact of head rotation (or any head posture) during either the fluoroscopic or endoscopic swallow examinations is helpful not only in identifying potential benefit from the posture, but also in identifying the degree of rotation (or flexion). The endoscopic swallow examination may have a slight advantage over the fluoroscopic study in the head-turn position in that the clinician can identify factors that may limit or negate potential benefit from the compensation. For example, years ago we evaluated a patient who had extensive left hemipharyngeal and laryngeal paralysis secondary to resection for a jugular foramen tumor. In addition to the tenth cranial nerve deficits extending from the velum to the larynx, this patient also had a twelfth cranial nerve paralysis that impaired movement and atrophy in the left side of the tongue. A head-turn position toward the left was attempted under endoscopic inspection. The technique failed as material was observed to collect in the posterior oral cavity on the left side, spill over the epiglottis, and enter the airway. Further evaluation of this examination revealed that the lingual atrophy in the left tongue created an anatomic deficit much like a small cup or bowl toward which all liquid (thin and thick) would flow. Subsequently, when a swallow was attempted, this material was already on the left side of the swallow mechanism and combined with a weakened left pharynx, liquids would simply pass over the epiglottis and migrate toward the airway. Fortunately, other compensations were beneficial for this patient.

reduced by compliance, cognitive factors, physical factors, or the presence of multiple swallowing deficits. Moreover, this postural adjustment may be combined with other compensations or maneuvers to improve swallow function.[2] Finally, the functional effects of a head-turn maneuver may be checked easily during either the fluoroscopic or endoscopic swallow examinations.

Thickening Liquids and Modifying Diets

Thickened Liquids: Pros and Cons

Alterations in liquid viscosity (specifically meaning "thickness") have been advocated in both the evaluation and treatment of patients with dysphagia.[27-29] Two major foci seem to emerge in relation to the use of thickened liquids: (1) thicker liquids result in less aspiration among patients with dysphagia and (2) thicker liquids have a physiologic impact on the swallow mechanism. In a 2005 survey of speech-language pathologists experienced in dysphagia intervention,[30] the most commonly reported reasons for the use of thickened liquids included delayed onset of swallowing and impaired oral control of thin liquids. Reduction of aspiration was not specifically reported among the most frequent reasons for use of thickened liquids. However, this lack of focus on aspiration seems to be the result of the survey questions, which did not include direct reference to aspiration reduction as a rationale for use of thickened liquids in adult patients with dysphagia. In this survey, the perception of patients' acceptance of thickened liquids was influenced by the degree of "thickness." Honey and spoon-thick liquids were considered less accepted (strong dislike) than nectar-thick liquids. Furthermore, these initial negative perceptions either worsened or remained the same with continued use over time. These patterns of patient acceptance also are reflected in the use patterns of thickened liquids among patients in skilled nursing facilities.[31] Results of a national review of thickened-liquid application in skilled nursing facilities indicated that approximately 8% of all patients (from a total sample of 25,470) received thickened liquids—60% received nectar-thick liquids, 33% received honey-thick liquids, and 6% received pudding or spoon-thick liquids. Thus thickened liquids are used frequently in the management of adult dysphagia with the most frequent being nectar or syrup consistency.

The frequent use of thickened liquids seems to occur in the relative absence of strong evidence that they provide significant clinical benefit to adult patients with dysphagia. In the 2005 survey,[30] nearly 85% of responding clinicians indicated that they believed thickening liquids was an effective management compared with only 5% who disagreed with this position. These opinions reflect clinicians' positive perception, but until recently, only scant empirical support existed for this clinical practice. Kuhlemeier, Palmer, and Rosenberg[32] studied bolus factors that influenced aspiration rates among 190 patients with dysphagia and reported that thickness of liquid (thin, thick, ultrathick) and manner of presentation (spoon versus cup) had a direct impact on the rates of aspiration during the fluoroscopic swallowing examination. Ultrathick liquids presented by spoon resulted in the lowest aspiration rates, followed by thick liquids presented by spoon, then by cup with thin liquids resulting in the highest rates of aspiration during the fluoroscopic study. To date, the strongest evidence that liquid viscosity affects aspiration during the fluoroscopic swallowing examination comes from a large randomization trial of techniques to reduce liquid aspiration in patients with dementia or Parkinson's disease.[20] The results of this study support those from the earlier report from Kuhlemeier, Palmer, and Rosenberg.[32] Aspiration rates were lowest for honey-thickened liquids (thickest liquid evaluated) and greatest for thin liquids (accompanied by a chin-down posture). Aspiration rates for nectar-thickened liquids were between the two other viscosities and significantly different from both. Interestingly, the reported benefit from honey-thick liquids was not maintained when this viscosity was presented last among the materials examined. The investigators suggested that patient fatigue may have been a factor in this result. Certainly, clinicians should consider patient endurance (converse of fatigue) when interpreting the results of the swallowing evaluation and in making clinical recommendations based on any evaluation.

The study by Kuhlemeier, Palmer, and Rosenberg[32] implied that manner of bolus presentation may influence the occurrence of aspiration in addition to viscosity. Other bolus characteristics also may affect aspiration rates. For example, in an unpublished study of aspiration and residue rates in adult patients evaluated in the acute care environment, we learned that bolus thickness and volume may interact. Table 14-1 summarizes the rates of aspiration and residue seen during fluoroscopic examination among 20 patients who swallowed 5 versus 10 mL of thin, nectar-thick, and pudding viscosities of barium sulfate contrast agent. Note that different clinical impressions result depending on both the thickness and the volume of the material swallowed. For example, the rates of aspiration and residue are the same for thin liquid across both volumes. However, although thickening material results in reduction or aspiration rates for 5 mL

TABLE 14-1

Potential Interaction Between Viscosity and Volume in Rates*

	ASPIRATION		
Amount	Thin	Nectar-Thick	Pudding
5 mL	20%	5%	5%
10 mL	20%	15%	20%

	RESIDUE		
Amount	Thin	Nectar-Thick	Pudding
5 mL	65%	70%	80%
10 mL	65%	80%	90%

*Percent of aspiration and residue during the fluoroscopic swallowing examination.

(20% to 5% to 5%), the benefit is not the same for 10 mL (20% to 15% to 20%). The rate of aspiration for 10 mL of pudding is as high as that for 5 or 10 mL of thin liquid. In addition, the rate of residue in the vallecullae increases more for the larger volume as the swallowed material is thickened. This type of pattern implicates the need to evaluate more than just thickness of swallowed material. Therapy and perhaps diet recommendations would differ based on the pattern presented by an individual patient.

Although studies such as those reviewed suggest that thickening liquids reduces aspiration rates in groups of patients, clinicians must remember that these are not *treatment* studies. These studies evaluate the immediate effect of thickening liquids during the fluoroscopic study and do not speak directly to the effectiveness of using thickened liquids as an intervention or longer-term management strategy. In fact, the single clinical trial[22] to date indicated no significant differences in pneumonia rates across patients who used thickened liquids versus a chin-down posture to reduce aspiration over a 3-month period. Thus the clinical benefits, especially long-term benefits from continued use of thickened liquids as a management strategy, are unclear. Morever, continued use of thickened liquids may impose other health risks to adult patients with dysphagia. A primary concern is the risk of dehydration from reduced fluid intake. Elderly patients, especially those with dysphagia, are considered at increased risk for dehydration secondary to reduced fluid intake.[33] Combining this potential risk with the results of surveys indicating a high rate of dislike of thickened liquids among adult patients with dysphagia suggests that reduced fluid intake, especially of thickened liquids, may further the risk of dehydration in this patient population. In one small randomized clinical trial,[34] stroke patients

with dysphagia were assigned to receive thickened liquids or thickened liquids plus water. Patients in the combination liquid condition (water plus thickened liquids) ingested less-thickened liquids and had greater daily fluid intake than those in the thickened-liquid–only condition. Neither group experienced significant respiratory complications. Related to this study are the clinical experiences of more than 20 years from the Frazier Rehabilitation Institute.[35] The Frazier Water Protocol has never been objectively evaluated, but in more than 20 years of application, this single rehabilitation hospital has allowed patients with dysphagia, including those considered to aspirate thin liquids, access to water between meals. They have experienced impressive outcomes with few instances of dehydration (5/234 or 2.1%) or chest infection (2/234 or 0.9%) among a large sample of patients ($N = 234$) who followed this protocol over an 18-month period. Despite the absence of more rigorous scientific evaluation, these long-term experiences from the Frazier Rehabilitation Institute provide a compelling argument for clinicians to consider access to water for patients with dysphagia, even those who may aspirate thin liquids. A note of caution, however—the Frazier Water Protocol is more complex that just providing water to patients with dysphagia. Clinicians are advised to review thoroughly the complete protocol before implementing this strategy.

These clinical and research examples are consistent in describing a reduced rate of aspiration as thickness of swallowed material is increased. In addition, the mode of presentation, volume, and patient fatigue may modify any clinical benefit from thickening liquids. Also important is that many of these studies are not therapeutic studies. Many are immediate effect studies that indicate a reduction of aspiration rates during the fluoroscopic swallowing examination. Thus clinicians should continually monitor patient compliance, potential benefit, and potential complications in patients in whom thickened liquids are used as a therapeutic intervention.

Additional Impact of Thickened Liquids on the Swallow Mechanism. Thickening liquids also may affect swallow physiology. For example, increasing liquid viscosity has been shown to increase lingual-palatal contact pressures during swallowing by healthy volunteers.[36] Furthermore, increasing liquid viscosity may slow the transit of a bolus[37,38] and increase pharyngeal pressure and upper esophageal sphincter relaxation.[38,39] These studies and others implicate the tendency of the healthy swallow mechanism to accommodate to different bolus characteristics—in this specific instance, liquid viscosity. However, aside from timing alterations, few studies have evaluated bolus accommodation to varying liquid viscosities in adults with dysphagia, and at least one study has suggested that increasing liquid viscosity did not affect the timing or bolus propulsive force of swallows performed by adults with neurogenic dysphagia.[40] Thus differences may exist in bolus accommodation between healthy adults and adults with dysphagia. Given the prevalence of liquid modifications in clinical management, the impact of thickening liquids on swallow physiology in adult patients seems an important area of clinical investigation.

Other Liquid Modifications

In the preceding section bolus volume, viscosity, and method of presentation were introduced as variables that may affect a patient's performance relative to aspiration of liquids during the fluoroscopic swallowing study. Another liquid variable was evaluated by Bülow et al.[41] These investigators evaluated the potential benefit of carbonated liquids in the rate of penetration/aspiration, the speed of swallowing (pharyngeal transit time), and post-swallow residue. Carbonated thin liquid resulted in less penetration into the airway than noncarbonated thin liquid, faster pharyngeal transit than thick liquid, and less residue than thick liquid. This finding is intriguing, but clinicians must remember that this is a study, like those described in the preceding section, of the immediate effect of carbonated liquids during the fluoroscopic swallowing examination and does not necessarily translate directly into a proven benefit from use of carbonation as a treatment approach.

Taste may be another bolus characteristic with the potential to affect swallowing performance. Logemann et al.[42] were among the first to evaluate the impact of taste on swallowing performance in adults with dysphagia. In a comparison of a sour bolus (50% lemon juice and 50% barium liquid) with a regular barium bolus they reported that patients with neurogenic dysphagia demonstrated faster oral onset of the swallow (all patients), decreased pharyngeal delay (stroke patients), and reduced frequency of aspiration (other neurogenic causes). Subsequently, Pelletier and Lawless[43] evaluated the impact of citric acid (a sour bolus) and citric acid plus sucrose (a sweet-sour bolus) on the swallowing performance of nursing home residents with dysphagia. They reported that the citric acid solution (2.7%) reduced aspiration and penetration compared with water and that both taste stimuli resulted in increased spontaneous dry swallows following the initial bolus swallow. Additional studies of the impact of taste stimuli on swallowing have focused on healthy volunteers. Chee et al.[44] reported that glucose (sweet), citrus (sour), and saline (salty) liquids reduced swallowing speed in healthy adults. Palmer et al.[45] compared swallows of sour liquid with water in healthy volunteers and reported that muscle contraction increased (greater **electromyographic** activity) with the sour bolus but that timing aspects of the swallow did not change across taste conditions. Finally, Pelletier and Dhanaraj[46] reported that moderate sucrose (sweet) and high citric acid (sour) and salt concentrations resulted in significantly higher lingual swallowing pressures compared with water. A different outcome is reported in a study from Miyaoka et al.[47] These investigators reported no motor changes in swallowing by healthy volunteers resulting from altering taste (sweet, salty, sour, bitter, umami).

Thickening liquids may alter the taste of the liquid. Matta et al.[48] reported that adding starch-based or gum-based thickeners to common liquids (coffee, milk, apple and orange juice) added either a starchy, grainy, or slick flavor or texture to the liquid and suppressed the base flavor of the beverage. These effects were more pronounced with thicker liquids such as honey-thick consistencies. This observation might help explain the dislike of thick liquids, especially thicker liquids, by adult patients with dysphagia.[30] At the least, such observations should encourage clinicians to consider taste and other sensory attributes when recommending thickened liquids for patients with dysphagia.

Thickening liquids is a common practice in the management of adult dysphagia. Common reasons for introduction of thicker liquids appear to revolve around clinician perceptions of the patient's ability to manage liquids orally and to protect the airway from aspiration of thin liquids. Unfortunately, little evidence exists to support this practice. Available evidence does indicate a reduction of aspiration rates in groups of patients when thin liquids are thickened to nectar or honey consistencies during the fluoroscopic swallowing study.[20,32] However, evidence also exists suggesting that thickening liquids as a management strategy does not necessarily reduce pneumonia rates.[22] Furthermore, evidence also exists that aspiration of thin liquids during the fluoroscopic swallowing study does not necessarily relate to the subsequent development of pneumonia in elderly patients with dysphagia.[49] Finally, growing experience with the Frazier Water Protocol[35] suggests that patients who aspirate thin liquids may be able to safely drink water with positive health benefit. These clinical and research observations emphasize the need for careful evaluation and continued monitoring of any patient for whom thickened liquids is recommended as a dysphagia management strategy. Clinicians should also consider other liquids modifications such as carbonation and taste variations when contemplating liquid modification as a component of dysphagia management.

Texture-Modified Diets

Similar to liquids, foods may be modified to accommodate perceived limitations in swallowing function in adults with dysphagia. Foods consumed by mouth may be modified for many reasons. Logemann[4] describes a study in which patient diet choices were examined. Patients who had been treated for oral cancer were monitored over a 6-month period. Patients tended to eliminate food consistencies that required too much time to eat or consistencies that they were prone to aspirate. These clinical observations suggest that patients will self-modify diet items that are difficult to swallow. Curran and Groher[50] described a strategy to modify a hospital's regular menu to reduce aspiration in patients with dysphagia. Similarly, O'Gara[27] and Pardoe[28] describe diet modifications intended to promote safe swallowing (minimize aspiration) and adequate nutrition. However, despite the optimism depicted in these early clinical descriptions, more recent clinical research has raised questions about the nutritional adequacy of modified diets. Wright et al.[51] reported that older hospital patients eating a texture-modified had lower nutritional intake (energy and protein) than patients consuming a normal diet. These investigators speculated further that other nutrients may also be deficient as a result of the texture-modified diet. Conversely, Germain et al.[52] reported nutritional benefit of texture-modified diets over traditional diets in institutionalized elderly patients. Although these two studies focused on different patient groups and evaluated nutritional intake over different periods, the apparent discrepancy between the results suggests that modifying diets for aspiration reduction should not be done in the absence of nutritional consultation. Thus dysphagia clinicians who recommend diet modifications should consult with nutritional specialists to ascertain the nutritional adequacy of the modified diet.

Few guidelines exist to aid dysphagia clinicians in making the recommendation for a texture-modified diet or in establishing the optimal level of diet modification. Groher and McKaig[53] evaluated swallowing abilities and the type of texture-modified diet in 212 residents in two skilled nursing facilities; 31% of these patients were using a mechanically altered diet. Based on a swallowing examination the investigators recommended changes to oral diets with patient follow-up for 30 days to evaluate response to the new diet level.

These investigators reported that 91% of patients examined had been consuming overly restrictive diets. Specifically, these patients could safely ingest diet levels higher (less modified) than they had been consuming on a regular basis; 4% of the patients were on diet levels above what they could safely tolerate, and only 5% were judged to be at the appropriate dietary level. These findings speak directly to two important program management points: (1) A qualified dysphagia clinician should be directly involved in any decision to modify an oral diet, and (2) patients should be monitored and reevaluated at regular intervals to ascertain whether they need diet modification or whether the prescribed level of diet modification remains optimal for the patient's swallowing abilities. Although this study indicates that modifying a diet level may be more complex than evaluation of airway protection, the results still do not offer clinical guidelines on selecting an appropriate modified diet level.

In an attempt to standardize menus and decision processes in the application of modified diets for adults with dysphagia, the National Dysphagia Diet was proposed in 2002.[54] The task force developing this diet suggested four standardized levels of diet modification based on assessment of food textures. These four levels are listed in Box 14-2. The task force developing these recommendations performed well in their attempt to recommend a standardized diet modification strategy. In their report they refer to the use of standard assessment tools, provide specific food recommendations for each diet level, describe foods to avoid at each level, describe food preparation approaches, and offer suggestions to enhance patient acceptance of modified diets. The task force also recommended a standard description of thickened

---

BOX 14-2 | **Four Levels in the National Dysphagia Diet**

LEVEL 1: DYSPHAGIA PUREED
Homogeneous, very cohesive, pudding-like; requires bolus control, no chewing required

LEVEL 2: DYSPHAGIA MECHANICALLY ALTERED
Cohesive, moist, semi-solid foods; requires chewing ability

LEVEL 3: DYSPHAGIA ADVANCED
Soft-solid foods that require more chewing ability

LEVEL 4: REGULAR
All foods allowed

liquids to include thin, nectar-like, honey-like, and spoon-thick. However, the efforts of this group did not include specific clinical strategies for use of thickened liquids.

Similar to the application of thickened liquids discussed previously, the National Dysphagia Diet represents a solid attempt to provide a standard approach to an important clinical problem, but it also lacks clinical research validation. To date, no significant study has compared the benefits of this standardized approach with other diet modification strategies. However, one study has raised an important question regarding the application of this standardized diet. Strowd et al.[55] reported a poor relation between dysphagia foods recommended in the National Dysphagia Diet and the barium materials used to assess patients with dysphagia. Specifically, the viscosity of barium test materials was much greater than the corresponding food recommendations in the National Dysphagia Diet. This observation questions, but does not invalidate, the apparent prescriptive value of National Dysphagia Diet recommendations. Until a high degree of correspondence is developed between the evaluation materials used to make diet recommendations and the food encompassed within those recommendations, clinicians are well advised to follow the advice of Groher and McKaig.[53] Patients receiving modified diets should be carefully monitored for acceptance and reevaluated periodically both for safety of the diet (here meaning airway protection) and nutritional adequacy. The core message is that diet modification for adults with dysphagia is not a simple adjustment. The decisions and processes inherent in diet modification demand input, cooperation, and ongoing communication from a team of qualified individuals.

One final point merits consideration. Like thickened liquids, texture-modified diets may not be pleasing or acceptable to adults with dysphagia. The National Dysphagia Diet task force acknowledged some of these issues and offered suggestions for improving acceptance. If food looks good, smells good, tastes good, and is presented at the appropriate temperature, it seems logical that patients will be more likely to eat it. The design of "altered foods" for adults with dysphagia is likely to become an important aspect of clinical science and practice. Studies evaluating food characteristics, such as particle size and other physical properties along with specific food content and other factors that may influence food quality, will likely be helpful in developing safe, nutritious, and pleasing diets for adult patients with dysphagia.[56]

CHANGING THE SWALLOW: ACTIVE THERAPY TECHNIQUES

Improving the Mechanism: Oral Motor Exercises

The concept of exercises to stretch, strengthen, or otherwise improve the basic motor properties of muscles in the speech/swallow mechanism is not new.[57] Logemann[4] indicates that if the patient is aspirating significantly, oral motor exercises may be a better strategy than directly working on swallow function. The rationale for this position is logical. If a patient is continually aspirating, swallow attempts are not maximized (and the patient experiences continued failure). Logemann terms this approach to swallow rehabilitation indirect therapy and offers three foci: (1) exercises to improve oral motor control, (2) stimulation of the swallow reflex, and (3) exercises to increase adduction of tissues at the top of the airway (airway closure). Oral motor exercises include tongue range of motion, tongue resistance, and bolus control activities. Swallow reflex stimulation is advocated via cold thermal-tactile stimulation of the faucial pillars. Airway closure activities incorporate various phonation and "pushing" activities.

Thermal-tactile stimulation to elicit a swallow response has generally fallen out of favor (see later in this chapter). However, oral motor exercises represent a frequent therapy approach used by dysphagia clinicians. In an unpublished 2007 survey, Crary and Carnaby-Mann used case problem-solving scenarios to describe therapy strategies for adult patients with dysphagia after stroke. Sixty clinicians were surveyed. Oral motor exercises were recommended for all of the cases presented and were the most frequently recommended technique for each case even though each case depicted a different swallowing problem. The results of this survey suggested that dysphagia clinicians may not be selective in applying therapy strategies to different patients and that oral motor exercises were frequently used, possibly because they posed little aspiration risk. This interpretation is speculative but does raise questions on the decision-making process used in selecting any therapy for patients with dysphagia.

Some available evidence does support the value of oral motor exercises. Lazarus et al.[58] demonstrated that tongue-pushing (resistance) exercises completed with either an Iowa Oral Performance Instrument (IOPI) or tongue blade produced strength increases in young healthy volunteers. Robbins et al.[59] reported that a systematic program of lingual resistance exercise improved lingual **isometric** and swallow pressures (e.g., strength) in a group of 10 healthy older adults. Subsequently, these investigators[60] demonstrated that a systematic program of lingual resistance exercise resulted in both increased lingual strength and swallowing ability in a group of 10 poststroke patients with dysphagia. Hagg and Anniko[61] demonstrated that a program of resistive lip training improved lip strength and swallow ability in stroke patients with dysphagia. These studies represent evidence that oral motor exercises, specifically lingual and labial resistance exercises, have the potential to strengthen weak swallowing musculature and improve swallow function. To date, little or no evidence has emerged to support other aspects of oral motor exercise. However, as described later in this chapter, exercise principles are being increasingly applied to dysphagia therapy in a variety of approaches.

PROTECTING THE AIRWAY: BREATH HOLD AND SUPRAGLOTTIC AND SUPER-SUPRAGLOTTIC SWALLOWS

The voluntary breath hold, supraglottic swallow, and super-supraglottic swallow maneuvers are techniques designed to protect the airway from aspiration of food and/or liquid by closing the airway before swallowing. In the case of the two supraglottic swallow techniques, a voluntary cough is executed after the swallow to clear any residue from the vocal folds. The difference between these two maneuvers is the degree of effort in the preswallow breath hold. As implied by the name, the *super-supraglottic swallow* requires an effortful breath hold, whereas the supraglottic swallow requires a breath hold with no extra effort. The extra effort in the super-supraglottic maneuver is needed to facilitate glottal closure. Glottal closure is one of the earliest aspects of the swallow[62]; thus techniques that facilitate glottal closure in patients who aspirate may contribute to reduced aspiration.

Endoscopic inspection has revealed that healthy adults may not completely close the glottis during a voluntary breath-hold maneuver. Estimates range from 57% to 82% of healthy volunteers who completely close the glottis with a voluntary breath hold.[63-65] Adding effort and/or vocalization to the voluntary breath-hold maneuver increases the likelihood that the glottis will be closed.[63,65,66] Figure 14-4 demonstrates the difference in glottal closure patterns between a simple breath-hold maneuver and a forced or effortful breath-hold maneuver. Figure 14-4, *A* demonstrates the glottal closure pattern associated with a simple breath-hold maneuver (e.g., voluntary breath hold or supraglottic swallow). The primary feature is the horizontal (right to left) movement of the arytenoid cartilages and vocal folds to close the airway. When complete, this pattern may be effective in accomplishing airway protection during swallowing attempts. Adding effort to the breath-hold maneuver increases the probability of complete glottal closure. Figure 14-4, *B* demonstrates the glottal closure pattern associated with a forceful breath-hold maneuver (e.g., super-supraglottic swallow). Note that in addition to the horizontal closure pattern observed in the supraglottic swallow, the arytenoids move anteriorly approximating the petiole of the epiglottis. This

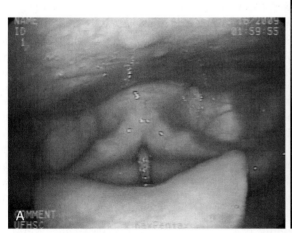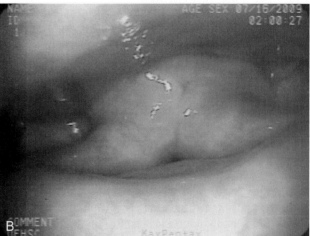

FIGURE 14-4. Laryngeal configurations associated with normal breath hold (**A**) and effortful breath hold (**B**).

movement results in more complete closure of the entire supraglottis rather than closure at the level of the vocal folds only. Of interest is the observation that these two glottal closure patterns (horizontal and anterior) reflect stages in glottal closure in the normal swallow. As demonstrated in Video 14-5, slow-motion analysis of the normal swallow reveals that the glottis is initially closed by the horizontal (medial) movement of the vocal folds. Subsequently, with laryngeal elevation the arytenoid cartilages move forward to approximately the petiole of the epiglottis. Magnetic resonance imaging has demonstrated that complete closure of the larynx is obtained at the point of maximum laryngeal elevation in the normal swallow.[67] These closure patterns are reflected respectively in the voluntary breath-hold, supraglottic, and super-supraglottic swallow maneuvers.

The physiologic effects of the supraglottic swallow maneuver have been assessed in both normal and dysphagic adults. Different studies report varied findings ranging from no difference between the supraglottic swallow and a control (normal) swallow to prolonged airway closure, increased anterior laryngeal movement, increased tongue base movement, and increased PES opening. In a study of eight healthy volunteers Bülow et al.[16] reported no movement or manometric pressure difference between the supraglottic swallow and normal swallows. These investigators noted that healthy volunteers varied in their ability to perform the supraglottic swallow and suggested that substantial training of this technique may be required for patients to perform this maneuver appropriately. This same clinical research team also reported no manometric alterations in peak amplitude or duration of intrabolus pressure[15] or number of misdirected swallows[14] among eight patients who used the supraglottic swallow. Furthermore, they noted that three of eight patients could not perform this technique. Bodén, Hallgren, and Hedström[68] reported a weaker peak contraction in the upper esophageal sphincter (also termed the PES) when healthy volunteers swallowed using the supraglottic swallow. These authors claimed that this decreased peak pressure is unlikely to improve swallow efficiency or decrease aspiration in patients with dysphagia. On the more positive side, Ohmae et al.[69] reported earlier and longer laryngeal closure, prolonged opening of the PES, and longer duration of hyoid and laryngeal movement in healthy volunteers who attempted the supraglottic and super-supraglottic swallow maneuvers. These observations were more pronounced in the super-supraglottic technique. Other research also supports increased physiologic effects of the super-supraglottic swallow

over the supraglottic swallow. For example, Miller and Watkin[70] reported longer duration of pharyngeal wall movement in healthy volunteers who swallowed with the super-supraglottic swallow technique. This finding implicates a longer swallow duration when this technique is used. This implication is supported by data from Bodén et al.,[68] who reported longer bolus transit time in healthy volunteers who performed the super-supraglottic swallow technique compared with normal or supraglottic swallows. These changes might be considered detrimental to some patients with dysphagia by increasing the duration of the swallow and post-swallow residue in patients with existing poor PES relaxation. However, the super-supraglottic swallow also has been reported to result in positive swallow changes in some patient groups. Lazarus et al.[71] reported longer base-of-tongue contact with the posterior pharyngeal wall in combination with higher manometric pressures at this contact point in three patients with dysphagia after treatment for head/neck cancer. Logemann et al.[72] reported earlier base-of-tongue movement, a higher position of the hyoid bone at swallow onset, and overall increased hyoid movement during swallowing in five patients with head/neck cancer after radiotherapy who used the super-supraglottic swallow. These same patients also demonstrated reduced maximum opening of the PES but little change in pharyngeal wall movement as a result of the maneuver.

Despite multiple studies evaluating the physiologic effect of these airway protection maneuvers on the swallow, few studies have documented clinical benefit. Hamlet et al.[73] identified reduced aspiration in a single patient who used this technique after supraglottic laryngectomy. However, the patient reported very prolonged mealtimes with this technique and thus modified the technique to reduce mealtimes. Lazarus et al.[74] reported that the supraglottic and super-supraglottic maneuvers prolonged airway closure but did not eliminate aspiration in a single patient after surgical treatment for head/neck cancer. The Mendelsohn maneuver (see next section), however, was successful for this patient. This case report emphasizes the importance of verifying the clinical impact of any maneuver before using it as a therapeutic technique. Lazarus[75] reported 100% elimination of aspiration using the super-supraglottic swallow during the fluoroscopic swallow examination in four patients who were within 6 months of completing radiotherapy intervention for head/neck cancer. However, she indicated that three of the four patients required multiple swallows per liquid bolus even with use of this swallow maneuver.

One of the few (if only) studies to evaluate these airway protection maneuvers on stroke patients reached a negative conclusion based on patient safety concerns. Chaudhuri et al.[76] evaluated the cardiovascular effects of the supraglottic and super-supraglottic swallow maneuver in stroke patients with dysphagia. Three groups of patients were evaluated during the poststroke period of inpatient rehabilitation. Group 1 included patients with dysphagia and a history of coronary artery disease. Group 2 patients had dysphagia but did not have a history of coronary artery disease. Group 3 patients were considered a control group and were selected from among orthopedic patients without dysphagia or a history of coronary artery disease. In all patients more than 1 week had passed since their stroke. All patients received training on the supraglottic and super-supraglottic swallow maneuvers and subsequently used these maneuvers in a dysphagia treatment session. Cardiac findings were monitored by a **Holter monitor** during treatment sessions and during subsequent routine daily activities. Results indicated cardiovascular abnormalities in 82% (9 of 11) of patients in group 1 and in 100% (4 of 4) of patients in group 2 during training/treatment sessions in which these airway protection maneuvers were used. No obvious cardiac differences were noted between the maneuvers. The authors attribute these cardiovascular changes to a modification of the Valsalva maneuver that occurs with physical exertion. They concluded that these maneuvers should not be used in stroke patients with dysphagia especially if they have a history of cardiac arrhythmia or coronary artery disease. These results raise many important questions regarding application of these maneuvers or, for that matter, any maneuver that might affect bodily functions beyond the swallow. Like all studies, questions may be raised about this research, but until additional research confirms or refutes the findings of the Chaudhuri study, clinicians should be cautious when applying these maneuvers in the acute stroke population.

Both variants of the supraglottic swallow maneuver appear to prolong airway closure and may have other physiologic effects on swallow performance. However, the available data on clinical benefit are restricted to small groups of patients; mostly those with dysphagia after treatment for head/neck cancer. An important study of clinical impact in stroke patients suggests that patients in acute stroke rehabilitation may be at risk for cardiovascular events from these maneuvers. These implications and suggestions that these techniques might require substantial clinical training warrant a focused look at potential clinical benefits compared with potential risks from these techniques.

These maneuvers would be considered compensatory in that they may contribute to improved swallowing function when applied correctly. Although, short-term physiologic change has been documented using these maneuvers, evidence of a lasting positive impact on swallowing once the maneuver is no longer applied (rehabilitative function) is limited.

Prolonging the Swallow: The Mendelsohn Maneuver

The *Mendelsohn maneuver* is achieved by asking the patient to suspend the swallow at the peak of hyolaryngeal excursion and pharyngeal constriction and to prolong this posture for a few seconds before relaxing and allowing the swallowing tract to return to the preswallow position. The result of this maneuver is to prolong and extend hyolaryngeal excursion.[77] Figure 14-5 presents a lateral fluoroscopic view of a swallow with the patient in the resting position and during the elevated and constricted position of the Mendelsohn maneuver. Video 14-6 depicts this maneuver performed by a healthy adult volunteer. Some investigators have suggested that, in addition to prolonged hyolaryngeal excursion, this maneuver also prolongs PES opening[77]; however, this is not a consistent finding across studies of normal swallowing.[78] Other physiologic changes in the normal swallow facilitated by this maneuver include (1) longer duration of lateral pharyngeal wall movement[70]; (2) increased pharyngeal peak contractions along with prolonged duration of pharyngeal peak contraction and increased bolus transit time[68]; and (3) increased amplitude and duration of surface electromyographic (sEMG) signals (increased effort and duration), especially in the submental muscle group (Clinical Corner 14-1).[79] Physiologic swallow changes in a small group ($N = 3$) of head/neck cancer patients include increased duration of base-of-tongue and posterior pharyngeal wall contact and increased pressure of this contact.[71]

This maneuver has been used extensively as a therapy technique and may serve both compensatory and rehabilitative functions. The compensatory function is indicated in studies that report reduced postswallow residue and/or aspiration with this maneuver.[71,74] The rehabilitative function is indicated in the studies that report improved swallowing function after use of this technique and without dependence on the technique. For example, Lazarus et al.[74] reported improved swallow timing coordination in a single patient who used this maneuver. Neumann et al.[80] reported successful therapy outcome (defined as total oral feeding) in two thirds of 58 tube-fed patients with neurologic defect as the primary cause for dysphagia. Nearly half of these patients used the

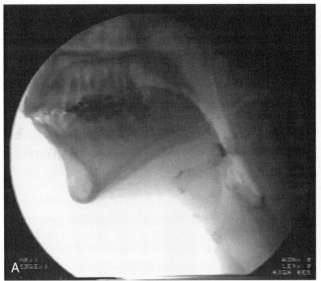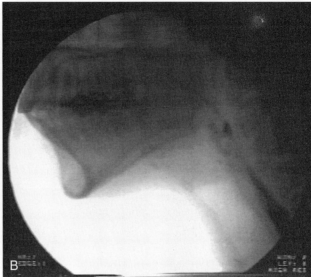

FIGURE 14-5. Pharyngolaryngeal configuration at rest (**A**) and with Mendelsohn maneuver (**B**).

CLINICAL CORNER 14-1

Whenever a clinician uses a therapy technique or approach, it is important to understand the expected physiologic and/or functional changes from that approach. In addition, a plan should be in place to address any "adverse events" that might arise from dysphagia therapy. Several years ago, I evaluated a patient with dysphagia after radiotherapy treatment for head/neck cancer. During the initial videofluoroscopic swallow evaluation, I instructed the patient in the use of a Mendelsohn maneuver and decided that this technique might be result in increased safe oral technique for this patient. Because this technique is difficult to monitor both for the patient and the clinician (and thus often difficult to learn), I decided to use adjunctive sEMG biofeedback to teach the technique to the patient and to monitor his performance. The patient did well during the first few days of therapy. By the end of the first week (5 sessions) he arrived with a fever and chest congestion. He was advised to check with his local physician immediately. The physician evaluated and admitted the patient for treatment of pneumonia. After a 10-day hospitalization and subsequent recuperation period this patient again requested therapy.

CRITICAL THINKING

1. What are the possible mechanisms that might have resulted in pneumonia in this patient?
2. What factors would you consider in deciding to restart therapy for this patient?

AND NOW ... THE REST OF THE STORY

After much discussion with the patient, his physician, and his family, we again enrolled this patient in swallow therapy. He used the same techniques as before the pneumonia episode. (Refer to Video sequence 6-9, *A-D*, to see his progress in learning the Mendelsohn maneuver. Note specifically the inconsistency in application of the maneuver.) This case teaches us that we have to fade the abnormal maneuvers used to rehabilitate swallowing as part of the therapy plan. In the end, this patient did very well. He returned to a total oral diet and lived an additional 5 years with no dysphagia-related health complications before he died of recurrent cancer.

Mendelsohn maneuver during therapy. Crary[81] used a technique termed *sustained pharyngeal contraction* (similar to the Mendelsohn maneuver) in an intensive therapy program with six tube-dependent brainstem stroke patients. This technique was taught to patients with the assistance of sEMG biofeedback. After an average of 3 weeks of daily treatment, 5 of the 6 patients with chronic, severe dysphagia returned to total oral feeding without complications. Changes in swallow physiology reflected improved coordination and effort during swallow attempts. In a follow-up paper, Crary et al.[82] reported increased safe oral intake in 87% of 45 patients with chronic dysphagia in an average of 10 therapy sessions. Huckabee and

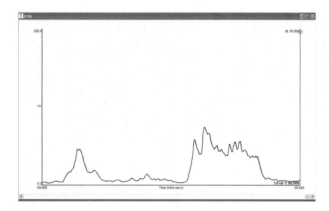

FIGURE 14-6. sEMG trace depicting a "normal" swallow *(left)* and a swallow using the Mendelsohn maneuver *(right)*.

Cannito[83] also reported significant improvement in swallowing function over 10 therapy sessions within a single week. These investigators used the Mendelsohn maneuver as part of their treatment regimen.

In general, positive outcomes in swallow function have been reported after use of the Mendelsohn maneuver in dysphagia therapy, (Refer to Video series 6-9, *B-D*, for an example of patient performance on this maneuver over time.) However, one clinical concern about this technique is that it can be difficult to teach patients to complete the maneuver. For example, in the study by Ding et al.,[79] healthy adult volunteers required between one and nine practice trials to adequately learn the Mendelsohn maneuver. Some clinical investigators have reported successful use of adjunctive biofeedback, primarily sEMG, to address the difficulty learning the Mendelsohn maneuver.[81-83] This adjunctive modality provides patients with immediate physiologic information on muscle activity during attempts at the maneuver. Figure 14-6 depicts a trace of sEMG activity from a normal swallow (left side or first event) compared with a swallow using the Mendelsohn maneuver (right side or second event). The different configurations are obvious and hence use of sEMG biofeedback may facilitate enhanced learning of this swallowing maneuver (see description later in this chapter). Another clinical concern with this maneuver is that, if done correctly, the prolongation of the swallow increases the apneic phase of the swallow. This prolonged cessation of respiration may be contraindicated in patients with respiratory disease or severe incoordination between swallowing activity and respiration.

Increasing Force: The Effortful Swallow

The *effortful swallow* technique, sometimes referred to as the *hard swallow* or the *forceful swallow*, represents a volitional attempt by the patient to increase the force applied to the bolus from structures within the swallowing mechanism. Pouderoux and Kahrilas[36] demonstrated a fourfold increase in tongue propulsive force in forceful swallows of healthy volunteers. Asking patients to "swallow harder" may induce several physiologic changes compared with a "normal" swallow. Bülow et al.[16] reported reduced hyoid/laryngeal-mandibular distances (hyoid and laryngeal elevation) before an effortful swallow completed by healthy volunteers ("swallow very hard while squeezing the tongue in an upward-backward motion toward the soft palate"). As a result of this preswallow posture, less hyoid and laryngeal elevation occurred during the effortful swallows. No pharyngeal pressure increases were observerd via manometry during effortful swallows produced by these healthy volunteers. Conversely, Hind et al.[84] reported that during effortful swallows healthy volunteers demonstrated increased elevation of the hyoid bone. These investigators also reported increased lingual pressures (pressure of tongue against hard palate during swallows) and increased swallow durations, including duration of hyoid excursion, duration of laryngeal closure, and duration of PES opening. Pressure increases combined with prolonged airway closure suggest that the effortful swallow technique may help certain patients clear a bolus through the swallow mechanism while reducing the risk of airway compromise via penetration or aspiration. Huckabee and colleagues[85-89] have completed a series of interesting investigations on the effortful swallow technique performed by healthy volunteers that expand the initial results of Pouderoux and Kahrilas[36] and Hind et al.[84] In the initial study,[85] this group reported greater pharyngeal pressures and lower PES pressures (more relaxation) during effortful swallows completed by healthy volunteers. In addition, sEMG amplitudes were higher with effortful swallows, implying greater overall effort during these swallow attempts. Hiss and Huckabee[86] compared the timing of pharyngeal and PES pressure onsets across effortful versus normal swallows. Their results indicated delayed onset of effortful swallows (delayed increase in pharyneal pressures or relaxation in PES) combined with an overall increased duration of these swallows. These results suggest that the effortful swallow technique may be contraindicated in patients with delayed onset of the pharyngeal component of the swallow, but it may help with pharyngeal clearance via increased pharyngeal pressures and greater PES relaxation. These initial results were further examined in a follow-up study by Witte et al.[89] These investigators evaluated the impact of a bolus (saliva versus 10 mL of water) on effortful versus normal swallows. In general, saliva swallows produced higher upper pharyngeal pressures during both types of swallows, but PES relaxation was greater for effortful swallows of saliva compared with water. Together, these two studies implicate a positive effect of the effortful swallow on PES relaxation—an effect that may be enhanced during saliva swallows.

In a pair of related reports Huckabee and Steele[87,88] evaluated the influence of orolingual pressure on amplitude and timing of pharyngeal pressures during normal and effortful swallows performed by healthy volunteers. These investigators reported that providing instructions that emphasize increased tongue-palate pressure during effortful swallows ("push hard with your tongue" versus "do not use your tongue to increase swallow force") resulted in increased sEMG amplitudes, tongue-palate pressures, and pharyngeal pressures. Conversely, only minimal timing differences were observed as a result of the effortful swallow with emphasis on tongue-palate pressure. These investigations support prior results and interpretations that the effortful swallow technique may be beneficial in facilitating pharyngeal bolus clearance in certain patients with oropharyngeal dysphagia.

One final study should be mentioned in reference to the physiologic impact of the effortful swallow in healthy volunteers. Lever et al.[90] reported increased peristaltic amplitudes in the distal, but not the proximal, esophagus during effortful swallows. In addition, lower esophageal sphincter (LES) residual pressure was lower for females but not males with the effortful swallow technique. Although the results are preliminary, this study has implications for pharyngoesophageal interactions including potential behavioral therapy strategies for patients who have reduced distal esophageal motility.

As reflected in the preceding paragraphs, the majority of investigations on the physiologic impact of the effortful swallow technique have been conducted with healthy adults, mostly young healthy adults. It is appropriate to make inferences on clinical applications from such investigations, but direct extension to performance in patients with dysphagia is considered overinterpretation. Thus it is important to study both the physiologic impact and treatment outcomes of this technique (or for that matter, any technique) in patients with dysphagia.

A presumption based on studies of healthy volunteers is that the effortful swallow technique increases movement and pharyngeal pressures during swallows. Potential benefits of these **kinematic** and physiologic changes are improved airway protection and less postswallow residue. However, few reports have addressed the physiologic impact of this "maneuver"

on swallowing in adults with dysphagia or documented the impact of this technique on swallowing change after therapy. In patients with pharyngeal dysfunction the effortful swallow reportedly had no impact on the number of misdirected swallows (frequencey of penetration or aspiration) or degree of pharyngeal residue, but it did reduce the depth of penetration of swallowed material into the larynx and trachea.[14] These same authors reported that four of the eight patients in this study had difficulty performing the technique, likely because of lingual weakness (though this was not studied directly in this study). In a separate study, this group of investigators examined manometric intrabolus pressure (defined as the manometric pressure when the pressure sensor was completely within the bolus) at the inferior pharyngeal constrictor in eight patients with pharyngeal dysphagia.[15] Results indicated no alteration in either peak pressure or duration of intrabolus pressure with use of the effortful swallow technique. Conversely, Lazarus et al.[71] reported increased swallow pressure (base of tongue to posterior pharyngeal wall) and increased duration of contact (base of tongue to posterior pharyngeal wall) in three patients with dysphagia secondary to treatment for head/neck cancer. These discrepant reports may result from a focus on different points in the swallow mechanism (upper pharynx versus lower pharynx) or from different causes contributing to dysphagia (six stroke patients and two patients with head/neckcancer versus three patients with head/neck cancer). Additionally, the variability noted across patients may exaggerate the findings from any small sample study of patient groups (Clinical Corner 14-2).

Treatment outcomes from use of the effortful swallow technique are more difficult to identify. Some clinical investigators have used the effortful swallow as part of a treatment program and thus the results from these treatment studies are not focused on the effortful swallow technique. Crary[81] used sEMG biofeedback to teach patients to swallow "harder and longer" during therapy. Five of six patients demonstrated dramatic functional improvement (feeding tube removal) and physiologic improvement in swallowing after therapy. Physiologic change in swallowing included increased amplitude and duration of the sEMG signal measured during bolus swallows. These changes mirror those reported in healthy volunteers who use this technique. Carnaby-Mann and Crary[91] reported significant clinical improvement and enhanced laryngeal elevation in five patients who completed a 3-week course of therapy using a technique that instructed them to swallow hard and fast for each bolus. These two studies suggest that the

CLINICAL CORNER 14-2

Lazarus et al.[71] reported on the effects of four voluntary swallowing maneuvers (effortful swallow, supra-superglottic swallow, Mendelsohn maneuver, and tongue-hold maneuver) in three patients who had been treated for head/neck cancer with various medical/surgical interventions. Their results suggest that all maneuvers increased both the duration and pressure of the base of tongue to posterior pharyngeal wall contact. They also reported less upper pharyngeal residue when using each maneuver. Their results are descriptive with no analytic statistical comparison.

CRITICAL THINKING

1. What is the benefit of small sample-size research in understanding the value of clinical techniques?
2. What are some limitations that must be considered when small samples are used to study clinical techniques?
3. How should clinical practitioners interpret/use this information?

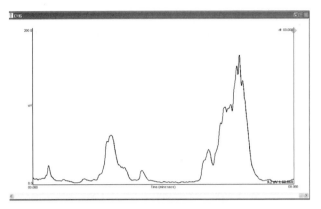

FIGURE 14-7. sEMG trace depicting a "normal" swallow *(left)* and an effortful swallow *(right)*.

effortful swallow technique may produce positive clinical and physiologic change in patients with dysphagia. Still, no study has examined this technique thoroughly from a clinical point of view.

The effortful swallow technique may facilitate improved swallowing by increasing force applied to the bolus and extending the duration of the swallow. Outcomes may include stronger and more coordinated swallows but this clinical effect requires more investigation. Available literature suggests that the nature of instructions given to the patient and the type and amount of material swallowed may have an impact on the immediate effect and the treatment outcome of this technique. Another variable to consider is the ability of the patient and the clincian to monitor the swallow performance using this technique. As mentioned for the Mendelsohn maneuver, sEMG biofeedback may be a valuable asset to help the patient use the technique effectively and to provide the clinician with immediate information on the patient's performance. Figure 14-7 depicts a normal dry swallow (right side of image) compared with an effortful dry swallow (left side of image). Like the Mendelsohn maneuver, the differences are obvious to even the untrained eye. Thus the visual display of sEMG biofeedback may be an important adjunct in teaching patients the proper application of this clini-

cal technique. More information on this modality is presented later in this chapter.

The therapy strategies just reviewed are considered more "traditional" strategies. Liquid and diet modifications, along with postural adjustments and swallow maneuvers. represent the large majority of dysphagia interventions used for several years. Table 14-2 summarizes the primary postural adjustments and swallow maneuvers with a brief description of how they are performed, their intended effects, the expected physiologic changes, and anticipated functional outcomes for each technique. Note that each postural adjustment and swallowing maneuver represents a form of "abnormal" swallowing. Thus, except in extreme situations, patients are not expected to use these swallowing interventions for long periods. Clinicians should view these techniques as either short-term compensations or as techniques used to change and hopefully improve an impaired swallow mechanism.

Additional Techniques to Change the Swallow

Multiple Swallows as a Therapy Technique

At one time or another most individuals engage in multiple swallows to clear a single bolus. Similarly, clinicians often ask patients with dysphagia to "swallow again." Presumably this strategy is used to clear residue from the initial swallow. However, little evidence exists to either support or refute the application of multiple swallows as a therapy strategy. Multiple swallows are frequently seen in adults with dysphagia[92-94] and may be more frequent in healthy adults with increasing age.[95] Also, multiple swallows may be elicited by texture[93,94] or taste[43] in both healthy adults and in adult patients with dysphagia.

No data are available to evaluate the effectiveness of a multiple-swallow strategy as a therapy technique.

TABLE 14-2

Summary of Behavioral Swallowing Maneuvers Commonly Used in Dysphagia Therapy

Technique	Performance	Intent	Physiology	Outcomes
Side-lying	Lie down with stronger side lower	Slows bolus Provides time to adjust and protect airway	Emphasizes pharyngeal contraction	Less aspiration
Chin-up	Elevate chin	Propel bolus to back of mouth	Widens oropharynx Increases PES pressure	Better oral transport
Chin-down	Lower chin	Improves airway protection	Narrow oropharynx	Reduced aspiration
Head-turn	Turn head to right or left	Reduces post-swallow residue and aspiration	Redirects bolus to stronger side of pharynx Lowers PES pressure	Increased amount swallowed Less residue and lower risk of aspiration
Supraglottic swallow	Hold breath ... swallow ... gentle cough ...	Reduces aspiration by increasing glottal closure	Horizontal glottal closure Increased movement of swallowing structures	Reduced aspiration Increased laryngeal excursion
Super-supraglottic swallow	Hold breath ... bear down ... swallow ... gentle cough ...	Reduces aspiration by increasing glottal closure	Horizontal and anteroposterior glottal closure Increased movement of swallowing structures	Reduced aspiration Increased laryngeal excursion
Mendelsohn maneuver	Squeeze swallow at apex	Improves swallowing coordination	Increased and prolonged hyolaryngeal excursion	Improved swallowing coordination Less post-swallow residue Less aspiration
Effortful swallow	Swallow harder	Increases lingual force on bolus	Increased tongue-palate pressures Increased duration of swallow Increased tongue base movement	Less residue

A common rationale for use of multiple swallows may be to clear residue from various points within the swallow mechanism after the initial bolus swallow. However, application of a multiple-swallow strategy, specifically excessive use of multiple swallows (either for a single bolus or after each bolus) may create a degree of inefficiency in a patient's functional eating ability. Logic dictates that using multiple swallows per bolus increases mealtime and thus may contribute to reduced oral intake. Also, excessive use of multiple swallows during functional eating may induce patient fatigue with negative consequences on oral intake or airway protection. Given the absence of objective data on the benefit or risk of a multiple-swallow strategy in dysphagia therapy, clinicians should take steps to evaluate the impact of this strategy on individual patients.

The Tongue-Hold Maneuver

The posterior pharyngeal wall has a tendency to "bulge" forward during swallowing, contacting the tongue base and thus creating a pressure source to help push the bolus through the pharynx. When the tongue base is not able to move posteriorly toward the pharyngeal wall, and if the pharyngeal wall is physiologically capable, it may increase the degree of anterior "bulge" in a presumed attempt to compensate for the reduction in tongue base–pharyngeal wall contact. This effect is demonstrated in Video 14-7. The patient in this video sustained neck trauma from a vehicle accident that increased the distance from the base of the tongue to the posterior wall. On swallowing, the posterior pharyngeal wall moves aggressively forward—presumably to increase contact with the base of tongue resulting in a functional swallow. The initial clinical observations of the tongue-hold maneuver were from a group of patients with oral cancer who demonstrated surgical anchoring of the anterior tongue, thereby limiting posterior tongue movement.[96] These individuals demonstrated anterior bulging of the posterior pharyngeal wall. Subsequently, healthy young adults were asked to perform

CLINICAL CORNER 14-3

Multiple Swallows

A common practice technique is to ask a patient to swallow again. Often this strategy is accompanied by the request to "swallow hard." During fluoroscopic or endoscopic swallow examinations this request is typically triggered by the observation of post-swallow residue. During therapy this request is typically triggered by clinical signs that the patient has post-swallow residue—often voice changes, throat clearing, or a cough. Despite these common practices the use of multiple swallows may introduce a degree of "inefficiency" into functional swallowing. As reviewed in this chapter, little evidence exists to either support or refute the use of multiple swallows as a therapy technique. This raises questions about the application of this strategy.

CRITICAL THINKING

1. What would be considered benefits from the application of a multiple-swallow technique in dysphagia therapy?
2. What difficulties or "inefficiencies" might be encountered by asking a patient to use a multiple-swallow strategy during functional eating?
3. What strategies might a clinician use during assessment or therapy in an attempt to decide whether a multiple-swallow strategy might help a patient?

Practice Note 14-3

THE TONGUE-HOLD MANEUVER AND EXERCISE

In discussing the potential benefits and risks to patients from application of the tongue-hold maneuver, clinicians often respond that they use this maneuver as a swallow exercise without a bolus. The problem with this point of view is that no data exist supporting potential exercise-related benefits of the tongue-hold maneuver. Clinicians have indicated that they feel the muscles working harder when patients swallow with the tongue-hold maneuver. Unfortunately, this feeling does not equate to acceptable exercise, and data such as those reported by Doeltgen et al.[99] seem to indicate a reduction in pharyngeal motor performance resulting from the tongue-hold maneuver. Thus the author's impression is that the tongue-hold maneuver may be a helpful technique, but currently there are no systematic data that support its clinical or physiologic benefit to adult patients with dysphagia.

---

a maneuver that attempted to mimic the anterior anchoring of the tongue.[97] These healthy subjects held the anterior tongue (slightly posterior to the tongue tip) between the teeth while swallowing. Fluoroscopic inspection indicated that with this swallow maneuver, healthy adults demonstrate an increased anterior bulging of the posterior pharyngeal wall.

Swallowing with this anterior tongue-hold maneuver does appear to contribute to increased anterior movement of the posterior pharyngeal wall during swallowing; however, at least three negative consequences of this maneuver during swallowing have been identified: (1) reduced duration of airway closure, (2) increased post-swallow residue, and (3) increase delay in the initiation of the pharyngeal component of the swallow.[98] In some patients each of these, alone or in combination, could contribute to an increased possibility of airway compromise (penetration or aspiration). This observation necessitates a cautionary

note for this maneuver; the Masako or tongue-hold maneuver should not be used with a bolus. Furthermore, no evidence currently exists supporting the clinical benefits of this swallow maneuver.

Physiologic swallow changes resulting from the tongue-hold maneuver are poorly studied. In a small sample of three patients with dysphagia secondary to treatment for head/neck cancer, Lazarus et al.[71] reported that the tongue-hold maneuver increased both the duration and pressure of tongue base–pharyngeal wall contact compared with swallowing with no maneuver. The tongue-hold maneuver also reportedly reduced post-swallow residue in these same patients. This observation is in direct contrast to those offered by Fujiu-Kurachi,[98] who identified increased postswallow residue. Although little relevant research on the tongue-hold maneuver has been conducted in patients with dysphagia, recent work has evaluated manometric changes associated with this maneuver in healthy adult volunteers. Doeltgen et al.[99] reported that swallows performed by 40 healthy young adults resulted in lower pharyngeal contraction pressures, shorter pharyngeal pressure durations, but greater relaxation in the upper esophageal sphincter than control swallows. These findings in part support the clinical observations of Fujiu-Kurachi.[98] Reduced pharyngeal pressures may contribute to increased postswallow residue.

The tongue-hold maneuver may have clinical application when an increased anterior bulging of the posterior pharyngeal wall at the level of the tongue base is desired. However, the type of patient, specific dysphagia characteristics, and specific anticipated outcomes need to be further detailed in reference to this technique. Without further study and clarification of effect and functional benefit, the tongue-hold manuever remains an unknown and potentially risky technique for use in dysphagia therapy.

The Head-Lift Exercise

The head-lift exercise, sometimes referred to as the *Shaker technique*, is an activity intended to improve opening of the PES by increasing the "strength" of muscle groups that contribute to PES opening. During swallowing, the suprahyoid (and other) muscle groups help the hyolaryngeal complex to move up and forward, exerting an upward and anterior pull on the PES. This is an important physiologic component of PES opening. Strengthening of weakened suprahyoid muscle groups would be expected to have a positive impact on PES opening via these mechanisms. The head-lift technique is intended to strengthen these muscles by having the patient lie supine and raise the head (but not the shoulders) sufficiently to see the toes. This head posture is maintained for a defined period and repeated on a prescribed schedule.[100] Briefly, patients are asked to lie in the supine position and complete three head lifts sustained for 1 minute each. A 1-minute rest period occurs between each sustained head lift. Immediately following the sustained head lifts, patients are asked to complete 30 consecutive head lifts without sustaining the lifted position. This series of head-lift exercises is completed 3 times each day for a period of 6 weeks. Contraindications for this activity may include cervical spine deficits, reduced movement capability of the neck (as in some patients with head and neck cancer), or cognitive limitations or other factors that might contribute to poor compliance with the prescribed routine.

Numerous studies have evaluated the clinical benefit and the physiologic bases of the head-lift technique. Shaker et al.[100] demonstrated increased anterior laryngeal excursion and upper esophageal sphincter opening during swallowing in a group of healthy elderly subjects who completed this exercise. Similar physiologic changes in swallowing were not observed in a group of adults performing a sham exercise. A follow-up study evaluated both physiologic and clinical changes resulting from the head-lift exercise in a group of adult patients who required tube feedings because of an abnormal upper esophageal sphincter opening.[101] After the head-lift exercise program,

patients demonstrated improved anterior laryngeal excursion, improved upper esophageal sphincter opening, and less post-swallow aspiration.

The main premise of the clinical improvements observed after the head-lift exercise is that this exercise program strengthens the suprahyoid muscles. Two small studies on this technique reported that both the suprahyoid and infrahyoid muscle groups fatigued after the head-lift exercise.[102,103] Muscle fatigue is accepted as evidence for muscle activity or exercise. Another study reported enhanced thyrohyoid shortening (less distance between the hyoid bone and thyroid cartilage) after the head-lift exercise.[104] Collectively, these results are interpreted as evidence that the head-lift exercise strengthens muscles that aid in opening of the upper esophageal sphincter by elevation and anterior excursion of the hyolaryngeal complex. The primary muscles considered responsible for this action are the suprahyoid muscles. The primary measurement techniques have been biokinematic measures from videofluoroscopy or physiologic measures from sEMG. A related study by Yoshida et al.[105] compared submental (suprahyoid) muscle activity measured with sEMG between the head-lift and the tongue-press (tongue pushed against hard palate) exercises. These investigators reported no differences in the amplitude of sEMG signals obtained between the two exercises from a group of 53 healthy young adults. In fact, in the sustained posture condition, submental sEMG activity was higher during the tongue-press exercise. These investigators suggested that perhaps the tongue-press activity may accomplish similar physiologic goals as the head-lift exercise but with fewer physical demands on patients.

The physical demands of the head-lift exercise should not be underestimated, especially in older or weaker patients with dysphagia. In a single study evaluating compliance with the demands of the head-lift exercise,[106] 26 older adults without dysphagia participated in the head-lift exercise as prescribed. Only 50% of these adults completed the **isokinetic** (repetitive lifts) portion of the exercise program, and 70% completed the **isometric** (sustained lift) portion. Most who withdrew from this exercise program did so within the first 2 weeks. These findings implicate the importance of compliance monitoring whenever the head-lift exercise program is used as a dysphagia therapy technique.

Thermal-Tactile Application

This therapy technique is perhaps one of the "grandparents" of dysphagia therapy. It has been used for years and has been revised and revisited in many treatment-related and swallow physiology studies.

Logemann[4] is credited with introducing this technique in her 1983 text as a technique to stimulate the swallow reflex. Her suggestion to stroke the anterior faucial pillar with a cold stimulus (#00 or #0 laryngeal mirror) is believed to originate from the work of Pommerenke,[107] who identified the anterior faucial pillars as one of the more sensitive oral areas for initiating the swallow reflex. The primary outcome measure of success for this technique is a reduction in the delay in the initiation of swallowing, primarily the pharyngeal phase. By logical reasoning then, this technique may be suitable for those patients who demonstrate delayed initiation of the pharyngeal aspect of swallowing. Lazzara et al.[108] reported faster pharyngeal and total transit times for swallows after thermal stimulation in patients with dysphagia from neurologic deficit. The change in swallow response time was evaluated fluoroscopically for single swallows. They concluded that their results support the position that thermal stimulation to the anterior faucial pillars triggers the swallow response. Rosenbek et al.[109] evaluated this technique (which they termed *thermal application*) as a therapy technique in seven adult patients with dysphagia after at least two strokes. Subjects received thermal application therapy daily for 1-week periods alternating with no treatment periods of a week. A total of 2 weeks of thermal application therapy was provided to each patient within this alternating treatment design. Despite an immediate effect of thermal application during the baseline fluoroscopic swallowing evaluation, these investigators did not find strong support for a therapy effect from this proposed intervention. Furthermore, aspiration and penetration were not improved as a result of thermal application, and any short-term therapy effects were not maintained at 1 month after therapy. In a follow-up study, Rosenbek et al.[110] reported that thermal application reduced the duration of stage transition in stroke patients with dysphagia. *Duration of stage transition* (DST) is the time interval between the arrival of the bolus at the posterior edge of the ramus of the mandible and the initiation of hyoid bone elevation. Smaller DST values represent less delay in the initiation of the pharyngeal component of the swallow. Thus, similar to the studies by Lazzara et al.[108] and earlier by Rosenbek et al.,[109] this study supports the presence of an immediate effect of cold application to the anterior faucial pillars—a reduction in the delay of the pharyngeal response during the swallow. Finally, Rosenbek and a large group of investigators[111] evaluated the intensity of treatment on the results of thermal application (which they now termed *tactile-thermal application*). Patients received 2 weeks of tactile-thermal application therapy and were ran-

domly assigned to 150, 300, 450, or 600 trials per week. A trial included three or more strokes of both faucial pillars with an ice stick (similar to a popsicle). This investigative team reported that no frequency of treatment was superior to any other. Furthermore, the higher intensity treatments (450 and 600 trials) were not fully completed during therapy (less than the target number of trials). Finally, changes in swallow timing and airway protection (penetration/aspiration) were observed but these were not consistent across different boluses evaluated in this study.

Studies of thermal stimulation in healthy adult volunteers have produced even more variable results than those in adult patients with dysphagia. Kaatzke-McDonald et al.[112] evaluated cold and taste (sugar versus salt) on swallow latency in healthy adult women. They reported that only the cold stimulus resulted in a reduction in swallow latency. Conversely, Sciortino et al.[113] reported that only the combination of mechanical, cold, and gustatory (sour) contributed to a reduction in swallow latency compared with a no-stimulation condition. Furthermore, this group reported that any stimulation effect lasted for only a single swallow. Finally, neither Knauer et al.[114] nor Ali et al.[115] identified any significant swallow changes resulting from application of a cold stimulus in healthy adult volunteers.

Studies evaluating functional benefits such as reduction in aspiration from application of a cold stimulus to the anterior faucial pillars have not provided positive results. The primary effect identified, but inconsistently, is reduced swallow delay. Thus this technique may be applicable for patients demonstrating delays in swallowing activity but not for patients who demonstrate airway compromise.

NEW DIRECTIONS: EXERCISE PRINCIPLES AND MODALITIES

Many of the techniques described in this chapter may be envisioned as forms of exercise for the muscles encompassing the swallowing mechanism. In fact, various forms of exercise have been used for years in the rehabilitation of speech and swallowing functions.[57] Yet, in recent years clinicians and clinical researchers have borrowed from exercise physiologists and related professions in an attempt to develop effective therapy programs based on systematic application of exercise principles. As noted below, this application is relatively new and not fully developed. Many suggestions exist but few feasible applications have been developed.

The use of adjunctive modalities also is growing in the area of dysphagia rehabilitation. Two adjunctive modalities that have received the most attention have been sEMG biofeedback and neuromuscular electrical stimulus (NMES). The term *adjunctive* specifies that the modality is used to support the benefits from the primary therapy. Neither sEMG biofeedback nor NMES provides maximum benefit to patients in the absence of a well-developed treatment program, but both modalities have the potential to enhance the benefits of good therapy.

Exercise Principles and Dysphagia Therapy

Reviews of exercise principles that may apply to dysphagia rehabiltation have focused primarily on strength training.[116,117] Although a comprehensive review of exercise principles is beyond the scope of this chapter, two common exercise principles frequently mentioned in discussion of strength training in dysphagia rehabilitation are *intensity* and *specificity*. Intensity may be increased in many ways. Increasing the resistance to movement is a common method to increase intensity. For example, lifting heavier weights adds increased resistance to a weight-lifting exercise. Intensity may also be increased by frequency of exercise. More repetitions of an exercise completed in a fixed period result in a more intense exercise. Increasing the intensity of exercise facilitates muscle change and results in greater strength. Conversely, when exercises are ceased or reduced in intensity, the principle of *reversibility* or a *detraining* effect may be seen. In simple terms, reversibility means that strength gains may be lost if exercise is reduced and if a maintainence program is not used.

The concept of *specificity* refers to the observation that certain exercises are more likely to benefit specific tasks. For example, extreme weight lifting would not be viewed as the most beneficial exercise routine for a long-distance runner. Different muscle groups are involved with different requirements to the neuromuscular system from the target activity (in this case, long-distance running). A common phrase used by dysphagia clinicians is paraphrased as follows— "the best way to rehabilitate swallowing is to have the patient swallow." This phrase represents the principle of specificity. However, a related concept should be mentioned—cross-system effect or transference. The *cross-system effect* occurs when exercise intended for one function produces benefits in a different function. Because muscles of the swallowing mechanism also are used in speech and voice production it seems logical that exercise directed at improving speech and/or voice functions may have a cross-system effect on swallowing function (or vice versa). Although this

cross-system effect has not been well studied in relation to dysphagia rehabilitation, published examples do support the potential for exercises involving the swallowing mechanism to affect other functions of the upper aerodigestive tract.[118-120]

Positive benefits have been reported from exercise-based dysphagia therapy. Robbins et al.[59,60] were among the first to use specific exercise-based criteria to establish a dysphagia rehabilitation program. The focus of the therapy was to increase tongue strength using a tongue-press activity in which the tongue was pressed against the hard palate. Robbins and her colleagues progressively increased the intensity of the tongue-press activity by using the Iowa Oral Performance Instrument (IOPI) to measure the force of the tongue push and to provide patients feedback on how hard they were pushing. She incorporated the concept of 1-RM (1 repetition maximum or the greatest effort the patient can exert) to systematically increase resistance in the exercise (e.g., 60%, 70%, 80% of 1-RM), She also used a fixed time period in which to complete therapy (8 weeks). Results from two studies showed increased tongue strength during volitional tongue-push activity and swallowing, improvement in airway protection during swallowing, and increased lingual muscle size. These results are encouraging because they demonstrate that a simple, swallow-related exercise can increase strength in key muscle groups used in swallowing with some functional benefit to patients.

The McNeill Dysphagia Therapy Program (MDTP)[91,121] incorporates the exercise principles of specificity and intensity with frequent therapy sessions and variety to facilitate enhanced coordination during swallowing. Patients receive daily therapy sessions that are structured to evoke mass practice of swallowing. Swallowed materials are introduced sequentially to facilitate progressive resistance and/or speed and coordination of swallowing. Clinicians follow specific rules to advance patients during treatment based on patient performance. Early results from this therapy program suggest that it is effective with patients with chronic dysphagia in whom other therapies have failed[91] and that MDTP produces clinical results superior to more traditional swallow maneuvers (e.g., Mendelsohn maneuver) taught with adjunctive biofeedback.[121] The MDTP approach requires further clinical investigation, but initial results are encouraging and the program does represent an exercise-based therapy incorporating more than strength training alone.

Exercise-based swallowing therapy also has been used in attempts to prevent the occurrence of dysphagia in patients receiving medical treatments that cause swallowing problems. Carroll et al.[122] reported improved swallowing mechanics after head/neck cancer treatment in patients who completed a simple program of swallowing exercises *before* receiving chemoradiotherapy. Carnaby-Mann et al.[123] reported preserved swallow function, less weight loss, preserved muscle mass, less xerostomia, and other health-related benefits in patients completing a simple swallow exercise program *during* the course of chemoradiation for head/neck cancer. These reports not only reflect the positive benefits to be gained from exercise-based swallowing therapy, but they also represent a shift in dysphagia treatment. These reports strongly suggest the potential for exercise-based swallowing therapy to prevent or minimize dysphagia in clinical populations who are at risk to develop significant swallowing difficulties.

What Do Adjunctive Modalities Offer the Patient?

Surface Electromyographic and Other Forms of Biofeedback

Many of the swallowing maneuvers discussed in this chapter require motor learning by the patient. Furthermore, many of these adjustments represent novel motor patterns that may be difficult to learn. Application of biofeedback as an adjunct to therapy may be valuable in enhancing the rate of motor learning, thereby resulting in reduced time in therapy. Biofeedback has been facilatory in teaching new movements, unfamiliar movements, or movements that are otherwise difficult to monitor.[124] Many swallowing therapy maneuvers fit into one or more of these categories. In addition, biofeeedback may be useful in helping a patient monitor swallow performance. A simple example of this involves the effortful swallow. Asking a patient to "swallow harder" may not result in a significant increase in swallow effort. However, use of sEMG biofeedback to monitor the amplitude of the sEMG signal increases the probability that the patient has increased the effort involved in the swallow (see Figure 14-7). sEMG biofeedback is the process of monitoring and displaying muscle activity to a patient. Not only does this feedback help the patient to monitor effort, it also is immediate to the patient and the treating clinician and thus facilitates support or reinstruction from the clinician to the patient. A more comprehensive review of the application of sEMG biofeedback to dysphagia rehabilitation is offered by Crary and Groher.[125]

Several reports have advocated the use of sEMG biofeedback as an adjunct to dysphagia therapy. This form of biofeedback has been used to teach relaxation, strengthening, and coordination activities. Studies specific to dysphagia therapy have suggested that this form of biofeedback can reduce the amount therapy time while producing favorable outcomes even in patients with chronic dysphagia.[81,126-129]

Other forms of biofeedback may be applicable to swallow therapy. Having the patient watch swallow attempts on the monitor during a fluoroscopic examination has been suggested as a way to teach certain

---

Practice Note 14-4

Many years ago I was asked to see a 4-year-old boy who had survived treatment for a brainstem tumor. Like many adults with brainstem difficulties he had a significant dysphagia. I was actively studying the application of sEMG biofeedback at that time and decided that because of good results with survivors of adult brainstem stroke, I would try a similar approach with this child. We used a laptop computer to provide visual feedback. The software program featured a car on a hill that would go up the hill to a familiar yellow "M," a common symbol for a popular food chain. The harder the child swallowed, the closer the car got to the "M." The longer he maintained his swallow contraction, the longer the car stayed at the restaurant.

Therapy started with a bang! This boy was doing much better than anyone would have expected. He hit his goals almost immediately. Then I realized a critical mistake on my part. I did not verify that the movement driving the sEMG biofeedback was, in fact, a *swallow*. As it turned out, this little man was simply pushing his tongue against his palate and figured out that this would make the "car go." Clever!

I realized I needed to find a way to link the boy's attempts at swallowing with the biofeedback signal, so I made a second biofeedback source. I took a stethoscope head from a toy medical kit and connected it to a small microphone using rubber tubing. Then I plugged the microphone into a portable battery-operated speaker. I put the stethoscope head against my throat and swallowed hard. The sounds were clearly audible from the speaker and I asked the boy to do what I did. After he was trying to swallow on request on a consistent basis, I reintroduced sEMG biofeedback. His success level was not as dramatic this time. Eventually he did gain some functional swallowing ability with the combined biofeedback approach.

The lesson? Be sure of the movement for which you are providing biofeedback.

maneuvers.[130] Obviously, this application is time limited but potentially valuable for certain patients. In a similar manner, endoscopic biofeedback has been suggested as a mechanism to teach appropriate breath-hold maneuvers such as the supraglottic and super-supraglottic swallows.[131] If available, endoscopic biofeedback may be a valuable adjunct in teaching certain maneuvers. Less invasive than either fluoroscopy or endoscopy is the use of cervical auscultation as a biofeedback approach (see Chapter 9). Although this approach has not been formally evaluated, having patients listen for specific sound patterns associated with the swallow or the respiratory pattern surrounding the swallow may facilitate more rapid change in the swallowing pattern.

Regardless of the biofeedback form that is chosen, it is important for clinical practitioners to remember that biofeedback alone is not therapeutic. As an adjunct to a well-conceived plan of therapy, judiciously applied biofeedback can have a positive impact. The key word is *adjunct*. The key concept is "What change is intended to be facilitated by biofeedback?" Clinicians should develop a strong therapy plan based on the individual characteristics of the patient, the problem, and the underlying disease and then decide whether and how to apply biofeedback to support this plan.

Neuromuscular Electrical Stimulation

NMES is a relatively new adjunctive modality in dysphagia rehabilitation. As a result of the novelty of NMES, many clinicians may not fully appreciate its implications or potential applications, An in-depth discussion of NMES principles is beyond the scope of this chapter, but a basic review of the principles and data addressing application to dysphagia rehabilitation is appropriate.

NMES is intended to facilitate improved contraction of weakened muscles when the peripheral nerve supply to those muscles is intact.[132] Electrical stimulation to muscles via NMES may be accomplished through electrodes placed on the skin (transcutaneous), with intramuscular placement (percutaneous), or with fully implanted devices. NMES may be viewed as a subset of functional electrical stimulation, which implies that electrical stimulation is applied during the performance of a functional movement or task. Multiple examples from various fields of physical rehabilitation indicate that NMES can enhance a functional activity, change physiology to support function without overt functional change, and contribute to a motor relearning effect.[132] Specific to dysphagia rehabilitation, NMES application has been studied primarily in reference to improved function

or physiologic impact on the muscle groups involved in swallowing.

Several published studies have reported functional improvement in swallowing ability after dysphagia therapy with adjunctive NMES.[91,133-139] These reports of functional gain are also reflected in a large national survey of electrical stimulation in dysphagia rehabilitation.[140] Results from that survey indicated that nearly 80% of responding clinicians believed more than half of the patients they treated with NMES showed swallowing improvement. The primary gains reported by these clinicians included advances in the oral diet, reduced aspiration, and reduced reliance on tube feedings. Conversely, two studies reported no significant differences between outcomes of dysphagia therapy with and without adjunctive NMES.[141,142]

A few studies have investigated nontherapeutic effects of NMES on both healthy and adults with dysphagia. Suiter, Leder, and Ruark[143] evaluated the effect of 2 weeks of daily NMES without exercise in 10 healthy adult men. The investigators measured sEMG activity from the submental muscles before and after the 2 weeks of NMES and found no differences in swallow-related muscular activity. Humbert et al.[144] reported laryngeal and hyoid descent at rest and reduced laryngeal and hyoid elevation during swallowing when healthy adult subjects received electrical stimulation to the anterior neck. In a related study,[145] patients with chronic poststroke dysphagia demonstrated hyoid—but not laryngeal—descent at rest with the introduction of electrical stimulation to the anterior neck. Interestingly, in that study the degree of hyoid lowering during rest was inversely related to scores of swallow function during a videofluoroscopic swallow examination. Thus greater hyoid descent during electrical stimulation at rest related to better swallowing. In a follow-up study,[146] these investigators reported no effect of transcutaneous electrical stimulation to the anterior neck on vocal fold adduction.

Each of these studies used a form of NMES with stimulating electrodes placed in various locations on the anterior neck. However, two additional studies evaluated different forms of electrical stimulation. Park et al.[147] placed stimulating electrodes within a palatal prosthesis to provide NMES to the soft palate during the videofluoroscopic swallowing examination. They reported that two of four stroke patients demonstrated improved swallowing with NMES during the radiographic procedure. Power et al.[148] reported no change in any swallowing measure during a videofluoroscopic swallowing study in stroke patients who received electrical stimulation to the anterior faucial pillar by a fingertip electrode.

As with many techniques, the available data on the potential benefits or risks associated with the application of NMES for dysphagia rehabilitation are not clear. Although many studies report positive gains, some report no benefit from the addition of NMES to traditional therapy. Whereas some studies suggest movement of swallowing structures during application of NMES, other structures do not appear to be influenced. All of these studies are limited by some common variables. With few exceptions, most studies have incorporated small numbers of subjects and many have weak scientific designs. Furthermore, many, if not most, have evaluated the impact of NMES using unvalidated measurement tools. Given the positive clinical outcomes reported across several studies in the absence of reported complications, the application of NMES for dysphagia rehabilitation should be classified as promising but unclear until future, more rigorous studies contribute to our knowledge of the potential for this adjunctive modality.

Potential Future Directions

Much information has been presented in this chapter. Unfortunately, even this amount of information is likely insufficient to address the rich and growing body of information that pertains to the treatment of dysphagia. Clinical and translational research continues to yield new ideas that may be relevant to dysphagia therapy. Three focus points for future efforts in research surrounding dysphagia therapy might include the following areas. First, researchers and clinicians need to continue to evaluate the benefits and risks of traditional therapy techniques. More knowledge about techniques such as the chin tuck, Mendelsohn maneuver, effortful swallow, and others will give practicing clinicians much needed ammunition to select and apply these techniques on a best-practice basis. Second, further evaluation of exercise-based strategies for dysphagia rehabilitation is needed. Many swallowing difficulties are related to muscle weakness, but it is unlikely that *all* problems will respond to a single therapy. A better understanding of the exercise principles best suited for specific swallowing difficulties will help clinicians select the best available interventions for individual patients. Third, the potential applications of adjunctive modalities need to be considered and evaluated. Use of modalities is a relatively new aspect of dysphagia rehabilitation. Thus there is much to learn about which modalities may (or may not) be helpful to different aspects of dysphagia rehabilitation.

Other avenues of clinical research will emerge to help clinicians provide the best possible care to patients with dysphagia. As the evidence base for various clinical tools increases, the clinicians' skills and clinical outcomes will improve for many patients with dysphagia.

FINAL COMMENTS ON USING EVIDENCE

Information is not the same as evidence. *Evidence* is information that has been filtered systematically through scientific processes and meets minimum standards of rigor. The term *evidence-based practice* has become commonplace in the field of dysphagia rehabilitation. Earlier in this chapter clinically relevant questions regarding application of evidence were discussed. The concept of levels of evidence is discussed in Chapter 12 with details in Box 12-1. Although levels of evidence were not provided for each technique discussed in this chapter, most techniques are supported by some degree of evidence: primarily case reports, case control studies, or small cohort studies. This is a start; as a profession speech-language pathologists are moving toward obtaining stronger evidence for therapeutic endeavors. Clinicians can focus on simple but important questions in helping to choose appropriate clinical interventions. Perhaps the first consideration is whether information is published in credible journals or other formats. If so, does more than one publication exist? Replication of clinical findings is an important component of building supportive evidence. If information is not obtained in a published format, is it based on credible publications? This initial step provides some indication of the degree of scientific review. The levels of evidence described in Chapter 12 can be referenced in determining the strength of evidence supporting a given technique. However, given the overt recognition that most techniques have not been subjected to the highest levels of evidence, clinical practitioners still need to rely on some system to evaluate whether a given technique might be appropriate for a specific patient. The following questions, adapted from Sackett et al.,[149] may help with this process. These questions are not meant to be exhaustive. Rather they are intended as a starting point from which clinicians may evaluate information/evidence on the appropriateness of therapy techniques for specific patients. When reading available literature the following questions may be helpful in choosing a therapy technique:

1. Are the patients in the study similar to my patient?
2. Is the technique described in sufficient detail that I may use it in the same way?

3. Is the technique applied in an environment similar to the environment in which I practice (hospital, outpatient clinic, long-term care facility, other)?
4. Does the technique require technology that is available (or unavailable) to me?
5. Are the outcomes obtained in the study the same as (or similar to) those I want to obtain for my patient? What were the benefits to patients?
6. Are failures and reasons for failure described in the study? What are the risks to my patient?
7. Do I have the clinical skills to apply this technique as it is described in the study or is specific training required?
8. Is the technique pragmatically appropriate for my patient and environment (e.g., does it have time demands or intensity demands that exceed the reality of my workload or my patient's endurance or compliance)?

TAKE HOME NOTES

1. Evidence-based practice offers practitioners a systematic approach to improve clinical practice and enhance the care of individual patients. This approach involves finding, evaluating, and using scientific information.
2. Although most evidence supporting dysphagia intervention is not at the strongest levels, evidence does exist that can guide clinical practice and facilitate improved individual patient care.
3. Compensatory techniques are those intended for short-term use and that provide an adjustment to the swallowing pattern that has an immediate positive impact on safe, efficient swallowing. Rehabilitative techniques may not have an immediate impact but they contribute to reorganization of the impaired swallow, leading to improved functional swallowing once the technique is no longer applied.
4. Many factors should be considered before applying a therapy technique, including the technique, the patient, the environment, and/or the clinician. Not all techniques have been studied to the point of providing information on all of these factors. Clinical practitioners should consider many factors even in the face of limited evidence before applying a given therapy technique.
5. The functional impact of some therapy maneuvers is overtly evaluated during imaging studies. Others may require additional, adjunctive procedures (such as biofeedback) to evaluate, teach, and/or monitor the impact of the technique.

CLINICAL CASE EXAMPLE 14-1

A 70-year-old man had a brainstem stroke 2 years ago. The patient is receiving all nutrition by percutaneous gastrostomy (PEG) tube but attempts to swallow some liquids with reported intermittent success. Fluoroscopic evaluation indicates reduced pharyngeal constriction, reduced hyolaryngeal movement, and reduced PES opening. No aspiration is noted, and the patient is able to clear residue effectively by throat clearing and expectoration.

In searching for information on how to best approach the chronic dysphagia in this patient, you discover three published articles describing therapeutic experiences with long-term dysphagia in brainstem stroke. Two of the articles are from different centers and use slightly different approaches, although both incorporate a modification of the Mendelsohn maneuver and both use sEMG biofeedback to teach this technique and monitor physiologic progress. The third article is a summary of a retrospective outcome study from one of the centers reporting on a larger number of patients. Not all of these patients had brainstem strokes.

INTERPRETATION
The strength of evidence in this case is a level IV. The first two studies are case series using the patients as historical controls. Both include a small number of patients and are retrospective. The fact that different centers reported similar results with similar patient groups reflects a degree of replication that strengthens the evidence.

An initial question is whether the patients described in these studies resemble your patient. This depends in large part on the detail of description of the patients in the articles and on the evaluation completed on your patient. This is essential if you are to apply the described techniques to your patient. Do the evaluation results, functional eating profile, chronicity, and other descriptive characteristics of the published patient groups resemble your patient? Also, was the technique applied in an environment similar to that of your patient? If your patient matches the published descriptions, the technique may be appropriate for your patient.

A second question might be whether the outcomes described in the articles are the same as those you want to achieve for your patient. How were these outcomes measured? Do you understand and can you use similar outcome measures? Did these outcome measures make sense in terms of the problems presented by your patient?

The next question might be, "Did I understand the treatment technique?" This depends on the details of the provided description in the publications. Did the therapy protocol make sense to you? Were specific steps described, including the frequency and number of repetitions for each application? In this instance, sEMG biofeedback was used. Therefore, is this equipment available to you? Do you have the skills to use this technology, or can you acquire them in a time frame that will allow you to use them with this specific patient? Was the application of the biofeedback to the therapy technique clearly explained in the articles? Can your patient use this technique as described in the articles?

A final consideration might be whether treatment failures were reported and described. Clinicians are acutely aware that not all treatments result in the same degree of improvement. It is important to know the characteristics of patients in whom therapy did not result in improvement and if possible, why there was no improvement.

It may not be possible to address all these questions based on the published literature. Practitioners face the task of addressing as many of these questions as possible before application of any technique. The closer the individual patient fits the profile of published descriptions, the stronger the argument in favor of applying that specific technique.

References

1. Okada S, Saitoh E, Palmer JB et al: What is the chin-down posture? A questionnaire survey of speech language pathologists in Japan and the United States, *Dysphagia* 22:204, 2007.

2. Logemann JA, Rademaker AW, Pauloski BR: Effects of postural change on aspiration in head and neck surgical patients, *Otolaryngol Head Neck Surg* 110:222, 1994.

3. Rasley A, Logemann JA, Kahrilas PJ et al: Prevention of barium aspiration during videofluorographic swallowing studies: value of change in posture, *AJR Am J Roentgenol* 160:1005, 1993.

4. Logemann J: *Evaluation and treatment of swallowing disorders*, San Diego, 1983, College Hill Press.

5. Ohmae Y, Karaho T, Hanyu Y et al: Effect of posture strategies on preventing aspiration, *Nippon Jibiinkoka Gakkai Kaiho* 100:220, 1997.

6. Johnsson F, Shaw D, Gabb M et al: Influence of gravity and body position on normal oropharyngeal swallowing, *Am J Physiol* 269:G653, 1995.

7. Bernhard A, Pohl D, Fried M et al: Influence of bolus consistency and position on esophageal high-resolution manometry findings, *Dig Dis Sci* 53:1198, 2008.

8. Tutuian R, Elton JP, Castell DO et al: Effects of position on oesophageal function: studies using combined manometry and multichannel intraluminal impedance, *Neurogastroenterol Motil* 15:63, 2003.

9. Portale G, Peters J, Hsieh CC et al: When are reflux episodes symptomatic? *Dis Esophagus* 20:47, 2007.

10. Johnson LF, DeMeester TR: Evaluation of elevation of the head of the bed, bethanechol, and antacid form tablets on gastroesophageal reflux, *Dig Dis Sci* 26:673, 1981.

11. Ekberg O: Posture of the head and pharyngeal swallowing, *Acta Radiol Diagn* 27:691, 1986.

12. Castell JA, Castell DO, Schultz AR et al: Effect of head position on the dynamics of the upper esophageal sphincter and pharynx, *Dysphagia* 8:1, 1993.

13. Welch MV, Logemann JA, Rademaker AW et al: Changes in pharyngeal dimensions effected by chin tuck, *Arch Phys Med Rehabil* 74:178, 1993.

14. Bülow M, Olsson R, Ekberg O: Videomanometric analysis of supraglottic swallow, effortful swallow and chin tuck in patients with pharyngeal dysfunction, *Dysphagia* 16:190, 2001.

15. Bülow M, Olsson R, Ekberg O: Supraglottic swallow, effortful swallow, and chin tuck did not alter hypopharyngeal intrabolus pressure in patients with pharyngeal dysfunction, *Dysphagia* 17:197, 2002.

16. Bülow M, Olsson R, Ekberg O: Videomanometric analysis of supraglottic swallow, effortful, and chin tuck in healthy volunteers, *Dysphagia* 14:67, 1999.

17. Ayuse T, Ayuse T, Ishitobi S et al: Effect of reclining and chin-tuck position on coordination between respiration and swallowing, *J Oral Rehabil* 33:402, 2006.

18. Shanahan TK, Logemann JA, Rademaker AW et al: Chin-down posture effect on aspiration in dysphagia patients, *Arch Phys Med Rehabil* 74:736, 1993.

19. Lewin JS, Hebert TM, Putnam JB Jr et al: Experience with the chin tuck maneuver in postesophagectomy aspirators, *Dysphagia* 16:216, 2001.

20. Logemann JA, Gensler G, Robbins J et al: A randomized study of three interventions for aspiration of thin liquids in patients with dementia or Parkinson's disease, *J Speech Lang Hear Res* 51:173, 2008.

21. Zuydam AC, Rogers SN, Brown JS et al: Swallowing rehabilitation after oro-pharyngeal resectoin for squa-

mous cell carcinoma, *Br J Oral Maxillofac Surg* 38:513, 2000.

22. Robbins J, Gensler G, Hind J et al: Comparison of 2 interventions for liquid aspiration on pneumonia incidence: a randomized trial, *Ann Intern Med* 148:509, 2008.

23. Kirchner JA: Pharyngeal and esophageal dysfunction: the diagnosis, *Minn Med* 50:921, 1967.

24. Logemann JA, Jahrilas PJ, Kobura M et al: The benefit of head rotation on pharyngoesophageal dysphagia, *Arch Phys Med Rehabil* 70:767, 1989.

25. Tsukamoto Y: CT study of closure of the hemipharynx with head rotation in a case of lateral medullary syndrome, *Dysphagia* 15:17, 2000.

26. Ohmae Y, Ogura M, Kitahara S et al: Effects of head rotation on pharyngeal function during normal swallow, *Ann Otol Rhinol Laryngol* 107:344, 1998.

27. O'Gara JA: Dietary adjustments and nutritional therapy during treatment for oral-pharyngeal dysphagia, *Dysphagia* 4:209, 1990.

28. Pardoe EM: Development of a multistage diet for dysphagia, *J Am Diet Assoc* 93:568, 1993.

29. Penman JP, Thomson M: A review of the textured diets developed for the management of dysphagia, *J Hum Nutr Diet* 11:51, 1998.

30. Garcia JM, Chambers E, Molander M: Thickened liquids: practice patterns of speech-language pathologists, *Am J Speech Lang Pathol* 14:4, 2005.

31. Castellanos VH, Butler E, Gluch L et al: Use of thickened liquids in skilled nursing facilities, *J Am Diet Assoc* 104:1222, 2004.

32. Kuhlemeier KV, Palmer JB, Rosenberg D: Effect of liquid bolus consistency and delivery method on aspiration and pharyngeal retention in dysphagia patients, *Dysphagia* 16:119, 2001.

33. Whelan K: Inadequate fluid intakes in dysphagic acute stoke, *Clin Nutr* 20:423, 2001.

34. Garon BR, Engle M, Ormiston C: A randomized control study to determine the effects of unlimited oral intake of water in patients with identified aspiration, *J Neurol Rehabil* 11:139, 1997.

35. Panther K: *Frazier Water Protocol: safety, hydration, and quality of life*, Rockville, MD, 2008, American Speech-Language-Hearing Association.

36. Pouderoux P, Kahrilas PJ: Deglutitive tongue force modulation by volition, volume, and viscosity in humans, *Gastroenterology* 108:1418, 1995.

37. Chi-Fishman G, Sonies BC: Effects of systematic bolus viscosity and volume change on hyoid movement kinematics, *Dysphagia* 17:278, 2002.

38. Dantas RO, Dodds WJ, Massey BT et al: The effect of high- vs low-density barium preparations in the quantitative features of swallowing, *AJR Am J Roentgenol* 153:1191, 1989.

39. Butler SG, Stuart A, Castell D et al: Effects of age, gender, bolus condition, viscosity, and volume on pharyngeal and upper esophageal sphincter pressure and temporal measurements during swallowing, *J Speech Lang Hear Res* December 8, 2008 [epub ahead of print].

40. Clavé P, de Kraa M, Arreola V et al: The effect of bolus viscosity on swallowing function in neurogenic dysphagia, *Aliment Pharmacol Ther* 24:1385, 2006.

41. Bülow M, Olsson R, Ekberg O: Videoradiographic analysis of how carbonated thin liquids and thickened liquids affect the physiology of swallowing in subjects with aspiration of thin liquids, *Acta Radiol* 44:366, 2004.

42. Logemann JA, Pauloski BR, Colangelo L et al: Effects of a sour bolus on oropharyngeal swallowing measures in patients with neurogenic dysphagia, *J Speech Hear Res* 38:556, 1995.

43. Pelletier CA, Lawless HT: Effect of citric acid and citric acid-sucrose mixtures on swallowing in neurogenic oropharyngeal dysphagia, *Dysphagia* 18:231, 2003.

44. Chee C, Arshad S, Singh S et al: The influence of chemical gustatory stimuli and oral anaesthesia on healthy human swallowing, *Chem Senses* 30:393, 2005.

45. Palmer PM, McCulloch TM, Jaffee D et al: Effects of sour bolus on the intramuscular electromyographic (EMG) activity of muscles in the submental region, *Dysphagia* 20:210, 2005.

46. Pelletier CA, Dhanaraj GE: The effect of taste and palatability on lingual swallowing pressure, *Dysphagia* 21:121, 2006.

47. Miyaoka Y, Haishima K, Takagi M et al: Influences of thermal and gustatory characteristics on sensory and motor aspects of swallowing, *Dysphagia* 21:38, 2005.

48. Matta Z, Changers E, Mertz Garcia J et al: Sensory characteristics of beverages prepared with commercial thickeners used for dysphagia diets, *J Am Diet Assoc* 106:1049, 2006.

49. Feinberg MJ, Kneble J, Tully J: Prandial aspiration and pneumonia in an elderly population followed over 3 years, *Dysphagia* 11:104, 1996.

50. Curran J, Groher ME: Development and dissemination of an aspiration risk reduction diet, *Dysphagia* 5:6, 1990.

51. Wright L, Cotter D, Hickson M et al: Comparison of energy and protein intakes of older people consuming a texture modified diet with a normal hospital diet, *J Hum Nutr Diet* 18:213, 2005.

52. Germain I, Dufresne T, Gray-Donald K: A novel dysphagia diet improves the nutritional intake of institutionalized elders, *J Am Diet Assoc* 106:1614, 2006.

53. Groher ME, McKaig N: Dysphagia and dietary levels in skilled nursing facilities, *J Am Geriatr Soc* 43:528, 1995.

54. National Dysphagia Diet Taskforce: *The National Dysphagia Diet: standardization for optimal tare*, Chicago, 2002, American Dietetic Association.

55. Strowd L, Kyzima J, Pillsbury D et al: Dysphagia dietary guidelines and the rheology of nutritional feeds and barium test feeds, *Chest* 133:1397, 2008.

56. Hall G, Wendin K: Sensory design of foods for the elderly, *Ann Nutr Metab* 52(Suppl 1):25, 2008.

57. Stathopoulos E, Duchan JF: History and principles of exercised-based therapy: how they inform our current treatment, *Semin Speech Lang* 27:227, 2006.

58. Lazarus C, Logemann JA, Huang CF et al: Effects of two types of tongue strengthening exercises in young normals, *Folia Phoniatr Logop* 55:199, 2003.

59. Robbins J, Gangnon RE, Theis SM et al: The effects of lingual exercise on swallowing in older adults, *J Am Geriatr Soc* 53:1483, 2005.

60. Robbins J, Kays SA, Gangnon RE et al: The effects of lingual exercise in stroke patients with dysphagia, *Arch Phys Med Rehabil* 88:150, 2007.

61. Hagg M, Anniko M: Lip muscle training in stroke patients with dysphagia, *Acta Otolaryngol* 128:1027, 2008.

62. Shaker R, Dodds W, Dantas R et al: Coordination of deglutitive glottic closure with oropharyngeal swallowing, *Gastroenterology* 98:1478, 1990.

63. Mendelsohn M, Martin RE: Airway protection during breath holding. *Ann Otol Rhinol Laryngol* 102:941, 1993.

64. Hirst LJ, Sama A, Carding PN et al: Is a "safe swallow" really safe? *Int J Lang Commun Disord* 33(Suppl):279, 1998.

65. Donzelli J, Brady S: The effects of breath-holding on vocal fold adduction: implications for safe swallowing, *Arch Otolaryngol Head Neck Surg* 130:208, 2004.

66. Martin BJ, Logemann JA, Shaker R et al: Normal laryngeal valving patterns during three breath hold maneuvers: a pilot investigation, *Dysphagia* 8:11, 1993.

67. Flaherty RF, Seltzer S, Campbell T et al: Dynamic magnetic resonance imaging of vocal cord closure during deglutition, *Gastroenterology* 109:843, 1995.

68. Bodén K, Hallgren A, Witt Hedström H: Effects of three different swallow maneuvers analyzed by videomanometry, *Acta Radiol* 47:628, 2006.

69. Ohmae Y, Logemann JA, Kaiser P et al: Effects of two breath-holding maneuvers on oropharyngeal swallow, *Ann Otol Rhinol Laryngol* 105:123, 1996.

70. Miller JL, Watkin KL: Lateral pharyngeal wall motion during swallowing using real time ultrasound, *Dysphagia* 12:125, 1997.

71. Lazarus C, Logemann JA, Song CW et al: Effects of voluntary maneuvers on tongue base function for swallowing, *Folia Phoniatr Logop* 54:171, 2002.

72. Logemann JA, Pauloski BR, Rademaker AW et al: Super-supraglottic swallow in irradiated head and neck cancer patients, *Head Neck* 19:535, 1997.

73. Hamlet S, Mathog R, Fleming S et al: Modification of compensatory swallowing in a supraglottic laryngectomy patient, *Head Neck* 12:131, 1990.

74. Lazarus C, Logemann JA, Gibbons P: Effects of maneuvers on swallowing function in a dysphagic oral cancer patient, *Head Neck* 15:419, 1993.

75. Lazarus C: Effects of radiation therapy and voluntary maneuvers on swallowing function in head and neck cancer patients, *Clin Commun Disord* 3:11, 1993.

76. Chaudhuri G, Hildner CD, Brady S et al: Cardiovascular effects on the supraglottic and super-supraglottic swallowing maneuvers in stroke patients with dysphagia, *Dysphagia* 17:19, 2002.

77. Kahrilas PJ, Logemann JA, Krugler C et al: Volitional augmentation of upper esophageal sphincter opening during swallowing, *Am J Physiol* 260:G450, 1991.

78. Jaffe DM, Van Daele DJ, Rao SSC et al: Contribution of cricopharyngeal muscle activity to upper esophageal sphincter manometry in the normal swallow and Mendelsohn's maneuver [abstract], *Dysphagia* 15:101, 2001.

79. Ding R, Larson CR, Logemann JA et al: Surface electromyographic and electroglottalgraphic studies in normal subjects under two swallow conditions: normal and during the Mendelsohn maneuver, *Dysphagia* 17:1, 2002.

80. Neumann S, Bartolome G, Buchholz D et al: Swallowing therapy of neurologic patients: correlation of outcome with pretreatment variables and therapeutic method, *Dysphagia* 10:1, 1995.

81. Crary MA: A direct intervention program for chronic neurogenic dysphagia secondary to brainstem stroke, *Dysphagia* 10:6, 1995.

82. Crary MA, Carnaby-Mann GD, Groher ME et al: Functional benefits of dysphagia therapy using adjunctive biofeedback, *Dysphagia* 19:160, 2004.

83. Huckabee ML, Cannito MP: Outcomes of swallowing rehabilitation in chronic brainstem dysphagia: a retrospective evaluation, *Dysphagia* 14:93, 1999.

84. Hind JA, Nicosia MA, Roecker EB et al: Comparison of effortful and noneffortful swallows in healthy middle-aged and older adults, *Arch Phys Med Rehabil* 82:1661, 2001.

85. Huckabee ML, Butler SG, Barclay M et al: Submental surface electromyographic measurement and pharyngeal pressures during normal and effortful swallowing, *Arch Phys Med Rehabil* 86:2144, 2005.

86. Hiss SG, Huckabee ML: Timing of pharyngeal and upper esophageal sphincter pressures as a function of normal and effortful swallowing in young healthy adults, *Dysphagia* 20:149, 2005.

87. Huckabee ML, Steele CM: An analysis of lingual contribution to submental surface electromyographic measures and pharyngeal pressure during effortful swallow, *Arch Phys Med Rehabil* 87:1067, 2006.

88. Steele CM, Huckabee ML: The influence of oralingual pressure on the timing of pharyngeal pressure events, *Dysphagia* 22:30, 2007.

89. Witte U, Huckabee ML, Doeltgen SH et al: The effect of effortful swallow on pharyngeal manometric measurements during saliva and water swallowing in healthy participants, *Arch Phys Med Rehabil* 89:822, 2008.

90. Lever TE, Cox KT, Holbert D et al: The effect of an effortful swallow on the normal adult esophagus, *Dysphagia* 22:312, 2007.

91. Carnaby-Mann GD, Crary MA: Adjunctive neuromuscular electrical stimulation for treatment-refractory dysphagia, *Ann Oto Rhinol Laryngol* 117:279, 2008.

92. Robbins JA, Logemann JA, Kirshner HS: Swallowing and speech production in Parkinson's disease, *Ann Neurol* 19:283, 1986.

93. Dziadziola J, Hamlet S, Michou G et al: Multiple swallows and piecemeal deglutition; observations from normal adults and patients with head and neck cancer, *Dysphagia* 7:8, 1992.

94. Leslie P, Drinnan MJ, Ford GA et al: Swallow respiration patterns in dysphagia patients following acute stroke, *Dysphagia* 17:202, 2002.

95. Nilsson H, Ekberg O, Olsson R et al: Quantitative aspects of swallowing in an elderly population, *Dysphagia* 11:180, 1996.

96. Fujiu M, Logemann JA, Pauloski BR: Increased postoperative posterior pharyngeal wall movement in patients with anterior oral cancer: preliminary findings and possible implications for treatment, *Am J Speech Lang Pathol* 4:24, 1995.

97. Fujui M, Logemann JA: Effect of a tongue holding maneuver on posterior pharyngeal wall movement during deglutition, *Am J Speech Lang Pathol* 5:23, 1996.

98. Fujui-Kurachi M: Developing the tongue holding maneuver, *Perspectives on Swallowing and Swallowing Disorders (Dysphagia)* 11:9, 2002.

99. Doeltgen SH, Witte U, Gumbley F et al: Evaluation of manometric measures during tongue-hold swallows, *Am J Speech Lang Pathol* 2008 Oct 9 [epub ahead of print].

100. Shaker R, Kern M, Bardan E et al: Augmentation of deglutitive upper esophageal sphincter opening in the elderly by exercise, *Am J Physiol* 272:G1518, 1997.

101. Shaker R, Easterling C, Kern M et al: Rehabilitation of swallowing by exercise in tube-fed patients with pharyngeal dysphagia secondary to abnormal UES opening, *Gastroenterology* 122:1314, 2002.

102. Ferdjallah M, Wertsch J, Shaker R: Spectral analysis of surface EMG of upper esophageal sphincter opening muscels during head lift exercise, *J Rehabil Res Dev* 37:335, 2000.

103. White KT, Easterling C, Roberts N et al: Fatigue analysis before and after shaker exercise: physiologic tool for exercise design, *Dysphagia* 23:385, 2008.

104. Mepani R, Antonik S, Massey B et al: Augmentation of deglutitive thyrohyoid muscle shortening by the shaker exercise, *Dysphagia* August 2008 [epub ahead of print].

105. Yoshida M, Groher ME, Crary MA et al: Comparison of surface electromyographic (sEMG) activity of submental muscles between the head lift and tongue press exercises as a therapeutic exercise for pharyngeal dysphagia, *Gerodontology* 24:111, 2007.

106. Easterling C, Grande B, Kern M et al: Attaining and maintaining isometric and isokinetic goals of the Shaker exercise, *Dysphagia* 20:133, 2005.

107. Pommerenke W: A study of the sensory areas eliciting the swallowing reflex, *Am J Physiology* 84:36, 1928.

108. Lazzara, GL, Lazarus C, Logemann JA: Impact of thermal stimulation on the triggering of the swallowing reflex, *Dysphagia* 1:73, 1986.

109. Rosenbek J, Robbins J, Fishback B et al: Effects of thermal application on dysphagia after stroke, *J Speech Hear Res* 34:1257, 1991.

110. Rosenbek J, Roecker EB, Wood JL et al: Thermal application reduces the duration of stage transition in dysphagia after stroke, *Dysphagia* 11:225, 1996.

111. Rosenbek J, Robbins J, Willford WO et al: Comparing treatment intensities of tactile-thermal application, *Dysphagia* 13:1, 1998.

112. Kaatzke-McDonald MN, Post E, Davis PJ et al: The effects of cold, touch, and chemical stimulation of the anterior faucial pillar on human swallowing, *Dysphagia* 11:198, 1996.

113. Sciortino K, Liss JM, Case JL et al: Effects of mechanical, cold, gustatory, and combined stimulation to the human anterior faucial pillars, *Dysphagia* 18:16, 2003.

114. Knauer CM, Castell JA, Dalton CB et al: Pharyngeal/upper esophageal sphincter pressure dynamics in humans: effects of pharmacologic agents and thermal stimulation, *Dig Dis Sci* 35:774, 1990.

115. Ali GN, Laundl TM, Wallace KL et al: Influence of cold stimulation on the normal pharyngeal swallow response, *Dysphagia* 11:2, 1996.

116. Clark HM: Neuromuscular treatments for speech and swallowing: a tutorial, *Am J Speech Lang Pathol* 12:400, 2003.

117. Burkhead LM, Sapienza C, Rosbenbek J: Strength-training exercise in dysphagia rehabilitation: principles, procedures, and directions for future research, *Dysphagia* 22:251, 2007.

118. LaGorio LA, Carnaby-Mann GD, Crary MA: Cross-system effecs of dysphagia treatment on dysphonia: a case report, *Cases J* 1:67, 2008.

119. Easterling C: Does exercise aimed at improving swallow function have an effect on vocal function in the healthy elderly? *Dysphagia* 23:317, 2008.

120. El Sharkawi A, Ramig L, Logemann J et al: Swallowing and voice effects of Lee Silverman Voice Treatment (LSVT): a pilot study, *J Neurol Neurosurg Psychiarty* 72:31, 2002.

121. Carnaby-Mann GD, Crary MA: A case-control evaluation of the McNeill Dysphagia Therapy Program (MDTP). Presented at the Dysphagia Research Society, New Orleans, March 2009.

122. Carroll WR, Locher JL, Canon CL et al: Pretreatment swallowing exercises improved swallow function after chemoradiation, *Laryngoscope* 118:39, 2008.

123. Carnaby-Mann GD, Crary MA, Amdur R et al: Preventative exercise for dysphagia following head/neck cancer, *Dysphagia* 22:381, 2007 (abstract).

124. Mulder T, Hulstyn W: Sensory feedback therapy and theoretical knowledge of motor control and learning, *Am J Phys Med* 63:226, 1984.

125. Crary MA, Groher ME: Basic concepts of surface electromyographic biofeedback in the treatment of dysphagia: a tutorial, *Am J Speech Lang Pathol* 9:116, 2000.

126. Haynes SN: Electromyographic biofeedback treatment of a woman with chronic dysphagia, *Biofeedback Self Regul* 1:121, 1976.

127. Lichstein KL, Eakin TL, Dunn ME: Combined psychological and medical treatment of oropharyngeal dysphagia, *Clin Biofeedback Health Int J* 9:9, 1986.

128. Bryant M: Biofeedback in the treatment of a selected dysphagic patient, *Dysphagia* 6:140, 1991.

129. Crary MA, Carnaby-Mann GD, Groher ME et al: Functional benefits of dysphagia therapy using adjunctive sEMG biofeedback, *Dysphagia* 19:160, 2004.

130. Logemann JA, Kahrilas PJ: Relearning to swallow after stroke—application of maneuvers and indirect biofeedback: a case study, *Neurology* 40:1136, 1990.

131. Denk DM, Kaider A: Videoendoscopic biofeedback: a simple method to improve the efficacy of swallowing rehabilitation of patients after head and neck surgery, *ORL J Otorhinolaryngol Relat Spec* 59:100, 1997.

132. Sheffler LR, Chae J: Neuromuscular electrical stimulation in neurorehabilitation, *Muscle Nerve* 35:562, 2007.

133. Freed ML, Freed L, Chatburn RL et al: Electrical stimulation for swallowing disorders caused by stroke, *Respir Care* 46:466, 2001.

134. Leelamint V, Limsakul C, Geater A: Sychronized electrical stimulation in treating pharyngeal dysphagia, *Laryngoscope* 112:2204, 2002.

135. Blumenfeld L, Hahn Y, LePage A et al: Transcutaneous electrical stimulation versus traditional dysphagia therapy: a noncurrent cohort study, *Otolaryngol Head Neck Surg* 135:754, 2006.

136. Shaw GY, Sechtem PR, Searl J et al: Transcutaneous neuromuscular electrical stimulation (VitalStim) curative therapy for severe dysphagia: myth or reality? *Ann Otol Rhinol Laryngol* 116:36, 2007.

137. Oh BM, Kim DY, Paik NJ: Recovery of swallowing function is accompanied by the expansion of the cortical map, *Int. J Neurosci* 117:1215, 2007.

138. Baijens LW, Speyer R, Roodenburg N et al: The effects of neuromuscular electrical stimulation for dysphagia in opercular syndrome: a case study, *Eur Arch Otorhinolaryngol* 265:825, 2008.

139. Ryu JS, Kang JY, Park JY et al: The effect of electrical stimulation therapy on dysphagia following treatment for head and neck cancer, *Oral Oncol* 2008 Dec. 16 [epub ahead of print].

140. Crary MA, Carnaby-Mann GD, Faunce A: Electrical stimulation therapy for dysphagia: descriptive results for two surveys, *Dysphagia* 22:165, 2007.

141. Kiger M, Brown CS, Watkins L: Dysphagia management: an analysis of patient outcomes using VitalStim therapy compared to traditional swallow therapy, *Dysphagia* 21:243, 2006.

142. Bülow M, Speyer R, Baijens L et al: Neuromuscular electrical stimulation (NMES) in stroke patients with oral and pharyneal dysphagia, *Dysphagia* 23:302, 2008.

143. Suiter DM, Leder SB, Ruark JL: Effects of neuromuscular electrical stimulation on submental muscle activity, *Dysphagia* 21:56, 2006.

144. Humbert IA, Poletto CJ, Saxon KG et al: The effect of surface electrical stimulation on hyolaryngeal movement in normal individuals at rest and during swallowing, *J Appl Physiol* 101:1657, 2006.

145. Ludlow CL, Humbert IA, Saxon K et al: Effects of surface electrical stimulation both at rest and during swallowing in chronic pharyngeal, *Dysphagia* 22:1, 2007.

146. Humbert IA, Poletto CJ, Samon KG et al: The effect of surface electrical stimulation on vocal fold position, *Laryngoscope* 118:14, 2007.

147. Park CL, O'Neill PA, Martin DF: A pilot exploratory study of oral electrical stimulation on swallow function following stroke: an innovative technique, *Dysphagia* 12:161, 1997.

148. Power ML, Fraser CH, Hobson A et al: Evaluating oral stimulation as a treatment for dysphagia after stroke, *Dysphagia* 21:49, 2006.

149. Sackett DL, Haynes RB, Guyatt GH et al: *Clinical epidemiology: a basic science for clinical medicine*, ed 2, Boston, 1991, Little, Brown.

Chapter 15

Ethical Considerations

MICHAEL E. GROHER

CHAPTER OUTLINE

CHAPTER OBJECTIVES

1. Present the basic principles of medical ethics as they relate to the swallowing-impaired patient.
2. Discuss the risks and benefits of alternative types of feeding.
3. Highlight the differences between factors that predict aspiration and those that predict aspiration pneumonia.
4. Present an approach for weaning from feeding tubes.
5. Present examples of ethical dilemmas resulting from the placement or retention of alternative forms of feeding.

MEDICAL ETHICS

The Patient Self-Determination Act took effect on December 1, 1991. The act established guidelines to allow patients to participate fully in decisions regarding their health care, particularly decisions made in circumstances of severe or terminal illness. The act strives to establish a patient-physician interaction that allows both parties to balance individual morals and values against the known risks and benefits of proposed medical care. For example, patients might want to decide under which circumstances they would want to be resuscitated or whether they would want to be nourished by a feeding tube to sustain life. Counseling patients, families, and caregivers on the risks and benefits of tube feeding may involve the expertise of the dysphagia specialist.[1] One study found that speech-language pathologists (SLPs) who manage patients with dementia are involved in the decision making in 65% of cases when the recommendation is made for some type of alternative nutrition.[2]

Medical ethics is a subspecialty of medical care that brings together patients, caregivers, and nonmedical and medical professionals in an effort to make the best decision regarding a health care issue. The decision rests on the understanding that it is finalized by balancing data from individual and societal morals and values, evidence-based medical knowledge, and legal precedent. Ethical dilemmas result when balance is not achieved—when one party is not in agreement with the plan of care. For example, a patient may not agree to the short-term use of a nasogastric feeding tube (NGT) because of religious objections, although the medical team is convinced that it may save or prolong the patient's life. These dilemmas need to be resolved and may be referred to the medical center's ethics committee. Solutions generally are possible with a rational analysis of (1) how the patient came to establish his or her health care preferences; (2) the medical risks and benefits of a proposed intervention; (3) the burdens that medical intervention might bear on the patient and family; (4) the effect on the patient's and family's quality of life; and (5) any legal constraints, such as the patient being incapable of making an informed decision.

Advance Directives

The advance directive (AD) is a statement made by a person with decision-making capacity indicating his or her preferences for receiving medical treatment or not receiving medical treatment under certain circumstances. When a person is admitted to a medical setting, the patient is automatically given the option to execute an AD. Admission is not contingent on signing an AD, and patients frequently do not. Any member of the health care team may initiate the document if he or she thinks it will facilitate the patient's care. If an AD has already been executed, either from another admission or as a document the patient executed in the past, it will be placed prominently in the medical record so the medical team can be guided by the patient's wishes in the event of a medical crisis. Most often an AD is specific to end-of-life decisions or circumstances when an individual's medical condition is futile. Typically, the AD has two parts: a living will and a durable power of attorney for health care. The *living will* is a written request to forego some type of medical treatment in a terminal or irreversible medical condition. The *durable power of attorney for health care* appoints a person (**surrogate**) to act in the patient's behalf on end-of-life or irreversible conditions should the patient be in a state that he or she is not competent to make an informed decision. It is understood that the surrogate will have prior knowledge of the patient's desires and therefore will act in the patient's best interest. Patients with terminal, progressive diseases should be encouraged to execute an AD while they are competent and free from severe disease to facilitate end-stage medical care. Making decisions about tube feeding when the patient is in a crisis often clouds a rational decision and may complicate medical care.

TUBE FEEDING

Because most ethical dilemmas that the swallowing specialist faces center on the use or denial of tube feeding, it is important to understand the risks and benefits of this intervention. Tube feeding entails psychological and medical risks and benefits.

CLINICAL CORNER 15-1

A patient's surrogate told the medical care team that she wants to discontinue her husband's oral feeding because she has noticed as she assists him at mealtime that he has considerable choking episodes. Based on the patient's clinical and instrumental swallowing evaluations, the treatment team believes that he should be able to continue eating orally.

CRITICAL THINKING

1. What would be the next step for the treatment team? What are some options?
2. If the wife and the treatment team disagree after reviewing the case, who will make the final decision?

CLINICAL CORNER 15-2

A 58-year-old man has a 3-year history of amyotropic lateral sclerosis. A swallowing study has shown that he aspirates with a weak cough on all consistencies. Although the patient does not have an advanced directive, he is adamant that he wants to continue eating orally.

CRITICAL THINKING

1. You are the SLP. Make a case for letting the patient continue to eat.
2. If the patient became ill in the future and took you to court for encouraging him to eat, what defense would you have, and how would you prove it?

There are two major categories of nonoral nutritional provision: **enteral** and **parenteral**. Nonoral parenteral feedings are sometimes collectively referred to as *hyperalimentation*.

Enteral Nutrition

The major types of enteral tube feeding include nasogastric, gastrostomy, and jejunostomy. Specially prepared high-calorie formulas are delivered through the tube into the feeding site. They are delivered from a syringe, a plastic bag that hangs above the level of the tube site, or a mechanical pump.

Nasogastric Tubes

Tubes that are inserted through the nose and into the stomach can be used to deliver nutrients or suction unwanted secretions. Tubes that provide nutrition are *nasogastric feeding tubes*. They range in diameter from 8 to 18 Fr. Usually the larger the diameter (18 Fr), the stiffer and more uncomfortable the tube is in the nose and throat. Larger nasogastric feeding tubes are necessary for passing medications and pureed foods. They do not clog as much with these materials as do smaller bore tubes. Smaller bore tubes take thin liquid formulas, sometimes are prone to clogging and dislodgment, and generally are more comfortable in the aerodigestive tract. Smaller bore tubes that are weighted on the tip for ease of passage are called *Dobhoff tubes*.

The nasogastric feeding tube is inserted through the nostril into the pharynx, through the pharyngoesophageal segment into the esophagus, and finally through the lower esophageal segment into the stomach. In some cases it is passed beyond the stomach, through the pyloric valve, and into the jejunum. A special radiograph (kidney-ureter-bladder)

is ordered to ensure that the tube is positioned correctly in the aerodigestive tract before feeding begins. NGTs are used in acute medical situations that render the individual unable to swallow or to sustain nutrition orally. A nasogastric feeding tube is used when the medical care team believes that the patient's medical status has a good chance to improve in a short period. Although the length of time for use of an NGT is not prescribed, if a patient requires enteral feeding for longer than 3 or 4 weeks another enteral feeding method usually is selected. More permanent options that are still reversible include gastrostomy or jejunostomy feeding tubes. These tubes can be placed surgically (usually requiring general anesthesia for the patient) or endoscopically (requiring light anesthesia). Endoscopic placements are called **percutaneous endoscopic gastrostomy** (PEG) or **percutaneous endoscopic jejunostomy** (PEJ).

Gastrostomy and Jejunostomy Tubes

The gastrostomy tube is placed directly into the stomach with the assumption that the digestive processes of the stomach are intact. Formula is passed through a catheter that sits on the outside of the stomach. If the stomach is not functioning, the feeding tube may need to be placed into the jejunum of the small intestine. Because the stomach is bypassed, specialized, predigested formulas are required for jejunal tube feedings. Some clinicians argue that jejunal placement reduces the risk of reflux of the tube-fed material into the pharynx because the pyloric valve provides an additional barrier to retropulsion of stomach contents into the esophagus. However, the experimental evidence does not clearly support this contention.[3] Table 15-1 summarizes the medical risks and benefits of enteral tube feeding.

Parenteral Nutrition

Parenteral nutrition is indicated when the gastrointestinal tract cannot be used because of medical complications such as **gastroparesis**, obstruction, or bleeding. *Total parenteral nutrition* (TPN) is a specialized formula that most commonly is delivered into a central vein (subclavian or internal jugular). Although there are potential medical complications from this therapy, such as **pneumothorax**, patients can be supported nutritionally with this formula for 4 to 6 weeks if necessary.[4] *Peripheral parenteral nutrition* (PPN) is a form of nutritional support delivered through a peripheral vein. Because of potential medical complications, this therapy can be used effectively for only 7 to 10 days.[4] *Intravenous feeding* is a common form of parenteral nutrition, usually providing hydration and medication only rather than more complex elements

TABLE 15-1

Medical Risks and Benefits Associated with Enteral Tube Feeding

Risks	Benefits
Nasogastric	
Uncomfortable	Easy insertion
Poor cosmesis	No anesthesia
Distends PES and UES; may promote reflux	Tube can be small bore; well tolerated
Nasal ulceration	Good short-term nutrition
Sinusitis	Patient can eat with tube in place
Delays swallow	
May trigger vagal bradycardia	
Gastrostomy	
Requires surgical placement	Good long-term option
Infection and care at tube site	Out of visual sight
Tube may fall out	Easy tube replacement
Reflux if stomach fills too fast	Easily removed
Diarrhea	Patient can eat with tube in place
Jejunostomy	
Requires surgical placement	May reduce reflux
Needs continuous drip feeding	Out of visual sight
Requires hospital visit if dislodged	Good nutrition if stomach not available
Intolerance of special formula	
PEG or Jejunostomy	
Aspiration during procedure	Inserted under local anesthesia
Infection at tube site	Generally well tolerated
Potential for reflux	Operating room time not needed

PES, Pharyngoesophageal segment; *UES*, upper esophageal sphincter.

such as amino acids. *Hypodermal clysis* is a form of parenteral nutrition that is given for hydration through the subcutaneous tissues in the chest, thigh, or abdomen. Table 15-2 summarizes parenteral and enteral alternative nutrition and hydration.

REASONS FOR TUBE FEEDING

The three most common reasons for placing a feeding tube include (1) the patient's inability to sustain nutrition orally, although the swallow response is safe; (2) the requirement for sufficient calories on a short-term basis to overcome an acute medical problem; and (3) the risk of tracheal aspiration if the patient is allowed to eat orally.

The decision to place a feeding tube can be controversial and may precipitate ethical dilemmas that involve the entire medical care team. In general, no clear guidelines exist for long-term feeding tube placement; in most cases, the wishes of the patient or family guide the decision. For patients who are too ill to swallow and whose medical status is expected to improve, the decision to provide enteral feeding is apparent and usually proceeds without controversy. The decision is more difficult for the patient who is eating safely but cannot eat enough, particularly if the patient has an AD that states an unwillingness to be tube fed. In this situation, the patient may be putting himself or herself at medical risk from the consequences of undernutrition and dehydration. Placing a feeding tube in a patient who is at risk for tracheal aspiration to avoid the consequences of aspiration (e.g., life-threatening aspiration pneumonia) also is controversial. The literature suggests that for patients with chronic, terminal diseases that gastrostomy or jejunostomy does not reduce the incidence of aspiration pneumonia.[3,5,6] Furthermore, these measures do not prolong life beyond expected limits.[7] For patients with longer life expectancies or patients with dementia who are not interested in eating, tube feeding may extend their lives without undo risk. The decision to place a feeding tube in a patient must be carefully considered, and the patient's or surrogate's wishes must be weighed against the medical risks and benefits.

CLINICAL CORNER 15-3

A 90-year-old woman has a history of multiple bilateral strokes with poor oral intake. She is difficult to evaluate formally with either a clinical or instrumental evaluation. The reason for her poor intake is not known. She is slightly below her ideal body weight and did not respond to behavioral efforts to improve her oral intake. The team decided she needed a gastrostomy tube to maintain nutrition. Her daughter, who was acting on her behalf, agreed that it was necessary but felt uncomfortable providing consent because in the past her mother told her she never wanted a feeding tube.

CRITICAL THINKING

1. Do you think the dysphagia team should press the daughter for an alternative feeding route when they know that the resident did not want such an intervention?
2. If the patient were your mother, what would you do?

TABLE 15-2

Summary of Potential Methods of Providing Nutrition

Type of Nutrition Delivery	Route of Delivery	Method of Delivery	Indications for Use	Types of Formula	Possible Complications
Simple IV/CTPN	IV (small vein; catheter inserted or surgically placed for CTPN in deep central vein)	Continuous or cyclic infusion by pump	Supplemental hydration; restoration of fluid and electrolyte balance; need for complete parenteral nutrition or long-term CTPN	Simple IV solutions (% dextrose and saline, electrolytes) Complete solutions: amino acids, dextrose, fatty acids, vitamins, minerals, trace elements, IV lipid solutions	Simple IV: Infection, edema, bleeding, burn at insertion site; weakened and collapsed veins Central line: Air embolism, pneumothorax, myocardial perforation, phlebitis, blood clot, infection, sepsis
Nasogastric tube	Catheter/tube placed transnasally to the stomach	Intermittent or continuous drip by pump	Short-term alternative to oral intake (approximately 2 weeks); transnasal insertion, easily removed	Commercial nutritionally complete (standard, hydrolyzed, modular) supplements; regular liquids	Misplacement into the airway; irritation to nasal, pharyngeal, esophageal mucosa; discomfort; negative cosmesis; may affect swallow function; may contribute to reflux and aspiration
G-tube/PEG	Feeding tube inserted directly into the stomach	Bolus or gravity (syringe); drip by infusion pump	Option for long-term alternative to oral intake; does not necessarily preclude oral intake in certain cases	Commercially prepared nutritionally complete enteral formulas; fiber supplements, supplemental and regular liquids, select medications; some individuals may liquefy table foods	Nausea, vomiting, diarrhea, constipation, reflux, clogged tube, skin irritation at gastrostomy site; aspiration
J-tube/PEG	Feeding tube inserted directly into the jejunum (small intestine)	Bolus or gravity syringe; drip by infusion pump	Does not require stomach for digestion; allows enteral nutrition earlier after stress or trauma; less risk of reflux and aspiration	Commercial prepared nutritionally complete enteral formulas; fiber supplements, supplemental liquids	Loss of controlled emptying of the stomach; misplacement; diarrhea, dehydration
Hypodermal clysis	Subcutaneous; common infusion sites are the chest, abdomen, thighs, and upper arms	Injection (3 L in 24 hours/two sites)	Hydration supplement for mild to moderate dehydration	Saline; half saline/glucose; potassium chloride can be added	Mild subcutaneous edema

CTPN, Central total parenteral nutrition; *IV*, intravenous; *PEG*, percutaneous endosopic gastrostomy.
Reprinted from Krival K, McGrail A, Kelchner L: *Frequently asked questions about alternate nutrition and hydration (ANH) in dysphagia care*, Rockville, MD, 2006, American Speech-Language-Hearing Association.

CLINICAL CORNER 15-4

The dysphagia team is in total agreement that a gastrostomy tube should be placed in a mentally incompetent poststroke patient who is 89 years old. The family member who is the legal surrogate is against placement and asks that his mother be fed despite the risks. Some of the nursing assistants who were helping feed her have refused because they believe they are hastening her death. The family member has threatened to sue the hospital for negligence because it is his perception that his mother is not receiving good care and that the team is "against him" for not taking their advice.

CRITICAL THINKING

1. What should be the next step in solving this dilemma, and who should initiate this step?
2. Can the medical care team continue to ethically provide care they feel is not warranted? What are their rights?

CLINICAL CORNER 15-5

A 64-year-old resident in a nursing home has a past history of multiple strokes with aphasia and dysphagia with multiple admissions to the hospital for aspiration pneumonia. After her treatments for pneumonia she returned to oral feeding. Periodic chest radiographs revealed some lung infiltrates, but she continue to eat her mechanical soft diet. The SLP watched the patient eat and noticed that for the first 10 minutes she appeared to be eating well but then started to choke on most items. The family refused an attempt to get a modified barium swallow study because their insurance would not pay for it. Because of the resident's prior history of aspiration pneumonia and the lack of a modified barium swallow study, the SLP believed the patient should not be eating orally. The physician disagreed with that recommendation, stating that tube feeding was not in the patient's best interest because of a lack of serious symptoms of dysphagia and her good appetite.

CRITICAL THINKING

1. Should the disagreement between the SLP and physician be addressed? Whose position is more valid? Make a case for each.
2. At what point in this patient's medical scenario might it be appropriate to place a feeding tube?

WEANING FROM FEEDING TUBES

Although much discussion and research have focused on patients who require feeding tubes, little effort has been directed toward which tube-fed patients can make the transition to oral feeding. At a minimum, tube-fed patients with dysphagia who are candidates to return to oral feeding must demonstrate a safe and efficient swallow on a consistent basis. In addition, they must be able to consume adequate amounts of food or liquid to support nutritional requirements. Their cognitive status also must be at a level at which they can follow single-stage commands and remain alert long enough to finish a meal. Respiratory stability is important because the work required during attempts at oral ingestion may induce fatigue. Fatigue may predispose patients to interruption between the required time needed to protect the airway during the swallow sequence, thereby increasing the possibility of aspiration (see Chapter 8). Finally, the ability to self-feed or cooperate fully with feeding assistance is desired.

Buchholz[8] has presented a clinical algorithm specific to patients with acquired brain injury or stroke that offers valuable suggestions for transition of tube-fed patients to oral feeding. The initial phase of weaning from tube feeding is termed the *preparatory phase*. This phase focuses on physiologic readiness for oral nutrition and incorporates medical and nutritional stability, implementation of intermittent attempts at tube feeding, and a complete swallowing assessment. The second phase, *weaning*, is described as a graduated increase in oral feeding with corresponding decreases in tube feeding. Placement of a nasogastric feeding tube does not preclude patients from attempts at oral feeding, although attempts at oral feeding should be done on a schedule when the patient has not recently been fed through the tube. Avoiding attempts at oral feeding with a full stomach helps stimulate the hunger drive, which, in turn, may facilitate oral intake. Once a patient is able to consume 75% or more of his or her nutritional requirements consistently by mouth for 3 days, all tube feedings are discontinued. Specific clinical parameters to evaluate weaning success include weight gain, adequate hydration, a normal swallow, and no respiratory complications. No data are presented to support the specifics of this weaning approach in this population. However, data are available from other populations that pursue different recommendations and criteria for tube removal.

Naik et al.[9] evaluated predictors of feeding tube removal (and return to oral feeding) in cancer patients before and after PEG tube placement. Four clinical variables predicted PEG removal and return to oral feeding in these patients: age greater than 65 years, localized head/neck cancer, serum **albumin** level 3.75 g/dL or higher, and a serum **creatinine** level of less than 1.1 mg/dL. In the **multivariate analyses**, only age and localized head/neck cancer predicted resumption of oral feeding with PEG removal.

Clinical reality dictates that patients vary in terms of the need for feeding tube placement and in terms of readiness and success of feeding tube removal. In fact, not all tube-fed patients seek feeding tube removal. In addition, the transition process from tube feeding to oral feeding can be cognitively and physically challenging. Patients with feeding tubes typically consider the removal of the tube to be their primary goal, although some patients prefer to continue tube feedings even if return to some degree of oral intake is deemed possible. For some, oral intake can become a burden, whereas the implementation of tube feedings requires little effort. However, the transition process from tube to oral feeding should be thoroughly discussed and a plan of action outlined. For example, patients may be too aggressive when returning to oral feeding, experience failure, and then cease any efforts to resume an oral diet. Others are less aggressive and require more guidance and structure until the transition is complete. Discussion of patient-specific goals (see Chapter 12) for transitioning to oral feeding is advisable. One example for the initial goal might be oral intake of a single material to the point of nutritional adequacy with that item. At this point, the feeding tube might be removed with subsequent goals focused on the expansion of the oral diet.

The choice of the initial materials to restart oral feeding in the tube-fed patient is complex and based on findings from the clinical and instrumental swallowing examinations. Key considerations focus on the patient's ability to control the material in the mouth and to move this material to the pharynx. For example, stroke patients with oral weakness may have difficulty controlling a liquid material, which may leak anteriorly from the lips or posterior to the pharynx and into an open airway. Conversely, patients recovering from treatment for head/neck cancer sometimes perform better with thin liquids as a result of xerostomia. Beyond the oral stage of swallow, the SLP is concerned with the patient's ability to protect the airway during the swallow and the potential for aspiration of post-swallow residue associated with ineffective transport. As a result of clinical and instrumental evaluations with various materials, the SLP is likely to recommend a specific initial material for oral intake as well as some basic intervention strategies, such as specific postures or swallowing adaptations that increase

---

BOX 15-1 Suggestions for the Transition of Tube-Fed Patients to Oral Feeding

1. Identify a safe oral bolus.
2. Provide intermittent tube feedings.
3. Ingest oral feedings before a tube feeding.
4. Reestablish a normal meal routine.
5. Provide a specific diet in the initial transition stages.
6. Document the type and amount of all materials taken orally.
7. Keep track of the time it takes to consume a meal.
8. Document any complications with the oral diet.
9. Involve the patient and family in preferences for advancing the diet.
10. Monitor swallow safety, nutrition, hydration, and respiratory status.

---

airway protection or reduce post-swallow residue (see Chapters 13 and 14).

Once nutritional goals and the appropriate behavioral interventions have been identified, the patient is ready for oral intake. The clinician must remember that swallow safety does not always predict whether the patient can ingest a sufficient number of calories for feeding tube removal. Therefore careful documentation of the amount of food the patient ingests orally is important. If the patient has been receiving continuous tube feedings (delivered by a bedside pump), an intermittent schedule should be instituted to reinvolve normal hunger cycles.[8] Ideally, these intermittent feedings should be well tolerated before attempts at oral ingestion.[10] Attempts at oral feeding should begin with the patient fully upright and alert. For patients with fluctuating mental status, attempts at oral ingestion should be timed when their pattern of alertness is at its best. It is common for the return to oral ingestion to involve only short periods of time, once or twice per day. The number and type of food items received on the patient's tray are established during the clinical and instrumental examination and communicated to the dietitian or other medical staff. As tolerance improves, more challenging items can be introduced in larger bolus sizes. Box 15-1 summarizes some simple considerations in developing a strategy for the transition of tube-fed patients to oral feeding.

ASPIRATION PNEUMONIA

Aspiration pneumonia is a lung infection that may result from three primary sources: aspiration during swallowing, including saliva; retention of swallowed contents that eventually are aspirated; or aspiration of gastroesophageal contents. Physical signs include shortness of breath with a rapid heart rate, acute mental confusion, incontinence, and infection. Some patients have a fever and an increase in sputum with cough. Elderly patients in skilled nursing facilities may have aspiration pneumonia with few of these overt signs.[11] Chest radiographs may show diffuse infiltrates, usually in the posterior and right lower segments of the lung. If the source of the infection is thought to be related to oropharyngeal dysphagia, the patient is kept from eating while antibiotics are used to treat the infection. If the source is believed to be in the gastrointestinal tract, medications and posturing may be used to reduce the threat of recurrence.

Risk Factors

Aspiration pneumonia does not develop in all patients who aspirate material into the lung. For example, some patients frequently aspirate their saliva and do not become ill. This may be explained by the fact that their oral hygiene is sufficient to not allow bacteria to colonize and, in turn, infect the lung tissue. An aggressive oral care program is important for any patient with oropharyngeal dysphagia. When material is misdirected into the upper airway during swallow attempts, the first line of defense is cough at the level of the vocal folds. If the cough is sufficiently strong, most of the material may be expelled back into the pharynx to be swallowed while only a small amount enters the trachea below the level of the vocal folds. Even if material does enter the lung, it may trigger a secondary cough response that further protects the lower airway spaces. Specialized cells in the tissue of the lung work to engulf, absorb, and transport foreign fluid and food from the lung spaces. Other cells produce a chemical reaction that neutralizes aspirants that are acidic. For example, the acid in gastric reflux is particularly virulent in the lungs. The upper and lower airway defense systems are most active when the patient's immune system is strong. Therefore patients with an acute medical problem or older patients with chronic, multiple medical problems, particularly if they are immobile, may be at increased risk for aspiration pneumonia.

No studies in human beings have been able to link the amount and type of an aspirant to the development of pneumonia. Clinical practice suggests that although some patients aspirate and do not develop pneumonia, other similar patients do contract pneumonia. The ability to differentiate patients in whom pneumonia might develop from their aspirants might allow the clinician more latitude to not restrict patients from eating even in the circumstance of doc-

umented aspiration. Silver and Van Nostrand[12] studied 15 poststroke patients who were restricted from eating because they showed signs of aspiration on videofluoroscopic examination. They were subsequently studied with a nuclear medicine test known as *scintigraphy*. During scintigraphy the patient swallows a large radionuclide-labeled bolus with scanning immediately after and at hourly intervals (typically up to 3 hours) for any residue in the lung fields or digestive tract. They found that although some patients did aspirate the marker, after a short period the residue in the lungs was not detected by the scanner. This suggested that the lung defense mechanisms were active and therefore diminished the chances for the development of pneumonia. Eight of the patients with positive lung clearance were fed despite the evidence of aspiration on videofluoroscopy.

Although the data are not strong, some preliminary evidence suggests certain clinical signs are predictive of aspiration, whereas other variables (mostly historical) are more predictive of those in whom aspiration pneumonia will develop. In other words, aspiration pneumonia does not develop in *all* patients who aspirate, either on the clinical or instrumental examination. Interestingly, no data exist to support that clinical indicators from the clinical examination (such as dysphonia, dysarthria, wet-hoarse voice after trial swallows, and failure on the 3-oz water test) that predict aspiration (see Chapter 9) also predict aspiration pneumonia.

Studies of the factors that predict those in whom aspiration pneumonia will develop have focused on those most at risk—the elderly. The following factors have emerged as predictive of development of aspiration pneumonia: diagnosis of congestive heart failure and chronic obstructive pulmonary disease; use of multiple medications, especially sedatives; feeding dependence; poor oral hygiene; smoking; prior history of aspiration pneumonia; neck hyperextension while eating; use of suctioning; bedbound state; and having a feeding tube in place.[13-15] Although not confirmed experimentally, it might be assumed that the greater the number of factors, the greater the risk for patients to develop pneumonia from their aspirants. Interestingly, although the presence of dysphagia was a predictor in some studies, it was not a strong predictor.

NONMEDICAL RISKS AND BENEFITS

In addition to being informed about the medical risks associated with tube feeding, clinicians, patients, and caregivers need to be informed of the nonmedical risks and benefits to make an informed decision regarding whether enteral feedings are in the patient's best interest.

Nonmedical Benefits

Some patients with dysphagia continually struggle to maintain sufficient oral nutrition and hydration. Similarly, caregivers who assist patients in their nutritional needs also may be challenged to maintain nutritional levels. Family members often are troubled that their loved one is losing weight. Weight loss leads to a decrease in energy levels and mobility may be decreased. Poor nutritional levels also may precipitate mental confusion. All these factors are viewed by the patient and family as a diminution in the quality of life. This realization often is accompanied by situational depression. Providing the patient with sufficient calories by enteral feeding may relieve the burden of trying to maintain nutrition orally. In turn, the quality of life for the patient and caregiver(s) improves. Lost functions may return because nutrition and hydration levels can return to normal. Although the patient and caregiver(s) may have to familiarize themselves with the mechanics and care of the enteral feeding route, in some instances enteral feeding can provide both physical and psychological relief from dysphagia.

Nonmedical Risks

Patients who no longer eat by mouth or must consider not eating by mouth may feel threatened because

they are losing one of life's basic pleasures. Thus social withdrawal and depression may be a consequence of their decision. Patients with dementia who require enteral feeding may need to be sedated and physically restrained because they attempt to dislodge the feeding tube. Sedation and restraint during enteral feedings often is considered as a risk because it further erodes the patient's quality of life.

ETHICAL DILEMMAS

Myriad ethical dilemmas may develop when physicians, patients, and families consider tube feeding. Ethical dilemmas usually result when the patient or caregiver does not agree with or fails to understand the medical care team's plan. In most cases dilemmas can be resolved by reviewing the circumstances that led to the decision. Such a review entails an in-depth discussion with the key members of the medical team, the patient, and the family. If the dilemma is not resolved in this meeting, a request for resolution is sent to the medical center's ethics committee. In general, this committee is composed of physicians, nurses, a psychologist or social worker, a chaplain, and a member from the community. Swallowing specialists or dietitians may be asked to be a part of the

---

Practice Note 15-1

I had been monitoring a patient with multiple sclerosis and dysphagia for 3 years. He had continued to eat orally, although mealtimes were prolonged and the special preparations required in his diet were becoming an unwanted burden. We had never discussed his thoughts about a feeding tube, but it seemed appropriate that this might be the time. I suggested that it was clear to me that oral feeding was becoming a burden and that a gastrostomy might be a choice because it would relieve the burden of the oral intake by providing calories to maintain his health. Food items that he enjoyed and did not require special preparation could be continued orally. This option brought an immediate smile to his face and a consultation request was sent to gastroenterology to evaluate him for a percutaneous gastrostomy. It is important for the clinician to assess the burden of oral alimentation because even though patients may want to maintain that level of function, offering options may be in their best interest.

CLINICAL CORNER 15-6

You are confronted with Patient 1, who has the following clinical signs from your evaluation and from the patient's medical history: terminal medical illness, family desires to prolong life, history of multiple cases of aspiration pneumonia, uncooperative with any testing, good cough response, no dysphonia, frequent choking episodes with meals, multiple medications, and pulling of feeding tube because of poor cognition. Patient 2 has the following clinical factors: trace aspiration on thin liquids; pharyngeal stasis on thicker materials with airway penetration, multiple, chronic medical conditions; no advance directive; prior history of aspiration pneumonia; good cognition, good oral hygiene; ongoing weight loss; and undernourishment.

CRITICAL THINKING

1. Would you orally feed Patient 1? Justify your answer based on how you evaluate the importance of each clinical finding.
2. Would you orally feed Patient 2? Justify your answer based on how you evaluate the importance of each clinical finding.

committee if the issues require their expertise. In some cases, a clinician who deals extensively with swallowing disorders is a member of the committee.

CLINICAL CASE EXAMPLE 15-1

A 55-year-old man had been in a skilled nursing facility for 10 years with an unknown, progressive disease of the basal ganglia. It affected all the muscles of the head, neck, and limbs. Because he was counseled early in the disease that it would progress and lead to a premature death, he signed an advance directive that stated he did not want any "heroic" measures when he became terminally ill. This included a statement that he did not want to be fed through a tube in his stomach. His disease progressed to the point where he could not produce intelligible speech because of weakness in the muscles of articulation. He used an electronic communication board to compensate for the loss of communication skills. He continued to eat orally but choked violently at every meal as the nurses were feeding him. At the time of the consultation to speech pathology, he had been treated for six episodes of aspiration pneumonia in the previous 18 months. His videofluorographic swallowing examination showed aspiration on all bolus volumes and types, ranging from thin liquid to a semisolid. He was capable of transferring the bolus from the mouth to the pharynx. He was asked numerous times if he wanted to change his mind regarding the possibility of feeding tube placement to perhaps lessen the risk of developing pneumonia, but he refused.

The patient's refusal of feeding tube became a serious issue when the nursing assistants banded together and said they did not want to continue to feed him because they believed they were contributing to his death. The patient did not have a family member in the vicinity who might have been available to provide feeding assistance. A consultation was sought from the ethics committee to resolve the dilemma.

The ethics committee reviewed the entire medical history and established that the patient fully understood his medical condition. They found him competent to make decisions about his health based on the medical care team communications regarding the risks and benefits of continued oral feeding and those of tube feeding.

It was clear from the SLP's report that dietary compensations and behavioral swallowing treatment strategies were not successful in reducing the patient's risk of aspiration. It also was apparent that the nurses were not willing to cooperate with his feeding, leaving the patient at nutritional risk. After extensive discussion, the surgeon on the committee asked if it would be prudent to perform an elective laryngectomy, effectively separating the airway and food way to avoid the risk of aspiration. This would sacrifice vocal fold function. Because his speech was already unintelligible, it seemed like a reasonable option to sacrifice voice for swallow safety. This option was explained to the patient, who agreed to the procedure.

CLINICAL CORNER 15-7

The patient has a history of repeated aspiration pneumonias for which he has a gastrostomy. Unfortunately, he continues to pull the tube out because of his mental confusion. The physician wants to try oral feeding and wants to know the risk of aspiration. Only under ideal conditions did the modified barium swallow study show that the patient was not aspirating. The physician is worried that the family will place blame for a subsequent bout of pneumonia if the patient returns to oral feeding.

CRITICAL THINKING

1. What advice would you give to the physician?
2. What things does the family need to know and respond to that might affect the final decision?

Ethical issues in medicine surface for a number of reasons. First, the patient or family member is not convinced that they have received sufficient evidence to support the conclusions. Second, determinations of the best course of care, as well as who is the final arbiter making that decision, may not be clear. For example, the patient may have been told the best course of care by the attending physician but also received an opposing opinion from an outside consultant whom the patient trusts. Third, the medical care team and the patient may have personal biases that interfere with rational decision making. Fourth, it may not be clear who is acting in the patient's behalf and whether that person is acting in accordance with the patient's best interest. Finally, it may not be clear what the patient or surrogate considers a desirable outcome to the dilemma.

CLINICAL CORNER 15-8

A patient attempted suicide 3 years ago and now has considerable frontal lobe injury. He stopped eating, has lost 16 pounds, and his health will deteriorate unless a feeding tube is placed. His is ambulatory and responsive but is considered incompetent to understand his situation. The medical care team believes that an NGT would improve his current condition, but the family refuses. Interestingly, his wife instructed the team to do everything possible to save his life at the time of the suicide attempt. Her refusal now is based on the fact that she says this is his way of saying he wants to die and she is honoring that wish.

CRITICAL THINKING

1. What other information might be gathered to solve this dilemma?
2. Should the medical care team follow the wife's wishes? Make a case for each answer.

It is the task of the medical ethics committee to resolve ethical dilemmas that surface when the medical team recommends a feeding tube and the patient or family refuses, or when the patient wants a feeding tube and the medical care team thinks it is not necessary. The committee performs a thorough, nonbiased review of the medical and nonmedical risks associated with tube feeding in an effort to resolve the dilemma. In most cases, the committee does its best to honor the patient's wishes within accepted legal and ethical boundaries.

ETHICAL DILEMMAS

One of the most commonly encountered dilemmas that the swallowing specialist faces is the patient who is known to aspirate and has decided that under no circumstances does he or she want a feeding tube. A dilemma may arise when the medical team has decided that the patient's risk of aspiration pneumonia during continued oral feeding is greater than the risk of aspiration pneumonia with enteral feeding. If the medical care team is convinced that the patient and family understand all the risks associated with continued oral feeding, they most likely will honor the patient's wishes under the Patient Self-Determination Act and allow the patient to continue to eat. At this point a number of dilemmas may surface. The physician may have allowed the patient to continue to eat, although convinced it was not in the patient's best interest and may believe he or she is sacrificing professional responsibility. Furthermore, the physician may feel liable for legal action if aspiration pneu-

monia develops and the patient dies. In this case, it is important that specific documentation be placed in the medical record regarding the medical team's recommendations and the patient's refusal of those recommendations. Some institutions require the patient to acknowledge that he or she has refused the medical team's advice in a separate written document. These documents have not been challenged in the courts, so their validity remains questionable. However, because the medical record is a legal document, it is crucial that all conversations with the family about the risks and benefits of tube feeding, and the patient education they received on those issues, be thoroughly documented. Impressions regarding whether the family fully understood the team's recommendations also should be recorded.

The swallowing specialist whose evaluation might have helped the team make the decision that oral feeding was contraindicated also may believe that his or her professional ethics are at risk, particularly if asked to continue to assist the patient by providing the "safest" way to feed. Some clinicians argue that they would be contributing to the patient's demise and would be liable to court action if the family chooses to pursue it. In this case clinicians have the right to sign off the case and pass it to another colleague who may have a different perspective.[16] Other colleagues may believe they can provide safe feeding instructions without compromising their professional or personal ethics. In most cases the swallowing specialist provides additional care if convinced that the patient and family were fully informed of the continued risk and it was properly documented in the medical record. Furthermore, staying involved with the family and patient can allow for reassessment during times of change that may alter the original decision for oral or enteral feeding.

CLINICAL CASE EXAMPLE 15-2

A 90-year-old man had bilateral strokes that left him dysphagic with dementia. During his last hospitalization he had respiratory distress and a tracheostomy was performed. Although his prognosis was poor, he steadily recovered to the point that his physician wondered if he could once again eat orally. The SLP completed a clinical evaluation that revealed (1) poor mental status, but the ability to follow simple commands and stay alert; (2) generalized weakness of the tongue, lips, and velum; and (3) a weak and hoarse voice when his tracheotomy tube was occluded. On swallowing trials of 5 and 10 mL of thin and thick liquid the patient coughed on each bolus. Pudding pooled in the oral cavity but was swallowed with delay and post-swallow cough. Because of his fragile medical status and based on the results of the clinical evaluation, the SLP recommended that the patient continue NGT feeding and suggested the family consider gastrostomy. The daughter, acting on the patient's behalf, objected to this recommendation, stating that eating was his only pleasure in life. The SLP explained that the examination suggested he was aspirating and could die from aspiration pneumonia if he tried to eat. After asking questions about the definitions of aspiration and aspiration pneumonia, the daughter was not convinced he was aspirating because it could not be seen on a physical examination. She pressed the physician for a modified barium swallow study that she attended (Video 15-1 on the Evolve site). The patient was given 10 mL of a thickened liquid that pooled in the vallecula with residue above the PES. Although the hyoid bone moved, vallecular pooling and PES residue were consistent with tongue weakness. On subsequent boluses, material penetrated the airway with evidence of cough. Some material eventually went below the vocal folds without cough. On multiple swallows penetration was noted; however, eventually the pharynx was cleared. On the final swallows of a pudding-thick bolus, the patient was able to swallow without delay or pharyngeal residue with only trace penetration. The SLP believed that this examination showed that the patient was still at risk of aspiration, although considering his age, the presence of a tracheotomy tube, and the patient's general health, attempts at oral ingestion seemed warranted. The final decision to start oral feeding was based on evidence from the clinical and instrumental examinations as well as the daughter's implied stance that she did not want her father to have a gastrostomy. The patient started a soft mechanical diet but on the third day developed signs and symptoms consistent with aspiration pneumonia. Oral feedings were stopped while he was treated for suspected aspiration pneumonia. The daughter continued to argue for oral feeding and the team agreed to try again. This time he ate successfully for 5 days, and the decision was made to remove the tracheotomy tube. The patient left the hospital eating a regular diet with no restrictions.

TAKE HOME NOTES

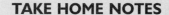

1. Medical ethics is a subspecialty of medical care that brings together patients, caregivers, and nonmedical and medical professionals in an effort to make the best decision on a health care issue. It is driven by a congressional mandate called *The Patient Self-Determination Act.*

2. An advance directive is a statement made by a patient that provides guidance to health care professionals regarding the patient's wishes for treatment or no treatment in certain medical circumstances.

3. The two broad categories of nonoral feeding include enteral and parenteral.

4. The major enteral feeding routes are nasogastric, gastrostomy, and jejunostomy.

5. Feeding tubes do not necessarily reduce the risk of aspiration pneumonia or prolong life.

6. Aspiration pneumonia does not develop in all patients who aspirate. Some clinical factors are more predictive than others in identifying aspirators in whom pneumonia will develop.

7. Ethical dilemmas regarding the use and acceptance of tube feeding may result in conflicts between the patient and the medical care team. Most of these dilemmas can be resolved with a review of the patient's wishes and a detailed review of the course of medical care.

8. Professional ethics can be threatened if a patient refuses to follow medical advice. Asking another professional to assume the care of the patient is within a practitioner's right.

References

1. Groher ME: Ethical dilemmas in providing nutrition, *Dysphagia* 9:12, 1990.

2. Sharp HM, Bryant KN: Ethical issues in dysphagia: when patients refuse assessment or treatment, *Semin Speech Lang Pathol* 24:285, 2003.

3. Lazarus BA, Murphy JB, Culpepper L: Aspiration associated with long-term gastric versus jejunal feeding: a critical analysis of the literature, *Arch Phys Med Rehabil* 70:46, 1990.

4. Griggs B: Nursing management of swallowing disorders. In Groher ME, editor: *Dysphagia: diagnosis and management*, Boston, 1997, Butterworth-Heinemann.

5. Feinberg MJ, Knebl J, Tully J et al: Aspiration in the elderly, *Dysphagia* 5:61, 1990.

6. Finucane TE, Christmas C: Aspiration pneumonia, *N Engl J Med* 44:1869, 2001.

7. Finucane TE, Christmas C, Travis K: Tube feeding in patients with advanced dementia: a review of the evidence, *JAMA* 13:1365, 1990.

8. Buchholz AC: Weaning patients with dysphagia from tube feeding to oral nutrition: a proposed algorithm, *Can J Diet Pract Res* 59:208, 1998.

9. Naik AD, Abraham NS, Roche VM et al: Predicting which patients can resume oral nutrition after percutaneous endoscopic gastrostomy tube placement, *Aliment Pharmacol Ther* 21:1155, 2005.

10. Groher ME, McKaig TN: Dysphagia and dietary levels in skilled nursing facilities, *J Am Geriatr Soc* 43:528, 1995.

11. Fein AM: Pneumonia in the elderly: special diagnostic and therapeutic considerations, *Med Clin North Am* 78:1015, 1994.

12. Silver KH, Van Nostrand D: The use of scintigraphy in the management of patients with pulmonary aspiration, *Dysphagia* 9:107, 1994.

13. Peck A, Cohen CE, Mulvibill MN: Long-term enteral feeding of aged demented nursing home patients, *J Am Geriatr Soc* 38:1195, 1990.

14. Langmore SE, Terpenning MS, Schork A et al: Predictors of aspiration pneumonia: how important is dysphagia? *Dysphagia* 13:69, 1998.

15. Langmore SE, Skarupski KA, Park PS et al: Predictors of aspiration pneumonia in nursing home residents, *Dysphagia* 17:298, 2002.

16. Beauchamp TL, Childress JF: *Principles of biomedical ethics*, ed 5, New York, 2001, Oxford University Press.

Index